Sexual Assault

Victimization Across the Life Span
A Clinical Guide

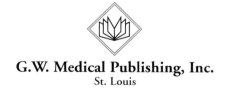

G.W. Medical Publishing, Inc.
St. Louis

To Bernadette Toner, whose tireless efforts in assisting me with both
my academic and administrative responsibilities made it possible
to effectively organize the massive effort it takes to produce a scholarly
publication such as this. Bernadette's attention to detail was invaluable
for getting everything done and her heart for all who suffer trauma was a
consistent confirmation of the necessity of this work.

— APG

To my husband, Sean Murphy, for his constant support and
creative criticism of my academic projects, and his humor without
which I would not enjoy each day so much.

— EMD

To my husband, David Kenty, whose love and support have shown
our daughters what a relationship should be.

— JBA

Sexual Assault

Victimization Across the Life Span
A Clinical Guide

Angelo P. Giardino, MD, PhD
Associate Chair – Pediatrics
Associate Physician-in-Chief
St. Christopher's Hospital for Children
Associate Professor in Pediatrics
Drexel University College of Medicine
Philadelphia, Pennsylvania

Elizabeth M. Datner, MD
Assistant Professor
University of Pennsylvania School of Medicine
Department of Emergency Medicine
Assistant Professor of Emergency Medicine in Pediatrics
Children's Hospital of Philadelphia
Philadelphia, Pennsylvania

Janice B. Asher, MD
Assistant Clinical Professor
Obstetrics and Gynecology
University of Pennsylvania Medical Center
Director
Women's Health Division of Student Health Service
University of Pennsylvania
Philadelphia, Pennsylvania

RA1141
S49
V.2
2003

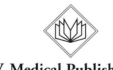

G.W. Medical Publishing, Inc.
St. Louis

Publishers: Glenn E. Whaley and Marianne V. Whaley

Design Director: Glenn E. Whaley

Managing Editors: Ann Przyzycki
Liz Stefaniak

Associate Editors: Christine Bauer
Kristine Feeherty

Book Design/Page Layout: G.W. Graphics
Kelly M. Brunie
Mark F. Fournier

Print/Production Coordinator: Charles J. Seibel, III

Cover Design: G.W. Graphics

Color PrePress Specialist: Terry L. Williams

Copy Editor: Susan Zahra

Developmental Editor: Elaine Steinborn

Indexer: Nelle Garrecht

Printed in the United States of America.

Publisher:
G.W. Medical Publishing, Inc.
77 Westport Plaza, Suite 366, St. Louis, Missouri, 63146-3124 U.S.A.
Phone: (314) 542-4213 Fax: (314) 542-4239 Toll Free: 1-800-600-0330
http://www.gwmedical.com

Library of Congress Cataloging-in-Publication Data

Sexual assault victimization across the life span : a clinical guide /
[edited by] Angelo P. Giardino, Elizabeth M. Datner, Janice B. Asher.--
1st ed.
p. ; cm.
Includes bibliographical references and index.
ISBN 1-878060-41-4 (hardcover : alk. paper)
1. Sexual abuse victims. 2. Sexually abused children. 3. Child
sexual abuse. 4. Sex crimes. I. Giardino, Angelo P. II. Datner,
Elizabeth M. III. Asher, Janice B. [DNLM: 1. Sex Offenses. 2.
Clinical Medicine. 3. Forensic Medicine. W 795 S5185 2003]
RC560 .S44 S495 2003
616.85'83--dc21
2002014237

CONTRIBUTORS

Randell Alexander, MD, PhD
Associate Professor
Clinical Pediatrics
Morehouse School of Medicine
Forensic Pediatrician
Department of Pediatrics
Morehouse School of Medicine
Atlanta, Georgia

Sarah Anderson, RN, MSN
University of Virginia
Department of Emergency Medicine (Registered Nurse)
School of Nursing (Doctoral Student)
Charlottesville, Virginia

Joanne Archambault
Training Director
Sexual Assault Training and Investigations (SATI, Inc.)
Retired Sergeant
San Diego Police Department
Sex Crimes Unit

Tracy Bahm, JD
Senior Attorney
Violence Against Women Program
American Prosecutors Research Institute (APRI)
Alexandria, Virginia

Kathy Bell, RN
Forensic Nurse Examiner
Tulsa Police Department
Tulsa, Oklahoma

Sandra L. Bloom, MD
CEO, Community Works
Philadelphia, Pennsylvania

Duncan T. Brown, JD
Staff Attorney
National Center for Prosecution of Child Abuse
American Prosecutors Research Institute (APRI)
Alexandria, Virginia

Mary-Ann Burkhart, JD
Senior Attorney
National Center for Prosecution of Child Abuse
American Prosecutors Research Institute (APRI)
Alexandria, Virginia

Michael Clark, MSN, CRNP
Nurse Practitioner
Department of Emergency Medicine
Hospital of the University of Pennsylvania
Clinical Lecturer
University of Pennsylvania School of Nursing
Philadelphia, Pennsylvania

Sharon W. Cooper, MD, FAAP
Adjunct Associate Professor of Pediatrics
University of North Carolina School of Medicine
Chapel Hill, North Carolina
Clinical Assistant Professor of Pediatrics
Uniformed Services University of Health Sciences
Bethesda, Maryland
Chief
Developmental Pediatric Service
Womack Army Medical Center
Fort Bragg, North Carolina

Thomas Ervin, RNC, FN, BSc †
Reception and Release Coordinator
California State Prison at Corcoran
Department of Corrections
State of California

Martin A. Finkel, DO, FACOP, FAAP
Professor of Pediatrics
Medical Director
Center for Children's Support
School of Osteopathic Medicine
University of Medicine and Dentistry of New Jersey
Stratford, New Jersey

Marla J. Friedman, DO
Fellow, Pediatric Emergency Medicine
Emergency Medicine
Alfred I. duPont Hospital for Children
Wilmington, Delaware

Donna Gaffney, RN, DNSc, FAAN
Associate Professor, Acute Care Nurse Practitioner Program
College of Nursing
Seton Hall University
South Orange, New Jersey

Ann E. Gaulin, MS, MFT
Director of Counseling Services
Women Organized Against Rape
Philadelphia, Pennsylvania

Eileen R. Giardino, PhD, RN, CRNP
Associate Professor
LaSalle University, School of Nursing
Nurse Practitioner
LaSalle University, Student Health Center
Philadelphia, Pennsylvania

Holly M. Harner, CRNP, PhD, MPH, SANE
Assistant Professor
William F. Connell School of Nursing
Boston College
Chestnut Hill, Massachusetts

†Deceased

Caren Harp, JD
Senior Attorney/Director
National Juvenile Justice Prosecution Center
American Prosecutors Research Institute (APRI)
Alexandria, Virginia

William C. Holmes, MD, MSCE
Assistant Professor of Medicine and Epidemiology
Philadelphia Veterans Affairs Medical Center
Center for Clinical Epidemiology and Biostatistics
University of Pennsylvania School of Medicine
Philadelphia, Pennsylvania

Jeffrey R. Jaeger, MD
Assistant Professor of Medicine
University of Pennsylvania Health System
Clinical Faculty, Institute for Safe Families
Philadelphia, Pennsylvania

Susan Bieber Kennedy, RN, JD
Senior Attorney
Violence Against Women Program
American Prosecutors Research Institute (APRI)
Alexandria, Virginia

Lisa Kreeger, JD
Senior Attorney
Violence Against Women Program Manager
DNA Forensics Program Manager
American Prosecutors Research Institute (APRI)
Alexandria, Virginia

Susan Kreston, JD
Deputy Director
National Center for Prosecution of Child Abuse
American Prosecutors Research Institute (APRI)
Alexandria, Virginia

Linda E. Ledray, RN, PhD, SANE-A, FAAN
Director
Sexual Assault Resource Service
Hennepin County Medical Center
Minneapolis, Minnesota

Patsy Rauton Lightle
Supervisory Special Agent
Lieutenant, Department of Child Fatalities
South Carolina Law Enforcement Division
Columbia, South Carolina

Judith A. Linden, MD, FACEP, SANE
Assistant Professor
Emergency Medicine
Boston University School of Medicine
Associate Residency Director
Boston University School of Medicine
Boston Medical Center
Boston, Massachusetts

John Loiselle, MD
Associate Professor of Pediatrics
Jefferson Medical College
Assistant Director, Emergency Medicine
Alfred I. duPont Hospital for Children
Wilmington, Delaware

Kathi Makoroff, MD
Mayerson Center for Safe and Healthy Children
Cincinnati Children's Hospital Medical Center
Cincinnati, Ohio

Jeanne Marrazzo, MD, MPH
Assistant Professor
Department of Medicine
Division of Allergy and Infectious Diseases
University of Washington
Seattle, Washington
Medical Director
Seattle STD/HIV Prevention Training Center
Seattle, Washington

Patrick O'Donnell, PhD
Supervising Criminalist, DNA Laboratory
San Diego Police Department
San Diego, California

Christine M. Peterson, MD
Director of Gynecology
Department of Student Health
Assistant Professor of Clinical Obstetrics and Gynecology
University of Virginia School of Medicine
Charlottesville, Virginia

Millicent Shaw Phipps, JD
Staff Attorney
Violence Against Women Program
American Prosecutors Research Institute (APRI)
Alexandria, Virginia

Hannah Ufberg Rabinowitz, MSN, CRNP

William J. Reed, MD, FAAP
Director of Behavioral/Development and Adolescent Medicine
for Medical Education
Assistant Professor of Pediatric
Texas A & M University College of Medicine

Iris Reyes, MD, FACEP
Assistant Professor
Emergency Medicine
Hospital of the University of Pennsylvania
Assistant Medical Director
Emergency Medicine
Hospital of the University of Pennsylvania
Philadelphia, Pennsylvania

Laura L. Rogers, JD
Senior Attorney
National Center for Prosecution of Child Abuse
American Prosecutors Research Institute (APRI)
Alexandria, Virginia

Mimi Rose, JD
Chief Assistant District Attorney
Family Violence and Sexual Assault Unit
Philadelphia District Attorney Office
Philadelphia, Pennsylvania

Pamela Ross, MD
Assistant Professor of Emergency Medicine & Pediatrics
University of Virginia Health System
Charlottesville, Virginia

Rena Rovere, MS, FNP
Sexual Assault Program Director
Clinical Nurse Specialist
Department of Emergency Medicine
Albany Medical Center
Albany, New York

Bruce D. Rubin, MD
Clinical Instructor
Department of Emergency Medicine
Hospital of the University of Pennsylvania
Philadelphia, Pennsylvania

Maureen S. Rush, MS
Vice President for Public Safety
University of Pennsylvania
Division of Public Safety
Philadelphia, Pennsylvania

Charles J. Schubert, MD
Associate Professor of Pediatrics
Division of Emergency Medicine
Cincinnati Children's Hospital Medical Center
Cincinnati, Ohio

Margot Schwartz, MD
Virginia Mason Medical Center
Infectious Diseases Section
Seattle, Washington
Clinical Instructor
Department of Medicine
University of Washington
Seattle, Washington

Philip Scribano, DO, MSCE
Assistant Professor
Pediatrics and Emergency Medicine
University of Connecticut School of Medicine
Director, Child Protection Program
Connecticut Children's Medical Center
Hartford, Connecticut

Christina Shaw, JD
Staff Attorney
National Center for Prosecution of Child Abuse
American Prosecutors Research Institute (APRI)
Alexandria, Virginia

Jeanne L. Stanley, PhD
Executive Director of Academic Services
Graduate School of Education
University of Pennsylvania
Philadelphia, Pennsylvania

Cari Michele Steele, JD
Staff Attorney
National Center for Prosecution of Child Abuse
American Prosecutors Research Institute (APRI)
Alexandria, Virginia

Jacqueline M. Sugarman, MD
Assistant Professor of Pediatrics
Department of Pediatrics
College of Medicine
University of Kentucky
Lexington, Kentucky

Kathryn M. Turman
Program Director
Office of Victim Assistance
Federal Bureau of Investigation
Washington, DC

Victor I. Vieth, JD
Director
National Center for Prosecution of Child Abuse
American Prosecutors Research Institute (APRI)
Alexandria, Virginia

J. M. Whitworth, MD
Professor of Pediatrics
University of Florida
State Medical Director
Child Protection Team Program
Children's Medical Services
Department of Health
State of Florida

Dawn Doran Wilsey, JD
Senior Attorney
National Center for Prosecution of Child Abuse
American Prosecutors Research Institute (APRI)
Alexandria, Virginia

Janet S. Young, MD
Assistant Professor
University of North Carolina-Chapel Hill
Department of Emergency Medicine
Chapel Hill, North Carolina

FOREWORD

Sexual assault is broadly defined as unwanted sexual contact of any kind. Among the acts included are rape, incest, molestation, fondling or grabbing, and forced viewing of or involvement in pornography. Drug-facilitated behavior was recently added in response to the recognition that pharmacologic agents can be used to make the victim more malleable. When sexual activity occurs between a significantly older person and a child, it is referred to as molestation or child sexual abuse rather than sexual assault. In children, there is often a "grooming" period where the perpetrator gradually escalates the type of sexual contact with the child and often does not use the force implied in the term sexual assault. But it is assault, both physically and emotionally, whether the victim is a child, an adolescent, or an adult.

The reported statistics are only an estimate of the problem's scope, with the actual reporting rate a mere fraction of the true incidence. Surveys of adults show as many as 18% of all women in the United States have been the victim of an attempted or completed rape over the course of their lives. The incidence of male victims is lower because of the reluctance of boys and men to report their victimization.

The financial costs of sexual assault are enormous; intangible costs, such as emotional suffering and risk of death from being victimized, are beyond measurement. Short term, there are healthcare consequences, such as unwanted pregnancy, sexually transmitted diseases, serious emotional upheavals, inability to carry out normal daily activities, decreased productivity, and, in some cases, loss of life. Longer-term disabilities can be both emotional and physical. It is well documented that survivors of sexual abuse have a much higher incidence of serious and chronic mental health problems than control populations of nonabused patients. Posttraumatic stress disorder, depression, suicidal ideation, and substance abuse are all over-represented among abused groups in case-control studies. Chronic physical symptoms, such as pain syndromes (pelvic, abdominal, chest, myalgias, headaches) and various somatization disorders, are reported in a wide variety of peer-reviewed medical specialty journals.

This book is the first to bring together the best information available concerning sexual victimization across the entire lifespan. Recognizing the radical differences required in approaching child, adolescent, and adult victims, the chapters are organized to present information from the medical and mental health literature specific to the various age groups. Victim and perpetrator characteristics are described. Most importantly, those who provide care for these victims and who handle the disposition of the perpetrators are given specific information to help them carry out their roles most effectively. This book offers information for all who care for the victims—the crisis hotline staff, law enforcement personnel, prehospital providers, specialized detectives, medical and mental health staff, specialized sexual assault examiners, and counselors. The information is as current, accurate, and specific as it can be in a rapidly evolving field. It will fill a need in many venues where sexual victimization is seen and care is given to victims.

Robert M. Reece, MD
Director, MSPCC Institute for Professional Education
Clinical Professor of Pediatrics, Tufts University School of Medicine
Executive Editor, the Quarterly Child Abuse Medical Update

FOREWORD

Sexual abuse is not just an epidemic — it is at pandemic proportions. In the United States, perhaps 20% to 25% of adults sustain some form of sexual abuse during their childhood. These numbers are somewhat higher or lower in other countries, but certainly do not vary by a factor of even 5. With such a high percentage of the world having been sexually abused, it may be legitimate to ask, is sexual abuse a "normal" behavior? Similarly, what is sexual abuse and why does it exist?

Anthropologically, concepts of appropriate sexual behaviors with young humans incorporate both biologically and culturally derived premises. Biologically, prepubertal animals are not frequent targets for sexual activity. This relative taboo is reasonably ubiquitous across species. Males and females of a given species usually wait until they achieve sexual maturity before they engage in sexual activity. This is utilitarian in that effort is not wasted on a non-reproductive member of the species. Besides olfactory, behavioral, and other cues that the individual is mature (and receptive), there are visual indicators of immaturity that seem to inhibit adults of most species. However, once having achieved sexual maturity an individual is fair game. Through most of human history, this biologic distinction of maturity has also apparently held. When the human life expectancy was a mere 30 years, however, one could not wait until the late teen years to begin reproduction.

In more recent historical times (and within certain cultures), a cultural overlay has developed that acknowledges a "delayed" maturity. Thus the age of consent is more likely to be 16 years or so, not age 10 or 11 years when some girls are having their first menstrual period. The concept especially derives from the notion that children need prolonged education and parental nurturance before they should have to compete with the adult population and its risks. The adult is supposed to ignore the development of secondary sexual characteristics (biologic maturity) and focus on chronological age with a somewhat arbitrary cutoff (e.g., what is the difference between a 15-year-old and a 16-year-old?).

Both the biologic cutoff and the chronological cutoff are respected by most adults in society. Yet some overlook the cultural cutoff and some even ignore the biologic cutoff (i.e., have sex with young children). For the latter, this is a violation of both cultural and biologic taboos.

Another biology-related taboo is having sex with close kin. The genetic implications could not have been consciously appreciated by humans through most of history, nor by some species, which also abide by this taboo. Yet nearly all human cultures respect the incest taboo—a sign of a relative biologic underpinning for this behavior. Nevertheless some adult humans also fail to respect this distinction and commit what we consider incest.

Views about appropriate and inappropriate sexual activity with younger humans have been codified into law and society as sexual abuse crimes. These are crimes about sex and reflect the perpetrator's sexual drive. While sexual drives help to maintain the species and are overall a necessary biologic imperative, sexual abuse incorporates biologically useless activity (i.e., sex with biologically immature children) and/or activity that is culturally shunned. In some instances the perpetrator may "love" the child and perhaps be the better caregiver. Yet the violation of taboos elicits a strong reaction by most members of society—reflecting a lack of concern for the child's well-being and trampling of the society's biologic and cultural ideations.

What can be done about this? One option would be to ignore the abuse. Yet this historically has not been done if the act becomes known, and it fails to meet the developmental needs of children. Another option would be to mount an aggressive prevention campaign aimed at potential perpetrators before they commit sexual abuse (primary and secondary prevention). This has not been done to any significant extent as yet. The third option is what most of this book is about—identifying sexual abuse when it has occurred and providing the types of interventions that might minimize its impact. We can treat the child and treat and/or incarcerate the offender. Considerable progress has occurred in the last three decades that enables us to better understand, identify, and intervene with child sexual abuse. The results of this progress are reflected in the state-of-the-art descriptions within this volume. These approaches make a real difference in children's lives and help us to respect the boundaries we place on sexual activity with our young.

One unanswered question remains: When will we as a society care enough about our children to make the substantial efforts required to implement the very best in primary, secondary, and tertiary prevention for our children? Until this becomes a cultural imperative of its own, we will continue to need books such as these, and the misery of lost childhoods will contribute to a sordid reality. Let us hope that some future generation can appreciate the brilliance of the work portrayed herein, but is also able to view child sexual abuse as an extinct historical oddity.

Randell Alexander, MD, PhD
Atlanta, Georgia

PREFACE

What is sexual assault? It is a crime of violence, where the assailant uses sexual contact as a weapon, seeking to gain power and control. Often youths and adolescents are disproportionately targeted, although sexual assault can occur at any age. Sexual assault is also an act of opportunity. Particularly vulnerable populations include children, especially young females, and individuals who are less able to care for themselves, such as the homeless or physically or mentally handicapped persons. Their vulnerability and ease of manipulation makes them prey.

Who commits these acts? While there is no classic profile of an offender, child sex abusers tend to be males who are known to the child's caregivers, and 80% of the women who are assaulted know their attackers as well—they are their ex-husbands, their stepfathers, their boyfriends, and other friends or relatives. Men may also experience victimization.

To protect victims from these offenders will require a change in the attitude of society toward its most vulnerable members. Society must value these individuals before anything will be done. Education plays a key role in accomplishing this change in attitude. This book was prepared with the goal of disseminating the information required to bring about change, to better protect and care for victims of sexual assault. Written for healthcare professionals and other mandated reporters, Sexual Assault Across the Life Span offers a complete approach to the topic. The problem is defined, all aspects are explored, and treatment and interventions are outlined. Victim characteristics are explored, especially those seen in children. But most importantly, useful information is offered to those who provide care for these victims and those who handle the disposition of the perpetrators. We see the problem through the eyes of many professionals: physicians, paramedics, law enforcement personnel, the judicial system, social workers, and people who work with children. This covers everyone from the crisis hotline staff, to police and law enforcement personnel, to prehospital providers, to specially trained detectives, to skilled medical staff, to trained sexual assault examiners, to rape crisis counselors. Finally, the text offers information on programs that are in place or are under consideration to aid in the prevention of sexual assault.

Knowledge gives us the power to intervene, and this book offers current, accurate, and specific data concerning the problem of sexual assault. With the information at hand, we can become empowered and participate in effective interventions to prevent sexual assault as well as care for its victims.

Angelo P. Giardino, MD, PhD
Philadelphia, Pennsylvania

G.W. Medical Publishing, Inc.

St. Louis

OUR MISSION

To become the world leader in publishing and

information services on child abuse, maltreatment and

diseases, and domestic violence. We seek to heighten

awareness of these issues and provide relevant

information to professionals and consumers.

*A portion of our profits is contributed to non-profit organizations dedicated to
the prevention of child abuse and the care of victims of abuse and other children
and family charities.*

TABLE OF CONTENTS

CHAPTER 3: EVALUATION OF CHILD SEXUAL ABUSE

CHAPTER 4: FORENSIC EVALUATIONS FOR SEXUAL ABUSE IN THE PREPUBESCENT CHILD

CHAPTER 17: SEXUALLY TRANSMITTED DISEASES AND PREGNANCY PROPHYLAXIS IN ADOLESCENTS AND ADULTS

Sexual Assault

Victimization Across the Life Span
A Clinical Guide

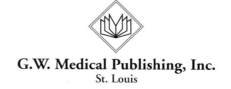

G.W. Medical Publishing, Inc.
St. Louis

OVERVIEW OF CHILD SEXUAL ABUSE

John Loiselle, MD
Marla J. Friedman, DO

HISTORICAL PERSPECTIVE

The sexual abuse of children has been discussed in writings dating back to the late 19th century. Freud (1961) publicly noted in 1896 that many of his patients with hysterical illnesses had a history of a sexual experience in their childhood. He thus theorized that hysteria was a direct result of childhood seduction. Unfortunately, he supported this seduction theory for only a short time, and by 1905 his belief had shifted. He renounced his previous views and stated that the sexual events recalled by his patients were unconscious fantasies rather than real events. He claimed that his patients' memories of sexual abuse were merely projections of their own desire for the parent of the opposite sex. Freud's adoption of this oedipal theory was a setback to the widespread acceptance of child sexual abuse because it caused others to question the existence of the problem as well as its psychologic effects (Cosentino & Collins, 1996; Whetsell-Mitchell, 1995b).

Over the next sixty years, child sexual abuse did receive occasional mention but almost always as it related to incest. Most of Freud's followers questioned the impact of sexual experiences on children as well as the role the children played in these activities. Between 1920 and 1950, investigators conceded that family members did sometimes involve children in sexual activities but that this contact did not have a damaging effect on the children (Cosentino & Collins, 1996; Whetsell-Mitchell, 1995a). Furthermore, some proposed that these experiences may even have had a beneficial effect on the children involved. Children were characterized as active participants in the sexual activities, often being labeled as the initiators of their own seduction (Bender & Blau, 1937).

In 1953 Kinsey et al. published the results of their study, which revealed that sexual abuse was indeed common in childhood. Even though they showed that almost 10% of women admitted to being sexually abused before age 18 years, their results received little attention (Whetsell-Mitchell, 1995a). It was not until the release of the landmark paper of "The Battered Child Syndrome," in 1962 that the medical profession began to take notice (Kempe et al.,1962). In 1971 the first child sexual abuse program was opened in San Jose, California. The Child Protective Movement began to campaign for legislation that would confront the problem of child sexual abuse on a national level. In 1974 the Child Abuse Prevention and Treatment Act was passed, which "mandated mental health professionals and educators to assist in the detection and reporting of child sexual abuse" (Cosentino & Collins, 1996; Whetsell-Mitchell, 1995b).

The publication of "Sexual Abuse, Another Hidden Pediatric Problem" by C. Henry Kempe (1978) forced the healthcare community to address the importance of the diagnosis and treatment of child sexual abuse. Works in the early 1980s focused on the child as the victim and the offender as the initiator. Blame

Key Point:
Sexual abuse of children is not a new problem, but has only been accepted as a bona fide problem deserving professional attention since the 1970s.

was put on the offender, not the child (Sgroi et al., 1982). At the same time, the publication of books by survivors of child sexual abuse and the release of television movies on the topic brought the issue of child sexual abuse to the public forefront (Whetsell-Mitchell, 1995b).

DEFINITION

The characterization of child sexual abuse is subject to interpretation on multiple levels. Institutional, societal, medical, and legal terminology all differ in their definition or emphasis. It is impossible to find a single universally accepted definition. Child sexual abuse encompasses a wide spectrum of activities ranging from the less serious to the more serious. Sexually abusive actions may or may not involve direct contact with the child. Kempe defined sexual abuse as "the involvement of dependent, developmentally immature children and adolescents in sexual activities that they do not fully comprehend, to which they are unable to give informed consent, or that violate the social taboos of family roles" (Kempe, 1978). Most legal definitions emphasize certain elements such as the age of the perpetrator and victim, description of specific acts or categories of sexual abuse, and who is considered a mandated reporter. The Child Abuse Prevention and Treatment Act (CAPTA) of 1974 provided a federal legal standard that all states were mandated to follow to be eligible for funds for child abuse programs. This act defined sexual abuse as "the employment, use, persuasion, inducement, enticement, or coercion of any child to engage in, or assist any other person to engage in, any sexually explicit conduct or simulation of such conduct for the purpose of producing a visual depiction of such conduct" (Child Abuse Prevention and Treatment Act, 1974). All 50 states have written statutes regarding sexual abuse based on this standard, but many differ in the specific wording. A child, in almost all instances, is defined as a person under age 18 years. Exceptions are made when that person is married. Certain laws are more specific with regard to the age of the perpetrator and victim when specific sexual acts are involved. Most statutes emphasize the discrepancy between the ages of the perpetrator and the victim. These laws also take into consideration the developmental level of the abused child. For purposes of reporting and involving specific legal agencies, laws distinguish who is considered a caretaker or guardian of the child. The involvement of a caretaker in the abuse necessitates the involvement of the local child protective services agency, as well as law enforcement. When the alleged perpetrator is considered a child, intervention may be limited to child protective services alone. When the assailant is unknown, unrelated, or not considered to be someone involved in the care of that child, the abuse may be a purely criminal case.

Key Point:
Sexual abuse is a term that covers a broad range of developmentally inappropriate sexual behaviors that span both contact and non-contact type activities.

Sexual abuse encompasses a large variety of actions. Whereas all states include a provision for rape or intercourse, some states use general terms in defining actions that constitute sexual abuse, while others are far more specific. The degree of detail can be crucial in certain cases; for example, medical and legal definitions do not require actual vaginal entry to occur for an act to be considered rape (Kempe, 1978). Genital fondling, oral-genital, genital-genital, and anal-genital contact are generally recognized forms of sexual abuse. The perpetrator does not need to have direct physical contact with the child for sexual abuse to occur. Exhibitionism, voyeurism, and viewing, producing, or distributing pornography are included under most definitions. Exposing a child to sexually explicit material or acts is also considered abuse. Laws making the use of computers and the Internet in producing, compiling, possessing, or disseminating child pornography a crime had been instituted by 27 stated and the District of Columbia as of December 31, 1999. Violations are included under the heading of sexual abuse or sexual exploitation of children. Other laws address the use of computers to seduce or attract children with the intent of sexual misuse. The failure to protect a child is an important component of many definitions of child abuse and is relevant to sexual abuse when a caretaker is aware that such abuse is occurring and takes no action to stop or prevent it.

Incest, or sexual relations between persons closely related by blood, is a category of sexual abuse that carries with it a different level of psychosocial problems, prognosis, and family dysfunction. Incest includes sexual relations with members of adoptive families and stepfamilies. For the purposes of reporting and meeting a legal definition of sexual abuse, the terms are the same.

Sexual play occurs between young children of similar developmental levels and frequently involves viewing or touching. Sexual play or exploration is considered a normal part of childhood development and curiosity. The distinction between sexual play and sexual abuse is not always clear. Most definitions focus on the discrepancy in age between the two participants, the level of control or authority the older child holds over the younger one, the degree of coercion, and the actual activity involved.

The variation in the definition of child sexual abuse and the wide spectrum of activities covered within these definitions lead to confusion in the minds of mandatory reporters. Those who have a responsibility for the welfare of children should be familiar with their own state statutes. Statistics regarding the incidence of child sexual abuse are also highly dependent on the definition used.

SCOPE

The true magnitude of child sexual abuse is unknown. Incidence rates are based on reports filed with central agencies or cases that otherwise come to the attention of professionals. These rates are generally considered to underestimate the actual number of cases of sexual abuse because they are subject to substantial underreporting. An unknown number of cases are never disclosed or detected. Other cases are disclosed by victims but never reported to authorities. Prevalence statistics are based on surveys of adults regarding childhood experiences of sexual abuse. These studies have their own set of limitations, including variations in study definitions and methodology.

In 1993 the US Department of Health and Human Services conducted the Third National Incidence Study of Child Abuse and Neglect (NIS-3). The findings were based on a nationally representative sample of community professionals and included children who were reported to child protective services agencies as well as those who came to the attention of other professionals. The estimated number of sexually abused children in 1993 was 217,700, a rate of 3.2 cases/1000 children (Sedlak & Broadhurst, 1996). This was almost a two-fold increase from NIS-2 figures from 1986, which reported 119,200 cases or 1.9 cases/1000 children.

The National Child Abuse and Neglect Data System (NCANDS) collects and analyzes data from reports made to individual state child protective services agencies on an annual basis. In 1998, 48 states reported a total of 99,000 cases of child sexual abuse for an overall rate of 1.6 cases/1000 children. Female victims had a higher rate (2.3/1000) than male victims (0.6/1000) (US Department of Health and Human Services, 2000).

Prevalence studies report much higher rates of child sexual abuse. A national survey conducted in 1985 by the Los Angeles Times Poll included a random sample of 2626 American men and women over age 18 years. Some form of child sexual abuse was reported by 27% of women and 16% of men. One third of victimized women and 40% of victimized men never disclosed the incident to anyone (Finkelhor et al., 1990).

In a survey of a random sample of 930 adult women in San Francisco, Russell (1983) reported that 38% experienced at least one form of sexual abuse before age 18 years. Less than 10% of cases were ever reported to the police.

Several obstacles limit the ability of current research to provide truly reliable numbers regarding child sexual abuse. Victims seldom disclose episodes of sexual abuse for reasons discussed later in this chapter. This fact is supported by the low disclosure rates found in adult surveys. Furthermore, cases that are disclosed or eventually recognized by others are not always reported. A broader awareness of child sexual abuse and the passage of mandated reporting laws have resulted in a higher reporting rate. The consistent percentage of reports that are substantiated suggests that this increase reflects actual cases rather than a higher number of unfounded cases.

Despite improved reporting, physicians and other mandated reporters fail to report all cases of sexual abuse (Kempe, 1978). Barriers to reporting are substantial and well documented. In one study fewer than half of the physicians surveyed stated they would report all cases of sexual abuse that came to their attention (James et al., 1978). A study of mandated reporters also found dramatic inconsistencies in reporting practices among pediatricians (Zellman, 1990). The most common reasons provided for not reporting sexual abuse were a perceived lack of sufficient evidence, concern that a report would disrupt the patient-physician relationship or would be harmful to the family, and distrust of the local child protective services agency.

Most practitioners and mandated reporters, as well as the general public, concede that child sexual abuse represents a significant problem in the United States (Tabachnick et al., 1997). Still, the misperception exists that "Child sexual abuse happens, but not in my neighborhood." This belief is contradicted by substantial evidence showing sexual abuse is not related to socioeconomic status or race (Feldman et al., 1991; Finkelhor, 1993; Hymel & Jenny, 1996; Kempe, 1978; Leventhal, 1998; Sedlak & Broadhurst 1996). As a result of misperceptions, the threshold for reporting potential cases remains unacceptably high. The estimated rate of child sexual abuse in the United States is equal to the rate of asthma in childhood, which is considered one of the leading medical disabilities in this age group and an affliction routinely diagnosed and treated in the average pediatric practice (Future directions, 1998).

A different set of potential biases influences prevalence statistics. Recall bias may affect the quoted prevalence in these studies in several ways. False childhood memories overestimate the true prevalence of child sexual abuse, while denial, repressed memories, and a continued unwillingness to disclose these traumatic events give an underestimate of the actual prevalence. Critics point out that many surveys are conducted among select populations limited to college students or specific geographic regions. This limits the ability to extrapolate results to the general population. The definition of sexual abuse, the acts that constitute sexual abuse, and the age at which such acts occur differ between studies.

Despite these limitations, comparative numbers between most studies remain consistent, and experts agree that approximately 20% of women and 9% of men experience some form of inappropriate sexual contact during childhood (Hymel & Jenny, 1996; Kerns et al., 1994). There is a wide discrepancy between the actual number of cases of child sexual abuse and the number of cases reported to authorities.

Child protective services agencies have noted a continued rise in the number of reported cases of child sexual abuse since the 1970s, when these numbers were first recorded. Researchers disagree as to whether this reflects improved recognition and reporting of cases, an actual increase in the occurrence of child sexual abuse, or both. The paucity of data before 1980 makes definitive conclusions difficult. To date there is no firm evidence that the rate of sexual abuse has, in fact, increased (Feldman et al., 1991; Leventhal, 1998).

The most recent data from the National Child Abuse and Neglect Data System and the Annual Fifty State Survey shows an actual decline in reports of child sexual abuse beginning in the early 1990s. These studies show a 26% reduction in child

Key Point:
A number of incidence and prevalence studies have been done over the past several decades and, despite their scientific limitations, both types of studies demonstrate that children in our society are at risk for sexual abuse.

sexual abuse reports and a 30% decline in the number of substantiated reports in the period from 1992 to 1998. It is not clear whether this decline represents a true decrease in the incidence of sexual abuse or changes in the policies or definitions used to tally these numbers. Jones and Finkelhor (2001) offer several possible explanations for the decline. Several theories are currently being investigated. The basis for this trend will have significant implications for future interventions.

Not all cases of reported child sexual abuse result in criminal charges. Cases are selectively prosecuted. This may depend on the particular acts involved in the case, the age of the child, and the age and relationship of the perpetrator. A high number of cases prosecuted end in guilty pleas, and 60% to 90% of cases that go to trial result in convictions (De Jong & Rose, 1991; Martone et al., 1996; San Lazaro, et al., 1996). Some reports show that three fourths of perpetrators convicted of child sexual abuse were sentenced to jail time (Martone et al., 1996; San Lazaro et al., 1996). All 50 states include laws requiring convicted sex offenders to register with the local law enforcement agency.

The media has been vilified as well as praised for its role in the area of child sexual abuse. Some experts argue that the increasing use of graphic images contributes to the problem. Movies and television have been accused of showing increasingly sexually explicit images. Advertisements have been accused of exploiting children by depicting them in adult, sexually stimulating poses and situations. The Internet has made possible on-line sharing of child pornography. Sexual predators have used the Internet as a means to gain access to young children. Highly publicized cases of child sexual abuse have increased public awareness and contributed to widespread recognition of the issue. In one survey, over 90% of respondents reported having seen or heard a news media report during the previous year regarding child sexual abuse (Tabachnick et al., 1997). A Dutch study demonstrated the ability of a mass media campaign to increase the rate of disclosure by sexually abused children by over 300% (Hoefnagels & Baartman, 1997).

False accusations or the fear of such complicates the investigation of reports. False allegations of sexual abuse are an uncommon, but existent, feature of custody battles. The American Bar Association reports that relatively few custody disputes involve sexual abuse allegations (Nicholson & Bulkley, 1988). One literature review found sexual abuse allegations were involved in only 2% of custody disputes, and only 8% to 16.5% of these were false (Penfold, 1995). One report found that 11 of 551 reported cases over a 1-year period involved false allegations of sexual abuse (Oates et al., 2000). These included three cases in which the allegation was made in collusion with a parent. In a survey of New York State teachers, 56% reported knowledge of a false allegation of abuse made against a teacher in their school district (Anderson & Levine, 1999). Differentiating false allegations from true cases can be exceedingly difficult, because most sexual abuse cases tend to be based on circumstantial or hearsay evidence. Investigators are faced with the difficult choice between the potential prosecution of an innocent person versus the devastating situation of not believing a victimized child and providing protection from future abuse. A detailed evaluation of each case by an experienced investigator seeking inconsistencies in the story or evidence that a child's responses have been coached is often necessary.

VICTIMS

Extensive research has been done on sexual abuse victims. The main conclusion from the literature is that there is no classic profile of a sexually abused child. Finkelhor (1993) states that "no identifiable demographic or family characteristics of a child may be used to exclude the possibility that a child has been sexually abused. Some characteristics are associated with greater risk…none of these factors bear a strong enough relationship to the occurrence of abuse that their presence could play a confirming or disconfirming role in the identification of actual cases." Although it is important to consider every child as a possible victim of sexual abuse, some consistencies have been established in the research.

Most literature has focused on females as the victim of sexual abuse. This is in part because female victims account for more than three times the number of male victims in reported cases of child sexual abuse (Finkelhor, 1993; Guidry, 1995). This discrepancy exists partly because of a boy's increased reticence to admit that he was a victim of sexual abuse. Although female victims are much more highly represented in the literature, the number of male victims is greater than once believed. A collaboration of eight studies revealed that girls are 2.5 times more likely to be victims of sexual abuse than boys (Finkelhor & Baron, 1986). It is imperative that healthcare workers acknowledge the problem of child sexual abuse and not overlook the potential victimization of any child, male or female.

Key Point:
Both boys and girls are at risk for sexual abuse, with male victims, on average, being younger than female victims.

Most experts agree that the risk for sexual abuse is highest during preadolescence, with a smaller peak in the early school-age years (Finkelhor, 1993; Nieves-Khouw, 1997; Pierce & Pierce, 1985). Pierce and Pierce (1985) demonstrated that sexually abused boys are, in general, younger than their female counterparts. The male victim averaged 8.6 years (mode = 7 years) and the female 10.6 years (mode = 14 years). Another study quoted a median age of 7 years for male victims and 10 years for females (Nieves-Khouw, 1997).

Although the number of reported cases of child sexual abuse shows a larger percentage of children from lower socioeconomic groups, the epidemiologic research to date does not support this. Similarly, race and ethnicity do not seem to be risk factors for abuse. Overall, no demographic feature has been identified to increase the risk of child sexual abuse (Finkelhor, 1993).

Conversely, certain victim and parenting characteristics have been associated with child sexual abuse. Studies show that most children who become victims of abuse have a tendency to be easily controlled. These children may be physically or mentally disabled and often have needs for love and belonging that are not being met at home.

In general, children living without one or both of their natural parents are at an increased risk of being abused. Females who live apart from their mothers or are not emotionally close to their mothers are at increased risk of sexual abuse (Finkelhor, 1982). Abused males were more likely to live with their mothers and have no father figure in the home (Pierce & Pierce, 1985). The single most important risk factor, for both females and males is the presence of a stepfather in the household (Finkelhor, 1982, 1993; Pierce & Pierce, 1985; Whetsell-Mitchell, 1995a). Other parenting impairments that pose a greater risk of abuse include a mother who is ill, disabled, or extensively out of the home. Substance abuse, parental conflict, or violence in the home are also risk factors for abuse (Finkelhor, 1982, 1993; Finkelhor & Baron, 1986; Whetsell-Mitchell, 1995a). Children of adolescent parents, foster parents, or parents who were sexually abused themselves are often at increased risk of abuse. Finally, siblings of abused children are at increased risk of being abused themselves (Herendeen, 1999).

OFFENDERS

Key Point:
No all-encompassing profile has emerged for describing sexual abuse perpetrators.

Much has been written on the epidemiology and psychopathology of child sex offenders, but one thing remains constant: there is no classic profile of an abuser. Studies have shown that child sex abusers are usually older men. However, one fourth to one third of male perpetrators are reported to be adolescents (Leventhal,

1998). Women have been found to be offenders in up to 5% of cases involving female children and 20% of cases involving male children (Guidry, 1995). Most often, the perpetrator is well known to the child. Male family members, such as the father, stepfather, and uncle, are the most common offenders (Guidry, 1995; Nieves-Khouw, 1997). Children living with a stepfather are at substantially greater risk of being abused than those living with a biologic father. Stepfathers molest girls more often than boys. However, biologic fathers reportedly molest a similar number of girls and boys (Kendall-Tackett & Simon, 1992; Leventhal, 1998; Pierce & Pierce, 1985; Whetsell-Mitchell, 1995a).

Incest is one of the most commonly reported types of abuse. It has been suggested that the occurrence of incestuous abuse may match or even exceed the incidence of physical child abuse. Experts agree that between 75% and 90% of incest victims are female children. Sexual contact between father and daughter and between stepfather and daughter is encountered most frequently (Guidry, 1995). Father-son abuse is revealed less often because it involves two social taboos: the incest taboo and the homosexual taboo. Mother-son abuse is a rare occurrence (Pierce & Pierce, 1985). Models of the incestuous family have been elucidated and typically involve a family in which multiple stressors exist. The father-daughter model illustrates many characteristics of the incestuous family (Justice & Justice, 1979). There is parental conflict leading to absence of sexual relations between the father and mother. The father longs for a source of physical intimacy, often looking to his daughter for comfort and love. The daughter may be depressed and withdrawn and have a poor self-image. She, too, yearns for attention and affection and may be happy to fill a need in her father's life. The mother feels completely dependent on her husband, to the point of being powerless. She subconsciously suggests and allows her daughter to assume her role of wife. She abandons her husband and daughter both emotionally and physically and finds a way to be increasingly absent from the home (Guidry, 1995).

Unfortunately, incestuous abuse is a difficult pattern to break. Commonly, the nonperpetrating parent does not believe the disclosure of abuse when it is revealed, thus allowing it to continue. Often, the nonperpetrating parent is physically or emotionally ill and is unable or unwilling to end the abuse. Some nonperpetrating parents fear violence from the perpetrator. Others are afraid of losing emotional or economic support. Pierce and Pierce (1985) reported that up to 15% of nonperpetrating parents actually encouraged the abuse.

Extrafamilial abuse is more common among boys than girls (Kendall-Tackett & Simon, 1992; Leventhal, 1998; Pierce & Pierce, 1985). Boys younger than age 6 years are at highest risk of abuse by family and friends. Boys older than age 12 years have a greater risk of being abused by strangers (Holmes & Slap, 1998). Extrafamilial abuse is two times more likely to be "very serious" (vaginal/anal intercourse, oral sex) than familial abuse (Leventhal, 1998). Pierce and Pierce (1985) showed that perpetrators of male sexual abuse engaged the boys in three or more sexual acts almost twice as often as perpetrators of female sexual abuse. However, the duration of molestation is shorter on the average for male than for female victims (3.9 years vs. 5.6 years) (Whetsell-Mitchell, 1995a). Kendall-Tackett and Simon (1992) propose several reasons for this. Perpetrators of sexual abuse of boys are more likely to be from outside the home, without continued access to the child; male victims sustain more physical injury, bringing them to medical attention sooner; and males are more likely to possess the physical strength to end the abuse.

Fewer than 50% of child sex offenders are mentally ill (Hilton & Mezey, 1996; Pierce & Pierce, 1985). However, the majority have an emotional disorder that prohibits them from forming intimate relationships with partners their own age. Most offenders feel a sense of excitement when anticipating the abuse of a child and experience both emotional and sexual gratification when the act is complete.

Perpetrators often view their abuse of a child as proof to themselves that they have the power to control one aspect of their lives (Hilton & Mezey, 1996). This partly explains the motivation of abusers who have been victims of sexual abuse themselves. The "victim-to-victimizer" cycle is particularly true of adolescent perpetrators and seems most frequently to involve male victims of male offenders. The characteristics of the chosen victim, including age and physical appearance, as well as the characteristics of the abuse often closely parallel the offender's own memory of abuse (Hilton & Mezey, 1996).

To help understand the events leading up to sexual abuse, Finkelhor (1984) proposed a set of four preconditions that must be overcome before the victimization of a child can occur. The first step is arousal, in which the abuser has sexual desires surrounding children. The perpetrator must then overcome his internal inhibitions relating to the abuse of children. This step is facilitated if the perpetrator experienced a traumatic childhood sexual event of his own (Hilton & Mezey, 1996). The offender must then find a way to have repeated physical contact with the child. This explains why perpetrators usually are people on whom the child depends for emotional, physical, financial, educational, or religious support. Finally, the abuser must overcome the child's resistance to the sexual interaction (Hilton & Mezey, 1996).

Key Point:
Finkelhor has described a set of four preconditions that are typically present in cases of sexual abuse. Sgroi has described a longitudinal model of how sexual abuse typically occurs over time, progressing from non-sexual contact to sexual abuse to the point at which the abuse is discovered.

The strategies employed by the perpetrator to gain the child's trust involve many forms of manipulation (Nieves-Khouw, 1997). This "engagement" is the first step in Sgroi's model, which describes the progression of sexual abuse. The abuser targets the child, and they begin to share nonsexual activities. The abuser may use bribery, including gifts, favors, or privileges to entice the child. He may shower the child with encouragement and compliments. He may use persuasion to deceive the child into believing that they share a special friendship. Over time there is an escalation of activity, with each subsequent interaction becoming more sexual in nature. Once the sexual intimacy occurs, the perpetrator focuses on maintaining the secret. He now uses a different form of manipulation to intimidate the child. Playing upon the child's guilt, he may threaten to stop loving the child. He may use threats of physical harm either to the child or to a family member. He may actually use force or violence. The child feels confused, alone, and betrayed and so perpetuates the secret. This progression of events details the next two steps in model developed by Sgroi et al. (1982): sexual interaction and secrecy (Hilton & Mezey, 1996)

INDICATORS OF SEXUAL ABUSE

The disclosure of sexual abuse, the next stage in the model, may be suppressed for a long time (Sgroi et al., 1982). There are many barriers to disclosure. Children may not reveal a history of sexual abuse because they fear that no one will believe them. Often the child feels guilt and shame surrounding the event and worries about being blamed for the abuse. Children often do not want to get the perpetrator in trouble, and they fear retaliation if they tell (Hilton & Mezey, 1996). For these reasons, children rarely provide a direct disclosure of sexual abuse. When they do, the disclosure may come at any time and to any of a multitude of people. It may occur in a place that reminds the child of the event or in a place where the child feels safe. Children may disclose a history of sexual abuse to a parent at bathtime or at bedtime. It may be made to a sibling to a playmate. The disclosure may be revealed to a teacher or guidance counselor after a sexual abuse prevention program in school. The disclosure may even be confided to the child's physician during a routine health examination (Guidry, 1995; Whetsell-Mitchell, 1995a). More commonly, a nonspecific indicator prompts an evaluation for sexual abuse. A common early warning sign is the use of broad general statements. These statements are used by the child to gauge the response of a trusted listener. Some statements might be relatively general, such as, "Date rape has been a common topic on the news lately." Other examples might be more specific: "Mr. Smith wears tight underwear." These subtle suggestions should alert the listener to the possibility of sexual abuse (Guidry, 1995; Whetsell-Mitchell, 1995a).

In a literature review, Friedrich (1993) concluded that, overall, the most consistent indicator of sexual abuse in all age groups is the demonstration of sexualized behavior. This is defined as age-inappropriate knowledge of both sexual language and behaviors. Victimized children often masturbate when stressed. They may unknowingly use seductive vocabulary or exhibit sexually aggressive intentions. Younger children may use dolls to portray sexual play, whereas older girls may demonstrate promiscuous sexual activity. Male victims have a high rate of cross-dressing (Friedrich, 1993; Sansonnett-Hayden et al., 1987; White et al., 1988). It is important to note that some sexual behavior is considered normative rather than pathognomonic for sexual abuse. The most frequent normative sexual behaviors appear to be self-stimulating behaviors, exhibitionism, and behaviors related to personal boundaries. There seems to be an inverse relationship between normal age and sexual curiosity and exploration, with the overall frequency peaking at 5 years for both boys and girls, then decreasing over the next 7 years. More intrusive or excessive sexual behavior seems to indicate a psychosocial problem. Some issues to consider include family sexuality, life stress, domestic violence, and sexual abuse (Friedrich et al., 1998).

There are many other broad, nonspecific indicators of child sexual abuse, and these can be divided into three categories: physical signs, behavioral signs, and psychiatric signs. In terms of physical indicators, few are diagnostic of sexual abuse. The presence of a sexually transmitted disease in a young child, including gonorrhea, chlamydia, syphilis, genital warts, and herpes simplex type 2, is strongly suggestive of abuse (Whetsell-Mitchell, 1995a). Still, fewer than 7% of cultures for sexually transmitted diseases are positive in suspected cases of sexual abuse (Atabaki & Paradise, 1999). The presence of sperm in or on the body or the discovery of a childhood/teenage pregnancy is a strong indicator of abuse, especially if there is no history of sexual interaction with a peer (Whetsell-Mitchell, 1995b). However, it is rare to find such blatant physical signs of assault (DeJong & Rose, 1991). More often the proof of sexual assault is in scars that are not visibly evident (Friedrich, 1993; Guidry, 1995; Whetsell-Mitchell, 1995a). Other broad indicators that may bring a child to medical attention include chronic abdominal pain, enuresis or encopresis, constipation secondary to anal discomfort, recurrent urinary tract infections, vaginal discharge, or the presence of a vaginal foreign body (Friedrich, 1993; Guidry 1995; Herendeen, 1999; Whetsell-Mitchell, 1995a).

Key Point:
Sexual abuse often presents with non-specific indicators that fall into three categories:
1. physical signs and symptoms
2. behavioral signs and symptoms
3. psychiatric signs and symptoms

Behavioral indicators of abuse are often the first signs noticed by people close to the child. However, these issues are not unique to victims of sexual abuse. They may also be seen in children experiencing other forms of severe stress (Whetsell-Mitchell, 1995a). Some of these behaviors include temper tantrums or running away from home. Children may begin to demonstrate developmentally regressive behaviors, such as thumbsucking or bedwetting. Victims may become fixated on obsessive cleanliness, or they may begin to neglect their bodies. They may engage in self-mutilating behaviors or self-stimulating behaviors such as excessive masturbation. Abused children often exhibit poor school attendance and performance. They may begin to experiment with delinquency or substance abuse. Finally, they may become involved in sexual relationships prematurely (Guidry, 1995; Herendeen, 1999; Hilton & Mezey, 1996; Whetsell-Mitchell, 1995a).

The psychiatric indicators of abuse must also be recognized. Victims of sexual abuse often become victims of depression. This may be exhibited as social withdrawal and the inability to form or maintain meaningful peer relations. Victims experience a profound grief in response to the many losses that they incur after the abuse. These include the loss of innocence and the loss of childhood, the loss of trust in oneself and the loss of trust in adults. The pain of the abuse may be expressed as a sleeping disorder, with fear of the dark and nightmares preventing rest. Children may adopt changes in their eating habits: anorexia, overeating, or avoiding certain foods, such as milk, which reminds them of semen. Victims may attempt suicide to rid themselves of their psychologic pain (Guidry, 1995; Herendeen, 1999; Hilton & Mezey, 1996; Whetsell-Mitchell, 1995b).

The final stage of the model developed by Sgroi et al. (1982) follows either purposeful or accidental disclosure of abuse. At this time the victim's caregivers and/or the offender attempt to suppress the allegation of abuse to restore the perceived state of peace that existed before the disclosure. This suppression accounts for many of the effects described by survivors of child sexual abuse. The short-term effects can range from physical to psychologic derangements, closely paralleling the aforementioned indicators of abuse. If unrecognized or untreated, these effects can lead to severe long-term issues (Guidry, 1995).

SUPPORT SYSTEMS

As the issue of child sexual abuse has come increasingly to the national forefront, support services have slowly been increasing. Specialty divisions have arisen in several areas. Special police units are trained specifically to deal with child sexual abuse victims. Social workers receive specialized training to deal with childhood sexual abuse cases. Multidisciplinary child abuse evaluation teams or Child Advocacy Centers consisting of social workers, nurses, and physicians assist in evaluating potential cases. A 1988 survey of 29 pediatric hospitals with accredited residency programs reported that 69% had a designated pediatric sexual assault center (Smith et al., 1988). Protocols have been developed to improve the accuracy and thoroughness of evaluation and the recommended management of the sexually abused child. Legal services for victims are available, including the appointment of a guardian ad litem when necessary.

Even with these expanded services and referral sources, the pediatrician and family practitioner play a key role in child sexual abuse assessment and evaluation. The practitioner is often the person a family feels most comfortable turning to when there are concerns regarding this issue. He or she may be the person to whom a child discloses the abuse. This person must remain vigilant about detecting subtle clues and recognizing signs and symptoms of sexual abuse. The physician is a mandatory reporter of child sexual abuse and must be familiar with local state law with regard to reportable offenses, as well as the process of reporting such suspicions (American Academy of Pediatrics, 1999; Botash, 1994; Kempe, 1978; Kerns et al., 1994). The primary care physician can provide emotional as well as medical support to the child and family. The physician must be familiar with potential resources in terms of referrals and consultants that deal with this problem in the community. The increasing number of reports suggests that a growing number of physicians are willing to consider sexual abuse a possibility. Primary care practitioners can provide parental education through anticipatory guidance. Young children can be taught to discriminate between "a good touch and a bad touch." Families can be alerted to behaviors or physical signs that are cause for concern or be reassured regarding normal childhood play and curiosity. The physician who routinely performs a genital examination continually reviews the normal anatomy and increases the likelihood that abnormal physical findings will be detected. Regardless of the sophistication and specialty resources eventually incorporated into the system, the primary care physician remains a crucial link. The extent of the evaluation performed by the pediatrician or family practitioner depends on the experience and competency of the physician, the availability of adequate time and equipment to perform an appropriate evaluation or obtain forensic specimens, and the accessibility of a referral site for performing the necessary examination.

Key Point:
Sexual abuse is a problem that could affect any child. Therefore, professionals who come in contact with children need to be aware of the problem, need to know how it presents, and need to know what resources exist in their communities to assist in the evaluation and investigation.

OUTCOMES

Finkelhor and Browne (1985) describe a set of four traumagenic dynamics as a framework for understanding the link between the experience of sexual abuse and its sequelae. *Traumatic sexualization* refers to the inappropriate and dysfunctional development of a victim's sexuality as a result of the abuse. These children are burdened with confusion and misconceptions surrounding their sexuality. They have distorted perceptions of sexual activities. They emerge from the abuse with sexual preoccupations, such as compulsive masturbation, sexualized play, sexual aggression, and seductive behaviors. They often suffer from gender identity conflict and may engage in cross-gender behavior. Several studies reveal a high rate of prostitution among sexual abuse victims. Adult survivors tend to question the role of sex in affectionate relationships and often complain of sexual dysfunction or disinterest. For most victims of sexual abuse, sexual contact will forever bear a negative connotation (Cosentino & Collins, 1996; Finkelhor & Browne, 1985; Guidry, 1995). Certain abuse experiences tend to result in more severe traumatic sexualization. Invasive abuse is probably more sexualizing than when the offender just uses the child to masturbate. Older children who can understand the implications of the abuse are more likely to suffer traumatic sexualization than younger victims (Finkelhor & Browne, 1985).

Key Point:
Finkelhor and Browne describe a conceptual framework that helps explain the damaging effects of sexual abuse on the developing child—the traumatogenic model.

A sense of betrayal emerges when victims realize that someone they trusted has caused them harm. This betrayal is often three-fold. First is the betrayal by the perpetrator in the form of manipulations and misconceptions about sex and love. Second is the child's betrayal by her own body. The child is often convinced that if her body responded to the sexual stimulation then she must have somehow wanted the abuse (Bass & Thornton, 1983). The third betrayal, committed by the victim's family, often confounds the other violations. A family who disbelieves the child's allegation or attempts to suppress it further violates the child's trust (Finkelhor & Browne, 1985).

Children respond to these betrayals in different ways. Some children express their betrayal as anger, with risk-taking behavior and delinquency representing attempts at retaliation (Finkelhor & Browne, 1985; Whetsell-Mitchell, 1995a). Other victims suffer from dissociation in which they separate themselves from their bodies and from the world (Briere & Runtz, 1988; Guidry, 1995). Yet other children display excessively clingy behavior in an effort to restore trust and security in their lives. Adult survivors describe a constant search for a redeeming relationship. Often these early betrayals are a lifelong deterrent to successful marriages. Intrafamilial sexual abuse can produce a more severe and long-lasting sense of betrayal than that involving strangers. Furthermore, the degree of betrayal is also related to the family's response to disclosure. A family who minimizes or blames the child for the abuse compounds the child's sense of betrayal. Finally, when an offender is not held accountable for his crime, the victim's sense of betrayal by the legal system and the norms of society is heightened (Finkelhor & Browne, 1985).

Powerlessness develops when a child feels that her will and her desires are continually superseded. In sexual abuse this occurs when the child's body is repeatedly misused or invaded without her consent. This loss of power is intensified with each manipulation to which the child falls victim. Each unsuccessful attempt by the child to end the abuse further magnifies her sense of disempowerment (Finkelhor & Browne, 1985). Many of the effects of sexual abuse are related to the fear and anxiety that stem from this loss of power. Nightmares, phobias, eating disorders, and somatic complaints all result from the excessive anxiety associated with the abuse (Finkelhor & Browne, 1985). *Somatization* refers to the preoccupation with bodily dysfunction that many victims of sexual abuse experience (Briere & Runtz, 1988). Some common manifestations of somatization include headaches, nausea and vomiting, heart palpitations, dizziness, fatigue, and muscle aches (Guidry, 1995; Whetsell-Mitchell, 1995a). Most survivors fear their susceptibility to repeat victimization and express their feelings of helplessness through runaway behavior, self-mutilation, and suicide attempts. Other victims display aggressive and dominating behaviors, often becoming abusive themselves, to compensate for frustration resulting from their powerlessness. If left untreated, many victims develop posttraumatic stress disorder (Cosentino & Collins, 1996; Hilton & Mezey, 1996). Frequent abusive interactions and lengthy duration of abuse both contribute to an increased sense of disempowerment. The use of force, threats, or excessive coercion by the perpetrator all create a greater degree of psychologic trauma. This is also true of a situation in which the child tries to end the abuse with a disclosure and is disbelieved (Finkelhor & Browne, 1985).

Stigmatization, the final dynamic, describes the negative connotations that become a part of the child's self-image after the abuse. This can happen in various ways. First are the demeaning comments made directly to the child by the offender. Furthermore, the pressure from the perpetrator to maintain secrecy sends a strong message of badness and shame to the child. Second, the child may know that this sort of sexual behavior is wrong, and thus, must deal with her own internal stigma of guilt. Finally, the stigmatization may be magnified if the family reacts with disgust or blames the child for the abuse. The victimized child feels different and alone and often associates with other stigmatized groups of society. This may explain why victims get involved with substance abuse, delinquency, and prostitution. Children often tend to alienate themselves from family and friends who may view them as "damaged goods" (Cosentino & Collins, 1996; Finkelhor & Browne, 1985). Their low self-esteem may contribute to the fact that many survivors of child sexual abuse develop multiple personality disorder (Cosentino & Collins, 1996; Guidry, 1995; Hilton & Mezey, 1996). Children who receive support from their families as well as from professional treatment programs often are less stigmatized than those who are made to feel different (Finkelhor & Browne, 1985).

It is well known that child sexual abuse leaves its victims with substantial psychologic trauma. Furthermore, the variability of abuse experiences seems to cause a wide range of outcomes. However, little is known about the effect of different coping mechanisms on the outcome of abuse. Chaffin et al. (1997) studied the strategies used by a group of sexual abuse victims to cope with their abuse, as well as their self-reported abuse-related symptoms. From the data, they developed a model of four coping mechanisms used by victims of sexual abuse and the group of characteristics associated with each. They defined the coping strategies as avoidant coping, internalized coping, angry coping, and active/social coping (Chaffin et al., 1997).

AVOIDANT COPING
Avoidant coping involved distraction, wishful thinking, and cognitive restructuring. Children who received greater social support after disclosure seemed to display more avoidant coping than others. It has been suggested that avoidant coping produces short-term benefits, but long-term problems. Victims who employed avoidant mechanisms seemed to have more negative attitudes and anxieties about sexuality. Their data revealed, however, that avoidant coping was associated with fewer behavioral problems than the other strategies (Chaffin et al., 1997).

INTERNALIZED COPING
Internalized coping included social withdrawal, self-blame, and resignation. This strategy seemed to be more common in children who received negative reactions from others after disclosure. Their data revealed that these victims displayed more hyperreactive behaviors after the abuse, perhaps leading to the development of post-traumatic stress reactions. Although their study did not differentiate between male and female behaviors, prior research has suggested a distinction (Friedrich et al.,

1986). Female victims seem to display internalized behaviors such as dissociation and depression more commonly than males. Furthermore, they (females) tend to develop phobias, regressive behaviors, and multiple somatic complaints. The research of Chaffin et al. (1997) demonstrated that children rated internalized coping the least helpful of the strategies.

ANGRY COPING

Angry coping involved the cathartic release of emotions and the tendency to blame others. Abuse situations in which the perpetrator had a more distant relationship to the child seemed to instigate angry behaviors. Similarly, a high frequency of abuse interactions and forceful abuse were noted to be antecedents of angry coping. Older victims seemed to react with anger more often than younger ones. This coping mechanism, termed externalization in other research, seems to be more common in male victims (Friedrich et al., 1986; Sansonnett-Hayden et al., 1987). The data of Chaffin et al. (1997) revealed that this strategy was associated with the greatest number of behavioral problems. Such behaviors include physical as well as sexual aggression used to prove their masculinity. Conversely, females demonstrate a greater tendency toward sexually reactive behaviors, which may put them at an increased risk of revictimization.

ACTIVE/SOCIAL COPING

Active/social coping consisted of the utilization of the child's problem-solving abilities as well as social support resources. Children who experienced less severe sexual experiences seemed to implement this coping strategy. The data demonstrated that active/social coping was the only strategy not associated with negative abuse-related behaviors. However, this coping mechanism did not produce any measured benefits either, suggesting that this was a neutral strategy (Chaffin et al., 1997).

There is a paucity of literature to date regarding guidelines for the intervention and treatment of child sexual abuse. The first intervention following disclosure is to ensure the child's safety from further abuse. The next intervention involves the family or nonperpetrating parent (Cosentino & Collins, 1996). The goal of family therapy is to facilitate a supportive and protective environment for the child (Cosentino & Collins, 1996). No available data delineate which type of personalized therapy is best for the child. The treatment, however, must be targeted to the appropriate developmental level of each child. Younger children may benefit from play therapy (Hilton & Mezey, 1996). Group therapy seems to be helpful with adolescent victims because it provides peer support and may reduce the sense of isolation and stigmatization that they feel (Cosentino & Collins, 1996; Hilton & Mezey, 1996). However, group treatment may be too threatening initially for some victims. They may be unable to openly discuss their experience or hear others' accounts of abuse in the early stages of healing. For these victims, individual therapy can help them regain trust and begin to achieve control in their lives once again (Hilton & Mezey, 1996). Recent research has focused on the success of directed abuse-specific therapy. Studies comparing abuse-specific cognitive behavioral therapy to nondirective supportive therapy reveal that both groups show improvement in posttraumatic stress symptoms, but those in cognitive behavioral therapy have significantly greater improvement. Furthermore, involving the nonoffending parent in the treatment of their sexually abused children has proved beneficial as well. Parents engaged in treatment describe a greater decline in their children's externalizing behaviors, as well as a greater improvement in their parenting skills. Cognitive behavioral therapy aims to instill in the nonoffending parent an increased level of confidence and encourages them to model appropriate coping mechanisms for their children. Subsequently, their children report a significantly greater reduction in their level of depression (Deblinger et al., 1996). One reason that this treatment modality may be helpful is its utilization of well-established treatment strategies to handle abuse specific symptoms. Furthermore, the treatment focuses on both amelioration of current symptoms and prevention of later behavioral problems and further victimization (Saywitz et al., 2000). The larger question is whether therapy has a beneficial effect on the well-documented long-term effects of child sexual abuse.

REFERENCES

American Academy of Pediatrics, Committee on Child Abuse and Neglect. Guidelines for the evaluation of sexual abuse of children. *Pediatrics.* 1999;103:186-191.

Anderson EM, Levine M. Concerns about allegations of child sexual abuse against teachers and the teaching environment. *Child Abuse Negl.* 1999;23:833-843.

Atabaki S, Paradise JE. The medical evaluation of the sexually abused child: lessons from a decade of research. *Pediatrics.* 1999;104:178-186.

Bass E, Thornton L, eds. *I never told anyone: writings by women survivors of sexual abuse.* New York, NY: Harper & Row; 1983.

Bender L, Blau A. The reaction of children to sexual relations with adults. *Am J Orthopsychiatry.* 1937;7:500-518.

Botash A. What office-based pediatricians need to know about child sexual abuse. *Contemp Pediatr.* 1994;11:83-100.

Briere J, Runtz M. Symptomatology associated with childhood sexual victimization in a nonclinical adult sample. *Child Abuse Negl.* 1988;12:51-59.

Chaffin M, Wherry JN, Dykman R. School age children's coping with sexual abuse: abuse stresses and symptoms associated with four coping strategies. *Child Abuse Negl.* 1997;21:227-240.

Child Abuse Prevention and Treatment Act (CAPTA).1974; PL 93-247.

Cosentino CE, Collins M. Sexual abuse of children: prevalence, effects, and treatment. *Ann NY Acad Sci.* 1996;789:45-65.

Deblinger E, Lippman J, Steer R. Sexually abused children suffering posttraumatic stress symptoms: initial treatment outcome findings. *Child Maltreatment.* 1996;1:310-321.

De Jong AR, Rose M. Legal proof of child sexual abuse in the absence of physical evidence. *Pediatrics.* 1991;88:506-511.

Feldman W, Feldman E, Goodman JT. Is childhood sexual abuse really increasing in prevalence? an analysis of the evidence. *Pediatrics.* 1991;88:29-33.

Finkelhor D. Sexual abuse: a sociological perspective. *Child Abuse Negl.* 1982;6:95-102.

Finkelhor D, ed. *Child Sexual Abuse: New Theory and Research.* New York, NY: Free Press; 1984.

Finkelhor D. Epidemiological factors in the clinical identification of child sexual abuse. *Child Abuse Negl.* 1993;17:67-70.

Finkelhor D, Baron L. High risk children. In Finkelhor D, ed. *Sourcebook on Child Sexual Abuse.* Beverly Hills, Calif: Sage; 1986:60-88.

Finkelhor D, Browne A. The traumatic impact of child sexual abuse: a conceptualization. *Am J Orthopsychiatry.* 1985;55:530-541.

Finkelhor D, Hotaling G, Lewis IA, Smith C. Sexual abuse in a national survey of adult men and women: prevalence, characteristics, and risk factors. *Child Abuse Negl.* 1990;14:19-28.

Freud S. The aetiology of hysteria. In: J. Strachey, trans-ed. *The Standard Edition of the Complete Psychological Works of Sigmund Freud*, Vol. 3. London: The Hogarth Press; 1961:189-221.

Friedrich WN. Sexual victimization and sexual behavior in children: a recent review of the literature. *Child Abuse Negl.* 1993;17:59-66.

Friedrich WN, Fisher J, Broughton D, et al. Normative sexual behavior in children: a contemporary sample. *Pediatrics.* 1998;101:1-13.

Friedrich WN, Urquiza AJ, Beilke R. Behavioral problems in sexually abused young children. *J Pediatr Psychol.* 1986;11:57-67.

Future directions for research on diseases of the lung: ATS update. *Am J Respir Crit Care Med.* 1998;158:320-334.

Guidry HM. Childhood sexual abuse: role of the family physician. *Am Fam Physician.* 1995;51:414.

Herendeen PM. Evaluating for child sexual abuse. *Adv Nurse Pract.* 1999;7:54-58.

Hilton MR, Mezey GC. Victims and perpetrators of child sexual abuse. *Br J Psychiatry.* 1996;169:408-415.

Hoefnagels C, Baartman H. On the threshold of disclosure: the effects of a mass media field experiment. *Child Abuse Negl.* 1997;21:557-573.

Holmes WC, Slap GB. Sexual abuse of boys. *JAMA.* 1998;280:1855-1860.

Hymel KP, Jenny C. Child Sexual Abuse. *Pediatr Rev.* 1996;17:236-249.

James J, Womack WM, Stauss F. Physician reporting of sexual abuse of children. *JAMA.* 1978;240:1145-1146.

Jones L, Finkelhor D. *The Decline in Child Sexual Abuse Cases.* Juvenile Justice Bulletin. Washington, DC: US Department of Justice, Office of Juvenile Justice and Delinquency Prevention, Office of Justice Programs; 2001.

Justice B, Justice R, eds. *The Broken Taboo: Sex in the Family.* New York, NY: Human Sciences, 1979:109-202.

Kempe CH. Sexual abuse, another hidden pediatric problem: The 1977 C. Anderson Aldrich Lecture. *Pediatrics.* 1978;62:382-389.

Kempe CH, Silverman FN, Steele BF, Droegemueller W, Silver HK. The battered child syndrome. *JAMA.* 1962;181:105-112.

Kendall-Tackett KA, Simon AF. A comparison of the abuse experiences of male and female adults molested as children. *J Fam Violence.* 1992;77:57-62.

Kerns DL, Terman DL, Larson CS. The role of physicians in reporting and evaluating child sexual abuse cases. *The Future of Children.* 1994;4:119-134.

Kinsey AC, Pomeroy WB, Martin CE, Gebhard PH. *Sexual behavior in the human female.* Philadelphia, Pa: Saunders; 1953.

Leventhal JM. Epidemiology of sexual abuse of children: old problems, new directions. *Child Abuse Negl.* 1998;22:481-491.

Martone M, Jaudes PK, Cavins MK. Criminal prosecution of child sexual abuse cases. *Child Abuse Negl.* 1996;20:457-464.

Nicholson EB, Bulkley J, eds. *Sexual Abuse Allegations in Custody and Visitation Cases: A Resource Book for Judges and Court Personnel.* Washington, DC: American Bar Association, National Legal Resource Center for Child Advocacy and Protection; 1988.

Nieves-Khouw FC. Recognizing victims of physical and sexual abuse. *Crit Care Nurs Clin North Am.* 1997;9:141-148.

Oates RK, Jones DP, Denson D, et al. Erroneous concerns about child sexual abuse. *Child Abuse Negl.* 2000;24:149-157.

Penfold PS. Mendacious moms or devious dads? Some perplexing issues in child custody/sexual abuse allegation disputes. *Can J Psychiatry.* 1995;40:337-341.

Pierce R, Pierce LH. The sexually abused child: a comparison of male and female victims. *Child Abuse Negl.* 1985;9:191-199.

Russell DEH. The incidence and prevalence of intrafamilial and extrafamilial sexual abuse of female children. *Child Abuse Negl.* 1983;7:133-136.

San Lazaro C, Steele AM, Donaldson LJ. Outcome of criminal investigation into allegations of sexual abuse. *Arch Dis Child.* 1996;75:149-152.

Sansonnett-Hayden H, Hakey G, Marriage C, Fine S. Sexual abuse and psychopathology in hospitalized adolescents. *J Am Acad Child Adolesc Psychiatry.* 1987;26:753-757.

Saywitz KJ, Mannarino AP, Berliner L, et al. Treatment for sexually abused children and adolescents. *Am Psychol.* 2000;55:1040-1049.

Sedlak AJ, Broadhurst DD. *Third National Incidence Study of Child Abuse and Neglect (NIS-3final Report).* US Department of Health and Human Services (contract #105-94-1840). 1996.

Sgroi SM, Blick LC, Porter FS. A conceptual framework for child sexual abuse. In Sgroi SM, ed. *Handbook of Clinical Intervention in Child Sexual Abuse.* Lexington, Mass: Lexington Books; 1982:9-37.

Smith D, Losek J, Glaeser P, Walsh-Kelly C. Pediatric sexual abuse management in a sample of children's hospitals. *Pediatr Emerg Care.* 1988;4:177-179.

Tabachnick J, Henry F, Denny L. Perceptions of child sexual abuse as a public health problem. *MMWR.* 1997;46:801-803.

US Department of Health and Human Services; Administration on Children, Youth and Families. *Child Maltreatment 1998: Reports From the States to the National Child Abuse and Neglect Data System*, Washington, DC: US Government Printing Office; 2000.

Whetsell-Mitchell J. Indicators of child sexual abuse: children at risk. *Issues Compr Pediatr Nurs.* 1995a;18:319-340.

Whetsell-Mitchell J. The many faces of child sexual abuse. *Issues Compr Pediatr Nurs.* 1995b;18:299-318.

White S, Halpin BM, Strom GA, Santilli G. Behavioral comparisons of young sexually abused, neglected, and nonreferred children. *J Clin Child Psychiatry.* 1988;17:53-61.

Zellman G. Child abuse reporting and failure to report among mandated reporters: prevalence, incidence and reasons. *J of Interpersonal Violence.* 1990;5:3-23.

ANOGENITAL ANATOMY: DEVELOPMENTAL, NORMAL, VARIANT, AND HEALING

William J. Reed, MD, FAAP

MEDICAL EMBRYOLOGY OF THE EXTERNAL GENITALIA

Genetic sex is determined at the time of fertilization of the ovum. The early genital system in the human fetus is undifferentiated and bipotential. That is, during the first 12 weeks of embryonic life both male and female primordial tracts are present and develop in unison (Moore, 1982). In the female the cortex develops into the ovary at 10 to 11 weeks, while the medulla regresses. In the male the medulla differentiates into the testis, and the cortex regresses. This gonadal development results from the migration of primitive germ cells to the urogenital ridge near the fetal kidney and adrenal gland. After fertilization, the undifferentiated gonad begins to change with the appearance of the mullerian ducts in the female at 6 weeks gestation. In the male, differentiation is present with the appearance of Sertoli cells at 6 to 7 weeks and Leydig cells at 8 weeks, respectively (Sadler, 1995). This phase of development of dual gonadal ducts then forms the phenotypic external genitalia.

The gonadal primordia are influenced by the sex-determining region (SRY) on the Y chromosome. If there is a deletion of the short arm (p-) of the Y chromosome or of the SRY gene, male differentiation does not occur. Deletions of the long arm (q-) of the Y chromosome result in normally developed males with short stature and azoospermia. The presence of an anti-müllerian hormone (AMH) or müllerian inhibitory factor (MIF) produced by the Sertoli cells in the testis causes the müllerian duct system to regress with dissolution of the female pelvic structures, that is, the uterus and fallopian tubes. This MIF is characterized as a glycoprotein whose gene locus has been localized to chromosome 19 (Simpson, 2000). Testosterone produced by the Leydig cells stabilizes the wolffian ducts and through 5-a reductase produces dihydrotestosterone, which virilizes the male external genitalia. The Sertoli and Leydig cell lines and their respective hormones function separately from the morphogenesis of the testis (Bhatnagar, 2000). Specifically, they direct gonadal development as opposed to being products of the testis. Therefore, if a functioning testis is present, the phenotype will be male. Conversely, in the absence of the sex determining region, whether or not an ovary is present, the phenotype will be female (Mittwoch et al., 1993). The uterus, fallopian tubes, and upper vagina will develop independently of the ovary. The female genital tract results from the müllerian ducts, urogenital sinus, and vaginal plate. In the male, the wolffian ducts, the genital tubercle, and the labioscrotal folds form the external genitalia. So, counterintuitively, M becomes female, and W becomes male.

Key Point:
Genetic sex is determined at the time the ovum is fertilized. The early genital system in the human fetus is undifferentiated and bipotential, meaning that during the first 12 weeks of embryonic life, both male and female primordial tracts are present and develop in unison.

DEVELOPMENT OF THE EXTERNAL GENITALIA IN BOYS

In boys, external genital development occurs between 10 and 16 weeks gestation and does not require high concentrations of testosterone, but does require the conversion of 6% to 8% of total testosterone to 5-dihydrotestosterone. The genital tubercle continues to grow to form the penis, and the urogenital folds fuse to enclose the penile urethra (Bukowski & Zeman, 2001). The distal head of the penis is the glans penis and the proximal shaft is joined at the corona. The opening of the penile urethra, which may be covered by the foreskin, is called the meatus. Where the foreskin attaches to the corona of the glans penis is termed the frenulum. Laterally, the labioscrotal folds develop and, in the presence of testosterone and 5-DHT, become fused in the midline to form the scrotum. This line may be very prominent on inspection and is referred to as the median raphe. At approximately 11 weeks, the processus vaginalis is present at the internal inguinal ring. It is contiguous with the gubernaculum, which inserts on the mesonephric (wolffian) duct. At 17 weeks the testis is now at the same site and begins to elongate along its vertical axis (Rohn, 1998). This phase of descent is androgen dependent. At 28 weeks the "inguinal scrotal" stage of descent begins. The testis descends into the scrotal sac between 28 and 32 weeks, depending on regression of the gubernaculum. The scrotal content may include fluid from a patent process vaginalis, intestine from a hernia defect, or a discolored and indurated mass caused by torsion of the testis, occasionally seen in breech presentations. The apparent clinical absence of one or both testes requires differentiating between an undescended or absent testis and the more common retractile testis. The spermatic cord and epididymis lie posteriorly to the testis, which is anchored to the scrotum by the gubernaculum, which now becomes a reticular strand.

Testosterone is responsible for the evolution of the mesonephric duct system into the vas deferens, epididymis, ejaculatory ducts, and seminal vesicle. Dihydrotestosterone results in the development of the male external genitalia, including the prostate gland, which arises from the urogenital sinus, and the bulbourethral glands of Cowper. At puberty, testosterone leads to spermatogenesis and the development of the secondary sexual characteristics as well as a five to seven-fold enlargement of the prostate gland, epidydimis, and testes (Moore, 1982).

ANATOMIC VARIATIONS IN BOYS

During examination of the male from infancy through puberty stage Tanner G5, many variations of normal as well as some previously unrecognized problems may be present. Many of these findings are frequent and easily noted and managed. Others are not so obvious and may be missed. The more common variations in genital findings are discussed throughout the following sections.

Leydig cell aplasia or hypoplasia (Rapaport, 2000) produces a phenotypic female with mild virilization. The testes, epididymis, and vas deferens are present. There is no uterus or fallopian tubes and no secondary sexual changes at puberty. Testosterone levels remain prepubertal, that is, at a serum level defined as less than 10ng/dL (Lee, 2002), but pubic hair can appear appropriately normal as a result of adrenal function. Abnormalities at this early stage also include congenital adrenal hyperplasia with subsequent virilization, or androgen receptor site/enzyme defects (5-a reductase) causing a lack of virilization and incomplete or normal development in the male (albeit eventually a large penis). It may lead to ambiguous genitalia in the female.

Partial androgen insensitivity produces the most common form of male pseudohermaphroditism. This occurs at a frequency of less than one in 20,000 genetic males and is an X-linked disorder with the androgen receptor gene locus at Xq11-12 (Simpson, 2000). All are 46XY and may appear with female genitalia, various male anomalies, or phenotypic albeit sterile males. Other reported androgen receptor site syndromes include Reifenstein's (severe hypospadias, hypogonadism and gynecomastia), Gilbert-Dreyfus, and Lub's syndromes.

Phimosis is present when the prepuce or "foreskin" remains tight and cannot be retracted to or over the corona of the glans penis by age 5 to 6 years. If recurrent balanitis or balanoposthitis occurs, circumcision is curative.

Paraphimosis refers to venous obstruction and pain caused by a tight and sometimes irreducible foreskin retracted behind the coronal sulcus. If manual reduction fails, a surgical slit in the dorsal prepuce may be required.

Hypospadias is caused by underdevelopment of the urogenital folds, resulting in a ventral (anterior) positioned urethral opening anywhere on a line between the corona of the glans penis and the perineal body (Bukowski & Zeman, 2001). Hypospadias is associated with an incomplete prepuce ventrally, which gives the appearance of a dorsal hood. Additionally, there is a curvature of the penis (chordee) ventrally toward the floor. Hypospadias occurs in one of 250 live male births, and may be associated with undescended testes (Elder, 2000). A karyotype should be obtained on any infant or child with a mid or proximal hypospadias and cryptorchidism. A voiding cystourethrogram may be indicated for penoscrotal hypospadias because 5% to 10% of cases have müllerian remnants. The incidence of hypospadias has been increasing over the past 26 years (20.3 to 39.7 per 10,000) because of either endocrine or polygenic reasons (Dolk, 1998). Hypospadias is the only absolute contraindication to circumcision. Relative contraindications include chordee without hypospadias, a small penis, or a dorsal hood anomaly. Dorsal hood/chordee occurs with a distal meatus. Circumcision is again contraindicated. This anomaly will require a urethroplasty.

Circumcision adhesions and bridging bands may cause penile curvature. These are rather easily separated in the first 9 to 12 months, but later may be tenacious and require surgery under analgesia.

Erythema or hyperpigmentation of the shaft immediately proximal to the glans may be caused by circumcision or occur from the natural friction produced by self-manipulation. It may also be noted in infection of the shaft of the penis (balanitis) in the circumcised male or as a purulent balanoposthitis in the uncircumcised male.

Smegma is a white creamy substance adherent to the coronal sulcus probably in all uncircumcised males and in 0.5% of circumcised males. It consists of desquamated epithelium, long chain fatty acids, sterols, and squalene. The etiology is probably the atypical organism Mycobacterium smegmatis.

Uric acid crystals in urine with a pH less than 7 may leave a pinkish red spot on the anterior diaper of an infant and should be easily discernible from blood after circumcision in the male newborn or withdrawal vaginal bleeding in the female newborn. The latter occurs following withdrawal from maternal estrogen and is discussed in the section on the effects of estrogen.

Pink pearly papules of the penis may be present in males ages 11 to 21 years and are discussed in the section on pubertal changes. They occur most often circumferentially and proximal to the corona of the glans. They appear monomorphic, homogeneous, and are in multiple rows. The do not blanch with acetic acid and do not yield positive for Human Papilloma Virus. They are essentially asymptomatic.

Urethral meatal stenosis is a complication that occurs in 5% to 10% of male infants who have been circumcised. It is likely the result of disruption of the arterial blood supply (frenular artery) to the distal frenulum (Elder, 2000).

Other anomalies of the glans penis in the male are exceedingly rare and include *epispadias*, in which the urethral meatus is found on the dorsum of the penis when the genital tubercle forms in the urorectal septum (Baskin 2000). The incidence is one in 30,000 to 40,000 live male births. It is more common in males (3.5:1) and is the least severe form of exstrophy.

Exstrophy of the bladder is a lack of primitive streak mesoderm, which results in externalization of the bladder mucosa. The prepuce is present only ventrally, and epispadias is always present in boys. In girls the clitoris is bifid and the urethra is split dorsally. The incidence is one in 117,000 boys and one in 148,000 girls, respectively (Canning & Gearhart, 1993).

Shawl Defect is a mild defect in masculinization due to a lack of complete migration of the labioscrotal folds. Ninety percent of these boys also have have cryptorchidism (Aarskog, 1970).

Micropenis is defined as a newborn penile stretch length less than 1.9 mm and is associated with the Prader-Willi, Kallmann, and Lawrence-Moon-Biedl syndromes. Agenesis of the penis has an XY genotype and an incidence of less than one in 1 million live male births.

Diphallia ranges from the presence of a small accessory penis to complete duplication.

Urethral duplication, atresia, fistula, parameatal cysts, and megalourethra are rare. When these are present, the diagnosis of prune belly (Eagle-Barrett) syndrome should be considered.

Penile torsion is rare and is usually rotated counterclockwise.

DEVELOPMENT OF THE EXTERNAL GENITALIA IN GIRLS

In the absence of the fetal testis, the female external genitalia develop from the genital groove and urogenital sinus. This begins at approximately 6 weeks in the embryo and is completed by the eleventh to twelfth week of gestation. In the XX female or the Xp-mosaic female, oocytes are present at 16 weeks. If two intact X chromosomes are not present, as in the case of Xp- deletion (Turner's syndrome), the ovarian follicles begin to degenerate by birth and become atretic variably thereafter. The missing second X is responsible for ovarian maintenance and not ovarian differentiation (Simpson, 2000).

Key Point:
In the absence of the fetal testis, female external genitalia develop from the genital groove and urogenital sinus. This begins at 6 weeks of gestation and is completed by the eleventh to twelfth week.

The *mons pubis* is derived from fusion at the anterior commissure and is formed inferiorly by the joining of the *labia minora*, which extend posteriorly and inferiorly, ending at the skin between the vagina and anus. It is the round and fleshy prominence created by the fat pad overlying the *symphysis pubis* in girls. The labia minora do not meet at this site. This structure is prominent in the newborn female because of maternal estrogen, and any pigmentation is directly related to those infants with darker skin colors. This includes the *linea nigra* extending cephalad or vertically from the mons to the umbilicus.

The *prepuce* (foreskin) is an anatomical structure formed by a midline collision of ectoderm, neuro-ectoderm, and mesenchyme creating a penta-laminar tissue covering both the male and female glans, as well as the male urethra (Moore, 1982). The clitoral prepuce develops independently of the urogenital and labioscrotal folds. The urogenital groove on the ventral surface or undersurface of the clitoris permits circumferential development and results in a hood-like appearance. Functionally, this hood is mucocutaneous tissue and seems to provide physiologic protection against irritation and perhaps bacterial contamination. The absence of the prepuce (aposthitis) is rare. It was reported in Jewish Law (1567 CE) in regard to a male "being born circumcised." Most likely, this represented hypospadias (Bukowski & Zeman, 2001). Canalization of the urethra requires complete development of the prepuce. However, both hypospadias and epispadias have been described with otherwise normal development (Baskin, 2000). As previously noted, virilization may cause partial or complete fusion of the labioscrotal folds, but there is no testis present. Often inguinal hernias or hydroceles (canal of Nuck) are present in the infant who is both a phenotypic and genotypic female.

The female pudendum or vulva is the remnant of the urogenital sinus and hymenal junction between the urogenital sinus and the canalized vaginal plate. The vaginal plate reforms from a tubular structure to a flat vestibule, with final canalization of the vagina occurring at 20 weeks. The latter occurs caudad to cephalad, and the distal portion of the sinovaginal bulb becomes the hymenal tissue. It is not completely clear if the epithelial proliferation, which begins in the dorsal lining of the urogenital sinus in the region of the sinovaginal bulb, is a derivative of the mesonephric duct or the genital tubercle (Bhatnagar, 2000). The development and normal variant anatomy of the hymen is well studied and will be presented later. The genital tubercle enlarges but slows in the female to form the clitoris, while the urogenital folds form the labia minora. The area within the labia minora where the urethra, vagina, paraurethral (Skene's) glands, and the greater posterior (Bartholin's) ducts open defines the vestibule. The labia minora encircle the clitoris anteriorly and form a hood posterior to the urethral and vaginal openings. Prepubertally, these do not join in the midline because they are not completely developed (Berek, Adashi, & Hillard, 1996). Where they join to enclose the vestibule inferiorly (posteriorly) is a frenulum of tissue known as the posterior fourchette. The concave space between the hymenal ring and the posterior fourchette is termed the fossa navicularis or posterior vestibule. Laterally, the labioscrotal folds develop and, in the absence of androgen, remain unfused, forming the labia majora, which appear flat and unpigmented until puberty when the effect of estrogen and androgen enlarges and pigments them.

ANATOMIC VARIATIONS IN GIRLS

Many anatomical and developmental variations are known to occur in girls. Some are present in the newborn, while others develop over time. An appreciable number of congenital abnormalities, notably vaginal agenesis, pass undetected in the newborn. Many eventually become clinically apparent, but some may only be partially expressed and found incidentally at the time of other procedures or surgery. The following is a compilation of the more prevalent entities, but others may be found through a search of the literature. The following have been chosen because of their frequent occurrence or because alert diagnosis and rapid intervention are necessary in certain cases. The treatment of these entities is not in the scope of this discussion.

Partial or complete virilization is usually caused by non–salt-losing congenital adrenal hyperplasia, which is the most common cause of female pseudohermaphroditism. This is most often the result of 21-hydroxylase deficiency. One should also suspect 11-hydroxylase and type II 3-beta hydroxysteroid dehydrogenase. Clinical expression in the female varies from no virilization or isolated clitoromegaly to ambiguous genitalia without palpable testes. The presence of palpable gonads excludes congenital adrenal hyperplasia and other forms of female pseudohermaphroditism. However, the clitoris can appear quite prominent in preterm females because of the immature development of the labia majora. With continued estrogenization, the labia will become more prominent while the growth of the clitoris will slow. Isolated enlargement of the clitoris may be familial and is sometimes a feature of neurofibromatosis or long-term phenytoin therapy (Rickwood & Godiwalla, 1998).

Partial androgen insensitivity syndromes include ***labial agglutination or fusion*** and ***premenarchal lichen sclerosis***. Both of these have been confused with or misdiagnosed as evidence of child sexual abuse. Labial agglutination or fusion is very common in a general pediatric practice and responds well to the gentle application of a topical estrogen cream such as dienestrol 0.01% (Ortho Dienestrol Cream). Lichen sclerosis becomes apparent over a wide age range. It is more common in girls but has been reported in boys. It has a predilection for the vulvar, perineal, and perianal skin. It most commonly appears in a figure-of-eight configuration and may be hypopigmented, hemorrhagic, or vesicular. It is most often confused with sexual assault, group A beta hemolytic streptococcal infections, and scleroderma. Premenarchal lichen sclerosis often improves spontaneously during puberty, although this is not the experience of all authors (Berth-Jones et al., 1989). It responds to 1% hydrocortisone (S. Pogorny, personal communication, August 1998) and more recently to clobetasol proprionate 0.05% ointment (Temovate, Glaxo) (Quint & Smith, 1999). It has also responded to topical progesterone and estrogen. The risk for cancer is not increased as is seen with postmenopausal lichen sclerosis et atrophicus. Much less commonly seen partial androgen insensitivity syndromes include blind vas deferens and the presence of testes in the labioscrotal folds in the 46XY girl (Fryer, 1998). In complete androgen insensitivity syndrome, 50% of girls presenting at puberty with amenorrhea and no secondary sexual characteristics will have an inguinal hernia present (Garden, 1998).

Labial hypertrophy is seen in children but is more evident after puberty. It may involve one or both labia minora and is generally noted during the inspection of the female pudendum. Very few patients request surgical reduction. This author has seen girls referred because of chronic irritation which is usually attributed to the hypertrophy but in most instances is not. Enlargement of the labia may also be caused by lymphangiomas and hemangiomas. Hypoplasia of the labia majora may be an isolated normal variant and has been described as a feature in trisomy 18.

Vulvar or vaginal variations most commonly seen include the following: In ***Hydrocolpos*** the vestibule appears tense and greyish white because of the hymen being imperforate. This may be present at birth. Treatment is by excision of the hymen or drainage of the fluid. It may also be found more often as hydrometrocolpos in young adolescent female as a bulging bluish vaginal mass associated with primary amenorrhea, abdominal pain, and sometimes a midline hypogastric mass. Rarely, hydrocolpos may present as part of an autosomal recessive syndrome (McKusick-Kaufman syndrome) with other anogenital anomalies, including a vaginal septum with absence of the cervix (McKusick et al., 1964; Westerhout et al., 1964).

Midline perineal fusion defect or groove includes mucosal exposure anywhere on a line from the fossa navicularis to the anus. This is mesodermal, resolves at puberty, and requires a note from the examiner so as to preclude any misdiagnosis of nonaccidental trauma.

Vaginal prolapse or procidentia has been reported in a newborn associated with paralysis of the pelvic floor and apparently resolved at age 6 months (Rickwood & Godiwalla, 1998). It is commonly seen in adolescents with spina bifida and meningomyelocele. Manual reduction is easily accomplished.

Vaginal agenesis or caudal müllerian agenesis is also known as the Von Mayer Rokitansky-Kuster-Hauser syndrome. The vagina is entirely absent or may resemble a smooth pit. There is hypoplasia or absence of the uterus and less often the proximal fallopian tubes. Isolated uterine agenesis is exceptionally rare, and 75% of these cases are associated with vaginal agenesis (Koram et al., 1979). The ovaries are normal. Because of the close embryologic approximation of the müllerian and wolffian systems, there may be associated upper urinary tract and renal anomalies. Müllerian agenesis is second only to Turner's syndrome as a genetic cause of primary amenorrhea.

Key Point:
The midline perineal fusion defect is mesodermal, resolves at puberty, and requires a note for the examiner so as to preclude any misdiagnosis of nonaccidental trauma.

Key Point:
Müllerian agenesis is second only to Turner's syndrome as a genetic cause of primary amenorrhea.

Vaginal atresia presumably results from maldevelopment of the vaginal plate. It is usually associated with an imperforate anus.

Vaginal duplication results from failure of the paired müllerian ducts to fuse. Partial fusion causes a longitudinal vaginal septum (see p. 18).

Linea vestibularis or midline sparing has been recognized since 1991 (Kellogg & Parra, 1991) and will be discussed in the section on hymenal variations.

Skene's duct cysts are located inferolateral to the urethra. The duct functions as a major contributor to vaginal lubrication. The duct usually does not occlude unless infected. Skene's duct is a derivative of the urogenital sinus and is embryologically homologous to the prostate gland in the male. Rare cancers in these ducts are associated with increased levels of prostate-specific antigen (PSA) (Berek et al., 1996). In the postpubertal teen and adult female, the posterior or inferior Bartholin's glands can become infected with gram-negative organisms or Neisseria gonorrhea.

URETHRAL VARIATIONS

Prolapse or the circular eversion of urethral mucosa through the urethral meatus may present as hematuria or blood stained panties in girls usually between ages 5 and 8 years. It may be misdiagnosed as vulvar bleeding if unrecognized and resolving (Anveden-Hertzberg et al., 1995). It is more commonly seen in girls of African-Caribbean descent and usually resolves with symptomatic therapy or the application of topical estrogen because the distal urethra is estrogen sensitive. Occasionally the mucosa may become friable or necrotic and require surgical resection. It has been previously reported in a newborn (Jenkins et al., 1984).

Paraurethral cysts are located dorsally or inferior to the lower urethra in the vaginal wall. They may be squamous or transitional epithelial invaginations of vaginal mucosa. Rarely, they may compress the urethra or obstruct the vagina. Marsupialization or excision may be required at puberty because of the frightening but benign prospect of rupturing during intercourse (Garden, 1998). The more frequently seen mesonephric duct cysts are located in the lateral vaginal wall. The most common of these, the Gartner duct canal cyst, may be associated with ectopic ureterocele and other upper urinary tract anomalies. These girls have the complaint of "always being wet" because of urinary incontinence. In addition, there may be paramesonephric (müllerian) cysts of the vaginal wall or cervix (Klein et al., 1986). Many of these retention cysts can present at birth as a swelling below the urethral meatus. Most resolve spontaneously (Garden, 1998). A few may require incision and drainage. On culdoscopic examination, congenital cysts are covered with capillaries, whereas imperforate hymen is not.

Urethral caruncle is mentioned for completeness but is less common than urethral prolapse.

VARIATIONS OF THE INTERNAL GENITALIA

OVARY

Bilateral absence of the ovaries is rare but has been associated with both sirenomelia and synpodia. Unilateral loss of an ovary occurs with absence of the ipsilateral fallopian tube (Sivanesaratum, 1968). Supernumerary ovaries may occur and are most often found in the mesovarium or broad ligament. Neonatal or fetal ovarian cysts are germinal or graffian in origin and may be simple, follicular, or theca lutein. These were considered rare or not readily recognized until the advent of ultrasonography (Ivarsson et al., 1983).

Tumors are very rare, and both granulosa cell and cystadenoma have been described (Garden, 1998). Streak ovaries occur in Turner's syndrome and mixed gonadal dysgenesis whereby there is a dysgenetic testis and the risk of gonadoblastoma.

UTERUS

Lack of union or fusion of the paired müllerian ducts may lead to anomalies such as duplication of the uterine body, incomplete or didelphys vagina and uterus, or bicornuate uterus with a single vagina and cervix. Epispadias in females is very rare, whereas hypospadias in females is diagnosed by finding the urethral meatus in the vagina (Bhatnagar 2000 and Simpson, 2000).

THE HYMEN

The hymen (Greek god of marriage) is a recessed structure at the entrance to the vaginal opening. Andreas Vesalius, the father of anatomy, first described it in 1561. It arises from the embryonal urogenital septum developing as mesenchymal tissue advances into the epithelial mass at the junction of the pelvic part of the urogenital sinus and the tubular vaginal plate. Absence of the hymen does not exist on an embryological basis as an isolated anomaly. It is present in all females even when other anomalies exist (Capraro & Capraro, 1971). Two separate studies in the United States and Israel examined 26,199 newborn females and found the hymen to be present in all instances (Jenny et al., 1987; Mor & Merlob, 1988). Even with vaginal agenesis, hymenal remnants have been found (Rock & Azziz, 1987).

Key Point:
Imperforate hymen is the only anatomic variation in configuration in which no functional opening is present. It is probably the most common obstructive anomaly of the female genitalia, is present in about 0.1% of females, and is reported to occur in families.

Imperforate hymen is the only anatomic variation in configuration in which no functional opening is present. It is probably the most common obstructive anomaly of the female genitalia, occurring in approximately 0.1% of females, and has been reported to occur in families (Usta et al., 1993). This should be diagnosed early in life once the effect of maternal estrogen on the female vestibule diminishes. Unfortunately, it often is not recognized until much later and can be associated with abdominal pain and amenorrhea (hydrometrocolpos). A clinical clue is the primary absence of menses in a Tanner 3-4 female with normal development of the breasts and secondary sexual hair. The vaginal orifice is obscured by a slightly bulging blue and ballotable or tense mass located in the vestibule inferior and midline to the urethra. There is no superficial vascularity with imperforate hymen as is present with congenital cysts. It has been reported in five girls after documented hymenal trauma (Berkowitz et al., 1987; Botash & Louis, 2001).

VARIATIONS IN CONFIGURATION

Key Point:
Factors that can influence the anatomic appearance of the hymen include internal factors (estrogenization, aging, and development) and external ones (the patient's position during the examination, the examiner's experience and/or bias, whether the patient is relaxed, and the use of labial traction or labial separation).

The hymen may have at least six well-described and anatomically differing configurations (Berenson, 1993, 1995; Berenson et al., 1991, 1992; McCann et al., 1990b; Pokorny, 1987; Pokorny & Kozinetz, 1988). Other factors that may influence the anatomical appearance of the hymen include estrogenization, aging, and development. Added factors include the patient's position during the examination, the examiner's experience and/or bias, relaxation by the patient, and the use of labial traction or labial separation (Adams & Wells, 1993; Brayden et al., 1991; McCann et al., 1990a; Paradise et al., 1997). Labial separation is no longer recommended in the genital examination of prepubertal girls for two reasons: it can frequently be the cause of iatrogenic tears to the posterior fossa navicularis and posterior fourchette; and exposure of the entire vestibule and hymenal opening is much better visualized using labial traction posterior and downward.

Pokorny (1987) and later Pokorny and Kozinetz (1988) studied the hymenal configuration in 265 girls and also reviewed the descriptions by six previous authors. *They proposed three basic hymenal types:*

1. ***Fimbriated*** (denticulate, sleeve-like, or scalloped)

2. ***Annular*** (concentric, symmetrical)

3. ***Posterior rim*** (crescentic, semilunar)

Pokorny (1987) noted redundant hymenal and paraurethral tissue such as hymenal tags in newborns through age 4 years. Other types of configurations, including septate, cribriform, microperforate with a small ventrally placed opening, and imperforate have all been well documented (Herman-Giddens & Frothingham, 1987). McCann et al. (1990b) categorized the hymen as being either crescentic or concentric and also noted the former was more common, particularly when examined in the knee-chest position. Berenson et al. (1991) examined 468 newborns and documented hymenal findings. Berenson (1992) followed 201 newborns over a 3-year period and described the changes after both the loss of maternal estrogen effect and the evolution of change over time. They noted that 79% of newborn hymens were annular in appearance. There was smooth tissue present 360 degrees circumferentially in 71%. The hymen appeared fimbriated with folded edges in 21% of the newborns while a ruffled appearance with three or more clefts was present in 35%. The annular configuration was more common in Caucasians, the fimbriated in African-Americans. There were no crescentic hymens noted in newborns. With the exception of the sleeve-like form, 65% of hymens changed morphologically by age 1 year, and all edges were sharply defined by age 3 years. As the newborn estrogen effect waned, there was an increase in crescentic (posterior rim predominant) shaped hymens. Seventy-seven percent of those noted as newborns to have a notch at the 12 o'clock position also became crescentic (Berenson 1993). By age 2 to 4 years, the crescentic configuration was the most common and 90% had developed a notch between the 11 and 1 o'clock positions (Berenson, 1995; McCann et al., 1992). The majority of hymenal studies have been cross sectional, not generalized to older girls, and probably fraught with racial, developmental, and anatomic differences (Berenson, 1995; Berenson, 1998).

There have been a total of five research papers published on normal hymenal anatomy in prepubertal girls chosen for study because of the absence of sexual abuse. (Berenson, 1992; Berenson et al., 1991; Gardner, 1992; McCann et al., 1990b; Pokorny, 1987). The studies included 296 girls and longitudinally followed 201 of 468 newborns.

HYMENAL CONFIGURATIONS

Fimbriated is also called denticular and is characterized by multiple projections and indentations along the edge of the hymen, creating a "ruffled" or flowery appearance. (**See Figure 2-1.**)

Annular shows equal amounts of hymenal tissue circumferentially encircling the entire vaginal opening. (**See Figures 2-2 and 2-3.**)

Redundant (sleevelike) presents with abundant circumferential tissue that folds back on itself or protrudes much like the neck of a turtleneck sweater. (**See Figures 2-4 and 2-5.**)

Crescentic has a predominantly posterior rim with hymenal attachments at the 11 and 1 o'clock positions and no tissue present between them. (**See Figures 2-6 and 2-7.**)

Septate is a band of tissue creating two openings and bisecting the hymenal opening. Estrogen may lyse this band, leaving opposing remnants. Although not always

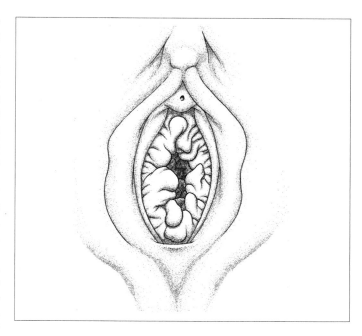

Figure 2-1. *A fimbriated or denticular hymen.*

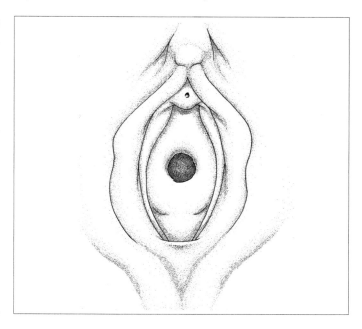

Figure 2-2. *The annular hymen.*

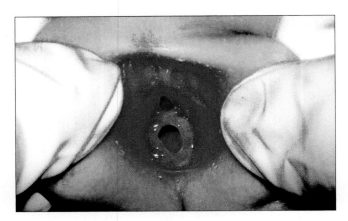

Figure 2-3. *An annular hymen.*

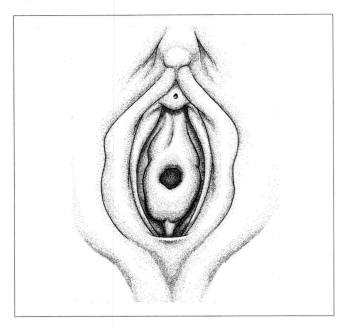

Figure 2-4. *The redundant or sleeve-like hymen.*

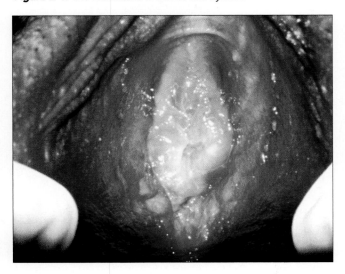

Figure 2-5. *A redundant or sleeve-like hymen.*

occurring together, a vaginal septum may also be present. **(See Figures 2-8, 2-9, and 2-10.)**

Cribriform describes a microperforate hymenal membrane with multiple small openings. There is usually, but not always, a thin layer of epithelium overlying the perforations.

Imperforate has no identifiable hymenal opening, although a microscopic orifice may be present. Obstruction still exists, and the tissue appears pale and avascular. This must be differentiated from agenesis of the vagina.

PREVALENCE IN STUDIES
As already described, the annular or fimbriated configuration is most common at birth. The fimbriated hymen is more frequently observed in African-American infants and decreases with age. The crescentic hymen increases with age to become the most prevalent by age 3 years. Septal remnants are common. Imperforate hymen is reported to occur in more than 1 in 1000 live female births (Usta et al., 1993).

CLINICAL FEATURES OF THE NORMAL HYMEN
The following is a list of the nonspecific clinical features of the normal and recognized variations of hymenal anatomy using terminology agreed on by the American Professional Society on the Abuse of Children (APSAC). A normal prepubertal hymen is seen in **Figure 2-11.**

Variations in Morphology
Flowery, fluted, ruffled, scalloped, sleeve-like with rolled edges are descriptive terms used by the pioneers in this field since early in the evolution of the written clinical observations on the hymen.

External Vaginal Ridge
The ***external vaginal ridge*** is a midline longitudinal ridge of tissue on the external surface of the hymen. It is usually located anteriorly and extends to the edge of the hymenal membrane. External vaginal ridges are observed in 82% of newborn females (Berenson et al., 1991). The incidence decreases with age, being present in 17% of girls at age 1 year and 7% at age 3 years.

Hymenal Tag
The ***hymenal tag*** is defined as an elongated projection of tissue arising from the rim of the hymenal membrane. They are commonly found in the midline at the six o'clock position and occasionally may be an extension of a posterior column. A hymenal tag can also be a septal remnant with opposing teat-like projections. They are common in the newborn (26%) but resolve once the estrogen effect is lost.

Longitudinal Intravaginal Ridge
Longitudinal intravaginal ridges are narrow mucosal tissue on the vaginal wall which may be attached to the inner surface of the hymen, often are multiple, and may be noted in all four quadrants of the vagina but appear to be more prevalent in the 4 and 8 o'clock positions. When prominent

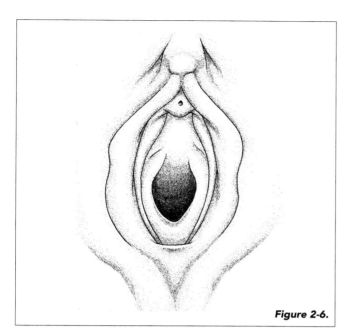

Figure 2-6.

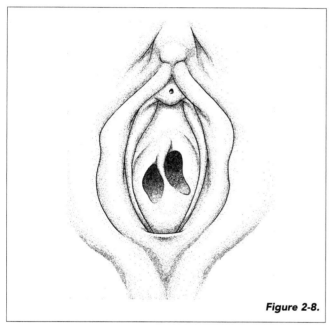

Figure 2-8.

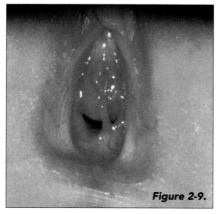

Figure 2-9.

Figure 2-6. *The Crescentic hymen.*

Figure 2-7. *A Crescentic hymen.*

Figure 2-8. *The septate hymen.*

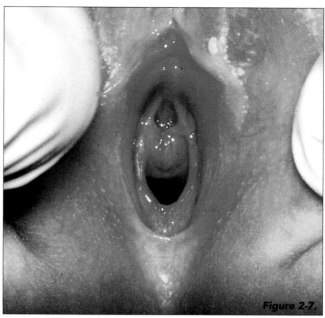

Figure 2-7.

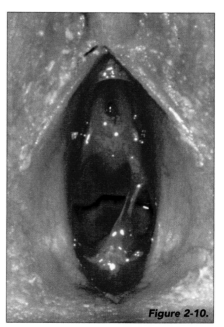

Figure 2-10.

Figure 2-9. *A septate hymen in knee-chest position.*

Figure 2-10. *A septate hymen.*

and located sagittally in the midline superiorly and posteriorly, they are termed the anterior and posterior columns. These are the "corduroy" or ribbing of the vagina. Their prevalence is 90% to 95% in preadolescent girls. Both McCann et al. (1990b) and Bays & Chadwick (1993) described these ridges as being covered by or arising from under the hymenal rim; that is, their exposure may be evidence of injury to the hymen.

Hymenal Notches or Clefts

A ***hymenal notch*** is defined as an angular or V-shaped indentation on the edge of the hymenal membrane. The V-shape occurs after injury as elastic fibers retract from the injured edge of the hymen. They have also been referred to as concavities when curved and smooth. A concavity does not extend to the junction of the hymenal ring and vestibule. A notch that extends to the junction of the hymen and vestibule is termed a transection ("complete tear"). These have been documented only in victims of sexual abuse or genital trauma and should be considered abnormal. Anterior notches are common between 11 and 1 o'clock and decrease with age. Both anterior and lateral notches (9 and 3 o'clock) occur frequently at birth (35%) (Berenson et al., 1991; Heger & Emans, 1992; Kerns et al., 1992). Berenson et al. (1991) suggest that these are part of the normal evolution of the hymen to the crescentic configuration. They further differentiate the single cleft at 12 o'clock position commonly found in annular hymens (24%) from the paired clefts seen laterally at 9 and 3 o'clock (6%). Posterior notches or clefts between 4 and 8 o'clock **(Figure 2-12)** increase in incidence with age and when complete have been considered markers for abuse and therefore abnormal. There is consensus on this issue by all national experts. Recently, Heger et al. (2002) in a study of 147 premenarchal girls chosen for nonabuse reported that partial notches/clefts occur in 360 degrees of the hymenal rim. Kerns et al. (1992) in a study of 1383 girls evaluated for sexual abuse found 174 (12.6%) girls had notches and 57.5% were posterior. Acute angle and irregular posterior notches were associated with acquired penile abuse (p <.001) and none were reported in studies on non-abused girls (McCann et al., 1990b).

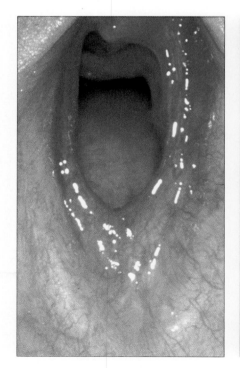

Figure 2-11. *A normal prepubertal hymen.*

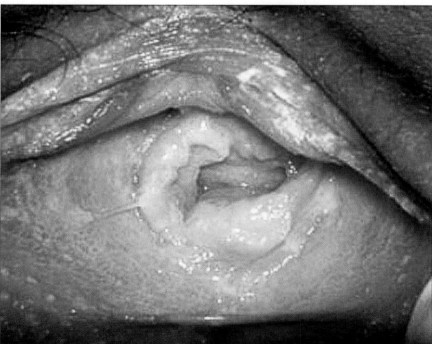

Figure 2-12. *Hymenal cleft at 8 o'clock.*

Vaginal Rugae

Vaginal rugae are defined as redundant epithelial folds in the vaginal wall running circumferentially from the vaginal columns. They apparently account in part for the ability of the vagina to distend (Heger & Emans, 1992). (**Figure 2-13.**)

Periurethral and Perihymenal Vestibular Bands

Periurethral and perihymenal vestibular bands are pubourethral support ligaments, which are lateral to the urethra and connect periurethral tissues to the wall of the vestibule. They are symmetrical in number most of the time and create semi-lunar spaces (ventricles) adjacent to the urethra. Berenson (1993) reported that newborns average 2.4 bands and that their number increases with age. They are present in 95% to 100% of girls. They may be located lateral to the hymen and connect to the lateral vestibular wall (pubovaginal bands).

Labial Agglutination/Adhesions

Labial agglutination/adhesions are superficial adhesions of the adjacent and outermost mucosal surfaces which are usually located posteriorly. They are very common (20% to 50%) between ages 2 months and 2 years (Berenson et al., 1992; Heger et al., 2002) and may present as complete labial fusion. Labial agglutination has been associated with diurnal enuresis from partial obstruction of the vestibule causing the trapping of already voided urine. Adhesions may occur after friction irritation or injury, including the outdated office practice of repeated labial separation. They now resolve much less painfully with the application of topical estrogen for 2 to 3 weeks or may be reduced with the use of a cotton-tipped swab soaked in a water-soluble lubricant and lidocaine viscous (Xylocaine Viscous). In the early 1980s the use of such oral mucosal treatments such as viscous xylocaine and diphenhydramine-antacids were used topically. Their application was used both for topical analgesia during examinations as well as the symptomatic relief of pain in prepubertal girls. (Cowell, 1981). Two studies in the literature noted that adhesions might be more common in girls suspected of being victims of sexual abuse (Berenson et al., 1993; McCann et al., 1988).

Erythema of the Vestibular Sulcus

Erythema is a common finding that results from the prominence of vascularity at this site. It is especially visible after the effect of estrogen has resolved. Vasodilatation and erythema increases with irritation or after a hot bath. No disruption of capillary vessels is seen using colposcopy with a green filter. Many nonspecific entities can increase the prominence of redness and vascularity, most notably vulvovaginitis. Erythema with induration is a very prominent feature with infections due to group A beta hemolytic streptococci and may be confused with sexual abuse.

Linea Vestibularis

Linea vestibularis was previously called midline sparing by several authors and when present, was readily noticeable using gentle labial traction In a study of 123 newborns, Kellogg and Parra (1991) described a white midline avascular structure and termed it linea vestibularisIt is defined as a vertical pale or avascular area in the midline of the posterior fourchette and/or the fossa navicularis. This linea was noted in the posterior vestibule in 12 infants (10%), whereas another 17 (14%) had a white spot, or "partial" linea vestibularis. This white line or spot was noted most often on "mature" genitalia, that is, in infants closer to term (38 weeks gestation). It was never asymmetrical, and had no associated neovascularization, vascular interruption, or scarring present. Its clinical prominence both increased and decreased during longitudinal followup (Kellogg & Parra, 1993). This might represent a variation of urogenital fold development (Reed, 2002).

Hymenal Bumps or Mounds

Hymenal bumps or mounds are defined as a firm elevation of hymenal tissue that

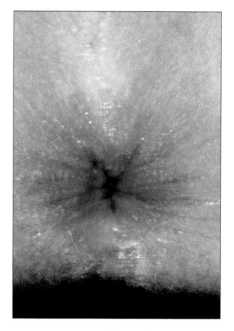

Figure 2-13. *Normal rugal folds.*

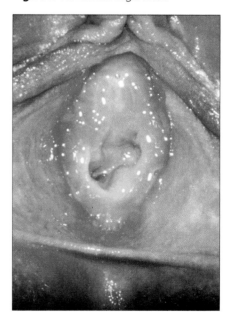

Figure 2-14. *A hymenal bump.*

are as wide as they are long (rounded), and located on the edge of the hymenal membrane primarily at the 3 and 9 o'clock positions. (**Figure 2-14.**) They are commonly associated with and attached to naturally occurring intravaginal ridges and, as noted above, their exposure, not existence, may prove meaningful. Prevalence is 11% to 34% and varies with both the examination position and techniques. (Gardner, 1992; Heger et al., 2002; McCann et al., 1990b). The incidence is the same in cross-sectional studies and histologically they are not scar tissue. Hymenal bumps were originally felt to be posttraumatic when uncovered in a normative study by McCann et al. (1992).

Lymphoid Follicles

Lymphoid follicles are defined as minute yellow-white, 1 to 2 mm prominences of follicular hyperplasia seen in the vestibule in approximately one third of girls. They are similar to the Fordyce's nodules seen most prominently on the mandibular aspect of the oral buccal mucosa.

Posterior Hymenal Measurement

The width of the posterior or inferior portion of the hymenal rim as viewed in the coronal plane, that is, from the edge of the hymen to the muscular portion of the vaginal introitus, and its relationship to sexual abuse continues to be a topic of controversy as well as redefining discussion. Several early studies suggested that narrowing of the posterior rim correlated with prior sexual misuse (Emans et al., 1987; McCann et al. 1988; Pokorny & Kozinetz, 1988). McCann et al., in their 1990 study of nonabused children stated that those children had a posterior rim exceeding 1 mm. Berenson et al. (1992), in a cross-sectional study of 211 prepubertal girls, reported that none had a posterior rim less than 0.9 mm. In a study of 22 girls age 1 through 3 years, Berenson (1995) later documented that this measurement was consistent over this same period of time. At age 3 years the mean measurement was slightly larger than 3 mm, with a range of 2.5 to 4 mm. Berenson (1998) cautioned that the available normative data neither support or refute the hypothesis that a width of less than 1 mm is a matter of concern for chronic sexual abuse. Heger et al. (2002) reported that 33 of 147 premenarchal girls with no history or findings of abuse had hymenal membrane widths estimated at 1 to 2 mm. 78.7% or 26/33 with narrow hymens were above the 75th percentile for weight ($c2=4.87, df:1, p<0.027$). This appears to confirm the anecdotal notion of "hymenal narrowing" in overweight girls. Heger notes how difficult it is to measure this parameter. Perhaps we need a micro-endoscopic device. She further noted an irregular hymenal rim in 51.7% of the 147 girls chosen for nonabuse versus McCann et al. 41.9% (1990a). Results from applying the "T-I-N-E" test training device (McCann, 1990) are presented in **Table 2-1.**

The previously noted variables in position, relaxation, examination techniques, and methods of measurement apply equally to the clinical observations on this aspect of normal hymenal anatomy. Of paramount importance may be the effect that pubertal estrogen plays in the correction of any injury to the posterior rim and what represents a normal external to internal thickness.

Transhymenal Diameter

This criterion was not mentioned in the literature on child abuse before Cantwell (1983, 1987). Many discussions, controversy, and a few studies have followed the notion that a transhymenal opening larger than 4 mm measured with "a slight spreading of the labia" was present in 80% of girls who described having been sexually abused. Huffman and colleagues (Huffman, 1974; Huffman et al., 1981) earlier noted that the size of the hymenal opening increased with age, and over the next 5 to 6 years several other studies agreed (Adams et al., 1988; Heger & Emans, 1990; Paradise, 1989). Woodling (1986) proposed a rule of thumb that after age 5 years, the normal transhymenal diameter equaled the child's age in millimeters.

Table 2-1. "T-I-N-E" Test Training Device Results

	McCann 1990	Heger 2002
Thinning	45.5%	53.8%
Irregularity	41.9 %	51.7%
Narrowing		22.4%
Exposure of Vaginal Vault	83%	93%

Several other investigators seemed to have confirmed this observation (Claytor et al., 1989; Emans et al., 1987; Hilton et al., 1988; White et al., 1989). Emans et al. (1987) noted that the hymenal diameters were significantly larger in abused girls, especially those who gave a clear history of penile-vaginal intercourse. Rimsza (1989) stated that measurement of the hymenal introitus was probably not useful because of a lack of both premenarchal and postmenarchal standards. McCann et al. (1990a) reported and compared the size of hymenal openings in prepubertal girls chosen for nonabuse using three different examination techniques. The colposcopic measurements were in line with previous studies and showed the greatest diameter in all age groups examined in the knee-chest position. Transhymenal diameters without standard deviations are listed in **Table 2-2**.

Data collected by Berenson et al. (1992) would seem to confirm the less than 4 mm rule below age 5 years and an increase of approximately 1 mm per year of age. They confirmed that the transhymenal diameter increases with age and, using labial traction, measured up to 8 mm at age 3 years. The size of the hymenal opening can vary depending on the embryologic development of the hymenal ring, type of hymenal opening, and degree of relaxation by the patient. Other factors are the amount of traction on the labia, the position of the patient during the examination, and probably the amount of time since any injury occurred, because healing has led to the misinterpretation of imperforate hymen (Berkowitz et al., 1987; Botash & Louis, 2001). The assessment of the hymenal diameter is also made more difficult by the alterations caused by estrogen (Rimsza, 1989). Elasticity varies from person

Table 2-2. Transhymenal Diameters

Age	Diameter
Preschool children (2 to 4 yrs 5 mos)	3.9–5.2 mm (range 1–8.5 mm)
Early school (5 to 7 yrs 11 mos)	4.2–5.6 mm (range 1–9 mm)
Preadolescent (8 yrs to Tanner 2)	5.7–7.3 mm (range 3–11 mm)

Modified from McCann et al., (1990b);428.

to person and there are no criteria or objective means to measure "stretching." Although it is difficult to quantify stretching or distensibility, blunt trauma or penetration of the hymenal opening may tear or "stretch" the hymen, or it may cause no injury. Because of this, the diagnosis of sexual abuse is not precluded by normal findings. Similarly, the diameter is also affected more by the knee-chest position than by the supine position, and more by labial traction than labial separation (McCann et al. 1990a). Between age 1 and 3 years the hymenal opening increases in size by 1 to 2 mm per year (Berenson, 1995). Maximum size in all studies available is 10 mm before puberty. Size alone (without evidence of injury) has a low predictability of abuse. In a 10-year survey of 1975 girls age 3 to 12 years (96% of 2058 girls evaluated for sexual abuse), Ingram et al., (2001) found that the maximized transhymenal orifice diameter by the separation technique alone is of no value in determining whether or not sexual abuse has occurred.

Finally, Berenson et al. (2002) compared the mean transhymenal diameter in 189 prepubertal girls with a history of digital or penile penetration and 197 controls who denied any sexual abuse. Comparison of the mean THDs showed that those girls with previous penetration were more likely to have a horizontal opening greater than 6.5 mm in the knee-chest position. Sensitivity was low (29%) as was specificity (86%). The presence of less than 1mm of hymenal tissue at the 6 o'clock position was detected in only 3 girls, all with a history of penetration (specificity 100%, sensitivity 1% to 2%).

Effect of Estrogen on the Hymen

The effect of estrogen is first noted in the newborn female and is caused by maternal estrogen crossing the placenta. It results in the prominence of the labia minora, clitoris, and paraurethral tissue. The hymenal tissue is also thickened, pale, and has fewer surface capillaries. Major changes occur at birth and again during puberty, including morphology and size, mucosa and secretions, environmental pH, and bacterial flora. Estrogen may cause pigmentation of the external genitalia, a thick white creamy discharge, and, occasionally, withdrawal vaginal bleeding in approximately 10% of newborn girls during the first 4 to 6 weeks of life.

By age 1 to 2 months the genitalia begin to appear prepubertal, although evidence of estrogenization is commonly seen on colposcopic examination for as long as 2 to 4 years. This clinician recently noted a robust estrogenic effect on the hymen and periurethral area in a 4 $^{7}/_{12}$ year old girl who continued to be breastfed. Heger & Emans (1990) suggested that as estrogen withdraws, there is a periurethral involution of tissue and that this accounts for the change in configuration of the hymen from annular to crescentic.

As the level of maternal estrogen decreases, the epithelium and mucosa begin to thin, secretions diminish, and the labia appear smaller. The entire vestibule appears more reddened and vascular. Because of vasodilatation, this redness increases with heat, irritation, and after hot baths.

At age 8 to 10 years, early changes in the hymen again show estrogen effect. There is maturation of the labia minora, an increase in periurethral tissue, as well as thickening of the hymen which may be the earliest sign of puberty (Heger & Emans, 1990; McCann et al., 1990; Styne, 2000).

FEMALE PUBERTY

Before 1997, normative pubertal data were extrapolated from European studies. Herman-Giddens et al. (1997) did a large-scale study involving more than 17,000 girls age 3 to 12 years. Although the study excluded "late" bloomers, it showed that a significant number of girls began puberty before age 8 years (**Table 2-3**).

The earliest age at onset of precocious sexual development has been reported in Puerto Rico (Anonymous, 1986; Bongiovanni, 1983; Ingle & Martin, 1986;

Montague-Brown, 1987; Ramirez de Arellano, 1986; Saenz de Rodriguez et al., 1985). Between 1978 and 1981, there was a three-fold increase in the number of children with premature thelarche. In boys and girls less than age 2 years, this was felt to result from the presence of phthalates in soy-based formula and various meat products with noncorn filler. Colon et al. (2000) identified phthalate and its major metabolite mono-(2-ethylhexyl) phthalate in 68% of 41 girls with premature thelarche and in only one of 35 controls. They reported that pesticides, plasticides, and phthalate esters may act as estrogen disrupting chemicals.

Michels et al. (1999) previously described early onset menarche in girls with high transplacental exposure to polybrominated biphenyls. Gladen et al. (2000) reported the effects of prenatal and lactational exposure to polychlorinated biphenyls and dichlorodiphenyl dichloroethene (DDE) on pubertal growth in both girls and boys. Larriuz-Serrano et al. (2001) reported on 2716 Puerto Rican children examined in the Sexual Development Registry for precocious puberty. Of this group, 1916 (70.5%) had isolated premature thelarche. This number represents an incidence of 6.2 per 1000 live births in children younger than age 2 years and 1.62 per 1000 live births in children age 2 to 8 years. This is the highest incidence ever reported and is 10 to 15 times that reported in Olmstead, Minnesota (Van Winter et al., 1990).

The earliest onset of thelarche and menarche occurs in individuals of African-American and Caribbean descent (age 6 to 7 years and 11 years 9 months, respectively, versus 6 to 8 years and 12 years 3 months in Caucasian girls).

THELARCHE

It has been traditionally taught that the first sign of puberty in the female is breast budding, which is produced by an increase in both the preadolescent alveolar system and the total amount of ductal fat (Bruni et al., 1990). There is, however, increasing anecdotal evidence that the first sign of puberty is found during examination of the hymen. The complete development of the breast through Tanner stage 5 requires approximately 4 years (Emans et al., 1997). A significant number of adolescent women will only develop to Tanner stage 3 or 4, but will rapidly increase the alveolar lobules during a first pregnancy. Developmental

Key Point:

Although the first sign of puberty in the female traditionally has been considered breast budding, which is produced by an increase in both the preadolescent alveolar system and the total amount of ductal fat, increasing anecdotal evidence indicates that the first sign of puberty is found in the hymen.

Table 2-3. Indications of Puberty in Girls Before Age 8 Years

INDICATOR	AGE	CAUCASIAN GIRLS	AFRICAN AMERICAN GIRLS
Tanner 2 breast	6 yrs	3%	6.4%
	7 yrs	5%	15.4%
	8 yrs	10.5%	37.8%
Tanner 2 pubic hair	6 yrs	1.4%	9.5%
	7 yrs	2.8%	17.7%
	8 yrs	7.7%	0 34.3%

Adapted from Herman-Giddens et al., (1997);505.

assessment may be difficult at times in young obese women because of lipomastia. Breast development is often asymmetrical, with one side initially larger because of end organ sensitivity to estrogen production and by age 17 to 18 years, any difference, although essentially negligible, is nonetheless clinically apparent in 25% of girls (Greydanus et al., 1989). Lack of breast development by 14 years of age or lack of any development by age 13 years is considered abnormal and deserves further evaluation.

Unilateral absence of breast tissue (amastia) may be seen in Poland's syndrome where the pectoralis muscles are absent and can be associated with rib deformities, syndactyly, and radial nerve agenesis. Athelia is the congenital absence of one or both nipples. It is very uncommon and may occur with or without the presence of breast tissue. Supernumerary breast (polymastia) and supernumerary nipples (polythelia) occur along the embryological milk line in 2% of children. (Greydanus et al., 1989). Polythelia has been associated with both cardiac and genitourinary anomalies. Other variations include the tuberous breast, inverted nipples, and the hyperplasia that occurs in newborns, at puberty, and associated with fibroadenomatosis.

PUBARCHE
The appearance of pubic hair occurs during Tanner stages 2 and 3, and usually accompanies the onset of breast development but may follow 6 months later. Axillary hair follows during Tanner stages 3 to 5. Both are controlled by adrenal androgen production. In the absence of normal ovarian function, the development of secondary sexual hair will still occur. Development of the breast will not. If breast maturation is Tanner stage 5 and there is no sexual hair development, partial androgen insensitivity should be considered. If pubic hair development is Tanner stages 3 to 5 and there is no progression from Tanner stage 1 to 2 breast, an estrogen-deficient state such as Kallmann syndrome with anosmia must be considered. Or, if virilized, an intersex problem may be present. Breast development will not occur in either case. In the presence of a functioning testis, there will be virilization of the external genitalia.

INTERNAL GENITALIA
In the prepubertal female the uterus/cervix ratio is 1:2 or 1:3. After puberty this reverses to 2:1. There is marked thickening of the myometrium during Tanner stages 2 to 3 (age 8 to 9 years) that is accomplished by both cellular hyperplasia and hypertrophy. Before puberty the uterine lining comprises a single layer of cuboidal epithelium. With the onset of estrogen production, this becomes multilayered columnar and mucocolumnar. A prepubertal uterine length greater than 1.8 cm on ultrasonography is specific for the onset of puberty (Tanner 2), with the average postpubertal length being 3.5 cm (Fleischer & Shawker, 1987). The ovaries are attached to the uterine cornu by the ovarian ligament. They are also attached at the hilum to the broad ligament and the mesovarian ligament, which serves as a conduit for arterial blood supply and nerves. There is an additional suspensory attachment in folds of peritoneum. Ovarian size increases from a prepubertal volume of 0.2 to 1.6 mL (not dissimilar to the male testis) to a postpubertal volume of 2.8 to 15 mL. The pelvic sonogram is quite sensitive for differentiating between premature thelarche and central precocious puberty in young girls (Haber et al., 1995).

CERVIX
The prepubertal cervix is flush with the vaginal vault and does not protrude into the vagina until puberty. During puberty, anteflexion occurs, putting the cervix in the posterior vaginal vault. The adolescent cervix is usually a healthy and homogeneous pink color, and is not painful or tender to motion unless the endocervix or endometrium is infected, as in pelvic inflammatory disease (PID). The cervix is small and oval. During adolescence, ectropion (ectopy) is present whereby the junction of squamous and columnar epithelium is located on the cervical portio instead of in its normal position within the endocervical canal

(Emans et al.,1997). It appears circumferentially red and is one reason sexually active teens develop pelvic inflammatory disease. This ectopy of columnar epithelium into the vaginal vault, which consists of squamous epithelium, may persist into late adolescence, especially in those young women taking combination oral contraceptive pills. The acidic environment produced by estrogen may encourage the process of metaplasia whereby squamous epithelium replaces the ectopy (Garden, 1998).

EXTERNAL GENITALIA

The development of the external genitalia in the female is estrogen dependent. The first sign of puberty is probably thickening of the hymen and tissue in the periurethral area, which has been reported to antedate other signs (Heger & Emans, 1990; McCann et al., 1990; Styne, 2000). There can be wide variation in size as well as asymmetry of the labia minora (see section on variations in the female). The vagina lengthens and the epithelial lining thickens. Mucus-secreting cells as well as the Skene's and Bartholin's glands produce watery mucus. This begins shortly after thelarche. Prepubertally, the vaginal epithelium is shiny red and quite thin. After puberty the epithelium is thicker and lighter pink in color, and there is increased tissue rugation and protrusion. There is maturation and cornification of the superficial squamous epithelium with an increase in elasticity and decreased sensitivity to pain. Functionally, there is an increase in cellular glycogen content and the flora of Döderlein's bacillus (Lactobacillus acidophilus). These lactobacilli break down the glycogen in desquamating cells, producing lactic acid. The vaginal pH of 6 to 7 before puberty then decreases to a pH of 3.5 to 5 after puberty. This is clinically felt to be protective against vulvovaginitis.

At age 8 to 10 years, there is rapid increase in linear height velocity and breast budding occurs. Pubarche occurs about 3 to 6 months after thelarche, and menarche follows 2 years later at Tanner stage 3 to 4. Early changes in the hymen again show estrogen effect, and this may be the earliest sign of puberty. Estrogen stimulation continues, and vaginal secretions thicken and become pearly white, usually 6 to 12 months before the onset of menses. This represents the physiologic leukorrhea that heralds menarche. This discharge may be copious and thick. It probably represents the sloughing of superficial cells, mostly from the mucus-producing columnar epithelium or as the result of fluid transudation through the vaginal wall. Some cervical component is also present. A vaginal smear will reveal 60% to 85% mature cells. This physiological leukorrhea of puberty is odorless and usually asymptomatic, but because of its daily volume, it may irritate the vulva and perineum. After menarche, a profuse clear or creamy vaginal discharge occurs during the late proliferative stage as well as during ovulation. Vaginal microscopic smears reveal "ferning." The discharge then thickens during the secretory phase. With progesterone production, this ferning is no longer present.

Occasionally a yellow stain is noted on the underwear of both prepubertal and postpubertal girls caused by the predominantly protein-containing debris being denatured by the lactic and acetic acid produced by *Lactobacillus* in the vaginal flora. When cotton fabric is heated during washing, a yellow stain appears similar to the stain of semen in boys. Many young girls are examined and cultured unnecessarily for vulvovaginitis. Remember that physiologic leukorrhea is more common in all age groups after age 9 to 10 years than is the leukorrhea of infection.

During puberty, both the labia majora and labia minora enlarge. The mucosa thickens and becomes pinker. The hymen becomes thicker, more elastic, and takes on a "scalloped" appearance. The hymenal opening also becomes less sensitive to pain. Adolescent females may have multiple monomorphic papillae that cover some or all of the entire surface of the mesial labia minora and vestibule. This papillomatosis often appears warty like condyloma acuminatum caused by several serovars of human papillomavirus, but it is uniform in appearance and does not blanch with acetic acid or stain with Lugol's iodine. These "vestibular growths" occur at Tanner stages 3 to 4 during peak maturation, and their embryologic location is quite similar to that in the male. Could this papillomatosis be the counterpart to pink pearly papules of the penis in males?

The age of onset and speed of pubertal changes vary individually, but the sequence is relatively constant. The normal clitoris is 2 to 4 mm wide. A measurement greater than 10 mm defines virilization. The mean transverse diameter of the glans clitoris is stated to be 3.4 +/- 1 mm (Bhatnagar, 2000). There is some variation noted in families, but isolated clitoromegaly should initially suggest the mild form of congenital adrenal hyperplasia.

PUBERTAL VARIATIONS IN GIRLS

In the female the fibromuscular vagina extends postero-superiorly from the vestibule to the uterine cervix. Size varies with age from 4 cm in length at birth, 8 cm between 8 and 10 years of age and 10 to 12 cm after puberty (Cowell 1981). The vagina becomes thickened, is more distensible, and produces thicker mucus. There is a marked variation in the tightness of the vaginal orifice via the pubovaginalis muscle. The elasticity of the hymen circumferentially increases during puberty. This anatomic change may be used along with Tanner staging as a measure of physiologic maturity (Pokorny et al., 1998). Findings that may be seen during inspection of the adolescent vulva include adolescent vestibular growths (previously described), elongation of the vestibule in obese girls, and intravaginal and paraurethral cysts. Myrtiform caruncles are hymenal remnants separated by complete clefts noted most often in sexually active girls. Before puberty or childbirth, these caruncles are felt to be the result of "stretch" trauma incurred during child sexual abuse involving penetration of the vagina.

PUBERTAL CHANGES AND VARIATIONS IN MALE SEXUAL DEVELOPMENT

Gonadal steroids exert a negative feedback on Gonadotrophin Releasing Hormone (GnRH) and the secretion of gonadotropins (FSH, LH). The level of testosterone continues to increase in the male. Free plasma testosterone levels are readily available in most regional laboratories as well as the alkaline phosphatase measurement which correlates better with sexual maturation than does age.

The first sign of puberty in the male is enlargement of the testes at a mean age 9.5 years. It is caused by formation of lumina in the seminal tubercles. *Testicular size is the most accurate method of assessing male puberty.* This is followed by Sertoli cell proliferation and sperm production. As the testes increase in size (puberty > 3ml), the scrotum becomes pink and smooth, then rugated and pigmented (Daniel, 1982). Concomitant with enlargement comes tenderness with referred pain to the ipsilateral lower quadrant. Spermarche is at Tanner 2 to 3, ejaculation occurs at Tanner 3, and fertility at Tanner 4. Average length of puberty is 2.5 to 3 years.

The penis then grows in length (mean age 11.6) and pubic hair appears at the base. The appearance of axillary hair occurs next followed by the peak height velocity which occurs at Tanner 4 (mean age 13.5). This sequence is followed by bone growth and lastly muscle mass. When calculating growth curve data, familial factors including midparental height expectation, mother's age at menarche, and the father's time and progress through puberty may figure prominently (Lee, 2002).

Body and breath odor, increases in arm, leg, and facial hair, acne, and oily scalp and skin usually precedes pubarche.

Isolated pubic hair development in the male may be isolated adrenarche or a normal variant of puberty. Premature pubarche is the appearance of pubic hair before age 9 in boys (age 8 in girls). Pubic hair may occur earlier in families and is noted to occur 6 to 12 months earlier in Afro-American girls—the latter usually at thelarche. This is attributed to early maturation of the normal adrenal secretory mechanism at puberty (Styne, 2000). Both DHEA and Androstenedione are weak androgenes and are converted peripherally to testosterone. The Hypothalamic-Pituitary-Gonadal Axis remains immature. While there is no breast development, normally (see below) height and height velocity both increase. One should always consider virilizing congenital adrenal hyperplasia and androgen secreting tumors.

PUBERTAL VARIATIONS IN MALES

Gynecomastia is defined as palpable subareolar enlargement of breast tissue in adolescent males. It occurs in 60% to 70% of boys during mid-puberty and may be firm, tender, unilateral (25% to 45%) and measure 1 to 5 cm in diameter (Strasburger & Brown, 1998). Estrogens strongly stimulate mammary gland growth while androgens weakly inhibit it (Braunstein, 1993). There is a temporary increase in the estrogen/testosterone ratio. In a study by Biro et al. (1990) the levels of free testosterone were lower and the testosterone/estrogen-binding globulin were higher. Late-onset 17-ketosteroid reductase deficiency produces greater conversion of androgens (1∞androstendione) to estrogen, which is proposed as one possible etiology (Rapaport, 2000).

Usually gynecomastia occurs during the newborn period, at puberty, and during senescence. Onset is usually between 10 to 12 years of age with a peak occurrence at age 13 to 14 during Tanner stage 3 to 5. Pubertal changes including wrinkling and pigmentation of the scrotal skin, pubic hair development, and greater than 6mL testicular volume are present 6 months before the breast enlargement.

The vast majority of cases are physiological (75%). In an earlier study of 1800 boy scouts, the overall incidence was 40% with a peak incidence of 65% in 14-year-olds. One fourth of cases were unilateral and 75% bilateral. Other studies have reported up to 45% cases being unilateral. Breast enlargement persisted up to two years in 25% and was noted at three years in only 7% (Nydik, 1961).

Marijuana and anabolic steroids are next in frequency as causative agents followed by chronic illnesses, chronic alcohol use, and psychopharmacologic medications (13%).

About 12% of cases are endocrine in origin and include: testicular failure, Klinefelter's syndrome, increased aromatase activity, defects in testosterone synthesis or action, true hermaphroditsm, ACTH deficiency, hyperthyroidism, prolactinoma, feminizing adrenal/testicular tumors, chronic disease and starvation, and zoster infection with paraplegia. Familial gynecomastia may be x-linked recessive or autosomal dominant (Sher et al., 1993).

Taller and heavier boys age 9 years and older with heights 1.4 SDs above the mean and weights 2.7 SDs above the mean represent most of the lipomastia or pseudo-gynecomastia (Sher et al., 1993).

In males, normal findings may include hyperpigmentation of the distal shaft of the penis proximal to the glans caused by recurrent and natural friction during self-stimulation. It has also followed circumcision.

A *spermatocele* is infrequently noted during examination of the scrotal contents. It is a cystic and nontender mass smaller than and attached to the upper pole of the testis.

A *varicocele* is an abnormal dilatation of the pampiniform venous plexus in the scrotal sac caused by valvular incompetence of the spermatic vein. The vast majority are located on the left and often present as a "bag of worms" during a pre-participation sports physical or by self-examination. This may be explained by the 90-degree angle at which the left spermatic vein empties into the renal vein. If right sided or bilateral (10%), a search for a retroperitoneal or intra-abdominal mass should be carried out. Varicoceles are common after age 10 years, occurring in 5% to 10% of Tanner stage 3 to 4 boys and present in up to 15% to 20% of adult men. Varicoceles are graded as subclinical (identified with Doppler); grade 1, palpable with Valsalva maneuver; grade 2, palpable and visible on inspection while standing or with Valsalva maneuver; and grade 3, visible to inspection (Hudson, 1988). The size of the left testis should be equal to or greater than the right. If not, there may be heat damage ultimately affecting spermatogenesis of both testes. This requires surgical intervention.

Pink pearly papules of the penis occur in 12% to 19% of boys age 11 to 21 years during Tanner stages 3 to 4 (Neinstein & Goldenring, 1984). They appear as 1 to 3 mm papillae along the coronal margin of the penis, usually anteriorly (ventrally), with one to five rows, uniform in size, and pearly white to pink in color. They do not blanch with acetic acid, like lesions of human papillomavirus do. They occur during the peak of pubertal development at a site embryologically similar to that of adolescent vestibular growth in females. While no scientific data confirm this suspicion, it is this author's suggestion that they are developmentally the same (Reed).

SEXUAL MATURITY RATING

A systematic classification of pubertal development in boys was first proposed by Greulich in 1942. Sexual maturity ratings came later and divided the process into five stages (Daniel, 1961), with Tanner stage 1 being prepubertal or childlike and stage 5 being adult. A child enters Tanner stage 2 of development when the first signs of puberty become apparent. In girls, breast budding and sparse labial hair characterize this stage (Marshall & Tanner, 1969). In boys, the first sign of puberty is testicular enlargement with the appearance of sparse pubic hair (Marshall & Tanner, 1970). The Tanner staging system does not include changes in the nipple to distinguish between Tanner 2 and 3 breast development. Recent studies have suggested using nipple papilla areolar staging, breast diameter/circumference, and even ultrasound to better assess actual glandular tissue (Biro et al., 1992; Rhone, 1982).

The alternative use of the Garn-Falkner system for breast changes includes the following:

Stage 1. Prepubertal
Stage 2. Palpable areola and increased pigmentation
Stage 3. Growth and separation of the areola with an increase in papillae
Stage 4. Regression of the areola as nipple papillae enlarge

Biro et al. (1992) noted that girls in Tanner Stage 2b were areolar stage 1 and that the system correlated well with Tanner staging (Spearman correlation coefficient 0.94). Changes that occur to the hymen during puberty are not currently part of a formal sexual maturity rating scale. Finally, changes in axillary hair (adrenarche) are not part of the rating system in either girls or boys.

The Tanner stages of maturity are strictly guidelines used in assessing the progression of pubertal development in adolescents (**Table 2-4**). They are not criteria for determining probable chronological age through video review by nurse examiners in child or adolescent pornography trials (Rosenbloom & Tanner, 1998).

DEVELOPMENT OF THE ANORECTUM

Theories of anorectal development are based on pig and human embryological investigations as well as postnatal histological studies of babies with anomalies. There is recent disagreement on all earlier theories of anorectal evolution (Van Der Putte, 1986). The principal event in normal development has proved to be a shift of the dorsal part of the cloaca and hindgut to the body surface of the tail groove (Moore, 1982). The hindgut develops at 4 weeks gestation and will ultimately form the spleen, bladder, descending colon, sigmoid, and rectum as far inferiorly as Hilton's white line (Gorsch, 1955). The allantoic diverticulum arises from the cloaca, which is then closed off. At 5 to 6 weeks gestation the anorectal bar of mesenchyme coronally bisects the cloaca into a dorsal anorectal compartment and ventral urogenital sinus. This area of fusion between the urorectal septum and the cloacal membrane forms the perineal body (tendinous part) of the perineum. At 6 weeks the dorsal anal fossa terminates the gastrointestinal tract and gives rise to the distal anal canal and anus. This anorectal septum divides the cloacal sphincter into an anterior part (ischiocavernosus and bulbocavernosus muscles) and a posterior part (external anal sphincter). Absence of the posterior or dorsal membrane leads to agenesis of the anus. Mesenchyme proliferates to produce an elevation of the surface ectoderm around the anal membrane. This is located centrally in an ectodermal depression termed the proctoderm or anal pit. At 8 weeks gestation the membrane ruptures, forming the anal canal. The superior two thirds of the hindgut (mesoderm) measures about 2.5 cm in adults. The inferior third arises from proctoderm and measures about 13 mm. The junction of these two at the inferior limits of the valves of Houston is called the pectinate line. Approximately 2 cm superior to the pectinate line is the anocutaneous line (Hilton's white line). This is where columnar epithelium from the embryological mesoderm meets the stratified squamous epithelium derived from the ectoderm.

NORMAL PERINEUM AND ANORECTUM

The perianal area in both males and females is fairly nondescript and less complex anatomically than the vestibule of the female. Additionally the anatomy is predictable both before and after nonaccidental trauma in that injury is easy to see (Wissow, 1990). Not all experts necessarily agree on this subject (Finkel, 1989; McCann & Voris, 1993). The anus is normally located in the middle of any pigmentation and has circumferential rugal folds formed by the corrugator cutis ani muscle. Ectopic anus would lie anteriorly and on the ventral edge of any pigmentation. The perianal tissue overlying the external anal sphincter at the most distal part of the anal canal is called the anal verge. This extends from the edge of the primitive proctoderm (or anoderm) to the margin of the anal canal. Where the anoderm meets the rectal ampulla is called the dentate or pectinate line. The pectinate line receives its name from the alternating columns and sinuses, which appear scalloped and less pink. The pectinate line is easily noted as the anal rugae flatten out post mortem (McCann et al., 1996). Circumferentially and deep to this tissue in the perianal space are the inferior or external hemorrhoidal veins. Because these veins have no valves, they are easily distended or obstructed. The finding of a hemorrhoid in children is considered rare and should initiate a search for an intra-abdominal mass or left renal vein obstruction. Hemorrhoids also occur with inflammatory bowel disease and with some deep perirectal infections.

Normative data have been well documented (Agnarsson et al., 1990; Berenson et al., 1993, 1998; Finkel & DeJong, 1994; McCann et al. 1989). McCann et al. (1989) described the following findings in children chosen for nonabuse.

COLOR CHANGES
Red

Erythema is noted in more than 40% of children. This is more noticeable with colposcopy (>50%) than with visual inspection (33%). It may include a radius or width of up to 1.5 cm. Perianal erythema with fever, sore throat, or nonspecific symptoms such as itching (80%), crying, painful defecation (50%), or blood-streaked stools without trauma should suggest infection with group A beta hemolytic streptococcus (GABHS) (Amren et al., 1966). Symptomatic pharyngitis occurs in about 10% of cases (Kokx et al., 1987). It is necessary to consider and do streptococcal antigen screening or culture on vaginal or anal erythema. The throat culture in perianal GABHS proctitis correlates in 50% to 65% of cases (Krol, 1999). Mogielnicki et al. (2001) counted 23 cases of GABHS in 4530 office visits in 1997; 13 cases were perianal, 8 were vulvovaginitis, and 2 cases involved both sites. All were T Types 28 and emm 28 streptococci. Infections with *Staphylococcus*

Table 2-4. Tanner Stages of Maturity

BREAST SEXUAL MATURITY RATING (SMR)

Stage 1 (prepubertal)	Elevation of the papilla
Stage 2	Breast budding with areolar enlargement and later tenderness
Stage 3	Enlargement with no separation of breast/nipple contour
Stage 4	Projection of the areola and papilla to form a clear mound (nipple)
Stage 5	The mature stage with areolar recession

PUBIC MATURITY RATING

Stage 1 (preadolescent)	Only vellus over the pubes, no pubic hair
Stage 2 (pubarche)	Sparse growth downy hair, straight, little curl, hairs easily counted
Stage 3	Hair darker, coarser, curlier, mainly over the pubes, still countable
Stage 4	Adult type hair over the mons and labia, counting now requires compulsive behavior
Stage 5	Mature stage spreads to medial thighs and forms the female escutcheon (inverted triangle)

BOYS SMR

Stage G1 (preadolescent)	Infantile, no enlargement of penis, testicular volume 1.5 mL
Stage G2	Testes enlarge (volume 1.6–6 mL), early sparse pubic hair

(continued)

Table 2-4. *(continued)*	
Stage G3	Hair increases, both testes (volume 6–12 mL) and penis grow
Stage G4	Hair now thickened, scrotum more rugated, volume of testes 12–20mL
Stage G5	Adult male hair on the thighs; penis and testes (volume >20 mL) full size; male escutcheon is triangular shaped

Testicular size may be measured by comparing the graduated sized testes on the orchidometer, developed by Austrian ephebiatrician and endocrinologist Dr. Andrea Prader.

aureus and methicillin-resistant *Saureus* (MRSA) have also been reported. The authors agree that the prevalence of GABHS seems to be lessening over the past 6 to 12 months. Its incidence is reported to be 1 in 218 to 1 in 1000. Erythema has been described in Kawasaki disease, hemolytic uremic syndrome, inflammatory bowel disease, and guttate psoriasis (Bays & Jenny, 1990).

Brown
Hyperpigmentation is common and increased in almost 30% of children, predominantly those with darker skin. The incidence increases after puberty.

Blue
Venous congestion is noted at mid-Valsalva maneuver in more than 50% of children, especially in the knee-chest position, and is believed to result from decreased outflow of the pelvic venous system. (**Figure 2-15**).

White
Pallor is associated with lichen sclerosis, which is probably the result of partial androgen insensitivity and may initially present with perivulvar and perianal hypopigmentation. Autoimmune disorders such as vitiligo may occasionally be diagnosed on the perianal skin and perineum.

ANATOMIC VARIATIONS

Diastasis ani is a congenital midline depression that may be V shaped or wedge shaped. It has been described as fanning, cupping, or funneling in appearance. It may be located anterior or posterior to the anus. It results from a congenital absence of the superficial division of the corrugator ani muscle, which serves as the external anal sphincter. Smooth areas occur near the anal verge in 26% of children. It is always midline and most often noted in the knee-chest position at 12 o'clock. A depression, dimple, or pit was seen in 47% of those examined by McCann et al. (1989).

Anal tags are a midline protrusion of anal verge tissue that interrupts the symmetry of perianal skin folds. They are present in the same proportion (11%) across all age groups. Skin tags have been noted more often on visual inspection than with colposcopy. They may represent redundancy or thickening of the perineal raphe. When located outside of the midline, they may be deflated hematomas or hemorrhoids and be associated with autoimmune disorders such as inflammatory bowel disease and perirectal infections.

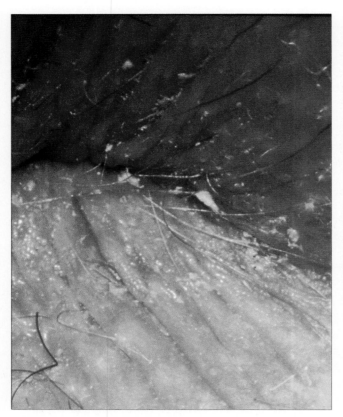

Figure 2-15. Perianal venous congestion.

Anal opening is symmetrical in 89% and irregular in 3% of children examined and reported by McCann et al. (1989). Radial folds or rugae are present in 81% and decrease to 37% at midpoint dilatation. Maximum dilatation of the anus without the presence of stool in the ampulla is less than 20 mm in almost 99% of children. Dilatation of the internal anal sphincter is probably caused by distension of the rectum, which disinhibits external anal constriction. Fixed irregularity or an anal opening larger than 20 mm should be considered abnormal and suspicious for sexual abuse. (**Figures 2-16 and 2-17.**)

Superficial fissures may be caused by hard stools, encopresis with or without constipation, or proctitis (Agnarsson et al., 1990). The prevalence of fissure ranges from 6% to 26% and is a common finding in a general pediatric practice.

VARIATIONS IN GENITOANAL DEVELOPMENT

Urogenital sinus anomalies are characterized by persistence in various forms of the urogenital sinus and primitive cloacae. They may exist as an isolated anomaly, as part of a cloacal deformity, or as part of an intersex state. These abnormalities of development usually present as a single and unusual vulvar orifice (Bhatnagar, 2000).

Imperforate anus may exist as an isolated anomaly. It is also associated with perianal, vestibular, or lower vaginal fistulae. Agenesis of the anorectum may present without ***fistulous*** formation. Imperforate anus is part of the VACTERL Association (DiGeorge, 1995). This is an acronym for the association of Vertebral anomalies, Anal Atresia, Cardiac disease, Tracheo-esophageal fistula, Renal anomalies, and Limb defects. The most common limb defect is radial dysplasia (Khoury, 1983). Other findings have been observed including deformations of the external ear, congenital deafness, and anal stenosis.

Cloacal exstrophy is more complex than either exstrophy of the bladder or epispadias. It consists of severe anomalies of the rectum and colon, including short bowel syndrome. It occurs in 1 of 400,000 live births, and there is a 50% incidence of both spina bifida and urinary tract anomalies (Rickwood & Godiwalla, 1998).

HEALING AFTER ANOGENITAL INJURY

It has long been recognized that evidence of tissue injury in childhood anogenital trauma heals rapidly (Finkel, 1989; McCann et al., 1992, 1993). Acute superficial injuries to the anogenital area may resolve and become unrecognizable because of the nature of the anatomy involved. These injuries heal rapidly and examples might include the biting of one's tongue or buccal mucosa or those minor and major injuries associated with controlled childbirth. Sexual misuse (fondling, licking) may result in no injury to the child victim; acute injury with rapid healing and no evident residual (abrasions, edema, hematomas); or evidence of chronic and recurrent abuse (hymenal notches, transections, and narrowing of the posterior rim) (Adams & Knudson, 1996; Cantwell, 1983; Cupoli & Sewell, 1988; Emans et al., 1987; Finkel, 1989; McCann et al., 1989; Teixeria, 1981). Repeated or ongoing friction can lead to a chronic inflammatory state with mucosal adhesions and wound hyperpigmentation. Serious tissue injury and deformation are more frequently seen in sexual assault cases than in child sexual abuse. This is not surprising because rape and aggravated assault are defined as the use of excessive force causing physical injury by both blunt and penetrating trauma to the hymenal

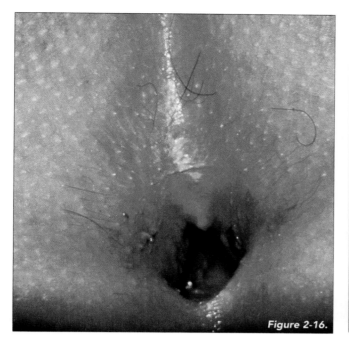
Figure 2-16.

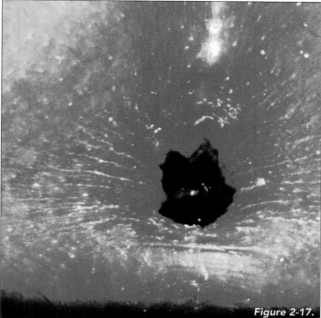
Figure 2-17.

orifice, vagina, or anorectum, whereas child sexual abuse may range from fondling, licking, kissing, voyeurism, or genital to genital touching without obvious injury as the molester encourages continued abuse. Scarring can distort the predicted clinical prognosis following a very complete evaluation of an acute injury. This sometimes has resulted in a later evaluation that has lead to a faulty conclusion in childhood genito-anal trauma cases, including those initially felt to be accidental in origin (Finkel & DeJong, 1994). Pain and bleeding correlate with an increased probability of finding evidence of significant injury in child sexual abuse (Kerns et al., 1993). Adams and Knudson (1996) reported findings from the examinations of 204 girls age 7 to 17 years with histories of vaginal penetration. Abnormalities were noted in 32% of cases without vaginal bleeding versus 50% of cases in those with vaginal bleeding at the time of assault (p <.004, c2). When the genital examination was performed within 72 hours of injury, 69% were abnormal, and 26% were normal (p <.001, c2). The authors concluded that a normal examination was a normal examination at the outset. Seemingly, the more protection from estrogenization, glycogen production, and secretion content, the less clinically observable the injury over time (Muram, 1989; McCann et al., 1992). Before the use of colposcopy, methylene or toluidine blue dye was used to identify the stained nuclei of abraded epithelial cells. With the colposcope and a green filter, even subtle interruptions in vascular supply are easily recognized. Also, any neovascularization that occurs during the healing process is readily visualized.

Wound healing requires inflammation, which is a nonspecific biochemical and cellular process that has been well described in the clinical literature (Cotran et al., 1999; Kissane, 1985). This is not antigen-specific with an autoimmune response memory, but is nonetheless autoimmune and automatic at the time of injury. This nonspecific inflammatory process lasts 8 to 10 days in various laboratory models and is considered chronic if it persists for more than 2 weeks.

Wound resolution is the reverse action of original structure and function. This is accomplished by two overlapping phases and is possible only if tissue damage is minor, complications do not ensue, and damaged or destroyed tissue has the capability to proliferate the remaining cells (McCausee & Huether, 1998). This cell proliferation is stimulated by tissue deformation and by cell injury and death. Early mediators facilitate the movement of plasma, multiple cytokines, the platelet cascade,

Figure 2-16. Anal dilation without stool.
Figure 2-17. Anal dilation without stool.

Key Point:
The more protection from estrogenization, glycogen production, and secretion content, the less clinically observable the injury becomes over time. Before colposcopy was used, methylene or toluidine blue dye identified the stained nuclei of abraded epithelial cells. Using a colposcope and a green filter, even subtle interruptions in vascular supply are easily recognized, along with any neovascularization that has occurred.

and multiple epithelial growth factors into the wound (Roit et al., 1996). Resolution may require up to 2 years, depending on the tissue injured.

Healing occurs in two ways (Edwards & Dunphy, 1958; Loeb, 1920). The first is **regeneration,** when injured cells are replaced by the same type of cells, and the second is **repair,** whereby a wound is filled in, covered, and additionally contracted by replacement with fibrous connective tissue.

The regeneration of superficial wounds occurs in the following four stages:

1. The generation of cellular debris as thrombosis, platelet degradation, and inflammation occur rapidly.
2. The regeneration of denuded epithelial cells.
3. The production of new immature cells.
4. The differentiation and maturation of those new cells (Dunphy, 1978).

This process occurs at a predictable albeit variable rate depending on the site of injury and the tissue injured. The mean rate of wound covering is 1 mm per 24 hours (Edwards & Dunphy, 1958). Cellular debris is noticeable within 24 hours, and healing may take place in 48 to 72 hours. There may be differentiation of new cells by 5 to 7 days and final resolution over several weeks (McCann et al., 1992). In fact, most superficial anogenital injuries cannot be seen with the unaided eye by 4 to 5 days (Finkel, 1989). (**Figures 2-18 and 2-19.**)

If there is extensive injury incapable of regeneration, wound infection, foreign body, or if fibrin persists in the lesion, repair must take place with replacement by connective tissue and subsequent scar formation (fibrosis). This results in a permanent albeit microscopic scar, such as is seen in transection of the hymen where a gap between the opposing wound sides exists.

The process of repair requires four main steps, as follows:

1. Angiogenesis of new capillaries
2. Migration and proliferation of fibroblasts
3. Synthesis of extracellular matrix by fibroblasts
4. Maturation and remodeling of the fibrous tissue scar (Cotran et al., 1999; Kissane, 1985)

Figure 2-18. *Acute hymenal bruising.*

Figure 2-19. *Subacute trauma, nine days post injury.*

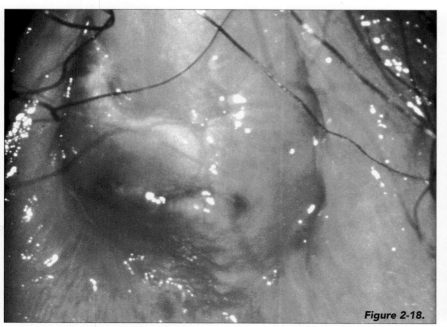

Figure 2-18.

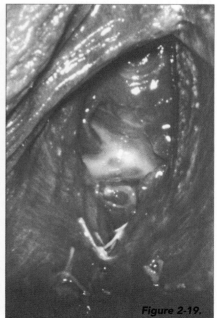

Figure 2-19.

The wound appears reddened from neovascularization, then contracts and pales as the scar matures at approximately 60 days. Very little repair healing occurs in the anogenital area, presumably because of mucosal surface qualities, but narrowing of the hymenal rim at the point of an injury is not uncommon. A V-shaped cleft or notch occurs when the elastic tissue in the separating edges of the hymen retracts during injury.

Only two studies investigating a total of 11 patients followed genital healing (Finkel, 1989; McCann et al., 1992). Only two papers followed perianal healing (Hobbs & Wynne, 1989; McCann & Voris, 1993). Serial colposcopic examinations revealed that all wounds healed rapidly and jagged edges smoothed off in 1 to 8 weeks. McCann et al. (1992) followed three patients (an infant, a preschooler, and a pre-adolescent) for up to 3 years. They noted that while all injuries resolved quickly, healing differed in each child. In the infant, injury to the hymen gradually formed a shallow concavity. In the preschool girl, the hymenal orifice enlarged as the torn edges of the hymen folded back on itself. In the pre-adolescent girl, injury to the hymenal ring disappeared into the folds of the estrogenized hymen.

McCann and Voris (1993) reported four children, ages 4 to 8 years, with varying degrees of perineal and direct anal trauma. These injuries usually healed by 24 hours, but anal laxity after penetrating injury persisted for 11 days in one child. Acute signs of trauma disappeared by 8 days, most between 1 and 5 days. Deeper first-degree injuries to the perianal skin folds healed by 8 days. Second-degree wounds healed at 1 to 5 weeks, and third-degree injuries requiring sutures healed at 8 days. The latter were replaced by pale fibrosis and curled narrow scars located outside of the midline and virtually disappeared by 12 to 14 months. The sutured injuries healed the fastest. McCann (1998) has also pointed out the possible hazards of extrapolating such limited data to scientific knowledge. In a review of 310 children (104 abnormal exams), Muram (2001) notes that "failure to document perianal injuries may be due to rapid healing."

There are many questions about healing that remain to be answered. New studies need to address such questions as precisely how the various types of genitoanal injuries are created and whether the rapidity of cellular turnover in the female genitalia causes the vast majority of tissue injury to disappear. Are all of the physical signs such as swelling or petechial hemorrhage part of the cascade of inflammation and platelet degradation? Does continued abuse during puberty erode the posterior barrier of the vestibule? Is puberty capable of repairing evidence of sexual trauma? Furthermore, how do estrogen and cellular glycogen content protect the tender yet resilient parts of the external portico of the pre-adolescent vestibule preparing to become the postpubertal birthing canal? And will suturing be found to be incremental in speedier healing of the hymen especially in complete or almost complete tears (transection)?

Several longitudinal studies to answer these questions and many others raised by McCann (1998) and Berenson (1998) would add to our knowledge of the normal course of wound healing after anogenital injury. Apparently, at least one study is in preparation (Heger et al., 2002). We must not create a situation of re-victimization for the alleged victims of child sexual abuse and their families (Berenson, 1998).

REFERENCES

Adams JA, Ahmad M, Phillips P. Anogenital findings and hymenal diameter in children referred for sexual abuse examinations. *Adolesc Pediatr Gynecol.* 1988;1:123-127.

Adams JA, Knudson S. Genital findings in adolescent girls referred for suspected sexual abuse. *Arch Pediatr Adolesc Med.* 1996;150:850-857.

Adams J, Wells R, Normal verses abnormal genital findings in children: how well do examiners agree. *Child Abuse Negl.* 1993;17:663-675.

Agnarsson U, Warde C, McCarthy G, Evans N. Perianal appearances associated with constipation. *Arch Dis Child.* 1990;65:1231-1234.

Amren DP, Anderson AS, Wannamaker LW. Perianal cellulitis associated with group A streptococci. *Am J Dis Child.* 1966;112:546.

Anonymous. Premature thelarche in Puerto Rico: a search for environmental factors. *Amer J Dis Child.* 1986;140:1263-1267.

Anveden-Hertzberg L, Gauderer MWL, Elder JS. Urethral prolapse: an often misdiagnosed cause of urogenital bleeding in girls. *Pediatr Emerg Care.* 1995;11:212.

Baskin LS. Hypospadias and urethral development. *J Urol.* 2000;163:851.

Bays J, Chadwick D. Medical diagnosis of the sexually abused child. *Child Abuse Negl.* 1993;17:91.

Bays J, Jenny C. Genital and anal conditions confused with child sexual abuse trauma. *AJDC.* 1990;144:1319-1322.

Berek JS, Adashi EY, Hillard PA. Molecular biology. In: *Novak's Gynecology,* 12th ed. Baltimore, Md: Williams & Wilkins; 1996:123-148.

Berenson AB. Appearance of the hymen at birth and one year of age, longitudinal study. *Pediatrics.* 1993;91:820-825.

Berenson AB. A longitudinal study of hymenal morphology in the first three years of life. *Pediatrics.* 1995;95:490-496.

Berenson AB. Normal anogenital anatomy. *Child Abuse Negl.* 1998;17:589-596.

Berenson AB, Chacko MR, Wiemann CR, et al. Use of hymenal measurements in the diagnosis of previous penetration. *Pediatrics.* 2002;109:228-235.

Berenson AB, Heger AH, Andrews SA. Appearance of the hymen in newborns. *Pediatrics.* 1991;87:458-465.

Berenson AB, Heger AH, Hayes JM, Baily RK, Emans SJ. Appearance of the hymen in prepubertal girls. *Pediatrics.* 1992;89:87.

Berenson AB, Somma-Garcia A, Barnett S. Perianal findings in infants 18 months of age or younger. *Pediatrics.* 1993;91:838.

Berkowitz CD, Elvik SL, Logan M. A simulated acquired "imperforate" hymen following the genital trauma of sexual abuse. *Clin Pediatr.* 1987;26:3007-3009.

Berth-Jones J, Graham Brown RAC, Burns DA. Lichen sclerosis. *Arch Dis Child.* 1989;64:1204-1206.

Bhatnagar KP. Embryology and normal anatomy. In: Sanfilippo JS, Muram D, Dewhurst J, Lee PA, eds. *Pediatric and Adolescent Gynecology.* 2nd ed. Philadelphia, Pa: WB Saunders; 2000:2-17.

Biro FM, Falkner F, Khoury P. Areolar and breast staging in adolescent girls. *Adolesc Pediatr Gynecol.* 1992;5:271.

Biro FM, Lucky AW, Huster GA, et al. Hormonal studies and physical maturation in adolescent gynecomastia. *J Pediatr.* 1990;116:450.

Bongiovanni AM. An epidemic of premature thelarche in Puerto Rico. *J Pediatr.* 1983;103:245-246.

Botash AS, Louis FJ. Imperforate hymen congenital or acquired from sexual abuse. *Pediatrics.* 2001;108:3.

Braunstein GD. Gynecomastia. *N Engl J Med.* 1993;328:490-495.

Brayden RM, Altemeier WA III, Yeager T, Muram D. Interpretation of colposcopic photographs: evidence for competence in assessing sexual abuse. *Child Abuse Negl.* 1991;15:69-76.

Bruni V, Dei M, Deligeoroglou E, et al. Breast development in adolescent girls. *Adolesc Pediatr Gynecol.* 1990;3:201-205.

Bukowski TP, Zeman PA. Hypospadias: of concern but correctable. *Pediatrics.* 2001;18:89-109.

Canning DA, Gearhart JP. Exstrophy of the bladder. In: Ashcroft KW, Holder TM, eds. *Pediatric Surgery.* 2nd ed. Philadelphia, Pa: WB Saunders; 1993:678-693.

Cantwell HB. Vaginal inspection as it relates to child sexual abuse in girls under thirteen. *Child Abuse Negl.* 1983;7:171-176.

Cantwell HB. Update on vaginal inspection as it relates to child sexual abuse in girls under thirteen. *Child Abuse Negl.* 1987;11:545-546.

Capraro VJ, Capraro EJ. Examination of the genital organ in the newborn, the child, and the adolescent. *Gynecol Pract.* 1971;22:169-177.

Christian CW, Lavelle JM, Delong AR, et al. Forensic evidence findings in prepubertal victims of sexual assault. *Pediatrics* 2000;106:100-104

Claytor RN, Barth KL, Shubin CI. Evaluating child abuse. Observations regarding anogenital injury. *Clin Pediatr.* 1989;28:418-422.

Colon I, Caro D, Bourdony CJ, Rosario O. Identification of phthalate esters in the serum of young Puerto Rican girls with premature breast development. *Environ Health Perspect.* 2000:108:895-900.

Cotran RS, Kumar V, Collins T. *Robbins Pathologic Basis of Disease.* 6th ed. Philadelphia, Pa: WB Saunders; 1999.

Cowell CA. The gynecological examination of infants, children, and young adolescents. *Pediatr Clin North Am.* 1981;28:247-266.

Cupoli JM, Sewell PM. 1059 Children with a complaint of sexual abuse. *Child Abuse Negl.* 1988;2:151-162.

Daniel WA, Feinstein RA, Howard-Peebles P, Baxley WD. Testicular volumes of adolescents. *J Pediatr.* 1982;101;1010.

Dewhurst Sir J. Rectovaginal fistulaes and associated anomalies. In: Garden AS, ed. *Paediatric & Adolescent Gynaecology.* London: Arnold; 1998:635-639.

DiGeorge AM. Genetic diseases and dysmorphic syndromes. In *Physicians Guide to Rare Diseases,* 2nd edition. Montvale NJ: Dowden Publishing;1995:156.

Dolk H. Rise in the prevalence of hypospadias. *Lancet.* 1998;351:770.

Dunphy JE. Wound healing. *Surg Clin North Am.* 1978;58:907-916.

Edwards LC, Dunphy JE. Wound healing in injury and normal repair. *New Engl J Med.* 1958;259:224-232.

Elder JS. Urologic disorders in infants and children. In: Behrman RE, Kliegmann RM, Jenson HB, eds. *Nelson Textbook of Pediatrics.* 16th ed. Philadelphia, Pa: WB Saunders; 2000:1645-1650.

Emans SJ, Laufer MR, Goldstein DP. *Pediatric and Adolescent Gynecology*. 4th ed. Philadelphia, Pa: Lippincott-Raven; 1997.

Emans SJ, Woods ER, Flagg NT, Freeman A. Genital findings in sexually abused, symptomatic and asymptomatic girls. *Pediatrics*. 1987;79:778-785.

Finkel MA. Anogenital trauma in sexually abused children. *Pediatrics*. 1989;84:317-322.

Finkel MA, DeJong AR. Medical findings in child sexual abuse. In: Reece RM, ed. *Child Abuse: Medical Diagnosis and Treatment*. Philadelphia, Pa: Lea Febiger; 1994:185-247.

Fleischer AC, Shawker TH. The role of sonography in pediatric gynecology. *Clin Obstet Gynecol*. 1987;30:735-746.

Fryer A. The XY girl. In: Garden AS, ed. *Paediatric and Adolescent Gynaecology*. London: Arnold; 1998:191-213.

Garden AS. Gynaecologic tumours. In: Garden AS, ed. *Paediatric & Adolescent Gynaecology*. London: Arnold; 1998: 242-252.

Gardner JJ. Descriptive study of genital variations in healthy non-abused menarchal girls. *J Pediatr*. 1992;120:257.

Gladen BC, Ragan NB, Rogan WJ. Pubertal growth and development in prenatal and lactational exposure to polychlorinated biphenyls and dichlorodiphenyl dichloroethene. *J Pediatr*. 2000;136:490-496.

Gorsch RV. *Proctological Anatomy*. Baltimore, Md: Williams &Wilkins; 1955:56-67.

Greydanus DE, Park DS, Faulk EG. Breast disorders in children and adolescents. *Pediatr Clin North Am*. 1989;36:601-638.

Haber HP, Wollmann HA, Ranke MB. Pelvic ultrasonography: early differentiation between isolated premature thelarche and central precocious puberty. *Eur J Pediatr*. 1995;1:182-186.

Heger A, Emans SJ. *Evaluation of the Sexually Abused Child. A Medical Textbook and Photographic Atlas*. New York, NY: Oxford University Press; 1992.

Heger A, Emans SJ. Introital diameter as the criterion for sexual abuse [commentaries]. *Pediatrics*. 1990;85:222-223.

Heger AH, Ticson L, Guerra L, et al. Appearance of the genitalia in girls selected for nonabuse: review of hymenal morphology and nonspecific findings. *J Pediatr Adolesc Gynecol*. 2002;15:27-35.

Herman-Giddens ME, Frothingham TE. Prepubertal genitalia: examination for evidence of sexual abuse. *Pediatrics*. 1987;80:203-208.

Herman-Giddens ME, Slora EJ, Wasserman BC. Secondary sexual characteristics and menses in young girls seen in office practice: a study from the pediatric research in office settings network. *Pediatrics*. 1997;99:505-512.

Hilton N, Williams J, Coulter K. Measurement of the hymenal diameter in pediatric sexual abuse exams. *Child Abuse Negl*. 1988;12:607-608.

Hobbs CJ, Wynne JM. Sexual abuse of English boys and girls: the importance of anal examination. *Child Abuse Negl*. 1989;13:195.

Hudson RW. The endocrinology of varicoceles. *Fertil Sterility*. 1988;49:199.

Huffman JW, Dewhurst CJ, Capraro VJ. *The Gynecology of Childhood and Adolescence*. Philadelphia, Pa: WB Saunders; 1981.

Ingle MB, Martin BW. Precocious puberty in Puerto Rico. *J Pediatr.* 1986;109:390-391.

Ingram DM, Everett VD, Ingram DL. The relationship between the transverse hymenal orifice diameter by the separation technique and other possible markers of sexual abuse. *Child Abuse Negl.* 2001;25:1109-1120.

Ivarsson SA, Nilsson KO, Persson PH. Ultrasonography of the pelvic organs in prepubertal and postpubertal girls. *Arch Dis Child.* 1983;58:352-354.

Jenny C, Kuhns M, Arakawa F. Hymens in newborn female infants. *Pediatrics.* 1987;80:399-400.

Jerkins GR, Verheeck K, Noe HN. Treatment of girls with urethral prolapse. *J Urol.* 1984;132:738-741.

Kellogg ND, Parra JM. Linea vestibularis: a previously undescribed normal genital structure in female neonates. *Pediatrics.* 1991;87:926-929.

Kellogg ND, Parra JM. Linea vestibularis: follow-up of a normal genital structure. *Pediatrics.* 1993;93:453-456.

Kerns DL, Ritter ML, Leong T, Brown WB. Clinical correlates to physical evidence of anogenital trauma in female suspected child abuse victims. *Amer J Dis Child.* 1993;147:422.

Kerns DL, Ritter ML, Thomas RG. Concave hymenal variations in suspected child sexual abuse victims. *Pediatrics.* 1992;90:265-272.

Khoury MJ, Codero JF, Greenberg F, James LM, Erickson JD. A population study of the VACTARL association: evidence for its etiology heterogenecity. *Pediatrics.* 1983;71(5):815-820

Kissane JM. Inflammation and healing. In: *Anderson's Pathology.* 8th ed. St. Louis, Mo: CV Mosby; 1985:47.

Klein FA, Vick CW, Broecker BH. Neonatal vaginal cysts: diagnosis and management. *J Urol.* 1986;135:371-373.

Kokx NP, Comstock JA, Flackam RR. Streptococcal perianal disease in children. *Pediatrics.* 1987;80:659.

Koram KS, Salti I, Haijj SN. Congenital absence of the uterus: clinicopathological and endocrine findings. *Obstet Gynecol.* 1979;50:531-533.

Krol AL. Perianal streptococcal dermatitis. *Pediatr Dermatol.* 1999;7:97.

Larriuz-Serrano MC, Perez-Cardona CM, Ramos-Valencia G, Bourdony CJ. Natural history and incidence of premature thelarche in Puerto Rican girls aged 6 months to 8 years diagnosed between 1990-1995. *P R Health Sci J.* 2001;20:13-18.

Lazala C, Saenger P. Pubertal gynecomastia. *J Pediatr Endocrinol Metab.* 2002;15:553-560.

Lee PA. Supplement to clinical update: *Pediatric Endocrinology.* 2002;5(2):1.

Loeb L. Comparison study of mechanisms of wound healing. *Med Res.* 1920;41:247-281.

Marshall WA, Tanner JM. Variations in the pattern of pubertal changes in girls. *Arch Dis Child.* 1969;44:291.

Marshall WA, Tanner JM. Variations in the pattern of pubertal changes in boys. *Arch Dis Child.* 1970;45:13-23.

McCann J. The appearance of acute, healing, and healed anogenital trauma. *Child Abuse Negl.* 1998;22:605-615.

McCann J, Reay D, Siebert J, et al. Postmortem perianal findings in children. *Amer J Forensic Pathol.* 1996;17:289-298.

McCann J, Voris J. Perianal injuries resulting from sexual abuse: a longitudinal study. *Pediatrics.* 1993;91:390-397.

McCann J, Voris J, Simon M. Labial adhesions and posterior fourchette injuries in childhood sexual abuse. *Amer J Dis Child.* 1988;142:659-663.

McCann J, Voris J, Simon M. Comparison of genital examination techniques in prepubertal girls. *Pediatrics.* 1990a;85:182-187.

McCann J, Voris J, Simon M. Genital injuries resulting from sexual abuse: a longitudinal study. *Pediatrics.* 1992;89:307-317.

McCann J, Voris J, Simon M, Wells R. Perianal findings in prepubertal children selected for non-abuse; a descriptive study. *Child Abuse Negl.* 1989;13:179-193.

McCann J, Wells R, Simon M, Voris J. Genital findings in prepubertal girls selected for non-abuse, a descriptive study. *Pediatrics.* 1990b;86:428-439.

McCausee KL, Huether SE. *Pathophysiology: The Biological Basis for Disease in Adults and Children.* 3rd ed. St. Louis, Mo: CV Mosby; 1998: 228-233.

McKusick V, Bauer R, Koop C. Hydrometrocolpos as a simply inherited malformation. *JAMA.* 1964;189:813-814.

Michels BH, Marcus M, Tolbert PE, et al. Age at menarche in girls exposed perinatally to polybrominated biphenyls. *Am J Epidemiol.* 1999;149:S21.

Mittwoch U, Burgess AMC, Baker PJ. Male development in a sea of oestrogen. *Lancet.* 1993;342(8863):123-124.

Mogielnicki NP, Schwartzman JD, Elliot JA. Perianal groups A streptococci disease in a pediatric practice. *Pediatrics.* 2001;108:820.

Montague-Brown K. Premature thelarche in Puerto Rico. *Amer J Dis Child.* 1987;141:1250-1251.

Moore KL. The urogenital system. In: *The Developing Human: Clinically Oriented Embryology.* 3rd ed. Philadelphia, Pa: WB Saunders; 1982:255-256.

Mor N, Merlob P. Congenital absence of the hymen only a rumor? *Pediatrics.* 1988;82:679.

Muram D. Anal and perianal abnormalities seen in prepubertal girls. *Amer J Obstet Gynecol.* 1989;161:278-281.

Muram D. Child sexual abuse. In: Sanfilippo JS, Muram D, Dewhurst J, Lee PA, eds. *Pediatric and Adolescent Gynecology.* 2nd ed. Philadelphia, Pa: WB Saunders; 2001:406.

Neinstein LS, Goldenring J. Pink pearly papules. An epidemiologic study. *J Pediatr.* 1984;105:594.

Paradise JE. Predictive accuracy and the diagnosis of sexual abuse, a big issue about a little tissue. *Child Abuse Negl.* 1989;13:169.

Paradise JE, Finkel MA, Beiser AS, et al. Assessment of girl's genital findings and the likelihood of sexual abuse: agreement among physicians self-rated as skilled. *Arch Pediatr Adolesc Med.* 1997;151:883-891.

Pokorny SF. Configuration of the prepubertal hymen. *Am J Obstet Gynecol.* 1987;157:950-956.

Pokorny S. Genital examination of prepubertal and peripubertal females. In: Sanfilippo JS, Muram D, Dewhurst J, Lee PA, eds. *Pediatric and Adolescent Gynecology.* 2nd ed. Philadelphia, Pa: WB Saunders; 2000:182-198.

Pokorny SF, Kozinetz CA. Configuration and other anatomic detail of the prepubertal hymen. *Adolesc Pediatr Gynecol.* 1988;1:97.

Pokorny SF, Murphy JG, Preminger MK. Circumferential hymen elasticity: a marker of physiologic maturity. *JReprod Med.* 1998;43(11):943-948.

Quint EH, Smith YR. The use of clobetasol in the treatment of premenarchal lichen sclerosis. Presented at: North American Society for Pediatric and Adolescent Gynecology (NASPAG); June 4, 1999; New Orleans, La.

Ramirez de Arellano AB. Incidence of premature sexual development in Puerto Rico. *J Public Health Policy.* 1986;7:543-545.

Rapaport R. Disorders of the gonads. In: Behrman RE, Kliegman RM, Jenson HB, eds. *Nelson Textbook of Pediatrics.* 16th ed. Philadelphia, Pa: WB Saunders; 2000:1760-1766.

Rapaport R. Gynecomastia. In: Behrman RE, Kliegman RM, Jenson HB, eds. *Nelson Textbook of Pediatrics.* 16th ed. Philadelphia, Pa: WB Saunders; 2000:1752.

Rickwood AMK, Godiwalla SY. Problems identified at birth and in the newborn. In: Garden AS, ed. *Paediatric and Adolescent Gynaecology.* London: Arnold; 1998:49-100.

Rimsza M. An illustrated guide to adolescent gynecology. *Pediatr Clin North Amer.* 1989;36:639-663.

Rimsza ME, Niggemann EH. Medical evaluation of sexually abused children: a review of 311 cases. *Pediatrics.* 1982;69:8-14.

Rock JA, Azziz R. Genital anomalies in childhood. *Clin Obstet Gynecol.* 1987;30:682-696.

Rohn RD. Papilla (nipple) development during female puberty. *J Adolesc Health Care.* 1982;2:217.

Rohn RD. Male genitalia: examination and findings. In: Friedman SB, ed. *Comprehensive Adolescent Health Care.* 2nd ed. St. Louis, Mo: Mosby-Yearbook; 1998:1079-1080.

Roit I, Brostoff J, Make D. *Immunology.* 4th ed. St. Louis, Mo: CV Mosby; 1996.

Rosenbloom A, Tanner JM. Misuse of Tanner puberty stages to estimate chronologic age [letter to the editor]. *Pediatrics.* 1998;102:6:1494.

Sadler TW. *Langman's Medical Embryology.* 7th ed. Baltimore, Md: Williams & Wilkins; 1995:286-301.

Saenz de Rodriguez CA, Bongiovanni AM, Conde de Borrega L. An epidemic of precocious development in Puerto Rican children. *J Pediatr.* 1985;107:393-396.

Sher ES, Migeon CJ, Berkovitz GD. Evaluation of boys with marked breast development at puberty. *Clinical Pediatrics.* 1998;37:367-372.

Simpson JL. Disorders of sexual differentiation. In: Sanfilippo JS, Muram D, Dewhurst J, Lee PA, eds. *Pediatric and Adolescent Gynecology.* 2nd ed. Philadelphia, Pa: WB Saunders; 2000:87-115.

Sivanesaratum V. Unilateral unexplained absence of the ovary and fallopian tubes. *Eur J Obstet Gynaecol Reprod Biol.* 1968;22:103-105.

Strasburger VC, Brown RT. Growth and development. *Adolescent Medicine: a Practical Guide.* 2nd ed. Philadelphia, Pa: Lippincott Raven; 1998:1-22.

Styne, DM. Normal growth and pubertal development. In: Sanfilippo JS, Muram D, Dewhurst J, Lee PA, eds. *Pediatric and Adolescent Gynecology.* 2nd ed. Philadelphia, Pa: WB Saunders; 2000:31.

Teixeria WR. Hymenal colposcopic examination in sexual abuse. *Am Med Pathol.* 1981;3:209-214.

Usta IM, Awwad JT, Usta JA, et al. Imperforation of the hymen: report of an unusual familial occurrencie. *Obstet Gynecol.* 1993;82:655-656.

Van der Putte SCJ. Normal and abnormal development of the anorectum. *J Pediatr Surg.* 1986;21:434-440.

Van Winter JT, Noller KL, Zimmerman D, Melton LJ. Natural history of premature thelarche in Olmsted County, Minnesota, 1940 to 1984. *J Pediatr.* 1990;2:278-280.

Vesalius A. De humanis corporis fabrica. In: Lyons AS, Petrucelli JR, eds. *Medicine, an Illustrated History.* 2nd ed. New York, NY: Harry Abrams; 1987:416-417.

Westerhout C, Hodgman JE, Anderson GV, Slack RA. Congenital hydrocolpos. *Amer J Obstet Gynecol.* 1964;89:957-961.

White ST, Ingram DL, Lyna PR. Vaginal introital diameter in the evaluation of sexual abuse. *Child Abuse Negl.* 1989;13:217-234.

Wissow LS. Injuries to the genitals and rectum. In: *Child Advocacy for the Clinician: An Approach to Child Abuse and Neglect.* Baltimore, Md: Williams & Wilkins; 1990:77-91.

Woodling BA. Sexual abuse and the child. *Emerg Med Serv.* 1986;15:17-25.

EVALUATION OF CHILD SEXUAL ABUSE

Jacqueline M. Sugarman, MD

The evaluation of the child who may have been sexually abused is multifaceted, containing components such as obtaining a history; conducting a physical examination; initiating diagnostic and forensic testing when deemed necessary; and making appropriate referrals. This chapter primarily focuses on evaluation of the child who comes to medical attention in the acute medical setting (emergency department or physician's office) because he or she has made a specific disclosure of developmentally inappropriate sexual contact (Hymel & Jenny, 1996). The chapter subsequently addresses the case of the child who has made no specific disclosure of sexual abuse but comes to medical attention because of either physical or behavioral symptoms about which a caregiver is concerned (Hymel & Jenny, 1996).

HISTORY

Physical evidence in child sexual abuse cases is often lacking because the majority of children who are sexually abused have normal examinations (Adams et al., 1994; Bays & Chadwick, 1993). When the examination is normal or nonspecific, the diagnosis of sexual abuse rests solely on the history, which is given by the child. Hence, obtaining and documenting an accurate account of what happened are crucial in diagnosing sexual abuse. If the child is deemed an ineffective witness, the state's ability to protect him or her through the legal system may be undermined (Meyers, 1986). The child's recitation of the abusive event or events to a physician treating the patient may be admissible in court as an exception to the laws restricting hearsay testimony (Meyers, 1986). When this situation occurs, preservation of verbal evidence through the proper questioning of the child and documentation of the child's history by the physician directly affects the state's ability to take legal action on behalf of the child (Meyers, 1986). Not only does the interview detail for the examiner what happened, it also provides the examiner an opportunity to establish rapport with the child, assess the child's developmental level and overall emotional status with regard to the abuse, and gauge how cooperative the child might be with further assessment (Faller, 1993; Poole & Lamb, 1998).

Key Point:
Because the physical examination of children who have been abused is often normal, the diagnosis may be based solely on the child's history. Thus, obtaining and accurately documenting the child's story are essential in diagnosing sexual abuse.

Every attempt should be made to interview the child separate from parents, guardians, or accompanying caregivers so that the presence of these individuals does not inhibit the child's full disclosure of the events. It should not be assumed that the child's caregiver believes the child and will protect the child from further abuse. Even a protective caregiver might inhibit a child's disclosure if the child perceives that the information might upset the caregiver. Furthermore, the absence of a caregiver during the interview helps negate the argument that the child is merely repeating what the caregiver told the child to say or what the child perceives the caregiver wants to hear.

It is often easier to first interview the accompanying caregiver separate from the child (Giardino et al., 1992). This allows the examiner to obtain a history from the caregiver as well as a better understanding of the child's world, which will aid in communication with the child. The examiner should obtain from the caregiver the child's names for his or her body parts, including genitalia. The examiner should try to ascertain how long ago the abuse took place and the possible extent of the abuse so as to be able to better tailor his examination. The examiner should discuss with the parent any unusual living situations (child lives at more than one home, child calls more than one person mom or dad) that might make the child's version of the history confusing. The child's past medical history should be addressed during the interview. Does the child have other medical problems that may mimic sexual abuse or make the diagnosis more suspicious? For example, lichen sclerosis is often misdiagnosed as sexual abuse. Genital warts can sometimes be acquired perinatally. Does the birth mother have a history of genital warts or abnormal PAP smears? Does the child have any physical signs and symptoms that are sometimes seen in children who are sexually abused, such as genital discharge or bleeding, recurrent urinary tract infections, chronic abdominal pain, sleep disturbances, bowel or bladder incontinence, or appetite disturbances (Jenny, 1996)? Has the child had any psychiatric or behavioral problems that might coincide with a history of ongoing abuse? For example, has the child been suicidal, socially withdrawn, depressed, or in trouble at school (Jenny, 1996)? Also suspicious would be a change in a child's behavior, such as, a child who was a straight A student and is now failing (Jenny, 1996). Has the child been manifesting sexualized play, trying to sexually abuse other children, or been masturbating excessively (Jenny, 1996)? Has the child been evaluated for sexual abuse before?

If the examination is consistent with old injuries, it may be impossible to determine when the injuries occurred. The interviewer should be cognizant of common presenting complaints of sexually abused children (Jenny, 1996)(**Table 3-1**). Medications the child is taking should also be documented. Antibiotics, for example, could alter culture results.

Finally, the interviewer should form his own impression as to whether the caregiver is protective of the child and if the child is at risk for being abused in the future. Is the child safe going home with the caregiver? Does the perpetrator reside at the home where the child lives? Are there other children at risk? The latter three questions must be addressed and discussed with child protective services before the child is discharged.

Key Point:
The child's interview should be appropriate for his or her developmental stage. It should not be hurried or threatening to the child.

Ideally, children should be interviewed in an unhurried manner and unthreatening environment. While some children may separate willingly, some may be more comfortable if an impartial third party, for example, a social worker, remains with the child when the parent leaves the room. It may be helpful if the parent remains for the beginning of the interview when the examiner is establishing rapport with the child but not asking questions directly related to the alleged abuse.

The establishment of rapport, as well as the subsequent interview, must be tailored to the child's developmental status. Appreciation of the developmental differences in children helps to achieve an optimal interview. Children as young as 2 years have been observed to give understandable information if properly questioned (Frasier, 1997). Very young children (age 0 to 3 years) have little or no ability to label time or sequence events; they may not even be able to identify body parts (Ludwig, 2000).

Preschoolers have better language skills, and although they still cannot tell time, they may be able to identify an event as occurring before or after another event or to sequence events. Interviewers must avoid long, complex questions, pronouns (instead use the name of the person), and be direct; for example, instead of "If you need to use the potty, let me know;" say, "Do you need to use the potty?" (Steward et al., 1993). School-age children may be uncomfortable about discussing their bodies, especially with strangers. The interviewer may want to give a reticent child a crayon or a pen so that he or she can draw or write what happened if verbalization is too difficult.

Initially the interviewer should introduce himself or herself and try to establish rapport with the child, asking questions such as, "What's your name? Do you have a nickname? How old are you? Do you go to school? Who lives in your house?" The interviewer should try to gauge the child's developmental level. Does the

---

Table 3-1. Common Presenting Complaints of Sexually Abused Children and Adolescents in the Medical Setting

Physical Signs and Symptoms

Genital discharge, bleeding	Genital skin lesions	Seizures
Genital pruritis (itching)	Genital or urethral trauma	Short stature
Pregnancy, including pregnancy with genetic disorders	STDs: typical, atypical, or disseminated	Appetite disturbance
Other genital infections	Recurrent urinary tract infections	Sleep disturbance
Muscle weakness	Drug overdose	Fatigue or exhaustion
Migraine headache	Abdominal pain	Enuresis and/or encopresis
	Numbing of body parts	

Psychosomatic Disorders

Diffuse somatic complaints
Hysterical or conversion reactions
Abdominal pain
Anorexia

Sexual Problems

Sexualized play	Promiscuity or prostitution
Sexual self-abuse	Sexual dysfunction
Excessive masturbation	Sexual revictimization
Sexual perpetration to others	Fear of intimacy

Social and Behavioral Problems

School adjustment problems	Suicidal ideation, gestures, or attempts	Family conflicts
Taking on parental roles	Neurotic or conduct disorders	Impulsive behavior
Phobias, avoidance behavior	Social withdrawal	Self-mutilating behavior
Temper tantrums	Aggressive behavior	Truancy or runaway behavior
Substance abuse		

Other Psychologic Problems

Excessive guilt	Altered states of consciousness	Anxiety
Irritability	Depression	Multiple personalities
Feelings of helplessness	Self-hate, self-blame	Identity diffusion
Low self-esteem	Mistrust	Dissociation
Amnesia	Hyperalertness	Obsessive ideas
Fear of criticism or praise	Terrified of rejection	Flashbacks
Rage		

Other

Asymptomatic sibling of a victim	Association with a known offender (Schmitt, 1982a)

Data from Hunter et al. (1983), Krugman (1986), and Massie & Johnson (1989).
Reprinted with permission from the publisher: Jenny C. Medical issues in sexual abuse. In: Briere J, Berliner L, Buckley JA, Jenny C, Reid T, eds.
The APSAC Handbook on Child Maltreatment. *Thousand Oaks, Calif: Sage Publications; 1996:197-199.*

child, for example, use prepositions (under, on, before, after) appropriately? What is the child's understanding of time? Does he or she know days of the week or only months of the year? Or is it better for the examiner to ask only if the abuse occurred, for example, "before Easter but after Christmas?"

The interviewer should then ask about daily living and intimate relationships with question such as, "Where do you sleep? Who gives you a bath?" The child should be asked to identify body parts by either pointing to them on a diagram or drawing a crude stick figure person. The examiner can ask the child to start from the head and work downward toward the genitalia.

Key Point:
The topic of abuse should only be introduced after the interviewer has established a rapport with the child. All questioning should be open-ended and nondirective to allow the child to respond spontaneously.

After establishing rapport with the child and assessing the child's daily routine, the interviewer might broach the subject of abuse. Initial questioning should be open-ended or as nondirective as possible to elicit spontaneous responses (American Professional Society on the Abuse of Children [APSAC], 1995). For example, the interviewer might begin by asking if the child knows why he or she is here. If open-ended questions are not productive, more direct questioning should follow (APSAC, 1995). A younger child might need a more specific or focused question, such as, "Did something happen to you?" Or, to be even more specific, the examiner could explain, "Sometimes children come to see me if someone has touched them in a way that made them feel uncomfortable. Has anything like that happened to you?" Faller (1990) has proposed a continuum of types of questions (generalized to leading) used in interviewing children alleged to have been sexually abused. Faller proposed that the amount of confidence one can place in the child's answer is related to the type of question asked to obtain that answer. One can place the most confidence in answers obtained as the result of open-ended questions and the least confidence in those answers obtained as the result of leading questions. The continuum of possible questions is reproduced in **Table 3-2**. Leading questions, such as, "He took your clothes off, didn't he?" should be avoided. Instead, the examiner might ask, "What happened to your clothes?" and if the child responds that they were off, the examiner might then ask, "How did they get that way?" Spontaneous responses regarding sexual details, for example, ejaculation, are important because most children have no knowledge of them unless they have experienced them (Frasier, 1997).

Not every child will be cooperative. Some children have been threatened by the perpetrator that something bad will happen to them or their loved ones if they disclose. Other children may feel guilty because they think the abuse was their fault. Other children may not want to betray the perpetrator, who may be a close friend or family member for whom they care. Some children fear that no one will believe them. Other children may be too embarrassed or shy to speak with an interviewer that they just met or just do not feel like talking at that particular time. If the child is uncooperative or does not want to discuss the abuse, it may be necessary to defer further interviewing and either proceed with the examination or reschedule the interview and examination for a later date, depending on the situation at hand. For example, if the abuse occurred years ago, the child has been removed from any potential danger, and the child is physically asymptomatic, the interview and examination may be deferred for another day if the child seems reluctant. On the other hand, if the abuse has occurred within the past 72 hours and there may be either physical findings or forensic evidence, it may be necessary to try to proceed with the examination (with the hope that the child will be more cooperative) despite the child's unwillingness to speak to the interviewer (American Academy of Pediatrics [AAP], 1999a).

Key Point:
The child should always be told that he or she did a good job and did the right thing by telling about the incident. The interviewer must always make it clear to the child that the abuse was not his or her fault.

At the conclusion of the interview, the child should be told that he or she did a good job and the right thing by telling (Frasier, 1997). He or she should be reassured that the abuse was not his or her fault. Also in conclusion of the interview the interviewer should tell the child what is going to happen next, for example,

Table 3-2. A Continuum of Types of Questions Used in Interviewing Children Alleged to Have Been Sexually Abused and Confidence in Responses (Faller, 1990)	
TYPE OF QUESTION	**EXAMPLE QUESTIONS AND CHILD RESPONSES**
Open-ended	*This type of question allows the child to respond with the most confidence* **Q:** How are you? **A:** Sad, 'cause my dad poked me in the pee-pee.
Focused	*Children respond with a little less confidence than the open ended questions* **Q:** How do you get along with your dad? **A:** OK, except when he pokes me in the pee-pee. **Q:** Did anything happen to your pee-pee? **A:** My daddy poked me there. **Q:** What did he poke you with? **A:** He poked me with his ding-dong.
Multiple Choice	*Children respond to this type of question with more confidence than the yes/no and leading questions, but with less confidence than a focused or open-ended question.* **Q:** Did he poke with his finger, his ding-dong, or something else? **A:** He used his ding-dong. **Q:** Did this happen in the daytime or nighttime? **A:** In the day and night.
Yes/No	**Q:** Did he tell you not to tell? **A:** No, he didn't say anything like that. **Q:** Did you have your clothes off? **A:** No, just my panties.
Leading	**Q:** He took your clothes, didn't he? **A:** Yes. **Q:** Didn't he make you suck his penis? **A:** Yes.

Reprinted with permission from The Advisor, *Vol. 3, No. 2 (Spring 1990). The Advisor is a quarterly publication of the American Professional Society on the Abuse of Children, Chicago, Ill.*

"Next I'm going to check you—listen to your heart and lungs, feel your tummy, and check your private parts" (Levitt & Martinez, 1998).

Care should be taken to document what history was obtained from each source and who was present during each interview. The affect of all interviewed should be noted. Whether a disclosure was made in response to questioning or whether it was spontaneous should be noted (Meyers, 1986). If the disclosure was made in response to questioning, the wording of the questions asked and the exact wording of the answers should be documented (Meyers, 1986). If the disclosure was spontaneous, the exact words should be documented (Meyers, 1986). If the child would not separate from the caregiver and the caregiver was present for the interview or a portion of it, this should be noted and why. If the caregiver was present but was able to sit behind the child where he or she could not be seen, this should be noted as well.

If the child has already been interviewed by law enforcement or social services and referred for an examination, the examiner may want to clarify with the authorities if another interview is necessary. Protocols vary in different states. Even if the interview is deferred, it is still important for the examiner to establish rapport with the child before examination, as well as discuss the past medical history, review of symptoms, medications, allergies, and family situation with the caregiver. A separate review of symptoms should be obtained from the older child, because he or she might have symptoms (for example, nightmares, school problems, or anorexia) of which the caregiver is unaware. Finally, it is important to assess whether the child feels that the caregiver is protective and supportive of him. **Table 3-3** describes an interview protocol for children suspected of being sexually abused.

Table 3-3. Interview Protocol

Initial procedure	Obtain information from caretaker or social worker Determine child's terminology for genitalia
Interview child alone in nonthreatening environment Establish rapport with child	What's your name? How old are you? Who lives at your house? Do you have any pets? What school do you attend?
Ask about daily living and intimate relationships Ask child to identify body parts/ascertain names for genitalia	Where do you sleep? Who gives you a bath? Identify hair, eyes, nose, belly button, private parts
Try to determine what happened Begin with open-ended questions (may need to ask more specific questions for younger children)	Why did you come to see the doctor? Did something happen to you? Did something happen to your bottom?
More specific questions	Where were you when it happened? Where was Mommy? Daddy? Who did it? What did he/she do? Where were your clothes? Did you tell anyone? Who did you tell? What did he or she say when you told?
Concluding the interview	Tell the child she did a good job. Reassure her that it was not her fault and nobody blames her.
Explain the examination	Now I'm going to check you out: listen to your heart, lungs, feel your tummy, and look at your private parts.
Document	Document questions asked and answers given. Try to record exact words and phrases.
Modifications for adolescents	Obtain more specific information: date and time of assault, history of assault (oral, rectal or vaginal penetration, oral contact by the offender, ejaculation [if known by the victim], digital penetration or penetration with foreign object). Obtain history of any self-cleaning activities (bathing, teeth brushing, urination, douching, changing clothes). Obtain menstrual history and whether patient uses contraceptives. Were any lubricants or a condom used?

Adapted with permission from Midwest Children's Resource Center Interview Protocol, Carolyn Levitt, MD, Director, Midwest Children's Resource Center

When the child is brought to medical attention by the child's caregiver because of behavior or physical symptoms that seem suspicious for sexual abuse, the physician must be able to distinguish what behavior and physical signs and symptoms are truly of concern for sexual abuse. Although many signs and symptoms occur in sexually abused children, most are nonspecific **(see Table 3-1)**. For example, sleep disturbances, dysuria, temper tantrums, school problems, and genital itching are all nonspecific problems in and of themselves. In these cases the physician must decide, first, whether sexual abuse might be the cause of these problems and, second, where and when an evaluation for sexual abuse should take place. There are physical signs that mimic sexual abuse, discussed in Chapter 6. When the behavior that is of concern to the caregiver is sexual, it is helpful for the physician to be aware of the broad range of sexual behaviors that are exhibited by children of the same developmental level who are not sexually abused, and conversely, those sexual behaviors that are not commonly exhibited in normal children (Friedrich et al., 1998). Sexual behaviors that appear most frequently in nonabused children include self-stimulating behaviors (touching sex parts at home, masturbating with hand), exhibitionism (trying to look at people when nude), and behaviors related to personal boundaries (standing too close, touching mother's breasts) (Friedrich et al., 1998). Infrequent behaviors in nonabused children are the more intrusive ones (putting the mouth on sex parts or putting objects in the vagina and/or rectum) (Friedrich et al., 1998). Thus, behavior (such as acting-out sexual scenarios) that suggests a child's explicit or inappropriate knowledge of adult sexual behavior and compulsive masturbation warrant further investigation to determine if the child was sexually abused (Ludwig, 2000).

In an all-too-frequent emergency department scenario, the child is brought for evaluation because one parent suspects that an estranged or divorced spouse is sexually abusing the child. Typically, the child is brought for evaluation after a visit with the accused adult. Often the grounds given for suspecting abuse are vague. Although these allegations may result from a bitter adult trying to "get back" at another adult, it is also possible that these allegations are true. They warrant either further evaluation by the examiner or appropriate referral to a specialty sexual abuse clinic where the concerns of the parent should be addressed and the child interviewed (AAP, 1999a).

PHYSICAL EXAMINATION

The purposes of the physical examination are to (1) document the condition of the patient; (2) diagnose and treat injuries and STDs; (3) collect and preserve evidence; and (4) reassure the patient and address concerns about her or his physical and psychologic well-being. Forensic evidence collection (if deemed necessary) should be integrated with medical testing and examination. For example, to minimize patient trauma, blood drawn for medical testing (rapid plasma reagin test [RPR], beta human chorionic gonadotropin [betaHCG], hepatitis serology) should be obtained concomitant with blood obtained for forensic evidence collection purposes (or deferred for another visit). Similarly, when evidence specimens are collected from oral, vaginal, and rectal orifices, cultures for sexually transmitted diseases (STDs) can be taken immediately afterward.

The examination is more likely to be successfully accomplished if the patient feels at ease with the examiner and can anticipate what the examination will entail. Certainly the degree of explanation regarding the examination depends on the patient's cognitive level. The patient's modesty should be respected, and gowns or drapes should be provided. The patient should be made to feel that she or he has some control over the examination. This may be achieved by allowing the patient to decide such things as what support person (if any) will be present for the examination, whether she wants her heart or lungs examined first, what book she would like to look at during the examination, etc. It may be helpful to show an

Key Point:
The physical examination is performed to document the patient's condition; diagnose and treat any injuries or infections; collect and preserve evidence; and reassure both patient and family concerning questions about the patient's physical and psychologic well-being.

older patient and accompanying caregivers of a child which instruments will be used to assuage some anxiety regarding the examination. The younger child may benefit from having a book read to him or watching a video or some other distraction during the examination. The younger child may also be examined while sitting in the caretaker's lap in the frog-leg supine position. All instruments, sexual assault kit swabs, culture material, etc. should be laid out and handy so that the examination can proceed smoothly. A list of recommended materials is provided in **Table 3-4.**

Table 3-4. Equipment for Sexual Assault Examination	
EQUIPMENT	COMMENTS
Drapes, gowns	Preserve patient's modesty
Books, videos, pictures	Distract young patient while exam is being performed
Small dacron swabs, sterile saline	May be needed to "float" hymen (see text)
Warmed *N. gonorrhea* culture plates (up to three for vaginal/urethral, anal, and pharyngeal specimens)	Culture is the gold standard for detecting *N. gonorrhea* in children
C. trachomatis culture tubes (for vaginal/urethral, anal and pharyngeal specimens)	Culture is the gold standard for detecting *C. trachomatis* in children
Saline solution for wet prep, microscope slides	When vaginal discharge needs to be tested for *T. vaginalis*
Viral culture media	If lesion is suspicious for herpes
Forensic evidence collection kit	If abuse occurred within last 72 hours and medical discretion determines need (see text). Available from police.
Additional sterile dacron swabs	May be necessary to collect additional forensic evidence
Colposcope with camera	Optional; magnification is helpful, not required. Photographs may help examiner describe findings; not essential.
Blood drawing supplies	If blood for serology or rape kit is to be obtained
Measuring tape	Should any lesions need to be measured

INITIAL ASSESSMENT AND EXAMINATION

No child should be forced to undergo an examination. Sexual abuse is by definition any sexual activity where consent is not or cannot be given (Finkelhor, 1979). The purpose of the examination is not only to look for injuries that may have been acquired as the result of sexual abuse, but to begin the healing process by reassuring the child and caregiver that the child will heal physically and by setting in motion mechanisms by which the child can be helped emotionally. If the child refuses an examination, the examiner must decide the urgency with which the examination can be performed. As noted earlier, if the abuse is old, the examination can be deferred; if the abuse occurred within the last 72 hours and forensic evidence may be lost by waiting, the risks and benefits of performing the examination with the aid of either conscious sedation or general anesthesia should be weighed (AAP, 1999a; Christian et al., 2000).

The sexually abused child should be treated as a victim of traumatic injury. Both nongenital and genital injuries should be identified. The examiner should begin, as in other examinations, with overall inspection of the patient. Most pediatric examinations begin with the part of the examination that is the least anxiety provoking (for example, the heart and lungs) and progress to the most sensitive (for example, the ears and pharynx). This rule works well for sexually abused children as well. In addition to giving the child time to get used to the examiner, it sends a message to the child that the purpose of the examination is to assess the well-being of the entire child and not just her genitals. Nongenital injuries such as contusions (where the child was held down), lacerations, petechiae, or bite marks may still be visible. Tethering could leave circumferential hypertrophy of the skin or ligature marks around the wrists, ankles, or neck (Richardson, 1994). The oral examination can be performed before or after the genital examination. Oral findings include condyloma, palatal petechiae, tooth dislocation, and a torn frenulum (AAP, 1999b; Donly & Nowak, 1994).

Persistent vaginal or rectal bleeding mandates consultation with either a pediatric gynecologist or surgeon who can examine the child under anesthesia.

A determination should be made as to when the alleged sexual abuse occurred. If the alleged sexual abuse occurred recently, it may still be possible to visualize an acute or healing injury. While the American Academy of Pediatrics recommends forensic evidence collection when sexual abuse occurred in the preceding 72 hours or when there is bleeding or acute injury, one recent study suggests that the yield of forensic evidence is negligible from the child's body after 24 hours and overall (from clothing and linens) after 48 hours (AAP, 1999a; Christian et al., 2000). Therefore, medical discretion is indicated related to the use or partial use of a sexual assault examination kit. Symptomatic children should be examined at the time of presentation regardless of the time of the alleged abuse. Asymptomatic victims whose most recent sexual contact was more than 72 hours before seeking medical attention can be referred to a specialty clinic dealing with child sexual abuse if one exists in the community and follow-up can be assured. The referral examination should take place as promptly as possible.

TYPICAL ANATOMY

The stages described by Tanner (1962) provide a sexual maturity rating system for the normal appearance and pattern of pubic hair in the male and female; testicle size, scrotum, and phallus development in the male; and breast development in the female (**Figure 3-1, a and b**). The Tanner stage is assessed by visual inspection and should be noted when reporting the examination findings.

Many clinics that evaluate children for suspected sexual abuse are equipped with a colposcope, which provides magnification for the examination and often has a camera attached for photographic documentation. Although it is helpful to use a

Figure 3-1-a.
Tanner stages in the female body.

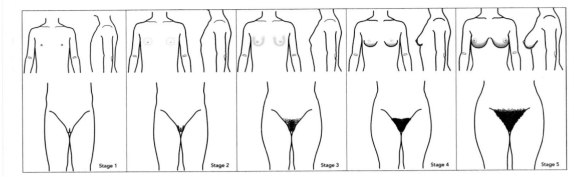

Figure 3-1-b.
Tanner stages in the male body.

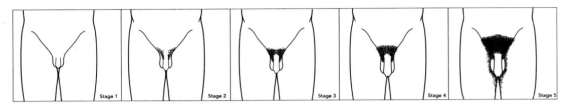

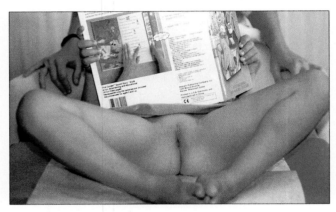

Figure 3-2. *Child in a frog leg supine position with a book on her abdomen to distract her attention away from the exam.*

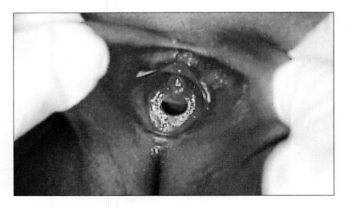

Figure 3-3. *Labial traction for a child in the supine frog leg position. Examiner is gently pulling outward and downward on labia majora with gloved hands. In view is a normal crescentic hymen of a Tanner stage 1 girl. Hymen has attachments at the 11 and 1 o'clock positions without tissue being present between the two attachments.*

colposcope, it is not absolutely essential. A careful examination with a good light source, such as an otoscope used for magnification, can be undertaken in the emergency department in the absence of a colposcope (Muram, 1989). Photographs can be taken with a macro lens 35 mm camera instead of a colposcope camera.

The prepubertal female genitalia are examined without a speculum. A speculum examination is only necessary if there is unexplained vaginal bleeding. In this case the child will most likely require examination under anesthesia, and a pediatric gynecologist or surgeon should be called. In most cases, thorough visual inspection of the external genitalia, vaginal vestibule, and hymenal structures is sufficient. Visual inspection may be accomplished while the prepubertal female is in the supine (**Figure 3-2**) or knee-chest position (McCann et al., 1990a). In the supine frog-leg position the hymen may best be visualized if the gentle traction is placed on the labia majora (**Figure 3-3**). The labia majora is pulled outward and downward. In the knee-chest position the labia majora is lifted upward and outward to bring the hymen into better view (**Figure 3-4**). This position allows for visualization of the posterior hymen, vagina, anus, and frequently the cervix. In circumstances where the hymen appears folded on itself or redundant, it may be necessary to tease the redundant hymenal tissue apart with a swab moistened with saline solution to avoid irritating the highly sensitive-to-touch unestrogenized hymen (touching the hymen with a dry swab may not be well tolerated by many patients) or by applying a few milliliters of warm saline solution on the hymen to make the hymenal edges "float." **Figure 3-7 a and b** illustrates the information that can be gleaned from this technique.

Figure 3-8 illustrates normal prepubertal vaginal vestibular structures and a normal hymen. The vulva is the external genitalia of the female and includes the clitoris, labia majora, labia minora, vaginal vestibule, urethral orifice, vaginal orifice, hymen, and posterior fourchette. The labia majora are

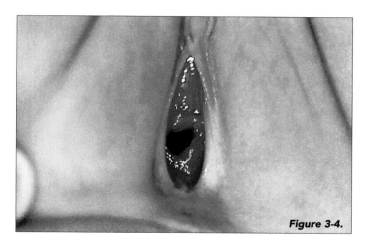

Figure 3-4.

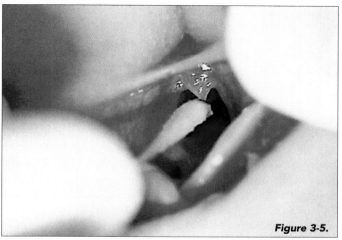

Figure 3-5.

Figure 3-4. *Labial traction for a child in the prone knee-chest position. Examiner is gently pushing the labia majora upward and outward.*

Figure 3-5. *The examiner is using a cotton swab moistened with saline solution to assess a bump (probably a septal remnant) on the hymen at 6 o'clock in the supine position.*

Figure 3-6. *Fimbriated or denticular hymen. Hymen with multiple projections and indentations along edge, creating a ruffled appearance (APSAC, 1995). A few milliliters of water were squirted on the hymen to make it float and to better assess its appearance.*

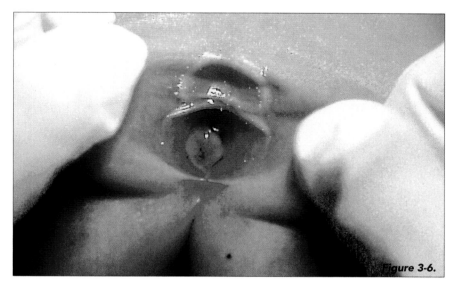

Figure 3-6.

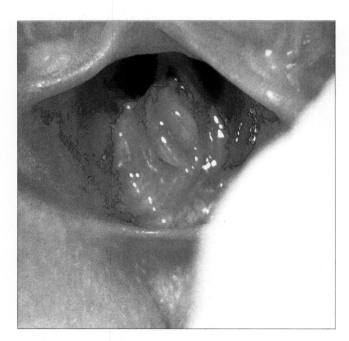

***Figure 3-7-a.** Supine view.*

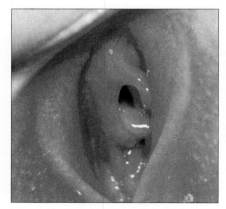

***Figure 3-7-b.** Knee-chest view.*

***Figure 3-7.** Supine and knee-chest views of a Tanner stage 1 hymen. It is difficult to assess the hymen supine. In the prone knee-chest position, however, the hymen is seen to be slightly redundant and annular, with a tag present at 6 o'clock. This is a normal examination. While the knee-chest position does not add much if the hymen is normal and well visualized in the supine position, it is helpful if results in the supine position are abnormal or equivocal. The knee-chest position is also helpful to assess whether the hymen is folded onto itself and therefore merely looks abnormal.*

rounded folds of skin that cover the vulva (APSAC, 1995). The labia minora are longitudinal thin folds of skin enclosed within the labia majora. In the prepubertal child, these folds extend from the clitoral hood to approximately the mid point on the lateral wall of the vaginal vestibule (APSAC, 1995). The hymen is the membrane that either partially or (rarely) completely covers the vaginal orifice. The posterior fourchette is the junction of the labia minora posteriorly (APSAC, 1995). In the prepubertal child, this area is referred to as the posterior commissure, because the labia minora are not completely developed to connect inferiorly until puberty (APSAC, 1995). The posterior fossa is the concavity that extends from the base of the vaginal vestibule to the posterior fourchette. It is frequently the site of positive findings for penetrating trauma resulting from sexual abuse. There are many normal hymenal variants, as illustrated in **Figures 3-6** and **Figures 3-9** to **3-11**. Because an imperforate hymen is rare, to say that the hymen is "perforate" has little meaning. The term "intact" should also be avoided when describing the hymen. Findings related to the hymen are usually described with relationship to the face of a clock, always noting whether the patient is prone or supine (**Figure 3-12**). Other normal findings include erythema of the vestibule, periurethral bands (**Figure 3-13**), labial adhesions (**Figure 3-14**), lymphoid follicles on the fossa navicularis, posterior fourchette midline avascular areas, urethral dilation with labial traction, hymenal mounds, septal remnants/midline hymenal tags (**see Figure 3-9**), and intravaginal ridges (McCann et al., 1990b). The size of the hymenal opening varies with the degree of patient relaxation, the amount of traction the examiner places on the labia, and the patient's age. A significantly enlarged hymenal opening is of concern in the presence of concomitant posterior hymenal abnormalities (Heger & Emans, 1990; Hymel & Jenny, 1996). Male genitalia can be examined while the patient is sitting or

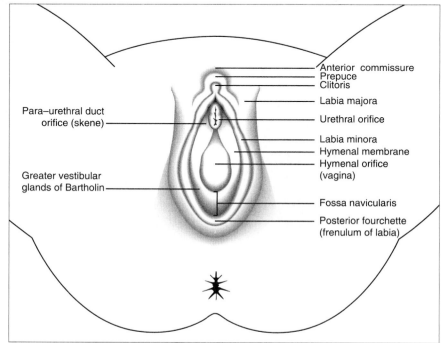

***Figure 3-8.** Normal structures.*

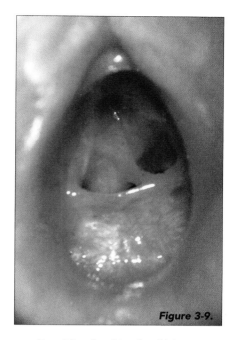

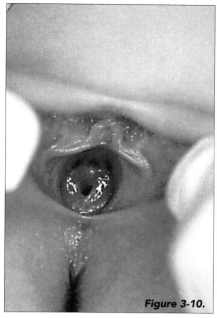

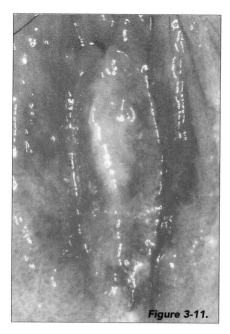

Figure 3-9.

Figure 3-10.

Figure 3-11.

standing. The foreskin should be retracted if possible and the glans examined. The scrotum and testes should be examined. Although injuries to the penis are uncommon, injuries may include petechiae, contusions, lacerations, and bite marks.

The anus in either sex can be examined while the child is supine (with knees drawn up to the chest), in the lateral decubitus position, or in the prone knee-chest position. The anus is visualized by spreading the gluteal folds. Rectal sphincter tone should be noted. Anal dilatation of more than 20 mm without the presence of stool in the rectum is unusual (McCann et al., 1989) (**Figure 3-15**). No digital rectal examination is necessary; however, when deeper rectal injury is suspected because of severe or unexplained bleeding, an endoscopic examination is indicated.

Figure 3-16 illustrates a normal anus. The external anal tissues have a symmetric appearance caused by the circumferentially radiating skin folds known as rugae. Wedge-shaped smooth areas in the midline are often seen in normal children, as is perianal erythema and venous congestion (McCann et al., 1989). Constipated children may develop superficial anal fissures.

Anal injuries are often difficult to detect (Adams et al., 1994; McCann et al., 1992). Acute anal injuries include abrasions (**Figure 3-17**), contusions, edema, and lacerations. Chronic and healed injuries from past abuse include skin tags outside of the midline, distorted or irregular anal folds, and dilatation of the anus greater than 15 mm within 30 seconds of examination and in the absence of stool in the rectal ampulla (Adams et al., 1994; Bays & Chadwick, 1993) (**Table 3-5**).

Most sexual abuse leaves no visible injury (Adams et al., 1994; Bays & Chadwick, 1993). Reasons for this are multiple: perpetrators may avoid physical injury to the child; injuries that occurred earlier may have healed by the time the child divulges the abuse; vaginal vestibular tissues are elastic and may stretch rather than tear; and digital fondling may not cause tissue damage (McCann et al., 1992; Bays & Chadwick, 1993). There is a spectrum of findings produced by molestation. Attempts have been made to provide classifications for these findings (Adams et al., 1994; Bays & Chadwick,1993). **Table 3-5** shows one of the frequently used classifications. Findings are often noted in the posterior hymen and vestibule in sexual assault, and specific attention during the examination should be focused there for abnormalities such as hymenal transections, absence of hymenal tissue,

Figure 3-9. Septate hymen. Hymen is bisected by band of hymenal tissue creating more than one opening.

Figure 3-10. Annular hymen in Tanner stage 1 girl. Hymenal tissue extends circumfer-entially around the entire vaginal orifice.

Figure 3-11. Imperforate hymen. (Courtesy of Dr. Mary Spencer, Escondido, Calif)

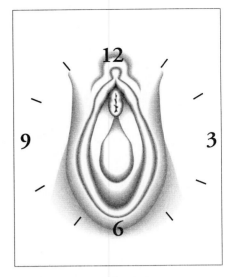

Figure 3-12. *Face of a clock.*

clefts to the base of the hymen, and scars) (**Figures 3-18 and 3-19**). Findings of concern for sexual abuse include fresh genital injuries in the absence of an adequate explanation (lacerations, contusions, transections, avulsions, hematomas, ecchymoses, petechiae, and bite marks), an enlarged hymenal opening with posterior hymenal abnormalities, and notches or clefts on the base of the hymen in the posterior region (between 3 and 9 o'clock with the patient in the supine position) (Adams et al., 1994). STDs in children may indicate sexual abuse if it is determined that they were not acquired in the perinatal period; these include gonorrhea, syphilis, and human immunodeficiency virus (HIV) infection (Centers for Disease Control and Prevention [CDC], 1998). The finding of trichomonas, chlamydia, condylomata acuminatum (**Figure 3-20**), and herpes simplex virus infection (**Figure 3-21**) warrants investigation into the mode of acquisition of the infection and possible referral to child protective services for further evaluation (CDC, 1998).

SEXUALLY TRANSMITTED DISEASES

Testing for STDs can be performed after the genitalia are inspected. If forensic evidence is collected, usually sexually transmitted disease testing is performed immediately afterward. Whereas adolescents should be treated as adults and undergo STD testing even if asymptomatic, the approach to STD testing in

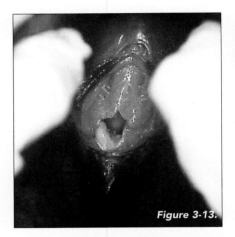

Figure 3-13.

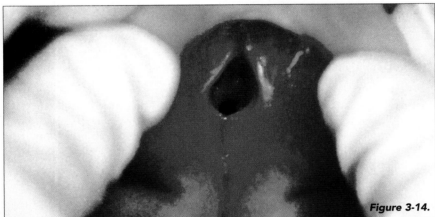

Figure 3-14.

Figure 3-13. *Thickened hymen as the result of estrogenization in a Tanner 3 girl. Hymen appears not only thickened but also pale in the patient as a result of estrogen changes. Clefts at 3 and 9 o'clock and periurethral bands are present here as well. Clefts anterior to 9 to 3 o'clock as well as periurethral bands are normal findings.*

Figure 3-14. *Labial agglutination posteriorly resulting from fusion of the adjacent edges of the mucosal surfaces of the labia minora.*

Figure 3-15. *Anal dilation without stool visible in rectum.*

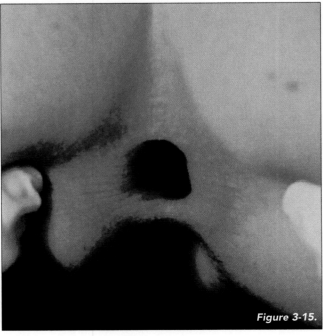

Figure 3-15.

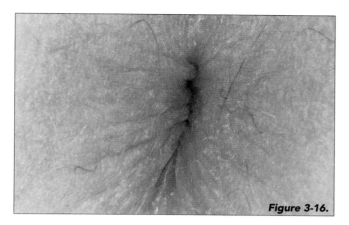

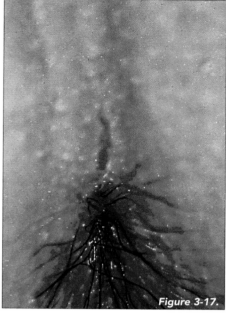

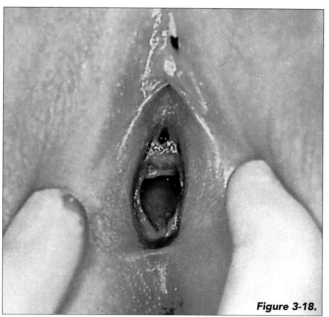

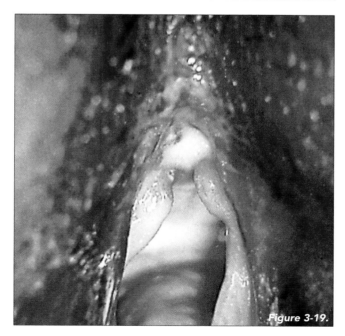

Figure 3-16. Normal anus of a 9-year-old girl. (Courtesy of Dr. Mary Spencer, Escondido, Calif)

Figure 3-17. Perianal superficial laceration that is healing at 12 o'clock in the prone knee-chest position.

Figure 3-18. A Tanner 1 girl several weeks after a rape. Note that there is absent hymenal tissue at 6 o'clock with the patient supine and very little hymenal tissue from 1 to 5 o'clock and from 7 to 11 o'clock.

Figure 3-19. Tanner 3 female a few days after rape. Note the healing tissue where the hymen was disrupted at 6 o'clock with the patient supine. Vaginal rugae (a normal finding) can be seen anteriorly.

Table 3-5. Revised Classification of Anogenital Findings in Suspect Sexual Abuse

CLASSIFICATION OF FINDINGS

Class 1: Normal
Found in newborns
— Periurethral or vestibular bands
— Longitudinal intravaginal ridges or columns
— Hymenal tags
— Hymenal bumps or mounds
— Hymenal clefts in the anterior (superior) half of hymenal rim, above the 3 to 9 o'clock line, with patient supine
— Estrogen changes, when hymenal tissue appears thickened, redundant, and pale
— Linea vestibularis (a flat, white, midline streak in posterior vestibule)

Class 2: Nonspecific
Findings that may result from sexual abuse, depending on timing of examination with respect to abuse, but that may also be normal variants or result from other causes
— Perianal skin tags
— Increased perianal skin pigmentation
— Diastasis ani, or a smooth area at 6 or 12 o'clock in perianal area, where there are no anal folds or wrinkles
— Erythema (redness) of vestibular or perianal tissues
— Increased vascularity, or dilation of existing blood vessels, in the vestibule
— Labial adhesions, or agglutination or fusion of labia minora in midline
— Hymenal rim that appears narrow, but is 1 mm wide or less, with measurements taken from magnified photographs by means of calibrated measuring device
— Vaginal discharge (this is a nonspecific finding unless appropriately obtained cultures confirm the presence of a sexually transmitted infection)
— Lesions of condyloma acuminata in child less than two years of age
— Anal fissures
— Flattened or thickened anal folds
— Anal dilatation, or the opening of internal and external anal sphincters, which demonstrates stool in the rectal vault
— Venous congestion or venous pooling in perianal tissues causing a purple coloration, which may be localized or diffuse

Class 3: Suspicious
Findings that have rarely been described in nonabused children, but have been noted in children with documented abuse, and would prompt examiner to investigate carefully the possibility of abuse
— Enlarged hymenal opening, with measurements more than 2 standard deviations above mean for age and examination method
— Hymenal notch/cleft/partial transection, which appears as sudden narrowing in hymenal rim to less than 1 mm in width, located on or below 3 to 9 o'clock line (patient supine)
— Acute abrasions, lacerations or bruising of labia or perihymenal tissue, with no history of accidental injury
— Apparent condyloma acuminata in child less than 2 years old
— Distorted anal folds, which are irregular in appearance and may have signs of edema of the tissues
— Immediate (within 30 seconds) anal dilation of 20 mm or more, with no stool visible or palpable in the rectal vault

Class 4: Suggestive of Abuse or Penetration
Findings, or combination of findings, that can be reasonably explained only by postulating abuse or penetrating injury of some type
— Combination of 2 or more suspicious genital findings or 2 or more suspicious anal findings
— Scar or fresh laceration of posterior fourchette, not involving the hymen
— Perianal scar

(continued)

Table 3-5. *(continued)*

Class 5: Clear Evidence of Blunt Force or Penetrating Trauma
Findings that can have no explanation other than trauma to hymen or perianal tissues
— Complete hymenal transection (healed): hymen has been torn through, to the base, so that there is no measurable hymenal tissue remaining between vaginal wall and fossa or vestibular wall
— Areas, more extensive than transections, where there is complete absence of hymenal tissue below the 3 to 9 o'clock line (patient supine)
— Acute laceration of hymen: recent tear through full thickness of hymenal tissue, which may also extend into the vagina and/or posterior fourchette
— Ecchymosis or bruising on the hymen
— Perianal lacerations extending deep to the external anal sphincter

OVERALL ASSESSMENT OF LIKELIHOOD OF ABUSE

Class 1: No Evidence of Abuse
— Normal results of examination, no history, no behavioral changes, no witnessed abuse
— Nonspecific findings with another known or likely explanation, and no history of abuse or behavior changes
— Child considered at risk for sexual abuse, but gives no history and has only nonspecific behavior changes
— Physical findings of injury consistent with history of accidental injury, which is clear and believable

Class 2: Possible Abuse
— Class 1 or 2 findings in combination with marked behavior changes, especially sexualized behaviors, but child unable to give history of abuse
— Presence of condyloma acuminata in a child less than 2 years old, or herpes type 1 genital lesions with history of abuse, and with otherwise normal results of examination
— Child has made a statement, but it is not sufficiently detailed or is not consistent
— Class 3 findings with no disclosure of abuse

Class 3: Probable Cause
— Child gives a clear, consistent, and detailed description of being molested, with or without physical findings
— Class 4 findings in a child with or without a history of abuse, and with no history of accidental penetrating injury
— Positive culture (not rapid antigen test) for C. trachomatis from genital area in child less than 2 years old
— Positive culture for herpes simplex type 2 from genital lesions
— Confirmed condyloma acuminata, when lesions first appeared in a child 2 years old or younger
— Trichomonas infection, diagnosed by wet mount or culture

Reprinted with permission from the publisher. Adams, J. Evolution of a classification scale: Appendix. Child Maltreatment. *Thousand Oaks, Calif: SAGE Publications, Inc. 2001;6(1):34-35.*

prepubertal children differs because prevalence rates of STDs among sexually abused children are low. In deciding whether to test and offer prophylaxis for STDs among prepubertal children, the physician must consider the following: the nature of the abuse (e.g., fondling on top of clothing versus vaginal penetration with a penis), the likelihood of the abuser having an STD, the examination findings in the child (vaginal discharge present, abnormal examination), and STD presence in the community (CDC, 1998).

Most experts would recommend STD testing for those children with a vaginal discharge, an abnormal examination, a close contact with an STD (e.g., an abused sibling with gonorrhea), or a perpetrator at high risk (Siegel et al., 1995). The only appropriate STD tests in children are cultures. Nonculture tests, such as direct fluorescent antibody, enzyme immunoassay, or DNA probe, should not be used because they lack adequate specificity and have not been well studied in children

Key Point:
The approach to STD testing must be geared toward the age and developmental level of the patient, with prepubertal children being handled differently from adolescents or adults.

(Hammerschlag, 1998). **Table 3-6** outlines STD screening recommendations. See Chapter 5 for further discussion of STDs in children.

DIFFERENTIAL DIAGNOSIS

The differential diagnosis of suspected child abuse injury is extensive and is discussed in another chapter. Emergency physicians commonly are asked to distinguish accidental trauma from child sexual abuse. It should be noted that accidental genital trauma (i.e., straddle injury) **(Figure 3-22)** is usually blunt force trauma as opposed to the penetrating trauma of sexual abuse and rarely causes hymenal injury (Bond et al., 1995). Blunt trauma to the genital area most often produces injury to the labia majora, labia minora, clitoris, and clitoral hood because these structures are pressed against the bony pelvis. If hymenal injury is noted, sexual abuse should carefully be ruled out. The physician should take a careful history and consider whether the mechanism of injury correlates with the physical findings in all cases of genital trauma.

Commonly seen conditions that are confused with sexual abuse include lichen sclerosis **(Figure 3-23)**, itching due to perivaginal or perineal group A beta hemolytic streptococcal infections **(Figures 3-24 and 3-25)** and pinworms **(Figure 3-26),** vaginal bleeding resulting from a foreign body (e.g., toilet paper) in the vagina or shigella vaginitis, and bleeding secondary to a prolapsed urethra (Bays, 1994). The differential diagnosis of suspected child abuse injury is extensive and is discussed in Chapter 6.

FORENSIC EVIDENCE

A sexual assault examination kit provides an organized means of collecting forensic evidence (American College of Obstetricians and Gynecologists [ACOG], 1987). Although kits vary from state to state, in general they provide the means to collect

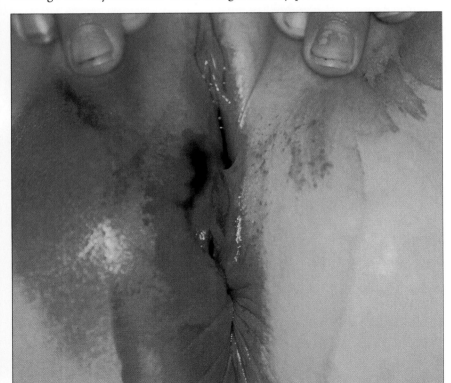

Figure 3-22. *Tanner stage 1 female with a straddle injury as a result of a fall on a bicycle. Note the large hematoma on the labia majora. There is no hymenal injury present.*

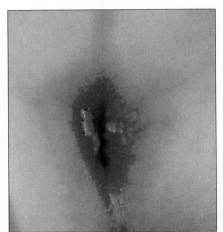

Figure 3-20. *Perianal condyloma.*

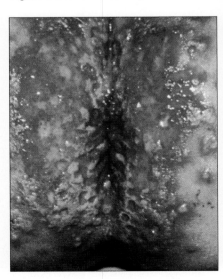

Figure 3-21. *Extensive Herpes simplex type II evident around the anus and on perineum and labia majora. (Courtesy of Dr. Mary Spencer, Escondido, Calif)*

Table 3-6. STD Screening Recommendations

Initial Examination

Prepubertal Children

Decision to evaluate for STDs must be made on an individual basis. Situations involving a high risk for STDs include symptomatic child, child with abnormal genital findings on examination, high STD prevalence in community, and suspected offender at high risk for having STD.

Cultures for *N. gonorrhoeae*
Cultures for *C. trachomatis*

Adolescents

Cultures should be obtained from any sites of penetration or attempted penetration.

Prepubertal Children

Cultures should be obtained from any sites of penetration or attempted penetration, including (when indicated): pharyngeal, anal, vaginal or urethral cultures. In evaluating for chlamydia a urethral specimen should be obtained only if urethral discharge is present. In evaluating for *N. gonorrhoeae,* a specimen of urethral meatal discharge can be substituted for intraurethral swab. Pharyngeal specimens not recommended for *C. trachomatis.*

Wet Mount and Culture for *T. vaginalis*

Adolescents and Prepubertal Children

Wet mount and culture of vaginal swab specimen for *T. vaginalis.* Examine wet mount for evidence of bacterial vaginosis and yeast infection if vaginal discharge or malodor is evident.

Serum for HIV, Syphilis, and Hepatitis B

Adolescents and Prepubertal Children

Preservation of a serum sample for subsequent analysis if follow-up serologic tests are positive.

Follow-up 2 Weeks after Assault

Adolescents

Repeat physical examination. Cultures should be repeated unless prophylaxis was given.

Prepubertal Children

Repeat physical examination. Cultures (if indicated) should be repeated unless prophylaxis was given. If abuse was chronic, testing for STDs once may suffice.

Follow-up 12 Weeks after Assault

Adolescents and Prepubertal Children

Serologic tests for HIV and syphilis.

Adapted from: Centers for Disease Control and Prevention. 1998 guidelines for treatment of sexually transmitted diseases. MMWR. 1998;47:1-116.

Table 3-7. Sexual Assault Exam Protocol and Evidence Collection

ADULTS/ADOLESCENTS	COMMENTS	MODIFICATIONS FOR PREPUBERTAL CHILDREN
— Examine for non-genital trauma — Inspect buccal cavity — Search hair for foreign material and blood — Inspect for bite marks — Inspect for bruises		
— Collect relevant clothing and underwear in a paper bag	— Avoid plastic bags because mold can form — Damaged or torn clothing may be significant — Clothing provides surface on which traces of foreign material may be found — Each garment should be placed in a separate bag to prevent cross contamination	— Collect underwear or diaper in a paper bag
— Examine genital area		— A speculum examination is not performed — If the examiner suspects a vaginal laceration or tear because the patient has unexplained vaginal bleeding, then a speculum examination will need to be done, most likely under anesthesia.
Specimen Collection: — Comb hair from pubic area	— May contain specimens from assailant and may, in some cases, help to identify race, sex, blood type, and hair color of suspect	— No pubic hair to comb — Debris can be collected from pubic area
— Pluck head and pubic hair from victim	— Must be plucked, not cut — Differentiates hair debris of assailant found on victim from victim's own — May choose to obtain these specimens after all other evidence is collected because many victims find this unpleasant — Patient may choose to pluck own hair	— Omit pubic hair, collect head hair
Specimen collection: — Vaginal fluid: wet mount of material from posterior fossa for motile sperm — Fixed smear from the vagina or vulva or both for sperm	— Wet mount may not be required in all states — If penetration to the anus or mouth occured, anal and/or oral swabs should be collected — For male victim or penile trauma, the external shaft and glans of the penis should be swabbed with cotton swabs that are slightly moistened with distilled water or saline solution	

(continued)

Table 3-7. *(continued)*

— Endocervical culture for *N. gonorrhea* and *C. trachomatis* — Swab from vaginal pool — Swab from any area that fluoresces with UV lamp (Wood's lamp) or appears to have dried secretions on it (vulva, rectum, inner thighs)	— State crime laboratory can analyze for acid phosphatase, ABO(H) antigen, and sperm precipitins	— Culture obtained by swabbing vagina for *N. gonorrhea* and *C. trachomatis*
— Collect debris from beneath fingernails if victim scratched assailant		
— Note dried secretions on skin by examination or fluorescing on Wood's lamp examination	— State crime laboratory can analyze for acid phosphatase, ABO(H) antigen, and sperm precipitins	
Serum: — Serology for hepatitis B, syphilis, and HIV — Beta HCG — Blood typing	— Repeat in 4 to 6 weeks	
— Collect saliva sample	— Sample will determine if the victim secretes blood group antigens in body fluids other than blood	

Adapted from: American College of Obstetricians and Gynecologists. Sexual assault. Tech Bull. *1987;(101):1-5.*

clothing worn by the victim, debris from the assaulted genital area, pubic hair (if the patient is pubertal), swabs for collecting dried secretions left on the genital area of the victim, head hair, saliva (to assess for ABO secretor status), and blood from the victim. (Chapter 4 offers a discussion of forensic evidence collection in children). Instructions are included in the kit. Modification is necessary for prepubertal children (**Table 3-7**). Collection, handling, and storage of specimens to maintain the "chain of evidence" is important to preserve the admissibility of the evidence in later court proceedings.

Definitive Care

Antibiotic prophylaxis for STDs should be offered to selected pubertal children. (CDC, 1998). **Table 3-8** provides antibiotic treatment regimens. In the case of an acute assault, the examiner may need to contemplate whether there is a need for HIV prophylaxis. Chapter 5 provides a discussion of this issue. Consultation with an infectious disease specialist may be necessary when HIV prophylaxis is being considered for a prepubertal child. A medical follow-up examination is warranted for those victims treated with antibiotics for infection to assure resolution of the infection and for acute injuries where adequate healing must be assured. Follow-up is generally recommended for all patients at 2 weeks and 12 weeks after an assault.

It is important not to neglect the patient's emotional as well as physical well-being. Examination findings should be discussed with the patient and accompanying caregivers. As noted already, the majority of children will have normal examinations. Although this may be a relief to most, some children may interpret the normal findings to mean that they will not be believed, and some caregivers

Key Point:
The likelihood of finding forensic evidence in cases of child sexual abuse is low and decreases markedly if the abuse occurred more than 72 hours prior to the time of examination.

Key Point:
The patient's emotional well-being should be addressed as well as his or her physical state. The examiner can offer reassurance that mental healing will be accomplished over time and make referrals as appropriate to resources available in the community.

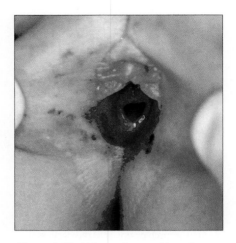

Figure 3-23. *Lichen sclerosis. Note the parchment-like epithelium and subepithelial hemorrhages.*

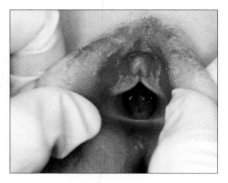

Figure 3-24. *Perivaginal group A beta hemolytic streptococcal infection.*

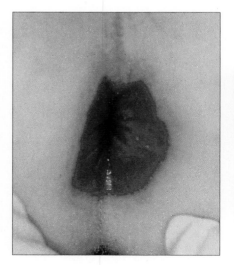

Figure 3-25. *Perianal group A beta hemolytic streptococcal infection. Child had no history of sexual abuse but positive history of perianal pruritus.*

may interpret the normal findings to mean that nothing really happened after all. This misinterpretation of a normal examination should be clarified. If the examination is abnormal, the child and caregiver should be reassured that the physical injuries will heal and that subsequent examinations of the healed tissue will only look abnormal to those who are experts in the evaluation of sexual abuse. The examiner should stress that mental health healing also must occur over time and assure that adequate follow-up with the resources available in the community (rape relief, psychiatry, sexual abuse clinic) is in place before the patient leaves the examination site (see the Sexual Assault Examination Checklist, **Table 3-9**).

DOCUMENTATION AND PHOTOGRAPHS

Documentation of the interview and examination should be done as carefully as possible. Documentation should include who was present for both the interview and examination, who was identified as the alleged perpetrator, what questions were asked, and what each person interviewed said (Meyers, 1986). The examination findings are documented, including the Tanner stage, position of the patient during the examination (supine, knee-chest), and configuration of the hymen. The emotional state of the child assault victim during both the interview and the examination should be noted. The child's exact words, in quotations, are documented as much as possible. State sexual assault examination forms are available in most states and are useful because they are comprehensive. Example state sexual assault examination forms can be viewed on most state health department websites. If the examiner encounters difficulty in describing examination findings in words, it may be helpful to draw a diagram to illustrate the findings. When writing a final assessment, the examiner should state what information, if any, supports the possibility that the abuse occurred (for example, child's statements or behavioral symptoms) (APSAC, 1995). The examiner should clearly delineate the physical findings and note whether they are consistent with the history given (Giardino et al., 1992). For example, if the examination is normal and the child gave a history of genital fondling, then the examiner might write that "the normal findings noted in this examination are consistent with the history as given by the child of genital fondling." If a camera is available and the patient consents, it may be helpful to document the examination with a photograph. Photography is helpful when the examiner is unsure of how to interpret the physical examination findings. Forensic photographic documentation is beyond the scope of this chapter but is discussed in an excellent article by Ricci (1994).

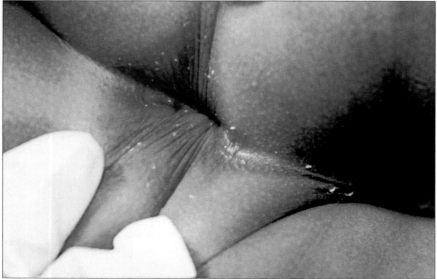

Figure 3-26. *Pinworms.*

Table 3-8. Prophylaxis

EMPIRIC REGIMENS	ADOLESCENTS PREPUBERTAL	CHILDREN*
Empiric regimen for chlamydial, gonococcal, and trichomonal infections and for bacterial vaginosis	Recommended regimen: Ceftriaxone 125 mg intra-muscularly or Cefixime 400 mg once orally or Spectinomycin 2 g intra-muscularly *PLUS* Metronidazole 2 g once orally *PLUS* Doxycycline 100 mg orally twice daily for 7 days or Azithromycin 1 g once orally	Recommended regimen: Ceftriaxone 125 mg IM or Spectinomycin 40 mg/kg IM *PLUS* Erythromycin base 50 mg/kg/d (max 2 g/day) orally 4 times/day for 10 to 14 days or (for children over 40 kg but under 8 years of age) Azithromycin 1 g once orally or (for children over 8 years of age) Azithromycin 1 g once orally or Doxycycline 100 mg orally twice daily for 7 days
Pregnancy	Please see chapter 10 for pregnancy prophylaxis information	
Hepatitis B	Postexposure hepatitis B vaccination (without hepatitis B immune globulin) should adequately protect against hepatitis B. Hepatitis B vaccine should be administered to victims of sexual assault at the time of the initial examination. Follow-up doses of vaccine should be administered 1-2 months and 4-6 months after the first dose if not previously vaccinated.	Consider vaccination if nonimmune

* Prophylaxis is generally offered to adolescents. Presumptive treatment for sexually abused children is not routinely done. (Often, they are not seen acutely or the nature of the abuse may make it unlikely that an STD has been transmitted; prepubertal girls appear to be at lower risk for ascending infections than are adolescent or adult women, and regular follow-up can usually be assured.) Treatment should be considered for prepubertal girls (after cultures for STDs are obtained) who are likely to have acquired an STD, have signs of a penetrating injury, are symptomatic (abdominal pain, vaginal discharge, or dysuria), or whose parents or guardians are very concerned about the possibility of contracting an STD (Muram, 1989).

Adapted from: Centers for Disease Control and Prevention (CDC). 1998 guidelines for treatment of sexually transmitted diseases. MMWR. 1998;47:110. Drug dosage recommendations listed herein are those of the authors and are not endorsed by the US Public Health Service or the US Department of Health and Human Services.

Table 3-9. Assault Examination Checklist

— History documented
— Physical examination documented (may use drawings)
— Documentation that photographs were taken (if indicated)
— Sexual assault evidence collection kit obtained, correctly labeled, sealed, locked up until retrieved by law enforcement
— Cultures and serologic tests for STDs obtained

— Prophylaxis for STDs and pregnancy discussed with patient and provided
— Mental health follow-up arranged
— Follow-up medical examination arranged
— Appropriate authorities (law enforcement, child protective services) notified
— Documentation of person to whom child was released

Table 3-10. Guidelines for Making the Decision to Report Sexual Abuse

DATA AVAILABLE			RESPONSE	
History	**Physical**	**Laboratory**	**Level of Concern About Abuse**	**Action**
None	Normal examination	None	None	None
Behavioral changes	Normal examination	None	Low (worry)	+/- report, *follow closely (possible mental health referral)
None	Nonspecific findings	None	Low (worry)	+/- report, *follow closely
Non-specific history by child or history by parent only	Nonspecific findings	None	Possible (suspect)	+/- report, *follow closely
None	Specific findings	None	Probable	Report
Clear statement	Normal examination	None	Probable	Report
None	Normal examination nonspecific or specific findings	Positive culture for gonorrhea; positive serologic test for syphilis; presence of semen, sperm, acid phosphatase	Definite	Report
Behavioral changes	Nonspecific	Other STDs	Probable	Report

From American Academy of Pediatrics Committee on Child Abuse and Neglect (1991).
* A report may or may not be indicated. The decision to report should be based on discussion with local or regional experts and/or child protective service agencies.

The American Academy of Pediatrics (1999a) has published guidelines for making the decision to report sexual abuse of children (**Table 3-10**). A physician is mandated by law to report all cases of suspected child abuse. Physicians should be familiar with the mechanism of making a report in their area.

CONCLUSION

In summary, the physician's role in the evaluation of the sexually abused child encompasses the areas of history taking, physical examination, diagnostic and forensic testing, and assuring appropriate referral and follow-up. All of these components are important not only to allow the state to take legal action on behalf of the child (Meyers, 1986), but also to allow the child to begin to heal. The long term psychologic effects of sexual abuse are discussed in Chapter 23.

REFERENCES

Adams, J. Evolution of a classification scale: Appendix. *Child Maltreatment.* Thousand Oaks, Calif: SAGE Publications, Inc. 2001;6(1):34-35.

Adams JA, Harper K, Knudson S, Revilla J. Examination findings in legally confirmed child sexual abuse: it's normal to be normal. *Pediatrics.* 1994;94:310-317.

American Academy of Pediatrics: Committee on Child Abuse and Neglect. Guidelines for the evaluation of sexual abuse of children. *Pediatrics.* 1999;103:186-191.

American Academy of Pediatrics. Oral and dental aspects of child abuse and neglect. *Policy Statement.* 1999;104(2);348-350.

American College of Obstetricians and Gynecologists. Sexual assault. *Tech Bull.* 1987;(101):1-5.

American Professional Society on the Abuse of Children (APSAC). *Guidelines for Psychosocial Evaluation of Suspected Child Abuse in Young Children.* San Diego, Calif: APSAC;1990.

American Professional Society on the Abuse of Children (APSAC). *Practice Guidelines, Descriptive Terminology in Child Sexual Abuse Evaluations.* San Diego, Calif: APSAC;1995.

Bays J. Conditions mistaken for child abuse. In: Reece R, ed. *Child Abuse Medical Diagnosis and Management.* Malvern, Pa: Lea & Febinger; 1994:386-403.

Bays J, Chadwick D. Medical diagnosis of the sexually abused child. *Child Abuse Negl.* 1993;17:91-110.

Bond GR, Dowd MD, Landsman I, Rimsza M. Unintentional perineal injury in prepubescent girls: a multicenter prospective report of 56 girls. *Pediatrics.* 1995;95:628-631.

Centers for Disease Control and Prevention (CDC). 1998 guidelines for treatment of sexually transmitted diseases. *MMWR.* 1998;47(No. RR-1):1-116.

Christian CW, Lavelle JM, DeJong AR, Loiselle J, Brenner L, Joffe M. Forensic evidence findings in prepubertal victims of sexual assault. *Pediatrics.* 2000;106(1):100-104.

Commonwealth of Kentucky. Child sexual abuse medical examination form. *Sexual Assault/Abuse: A Hospital/Community Protocol for Forensic and Medical Examination.* Frankfort, Ky: Office of the Attorney General, Victims Advocacy Division; 1989; Appendix A:23-27.

Donly KJ, Nowak AJ. Maxillofacial, neck and dental lesions in child abuse. In: Reece R, ed. *Child Abuse Medical Diagnosis and Management.* Malvern, Pa: Lea & Febinger; 1994:150-166.

Faller KC. Types of questions for children alleged to have been sexually abused. *Advisor.* 1990;3:3-5.

Faller KC. *Child Sexual Abuse: Intervention and Treatment Issues.* Washington, DC: US Department of Health and Human Services, National Center on Child Abuse and Neglect; 1993.

Finkelhor, D. What's wrong with sex between adults and children? ethics and the problem of sexual abuse. *Am J Orthopsychiatry.* 1979;49(4):692-697.

Frasier LD. The pediatrician's role in child abuse interviewing. *Pediatr Ann.* 1997;26:306-311.

Friedrich WN, Fisher J, Broughton D, Houston M, Shafran CR. Normative sexual behavior in children: a contemporary sample. *Pediatrics.* 1998;101(4):E9.

Giardino AP, Finkel MA, Giardino ER, Seidl T, Ludwig S. *A Practical Guide to the Evaluation of Sexual Abuse in the Prepubertal Child.* Thousand Oaks, Calif: Sage Publications; 1992.

Hammerschlag MR. The transmissibility of sexually transmitted diseases in sexually abused children. *Child Abuse Negl.* 1998;22:623-626.

Heger A, Emans SJ. Introital diameter as the criterion for sexual abuse. *Pediatrics.* 1990;85(2):222-223.

Hunter RS, Kilstrom N, Loda F. Sexually abused children: identifying masked presentation in a medical setting. *Child Abuse Negl.* 1985;9:7-25.

Hymel KP, Jenny C. Child sexual abuse. *Pediatr Rev.* 1996;17:236-250.

Jenny C. Medical issues in sexual abuse. In: Briere J, Berliner L, Buckley JA, Jenny C, Reid T, eds. *The APSAC Handbook on Child Maltreatment.* Thousand Oaks, Calif: Sage Publications; 1996:197-199.

Krugman RD. Recognition of sexual abuse in children. *Pediatr Rev.* 1986;8:25-30.

Levitt C, Martinez K. Midwest children's resource center interview protocol. Recognizing and reporting child abuse: medical and legal perspectives. *Medical Journal of Allina.* 1998;7:2-5.

Ludwig S. Child abuse. In: Fleisher G, Ludwig S, eds. *Textbook of Pediatric Emergency Medicine.* 4th ed. Philadelphia, Pa: Lippincott Williams & Wilkins; 2000:1669-1704.

Massie ME, Johnson SM. The importance of recognizing a history of sexual abuse in female adolescents. *J Adolesc Health Care.* 1989;10:184-191.

McCann J, Voris J, Simon M. Genital injuries resulting from sexual abuse: a longitudinal study. *Pediatrics.* 1992;89:307-317.

McCann J, Voris J, Simon M, Wells R. Perianal findings in prepubertal children selected for nonabuse: a descriptive study. *Child Abuse Negl.* 1989;13:180-193.

McCann J, Voris J, Simon M, Wells R. Comparison of genital examination techniques in prepubertal girls. *Pediatrics.* 1990a;85:182-187.

McCann J, Wells R, Simon MD, Voris J. Genital findings in prepubertal girls selected for nonabuse: a descriptive study. *Pediatrics.* 1990b;86:428-438.

Meyers JEB. Role of physician in preserving verbal evidence of child abuse. *J Pediatr.* 1986;109:409-411.

Muram D. Child sexual abuse – genital tract findings in prepubertal girls: comparison of colposcopic and unaided examinations. *Am J Obstet Gynecol.* 1989;160:333-335.

Poole DA, Lamb ME. *Investigative Interviews of Children: A Guide for Helping Professionals.* Washington, DC: American Psychological Association; 1998.

Ricci LR. Photodocumentation of the abused child. In: Reece R, ed. *Child Abuse Medical Diagnosis and Management.* Malvern, Pa: Lea & Febiger; 1994:248-265.

Richardson A. Cutaneous manifestations of abuse. In: Reece R, ed. *Child Abuse Medical Diagnosis and Management.* Malvern, Pa: Lea & Febiger; 1994:167-184.

Schmitt BD. Daytime wetting (diurnal enuresis). *Pediatr Clin North Am.* 1982;29:9-20.

Siegel RM, Schubert CJ, Meyers PA, Shapiro RA. The prevalence of sexually transmitted diseases in children and adolescents evaluated for sexual abuse in Cincinnati: rationale for limited STD testing in prepubertal girls. *Pediatrics.* 1995;96:1090-1094.

Steward MS, Bussey K, Goodmail GS, Saywitz KJ. Implications of developmental research for interviewing children. *Child Abuse Negl.* 1993;17:25-37.

Tanner JM. *Growth at Adolescence.* 2nd ed. Oxford: Blackwell Scientific Publications; 1962.

FORENSIC EVALUATIONS FOR SEXUAL ABUSE IN THE PREPUBESCENT CHILD

Sarah Anderson, RN, MSN
Pamela Ross, MD

The purpose of the forensic evaluation in the prepubescent child is to collect, document, and preserve evidence in a law enforcement investigation of a crime or possible crime. In the event of a crime, the systematic manner of collecting, documenting, and preserving evidence is referred to as ***processing the scene***. Healthcare providers also should be trained to perform careful, systematic evaluation of the prepubertal patient and to appropriately document the findings. The evidence collection required for the forensic evaluation in a prepubertal patient requires objectivity and accuracy. Caregivers and forensic evaluators must recognize the need for patience, compassion, and objectivity. The goal in forensic evaluation of prepubertal children is to obtain a history and to collect data that are as complete and accurate as possible (AAP Practice Guidelines, 1991). While obtaining the information, caregivers also should identify injuries that require treatment, screen for sexually transmitted infections, and evaluate for the possible risk of pregnancy. A systematic approach to evidence collection is the key, however, and the "crime scene" the healthcare provider is being asked to "process" is a child. It is necessary to be empathetic and attentive to the child's needs without contaminating the findings. Errors in judgment may lead to a false diagnosis of abuse with potentially serious consequences for a falsely accused perpetrator, whereas a false negative diagnosis can leave an abused child unprotected. Objectivity is required, as well as diagnostic certainty (Hymel & Jenny, 1996). For "evidence collectors" in the healthcare profession, the limitation of bias is of critical importance. The caregiver as evidence collector also must be sensitive to the patient's needs. This chapter outlines the elements of systematic evidence collection, documentation, and preservation and specific techniques that can be used in evidence collection for the prepubertal child.

Key Point:

The goals of forensic evaluation in prepubertal children are to obtain a history and to collect data that are as complete and accurate as possible under the circumstances. This involves careful, systematic evaluation of the patient and appropriate documentation of findings.

PRINCIPLES OF EVIDENCE COLLECTION

There are five principles to follow in processing the scene:

1. Determination of team composition
2. Contamination control
3. Documentation
4. Prioritization of evidence collection
5. Collection and preservation of evidence

First, a team of trained individuals must be established. These individuals should be able to provide contamination control, document accurately, prioritize the collection of evidence, and collect, preserve, package, transport, and submit the evidence by established protocols (US Department of Justice, 2000).

DETERMINATION OF TEAM COMPOSITION

Each team member should have adequate training in an assigned role and responsibility. During every forensic evaluation, the documentation of team members involved and their roles in the process is very important. The team members may come from the following disciplines: law enforcement, child protective services, social work, medical personnel, psychologists, forensic interviewers, and district attorneys' office. All of the team members should have specialized training in pediatric sexual abuse.

CONTAMINATION CONTROL

Contamination control is needed to ensure that the integrity of the evidence is maintained. Limiting the number of people with access to the patient and the evidence helps prevent contamination of the evidence. Nonreusable items for collection are preferred. Items such as specimen cups or tubes and cotton-tipped applicators that are sterile and prepackaged for one-time use are commonly found in medical areas. It is important not to use nonsterile items because contamination could occur. Using universal precautions decreases the risk for contamination and protects the healthcare provider.

Key Point:
Nonsterile items should not be used because contamination may occur. Following universal precautions not only reduces the risk of contamination but provides protection for the healthcare provider.

DOCUMENTATION

A careful assessment of what to document and how to document it is very important. Establishing the types of equipment that will be needed for documentation before starting evidence collection is essential. Things to consider include photography, video, diagrams, measurements, and notes to coordinate the documentation.

Photographs of evidence collected should be taken with and without scale and evidence identifiers. Videotaping can supplement photographs by giving a broader perspective and can be used to demonstrate correct technique during the evidence collection. Preliminary sketches with measurements can be used to note the location of injuries and evidence collected in relation to the body. Sketches may indicate which injuries or evidence are documented by photographs as well. It is important to document the location of the examination, the times of arrival and completion of the examination, general information noted on arrival before any evidence collection is started, and any transient evidence noted, such as smells, sights, or conditions. Circumstances that require any deviation from the usual standards of practice and care should be documented. By providing accurate documentation of the forensic evaluation and the evidence collection, the accuracy of the permanent record is ensured for later evaluation and interpretation.

PRIORITIZATION OF EVIDENCE COLLECTION

By prioritizing the collection of evidence, loss, destruction, and contamination of evidence are prevented. The clinician should determine the order in which the evidence should be collected. A careful and methodical evaluation is conducted, considering all physical evidence possibilities. The clinician should first focus on the easily accessible areas in open view and proceed to out-of-view locations. A systematic search pattern is selected for evidence collection based on the size, type, and location of the evidence. A progression of processing and collection methods is chosen so that initial techniques do not compromise subsequent processing and collection methods. The clinician should move from the least intrusive to the most intrusive processing and collection methods. It is important to continually assess environmental and other factors that may affect the evidence. The clinician should be aware of multiple scenes (such as other children in the house or neighborhood). Other methods that are available to locate, technically document, and collect evidence should be recognized (i.e., alternate light source, bite mark impressions). Prioritization provides for the timely and methodical preservation and collection of evidence.

Key Point:
Follow a systematic approach in searching for evidence. First, focus on easily accessible areas in open view (what is obvious) and then proceed to out-of-view locations (what is obscure).

COLLECTION AND PRESERVATION OF EVIDENCE

Handling the physical evidence is one of the most important factors in the investigation. Evidence security should be maintained throughout the process. This includes effective collection, preservation, packaging, and transport of evidence. The documentation of evidence collection provides the location of the evidence collection, date and time of evidence collection, who collected it, and who had access to the evidence. It is important to collect each item identified as evidence and to establish chain of custody. **Chain of custody** refers to the procedure of handling and accounting for all specimens through each step of the evidence processing. The chain of custody begins with the initial collection of evidence all the way to the courtroom. Usually, there is a standardized form or evidence collection label that documents the transfer of the evidence from the medical staff to the police officer. Maintaining the chain of custody will ensure the validity and admissibility of the forensic evidence in court.

In addition, reference and control samples must be obtained. It is also good to consider obtaining elimination samples. Any electronically recorded evidence should be secured immediately. Policies and procedures must be established and maintained. All evidence should be identified and secured as it is collected with a label that includes the date and initials of the collector. It is important to use the correct type of evidence container (porous, nonporous, crushproof, etc.). All items are packaged to avoid contamination and cross contamination. The clinician should avoid excessive handling of evidence after it is collected and maintain evidence at the scene in a way that diminishes degradation or loss. The evidence must be transported and submitted to law enforcement for secure storage. All evidence should be handled with special attention to integrity, including documentation, collection, preservation, or packaging, and, in addition, should be protected from contamination. During the processing and documentation of the evidence, it should be appropriately packaged, labeled, and maintained in a secure manner until it has been submitted to a secured evidence storage facility or the crime laboratory.

LIMITATIONS OF THE FORENSIC EVALUATION

The history given by the child is one of the most important factors in assessing possible abuse because the results of the physical examination are shown to be nonspecific in 83.5% to 94.4% of the cases. Of the patients referred by physicians for further physical evaluation without any history of sexual abuse, only 14.3% of patients actually had suspicious genital or anal changes on examination (Adams, 1999). Physical findings, which are rarely diagnostic of sexual contact or penetrating trauma, are given great weight by law enforcement, social work, courts, parents, and physicians. Abnormal findings from sexual abuse are uncommon, and many sexually abused children do not have any corroborating physical evidence (AAP Practice Guidelines, 1991; Adams et al., 1994, Berenson et al., 2000; Hymel & Jenny, 1996). With this basic knowledge, care must be taken not to over-interpret genital or anal anomalies, because the percentage of changes attributable to sexual abuse is so low. The forensic evaluation and report of the findings has social and legal consequences for the child and family.

FORENSIC EVIDENCE COLLECTION: WHEN DO YOU COLLECT EVIDENCE?

When should forensic evidence be collected? An investigation by a law enforcement or child protective service agency should be initiated first. If the healthcare provider collects evidence without involvement of these other agencies, there will be no place to process or securely store the evidence. The American Academy of Pediatrics recommends forensic evidence collection when sexual abuse is believed to have occurred within the previous 72 hours or when there is bleeding or acute injury. A recent but controversial clinical study indicated that physical examination of the

Key Point:
Handling physical evidence is a vital part of the investigation, and security for the evidence must be ensured. This includes effective collection, preservation, packaging, and transport of evidence. The chain of custody must be maintained to ensure the validity and admissibility of forensic evidence in court.

Key Point:
When the assault occurred less than 72 hours before an examination, a forensic evaluation with evidence collection should be performed.

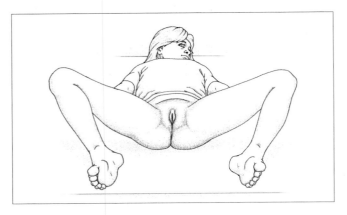

Figure 4-1-a. *A child examined in the supine frog-leg position.*

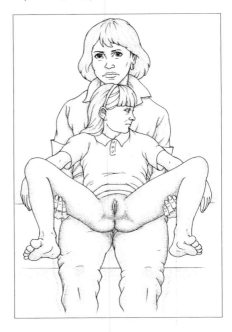

Figure 4-1-b. *A genital examination can also be performed with the patient in the frog-leg position while sitting on the caretaker's lap.*

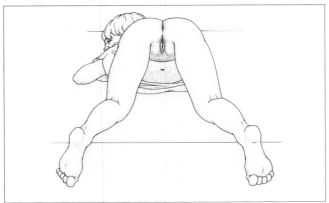

Figure 4-2. *A child examined in the prone knee-chest position.*

child's body yields little evidence if performed after 24 hours, and the processing of clothing and linen yields the majority of evidence (Christian et al., 2000). Nevertheless, most current standards of practice recommend performing an acute physical examination up to 72 hours after the event. Evidence of sexual trauma is rare but may be present. The American Academy of Pediatrics (1991) also recommends that if the event occurred more that 72 hours before presentation and there is no evidence of injury or history of ejaculation, the child should be referred to a regional specialist. Sexual assault evaluation protocols must be established to provide a consistent, high-quality response from forensic teams.

THE PROCESS OF COLLECTION

Generally, if the reported assault occurred less than 72 hours before the examination, a forensic evaluation with evidence collection should be performed. A head to toe physical examination with a detailed genital examination should be performed with the patient both in the frog-leg position (**Figure 4-1 a** and **b**), either supine or with the patient on caregiver's lap, and in the prone knee-chest position (**Figure 4-2**). Written documentation of evidence and diagrams should be provided. The provision of photographic evidence is also highly recommended.

The prepubertal child may be uncooperative in the collection of vaginal, anal, or oral swabs, especially after a traumatic assault. Depending on the individual circumstances, it may be necessary to evaluate the child by using conscious sedation or general anesthesia in the appropriate medical environment.

Physical evidence recovery kits specifically for sexual assaults are usually supplied by law enforcement agencies or can be obtained through a state forensics laboratory. Most physical evidence recovery kits are designed for adults and are routinely modified for pediatric use. It is important to be familiar with the contents and basic evidence collection techniques. Each kit contains instructions on how the evidence should be collected and how to handle the used and unused supplies. **Table 4-1** lists forensic collection methods and containers.

For the evidence to be considered free of contamination, the chain of custody must be maintained. This requires documentation of all personnel handling the specimens and careful accounting of each step of the evidence processing from collection to the courtroom. Once the evidence kit has been opened, it must remain within sight and possession of the evidence collector until it is turned over to law enforcement. If the collector loses sight or possession of the evidence, the validity of the collected evidence can be challenged.

Each kit contains swabs, slides, envelopes, and other containers designed to preserve evidence with the least amount of degradation (**Figure 4-3**). Swabs of genitals, anus, oral cavity, and stained skin can be collected and tested for the presence of biological fluids by the forensic laboratory. Hair samples and foreign debris can also be collected and analyzed.

BASIC EVIDENCE COLLECTION TECHNIQUES

Normal saline solution, distilled water, or sterile water, based on the recommendations of the local forensic laboratory, should be used to collect evidence for the evidence kit. A sealed bottle of normal saline solution, distilled water, or sterile water should be opened during the actual evidence

Table 4-1. Forensic Evidence Collection and Preservation

SPECIMEN TYPES	EVIDENCE COLLECTION ITEMS	METHOD OF PRESERVATION	RATIONALE
Clothing — Garments — Bedding (includes sheets piece and paper drapes used to lay clothing on) — Diaper	— Paper envelopes— various sizes — Evidence tape — Permanent marker — Examination table paper	— Remove clothing one piece at a time. — Avoid cutting through any holes, tears, or stained areas. — If clothing is damp or wet, place a piece of paper in between sides. — Place each item in its own paper envelope or package. — Seal with a piece of evidence tape labeled with he date, time, and initials. — If items are saturated and are soaking through the package, the package can be placed in a plastic bag, but it must be left open.	— Blood and body fluids, if not allowed to dry, will cause the fabric to break down. — If clothing is packaged together, the trace evidence may be transferred to other — If the items are placed in a sealed plastic bag, bacteria and fungus growth will be increased.
Debris — Hair — Paint chips — Grass, leaves, vegetation — Fibers	— Paper envelopes— various sizes — Evidence tape — Permanent marker	— Collect and place in separate envelopes. — Write a description of the item and where is was collected on the outside of the envelope before placing the item inside. — Seal the envelope with evidence tape labeled with the date, time, and initials.	— These items may connect the suspect with the child or the child and/or suspect with the crime scene.

(continued)

Table 4-1. Forensic Evidence Collection and Preservation *(continued)*			
SPECIMEN TYPES	EVIDENCE COLLECTION ITEMS	METHOD OF PRESERVATION	RATIONALE
Body Fluids — Seminal fluid — Blood — Urine — Gastric contents	— Specimen containers and tubes — Sterile cotton swabs — Sterile water — Paper envelopes— various sizes — Evidence tape — Permanent marker	— If large quantities, collect in specimen containers or tubes. The containers should be sealed with evidence tape that has been initialed with date, time, location collected. The container should be placed in a plastic bag. The fluid specimens must be refrigerated. — Areas of suspected body fluids or stains should be collected using the double swab technique. Swabs need to be either dried before packaging or placed in air-dry boxes. The swabs are placed in a paper envelope sealed with evidence tape labled with. date, time, and initials. — If clothing is damp or wet, place a piece of paper in between sides.	— These items may connect the suspect with child or the child and/or the suspect with the crime scene.

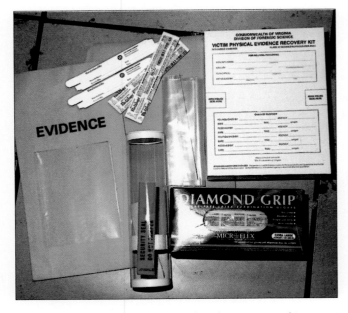

Figure 4-3. *The contents of a physical evidence recovery kit.*

collection, and a control sample should be taken to ensure that nothing was added to the evidence collected.

All clothing worn during and immediately after the assault should be collected and packaged individually in paper bags. If the child is still wearing the original clothes, the child should be undressed over a paper sheet placed on a clean hospital bed sheet. If the clothing is damp or wet, examination table paper should be placed between the layers and the police should be notified so that the articles of clothing are stored correctly without destroying evidence. Only one item of clothing or evidence should be placed in each paper package. Each package should be labeled to identify the child, date, time, and signature of the examiner (**Figures** 4-4 and 4-5). The package should then be sealed securely. All seals should be initialed through the seal. Linens and bedding must be collected because they recently have been identified as having a high yield in pediatric forensic evidence collection (Christian et al., 2000). If bedding and linens are brought to the emergency department, they can be packaged individually in paper bags, sealed, and turned over to the police. If bedding and linens are still at the scene, the police should be encouraged to return to the scene to collect these items. It is important to decrease the amount of handling of each item. Certain activities decrease the yield of positive evidence; these include bathing, brushing teeth, voiding, defecating, vomiting, eating, drinking, and changing clothes. If at all possible, the child's caregivers must minimize these activities following an acute assault. Instructions should be given to the child and/or caregivers about not bathing the child or changing clothes or diapers before the examination.

FORENSIC EVALUATIONS

MORE THAN 72 HOURS LATER OR WITH CHRONIC ABUSE

With nonacute sexual abuse (reported event occurred more than 72 hours before presentation), a forensic evidence collection kit is not used. A head-to-toe physical examination with a detailed genital examination should be performed with the patient both in the frog-leg position, either supine or with the patient on caregiver's lap, and in the prone knee-chest position. Written documentation of evidence and diagrams should be provided. The provision of photographic evidence is also highly recommended.

If a child is unable to cooperate, it is appropriate to reschedule, if possible, or use sedation, if necessary. The goal should be to do everything possible to avoid the child's perception that the forensic evaluation represents another "assault" by medical personnel.

CHRONIC ABUSE WITH THE MOST RECENT OCCURRENCE WITHIN 72 HOURS

Sometimes, a child will report that he or she has been abused over a period of time and that the latest event was less than 72 hours previously. In this case, forensic evidence collection and a full evaluation looking for both physical evidence of acute injuries and evidence of old injuries are performed.

INTERVIEW PROCESS

During the forensic physical examination, a portion of the process must include a brief interview. This is not to be confused with a forensic interview. The purpose of the brief interview is to establish a rapport with the child and to direct the evidence collection. If at all possible, the clinician should talk to the child alone. If it is not possible to interview the child alone, it is essential that the alleged perpetrator is not the supportive adult in the room with the child. The most critical component of the evaluation for suspected abuse is an interview of the child that is designed to avoid leading the child to particular responses. Asking open-ended questions, such as, "Has anyone ever touched you in a way that you didn't like?" as opposed to a leading question, such as a "Has Daddy ever touched you in a way that you didn't like?" avoids tainting the child's response. It is important for the interviewer to keep the tone of voice and manner neutral as the child responds. When the child responds, the interviewer should then ask the child to elaborate without suggesting possibilities or implying what answers might be acceptable. Because the medical interview may be admissible in court as an exception to hearsay, the importance of careful documentation of questions and responses is critical. Questions and answers should be recorded exactly as a quotation (Hanes & McAuliff, 1997; Lahoti et al., 2001).

Verbal children already have a set of terms they use to describe the different parts of their bodies. It is important to clarify the terms and to use terminology that they will understand. Again, using open-ended questions is essential.

Before the interview, it is also important to have information about the child regarding past medical problems, social and developmental history, any behavioral changes noted, and any physical complaints. Other information to consider is a

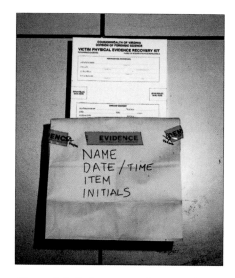

Figure 4-4. *Each paper package used to collect evidence should be labeled to identify the child, date, time, and signature of the examiner. The package should be sealed securely, and all seals should be initialed through the seal.*

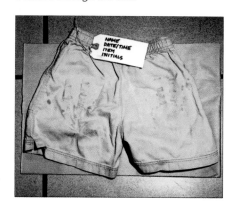

Figure 4-5. *Only one item of clothing or evidence should be placed in each paper package during evidence collection.*

Key Point:

Because the medical interview may be admissible in court as an exception to the hearsay rule, questions and responses must be carefully documented. Before beginning the interview, it is important to obtain information about the child, including past medical problems, social and developmental history, behavioral changes that have occurred, and any physical complaints.

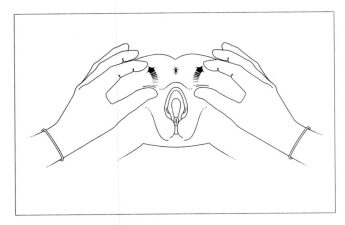

Figure 4-6-a. *Labial separation and traction in the genital examination of the female in the prone knee-chest position.*

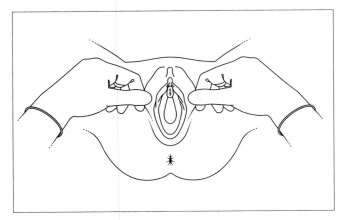

Figure 4-6-b. *Genital examination of the female in the supine frog-leg position with labial separation and traction.*

previous history of sexual abuse of the child or other family members and whether there has been any history of accidental injury or surgical procedures to the genital area (McClain et al., 2000).

PHYSICAL EXAMINATION

The physical examination and evidence collection are performed at the same time. During the physical examination, it is important to look for signs of injury from abuse (acute, healing, and chronic). Evidence must not be destroyed or created by accidental injury. The child should be examined from head to toe, with the genital examination last. The goal is to help the child feel that the examiner is just as interested in the scratch on the knee as in the genital examination. Extreme care should be taken to avoid retraumatizing the child.

The genital examination should be performed with the child in the frog-leg (supine) position, in the frog-leg position on the caregiver's lap, and in the knee-chest (prone) position. These positions are necessary to confirm injuries or noninjuries. In the female child the genital examination should include direct visualization initially, then gentle labial separation, and finally labial traction (**Figure 4-6, a and b**). During the visualization process the medial thighs, mons pubis, labia minora, labia majora, clitoris, urethra, periurethral tissue, hymenal opening, hymen, fossa navicularis, and posterior commissure/fourchette must be identified and inspected. The anus should also be viewed with and without traction. The presence or absence of stool in the rectal vault should be documented. In the male child, careful inspection of the medial thighs, scrotum, testicles, penis, and urethra should be done along with the anal examination (**Figure 4-7, a** and **b**). Speculum and digital examinations of prepubertal children are not necessary unless they facilitate the removal of a foreign body.

SPECIAL EVIDENCE COLLECTION TECHNIQUES IN THE EVALUATION OF SEXUAL ABUSE

Established protocols for the use of specialized techniques in the evidence collection process help to increase the consistency and yield of evidence.

FORENSIC PHOTOGRAPHY

Photographs can be taken with many different types of cameras. A 35 mm camera with a macro lens provides the best resolution; however, pictures cannot be viewed immediately for accuracy and technique. Polaroid or digital cameras allow immediate review and reduce the risk of returning inadequate photographs or no photographs at all. When taking pictures, it is important to take an overview or full body picture, an orientation or medium range shot, and then a close-up of the area to be emphasized. All of the close-up photographs should be taken with and without a scale. The scale should be held parallel to and in the same plane as the injury and camera.

Sometimes it may be necessary to have the child return several days later to repeat the photographs. Often, bruises are more pronounced and patterns are easier to identify. When acute genital trauma is suspected, a repeat examination can help to discern whether anomalies observed during the initial examination have changed or remained the same after allowing time for healing.

Colposcopy

Colposcopy is used to magnify the genitalia. It can increase the examiner's ability to identify genital and perineal abnormalities. Magnification, illumination, and photographic capabilities can increase the accuracy of the examiner's descriptions. The photographs of colposcopy findings can be used to facilitate consultation between examiners for the purpose of peer review and with a child abuse expert and for court purposes. All photographs should be taken with and without a scale. As a routine, photographs should be obtained with the child in both the frog-leg and the knee-chest positions.

Alternate Light Sources

Wood's lamp, an alterative light source, is a source of ultraviolet radiation, emitting wavelengths of approximately 320 to 400 nm. Alternate light source supplies are shown in **Figure 4-8**. Most Wood's lamps used in the medical profession emit wavelengths of approximately 360 nm. Data suggest that a longer wavelength is optimal for identifying semen (Santucci, Nelson, McQuillen, Duffy, & Linakis, 1999). Therefore a Wood's lamp is not used to confirm the presence of seminal fluid, but can be used to identify suspicious areas for more definitive testing (Gabby et al., 1992). Semen, urine, and other oily substances "fluoresce" a blue-green to orange color. The child's body should be completely examined with a Wood's lamp in a darkened room. Areas of fluorescence can be swabbed, packaged, and sent to the laboratory for further analysis (Hymel & Jenny, 1996).

Using an alternate light source with photography can help identify old, healed bruises and bite marks. Evidence of bruising has been identified up to a year after the injury. This is a highly technical procedure that requires specialized equipment and lighting, but it can be worthwhile if other evidence could not be obtained. The best place to find such photographic capabilities is either the forensic laboratory or a law enforcement agency.

DOUBLE SWAB TECHNIQUE

Areas that fluoresce when using the alternate light source or where the examiner suspects that a body fluid (such as saliva, blood, or seminal fluid) is present should be swabbed using the double swab technique to maximize the quantity of cells recovered and to minimize any potential contamination from cells of the victim's skin. The double swab technique showed the highest percentage recovery of saliva from human skin among the three methods studied by Sweet et al. (1997).

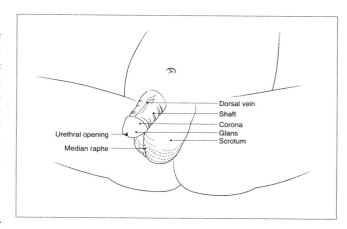

Figure 4-7-a. Anatomy of the circumcised prepubertal male.

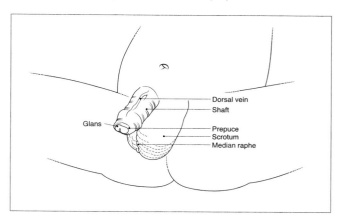

Figure 4-7-b. Anatomy of the uncircumcised prepubertal male.

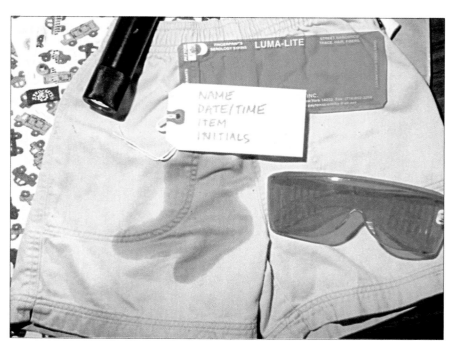

Figure 4-8. Alternate light source supplies.

In the double swab method the first swab should be obtained with a damped cotton-tipped applicator, followed by a dry cotton-tipped applicator. The swabs should then be placed on a slide and allowed to air dry. This technique should also be used on bite marks or areas of possible saliva or other body fluid contact that the child identifies.

SALINE FLOAT/IRRIGATION OF HYMENAL TISSUE

If hymenal tissue is folded over and the edges are not easily identified, even after placing the child in the frog-leg and knee-chest positions, saline solution can be gently dribbled over the edges of the hymen. The child should be informed before the application of saline solution because the prepubescent hymen is extremely sensitive and any type of contact may be painful. After the saline solution is dribbled over the hymenal edges, the child should be re-examined in both the frog-leg and knee-chest positions.

FOLEY CATHETER TECHNIQUE

The Foley catheter technique is only used in pubertal and postpubertal girls. It allows the identification of forensically significant abnormalities in the hymenal tissue by facilitating the visualization of the floppy, redundant edges through the insertion of a Foley catheter just past the vaginal opening, inflating the balloon with 10 mL of sterile water, and gently applying traction to help spread hymenal tissue edges for better inspection (Ferrell, 1995). This is not recommended for the prepubertal child because the hymen is very thin and sensitive before estrogenation and may be torn (Starling & Jenny, 1997).

TOLUIDINE BLUE

Toluidine blue dye is used as an adjunct for identifying acute lacerations and abrasions. By applying toluidine blue dye, a nuclear stain, to the external genitalia, there is an increase in the detection rate of perineal lacerations in rape cases (Lauber & Souma, 1982; McCauley et al., 1987). The dye should be applied sparingly to the external genitalia with a cotton swab or piece of gauze. After a few seconds, the dye can be removed with lubricating jelly and the areas examined for lacerations. Only damaged skin cells take up the dye, making it possible to identify abrasions or lacerations that may not be visible to the naked eye and to aid in photographic documentation. All DNA swabs of the external genitalia should be done before applying toluidine blue dye.

BITE MARK IMPRESSIONS AND EVIDENCE COLLECTION

Bite marks may take numerous shapes and forms. They may be easily misdiagnosed as a bruise or a normal childhood mishap (Jessee, 1994). The shape is usually oval or circular bruising, but the shape can vary depending on the amount of force, the surface area, and the amount of contact made with the area involved. Breaks in the skin are more common with animal bites than with human bites (Butts, 1994).

If the bite mark is suspected to be acute, the area should be tested using the double swab technique and should be dried or packaged in a self-drying box. In addition to swabbing, if indentations are noted in the skin, a bite mark impression can be made with a casting compound. All suspected bite marks should be photographed with and without a scale.

DOCUMENTATION

Documentation of the forensic evaluation should be done on a form that allows for the following information: basic demographic information; history received from the child; data collected during the physical examination; and evidence collected in written form along with schematic diagrams of the whole child and the genitalia. Photographs should be labeled on the back with the following information: child's name, date, time, and the examiner's initials. The position of the child during the examination should be noted on the back of the photograph. In addition, the photographs should be numbered to correspond with their locations on the diagrams.

PEER REVIEW OF CASES

As part of the forensic evaluation process, all cases should be reviewed by the team members to ensure consistency in the interpretation of the findings and as a continued learning experience. Feedback is also given regarding the written and photographic documentation of examinations.

TESTING FOR SEXUALLY TRANSMITTED DISEASES (STDs)

During the forensic evaluation in the prepubescent child, STD testing is reserved for cases in which vaginal or penile discharge is evident. The decision to obtain cultures and to perform serologic testing should be based on the likelihood of oral, genital, or anal penetration and the presence of symptoms. Prepubertal females are more likely to be symptomatic if they have *Chlamydia* infection or gonorrhea. Local prevalence of STDs and risk factors of the child and the alleged perpetrator of abuse should also be taken into consideration.

Asymptomatic children who disclose only fondling have a very low incidence of STDs (Sigel et al., 1995). In cases of acute sexual assault, performing tests for gonorrhea, *Chlamydia*, *Trichomonas*, and bacterial vaginosis should occur 2 weeks after the assault if the patient did not receive prophylactic treatment at the time of the initial examination. Serologic testing may be performed for syphilis, human immunodeficiency virus (HIV) infection, and hepatitis B (depending on immunization status) 6, 12, and 24 weeks after the assault (Centers for Disease Control and Prevention, 2002). When testing for *Chlamydia* and gonorrhea, it is vital that true cultures be obtained. If only nonculture methods (eg, antigen detection or nucleic acid detection methods) are available, patients must be referred to a location where true cultures can be obtained. Antimicrobial treatment should not be initiated before cultures are obtained. In most states, results of nonculture methods are not admissible in court (Hammerschlag et al., 1999). A positive culture for gonorrhea or *Chlamydia* and a positive serologic test for syphilis or HIV provide the basis for medical certainty for sexual abuse, even in the absence of a disclosure or history, once the possibility for neonatal transmission has been eliminated (AAP, 1999). For a complete discussion of STD testing and prophylaxis for prepubertal children, see Chapter 5.

CONCLUSION

Forensic evidence collection in the prepubescent child in cases of child sexual assault can be intimidating for many care providers. Healthcare providers are required by state statute to report suspected child physical and sexual abuse. By establishing standards of care and practice for evidence collection, educating staff, and knowing the resources available to the team, evidence collection can be done with accuracy and objectivity. By combining the techniques recognized by law enforcement to "process the scene" with the patience, compassion, and objectivity of the physical examination, a child and family can be assisted through a crisis event in their lives.

REFERENCES

Adams JA. Medical evaluation of suspected child sexual abuse. *Pediatr Adolesc Med Arch*. 1999;153(11):1121-1122.

Adams JA, Harper K, Knudson S, Revilla J. Examination findings in legally confirmed child sexual abuse: it's normal to be normal. *Pediatrics*. 1994;94:310-317.

American Academy of Pediatrics. Guidelines for the evaluation of sexual abuse of children. *Pediatrics*. 1991;87:254-260.

American Academy of Pediatrics Committee on Child Abuse and Neglect. Guidelines for the evaluation of sexual abuse of children: subject review. *Pediatrics*. 1999;103:186-191.

Berenson AB, Chacko MR, Wiemann CM, Mishaw CO, Friedrich WN, Grady JJ. A case-control study of anatomic changes resulting from sexual abuse. *Am J Obstet Gynecol.* 2000;182:820-834.

Butts JD. Injuries: description, documentation, and evidence issues. *North Carolina Med J.* 1994;55:423-427.

Centers for Disease Control and Prevention (CDC). 2002 guidelines for treatment of sexually transmitted diseases. *MMWR.* 10 May 2002;51(RR-6).

Christian CW, Lavell JM, De Jong AR, Loiselle J, Brenner L, Joffee M. Forensic evidence findings in prepuberal victims of sexual assault. *Pediatrics.* 2000;106:100-104.

Ferrell J. Foley catheter balloon technique for visualizing the hymen in female adolescent sexual abuse victims. *J Emerg Nurs.* 1995;21:585-586.

Gabby T, Winkleby MA, Boyce WT, Fisher DL, Lancaster A, Sensabaugh GF. Sexual abuse of children: the detection of semen on skin. *Am J Dis Child.* 1992;146:700-703.

Hammerschlag MR, Ajl S, Larague D. Inappropriate use of nonculture tests for the detection of Chlamydia trachomatis in suspected victims of child sexual abuse: a continuing problem. *Pediatrics.* 1999;104:1137-1139.

Hanes M, McAuliff T. Preparation for child abuse litigation: perspectives of the prosecutor and the pediatrician. *Pediatr Ann.* 1997;26:288-295.

Hymel KP, Jenny C. Child sexual abuse. *Pediatr Rev.* 1996;17:236-255.

Jessee SA. Recognition of bite marks in child abuse cases. *Pediatr Dent.* 1994;16:336-339.

Lahoti SL, McClain N, Girardet R, McNeese M, Cheung K. Evaluating the child for sexual abuse. *Am Fam Physician.* 2001;63:883-892.

Lauber AA, Souma ML. Use of toluidine blue for documentation of traumatic intercourse. *Obstetr Gynecol.* 1982;60:644-648.

McCauley J, Gysinski G, Welch R, Gorman R, Osmers F. Toluidine blue in the corroboration of rape in the adult victim. *Am J Emerg Med.* 1987;5:105-108.

McClain N, Girardet R, Lahoti S, Cheung K, Berger K, McNeese M. Evaluation of sexual abuse in the pediatric patient. *J Ped Health Care.* 2000;14:93-102.

Santucci KA, Nelson DG, McQuillen KK, Duffy SJ, Linakis JG. Wood's lamp utility in the identification of semen. *Pediatrics.* 1999;104:1342-1344.

Sigel RM, Schubert CJ, Myers PA, Shapiro RA. The prevalence of sexually transmitted diseases in children and adolescents evaluated for sexual abuse in Cincinnati: rationale for limited STD testing in pre-pubertal girls. *Pediatrics.* 1995;96:1090-1094.

Starling SP, Jenny C. Forensic examination of adolescent female genitalia: the Foley catheter technique. *Arch Pediatr Adolesc Med.* 1997;151:102-103.

Sweet D, Lorente JA, Valenzuela A, Lorente M, Villanueva E. PCR-based DNA typing of saliva stains recovered from human skin. *J Forensic Sci.* 1997;42:320-322.

US Department of Justice. Crime scene investigation: a guide to law enforcement. Washington, DC: US Department of Justice Publication; January 2000.

Sexually Transmitted Diseases in Sexually Abused Children

Charles J. Schubert, MD
Kathi Makoroff, MD

Overview

The relationship between sexually transmitted diseases (STDs) and sexual abuse is not as straightforward as one may assume. Even if a perpetrator of a sexual assault has an STD, there is no assurance that the victim will be infected. Perpetrators have a high incidence of sexual dysfunction, and in many cases there may not be the intimate contact required to transmit an STD (Groth & Burgess, 1977). In addition, there is a wide range in the type of sexual abuse that occurs, with some children being inappropriately fondled while others are violently raped. The likelihood of infecting a victim also depends on which organism is carried by the perpetrator. Gonorrheal and chlamydial infections are much more likely to be transmitted to the victim than genital warts. Because of these and other factors, the incidence of STDs in victims of child abuse is relatively low (Schwarcz & Whittington, 1990; Siegel et al., 1995).

As implied by the term, a ***sexually transmitted infection*** is generally transmitted by sexual contact. However, depending on the organism, other routes of transmission are possible **(Table 5-1)**. These include vertical transmission, auto or digital inoculation, and fomite or casual contact. Cases in the literature document transmission of an STD to a child when fomite or casual contact is thought to have occurred, although the bulk of scientific evidence does not support these accounts. Numerous studies support the view that sexual contact is necessary to transmit the majority of STDs (Branch & Paxton, 1965; Farrell et al., 1981; Neinstein et al., 1984).

Key Point:
The majority of STDs require sexual contact to be transmitted; other exposures account for only a few cases.

It is important to note that the vagina of a prepubertal girl is much different from the vagina of a female who has matured through puberty. The prepubertal vagina is lined by columnar epithelium with an alkaline pH, whereas the adult or pubertal vagina is a more acidic environment lined with squamous epithelium. These differences affect the transmission of STDs. This is reflected in the lower incidence of STDs in sexually abused prepubertal girls, where the incidence is less than 5%, compared to pubertal girls, where the incidence is around 15%. In addition, the clinical symptoms of STDs may differ between prepubertal and postpubertal females. For example, gonorrhea may be asymptomatic in adult females, whereas it is likely to cause a vaginal discharge in prepubertal girls. Few data outline the differences between the genital tracts of adult males and prepubertal males in relationship to STDs.

Other important considerations must be kept in mind when examining the relationship of an STD to sexual abuse. Disclosure of an episode of sexual abuse often occurs months to years after the abuse, which may affect the presentation of various STDs. Some infections may spontaneously resolve, whereas others may be

Table 5-1. Modes of Transmission of STDs in Children

ORGANISM BODY	SEXUAL ASSAULT	AUTOINOCULATION/ HETEROINOCULATION	FOMITES	INFECTED FLUIDS†
Bacterial vaginosis	X			
Chlamydia trachomatis	X			
Gonorrhea	X		?*	
Hepatitis B	X			X
HIV	X			X
HPV	X	X		
HSV	X	X		
Syphilis	X			
Trichomonas vaginalis	X		?*	

* No study has directly documented this in children.
† Excluding genital secretions.
Abbreviations: HIV, human immunodeficiency virus; HPV, human papillomavirus; HSV, herpes simplex virus.

asymptomatic. If a child is examined immediately after a sexual assault, the STD cultures may reveal the infections of the perpetrator instead of the victim (Schwarcz & Whittington, 1990). In evaluating children who have been sexually abused, it is important to consider potential STDs on an individual basis and proceed with the workup accordingly **(Table 5-2)**.

EPIDEMIOLOGY

The epidemiology of STDs in sexually abused children depends on the specific STD and the type of abuse that occurred. All STDs have been described in the victims of sexual assault. STD-specific factors are discussed in reference to each organism.

It is often difficult to differentiate preexisting diseases from those acquired during a sexual assault. When testing for STDs in a child within 72 hours of an assault, some positive cultures (e.g. gonorrhea and *Chlamydia*) may represent disease in the perpetrator (Schwarcz & Whittington, 1990). The underlying regional prevalence of STDs also affects the number of STDs diagnosed in the victim. In a large study, sexually abused pubertal females had a much higher incidence of STDs than younger girls (14.6% vs. 3.2%) (Siegel et al., 1995). This higher incidence is

Key Point:
It is essential to consider the following factors in determining what degree of workup is needed:
— Regional prevalence
— Likelihood of preexisting disease in the perpetrator
— How recently the episode occurred
— Type of abuse

Table 5-2. STD Testing in Children Evaluated for Sexual Assault

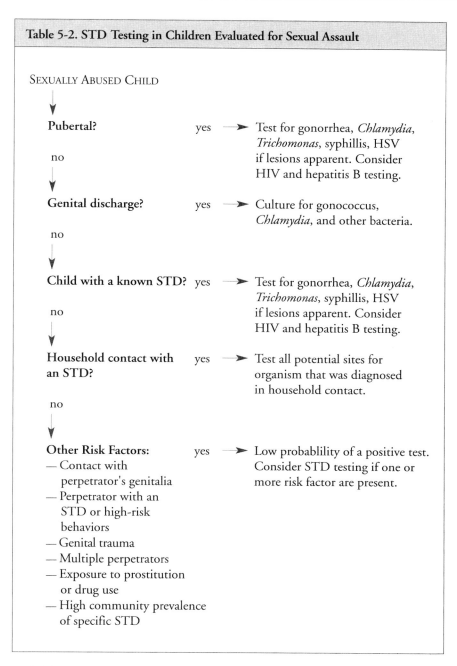

Sᴇxᴜᴀʟʟʏ Aʙᴜsᴇᴅ Cʜɪʟᴅ

Pubertal?   yes → Test for gonorrhea, *Chlamydia*, *Trichomonas*, syphillis, HSV if lesions apparent. Consider HIV and hepatitis B testing.

no

Genital discharge?   yes → Culture for gonococcus, *Chlamydia*, and other bacteria.

no

Child with a known STD? yes → Test for gonorrhea, *Chlamydia*, *Trichomonas*, syphillis, HSV if lesions apparent. Consider HIV and hepatitis B testing.

no

Household contact with an STD?   yes → Test all potential sites for organism that was diagnosed in household contact.

no

Other Risk Factors: yes → Low probablility of a positive test. Consider STD testing if one or more risk factor are present.
— Contact with perpetrator's genitalia
— Perpetrator with an STD or high-risk behaviors
— Genital trauma
— Multiple perpetrators
— Exposure to prostitution or drug use
— High community prevalence of specific STD

probably explained by preexisting disease in the older population. Other studies have also documented a similarly low prevalence of STDs in females after sexual assault, with even lower numbers for abused males (DeJong et al., 1982). Therefore it is important to consider regional prevalence, likelihood of preexisting disease in the perpetrator, the acuity of the episode, and the type of abuse when determining the extent of the work up required for different STDs.

The implications of finding an STD in a child depend on a number of factors. The most important aspects to consider are the child's age or Tanner stage and the specific organism. **Table 5-3** lists the likelihood that a specific infection is caused by sexual contact. In considering the child's age and Tanner stage it is important to note that in many jurisdictions, any child less than age 13 years cannot have consensual sexual relations. Therefore, if an STD is diagnosed, an evaluation for sexual abuse must be undertaken. This is true even in younger children who may

Table 5-3. Likelihood of Sexual Transmission-Specific Sexually Transmitted Diseases	
SEXUALLY TRANSMITTED DISEASE	LIKELIHOOD OF SEXUAL TRANSMISSION
Gonorrhea	Very high
Chlamydia infection	Very high
Syphilis	Very high
HPV	Possible
Trichomonas infection	High
HSV	Possible
HIV	Very high
Bacterial vaginosis	Low
Hepatitis B	Possible

Abbreviations: HIV, human immunodeficiency virus; HPV, human papillomavirus; HSV, herpes simplex virus.

not be able to give a clear history of the abusive episode(s). When a pubertal child with an STD claims a consensual relationship, it is critical to determine the age of the partner. If the partner is more than 4 years older than the patient or the partner is an adult (at least age 18 years), it is mandated to report these cases to the appropriate authorities in most jurisdictions.

SPECIFIC DISORDERS

Table 5-4 offers an overview of the laboratory investigations undertaken to evaluate sexually abused children, and **Table 5-5** lists recommended treatment options.

CHLAMYDIA TRACHOMATIS

Chlamydia trachomatis is a bacterial agent that is an obligate intracellular parasite. *C. trachomatis* infection is currently the most common sexually transmitted infection in the United States, with the highest rates among sexually active adolescents.

Infants can acquire *Chlamydia* infection via vertical transmission. Approximately 50% to 75% of infants born to women with active *Chlamydia* infection will become infected at one or more anatomical sites (Hammerschlag, 1994). These sites include the conjunctiva, nasopharynx, rectum, and vagina. Infection of the rectum and vagina in infants is usually asymptomatic, and cultures can remain positive for extended periods. Bell et al. (1992) followed infants who were born to women with culture-proven chlamydial infections. Positive cultures were detected in the nasopharynx and oropharynx of these children as late as 28½ months after birth, and positive cultures from the rectum and vagina were detected for over 12 months. There are also some case reports of perinatally acquired rectal and vaginal chlamydial infections persisting for 3 years (Hammerschlag, 1998).

Chlamydial infection in children that is not perinatally acquired is thought to have occurred through intimate sexual contact and therefore is a marker of sexual abuse.

Table 5-4. Laboratory Investigation for STDs in the Evaluation of Sexually Abused Children

SEXUALLY TRANSMITTED DISEASE	DIAGNOSTIC TEST
Gonorrhea	— Only acceptable method is a bacterial culture — A positive culture must be confirmed by two other identifying tests of different biologic principals — NAA tests (LCR, PCR)*
Chlamydia **infection**	— Only acceptable method is a bacterial culture — NAA tests (LCR, PCR)*

Syphilis	Serologic blood tests:
	   Positive nontreponemal test
	— RPR
	— VDRL
	— ART
	— In addition to:
	    Postive treponemal tests
	    Fluorescent treponemal
	       antibody absorbtion
	    Microhemagglutination test
	       for *T. pallidum*

HPV	— Usually made by appearance on physical examination — Virus type can be determined, but identification of virus type does not differentiate sexual from nonsexual transmission
Trichomonas **infection**	— Microscopic identification — Bacterial culture of vaginal secretions — Must differentiate from other types of *Trichomonas* organisms if identified in urine of stool
HSV	— Usually made by appearance on physical examination — Virus can be cultured if diagnosis is in question — Virus type can be determined, but identification of virus type does not differentiate sexual from nonsexual transmission

(continued)

Table 5-4. *(continued)*

HIV	Serologic blood tests — EIA — If EIA is positive: Western blot or immunofluorescence antibody test is used for confirmation
Bacterial vaginosis	Diagnosis made clinically by presence of three of following symptoms or signs: — Homogenous gray or white discharge on examination — Vaginal fluid pH > 4.5 — Positive amine test: mixing vaginal fluid with 10% postassium hydroxide results in a fishy odor — Presence of "clue cells": vaginal epithelial cells massively coated with coccobacilli
Hepatitis B	Serologic blood tests — HbsAg detects acutely or chronically infected individuals — Anti-HBs identifies individuals who have had infections with HBV; determines immunity after vaccination — Anti-HBc identifies individuals with acute past HBV infection; is *not* present after immunization

* NAA tests are not approved for use in prepubertal children or for medicolegal purposes.
Abbreviations: ART, automated reagin test; EIA, enzyme immunoassay; HBV, hepatitis B virus; HIV, human immunodeficiency virus; HPV, human papillomavirus; HSV, herpes simplex virus; LCR, ligase chain reaction; NAA, nucleic acid amplification; PCR, polymerase chain reaction; RPR, rapid plasma reagin test.

Key Point:
When chlamydial infection is found in children and it was not acquired perinatally, it is considered a marker of sexual abuse, having most likely been transmitted through intimate sexual contact.

There is no evidence that nonsexual postnatal acquisition of *Chlamydia* infection occurs. The possibility of perinatal transmission is often a confounding variable in younger children, and it is difficult to differentiate whether infection occurred through vertical contact or sexual contact. In these cases the history, physical examination findings, and other laboratory findings may be helpful. Rectal and vaginal chlamydial infections in children are often asymptomatic. In postpubertal individuals, however, epididymitis, urethritis, and vaginitis can occur and, in females, can lead to pelvic inflammatory disease, ectopic pregnancy, or infertility.

The diagnosis of chlamydial infection is made by isolating the organism in tissue culture. Cell culture remains the gold standard for the evaluation of *Chlamydia* infection in children with suspected sexual abuse, and it is the only evidence allowed in forensic cases. Because *Chlamydia* species are obligate intracellular organisms, culture specimens must contain epithelial cells and not just exudate. Several nucleic acid amplification tests (NAAs), such as polymerase chain reaction (PCR) and ligase chain reaction (LCR), are used to diagnose *Chlamydia* infections in adults and older adolescents. These tests are extremely sensitive and highly specific and allow the use of noninvasive sampling such as urine testing. NAAs are more sensitive than culture for the detection of *C. trachomatis* in genital specimens in adults, but

Table 5-5. Treatment Options for STDs in Children

ORGANISM	TREATMENT OPTIONS
Gonorrhea[a] Uncomplicated vulvovaginitis, cervicitis, urethritis, proctitis, or pharyngitis	— Prepubertal children who weigh <100 lb Ceftriaxone 125 mg IM in a single dose or spectinomycin 40 mg/kg IM in a single dose (maximum 2 g)[b] — Prepubertal children who weigh >100 lb and are 8 years old or older Cetriaxone 125 mg IM in a single dose or cefixime 400 mg orally in a single dose or ciprofoxacin 500 mg orally in a single dose
Chlamydia Uncomplicated genital tract infection	— Prebubertal children Erythromycin 50 mg/kg orally in divided doses for 14 days (maximum daily dose 2 g) or azithromycin 20 mg/kg orally as a single dose (maximum 1 g) — Adolescents Doxycycline 100 mg orally twice daily for 7 days or azithromycin 1 g orally as a single dose
Syphilis	— Primary, secondary, and early latent disease in children Benzathine penicillin G 50,00 U/kg IM in a single dose (not to exceed the adult dose of 2.4 million U) — Late latent syphillis in children Benzathine penicillin G 50,000 U/kg IM weekly for 3 weeks (not to exceed the adult dose of 7.2 million U)
Trichomonas infection	— Prepubertal children Metronidazole 15 mg/kg orally in three divided doses for 7 days (maximum daily dose 2 g) — Adolescents Metronidazole 2 g orally as a single dose
HPV	— Consultation with a dermatology specialist is recommended
HSV	— Consultation with an infectious disease specialist is recommended[c]

(continued)

Table 5-5. *(continued)*

HIV	— Consultation with an infectious disease specialist is recommended
Bacterial vaginosis	— Metronidazole 1 g orally in two divided doses for 7 days
Hepatitis B	— No specific therapy for acute HBV infection is available

a) Patients should also receive concurrent treatment for presumptive chlamydial infection.
b) Spectinomycin is not effective for the treatment of pharyngeal gonorrhea.
c) Acylovir is the only approved antiviral drug for children.
Adapted from: American Academy of Pediatrics (AAP). In: Pickering LK, ed. 2000 Red Book: Report of the Committee on Infectious Diseases. *25th ed. Elk Grove Village, Ill: American Academy of Pediatrics; 2000. Centers for Disease Control and Prevention (CDC). 2002 guidelines for treatment of sexually transmitted diseases. MMWR. 2002;47:110.*

Drug dosage recommendations listed herein are those of the authors and are not endorsed by the US Public Health Service or the US Department of Health and Human Services.

the overwhelming majority of these studies have been performed in high-prevalence populations (Black, 1997). Data on the use of NAAs in low-prevalence populations, such as with children, are limited. Girardet et al. (2001) tested the use of urine-based ligase chain reaction in 164 pediatric sexual abuse victims for the detection of *C. trachomatis* and *Neisseria gonorrhoeae*. The authors concluded that the low prevalence of disease in this study population precluded statistical analysis. Because the positive predictive value depends on both the specificity of the test and the prevalence of the disease, NAA testing may not be appropriate to detect *C. trachomatis* in low-prevalence populations, such as children.

If *Chlamydia* infection is detected in a child and is not thought to be the result of perinatal transmission, an investigation for suspected sexual abuse must be undertaken. Evaluation for other sexually transmitted diseases should also be performed.

C. trachomatis infections may be treated with doxycycline or, in younger children, oral erythromycin. Azithromycin has also been approved as a single-dose treatment for uncomplicated chlamydial urethral and cervical infections in males and nonpregnant women.

NEISSERIA GONORRHOEAE

Neisseria gonorrhoeae is a gram-negative diplococcus. Gonococcal infections can be transmitted vertically to the newborn infant and usually involve the eye, although disseminated disease can occur in infants and result in bacteremia, meningitis, endocarditis, or arthritis. When gonococcal infection presents in prepubertal children beyond the newborn period, sexual abuse must be strongly considered.

The organism is found in secretions of infected mucosal surfaces, and transmission occurs from intimate contact such as sexual activity and parturition. The transmission of gonorrhea to children from nonsexual household exposure has been debated. *N. gonorrhoeae* has been reported to survive up to 24 hours on toilet seats and towels. Yet the organism is very susceptible to drying and to cool temperatures, which would make transmission from fomites unlikely (Jenny, 1992). This is more consistent with studies that have shown that random toilet seat sampling in community and STD clinic bathrooms have failed to yield organisms (Gilbaugh, 1979).

Multiple studies in prepubertal children with gonococcal infections have found a history of sexual contact in almost all of the children. Ingram et al. (1992) found a

Key Point:
Usually, gonococcal infections that are transmitted vertically to the newborn infant involve the eye, although disseminated disease is seen in some cases. N. gonorrhoeae is highly susceptible to drying and cool temperatures, so fomite transmission is unlikely. Almost all of the children in a variety of studies contracted the disease via sexual contact.

history of sexual contact in 34 of 41 (83%) children with *N. gonorrhoeae* infection. Of the seven who did not have a history of sexual contact, three were "nonverbal." One limitation to studies such as this is that not all children will reveal a history of sexual abuse when it has, if fact, occurred. Most evidence strongly suggests that, as in adults, gonorrhea in children is sexually transmitted. If a child is diagnosed with a gonococcal infection, further investigations, including a forensic interview, physical examination, and evaluation for other STDs, are warranted.

Children with gonococcal infection are usually symptomatic. The most common symptom is vaginal discharge (**Figure 5-1**). Shapiro et al. (1993) reported that all 22 prepubertal girls who were diagnosed with gonococcal infection had a vaginal discharge present on examination. Similarly, Sicoli et al. (1995) showed that vaginal or urethral discharge on physical examination was the best predictor of *N. gonorrhoeae* infection. Disseminated disease is rare in childhood, but adolescents can have more ascending disease, such as pelvic inflammatory disease or gonorrheal perihepatitis (Fitz-Hugh-Curtis syndrome). Asymptomatic presentation has also been described, but in most cases, the gonococcal organism was isolated from the throat (Nair et al., 1986).

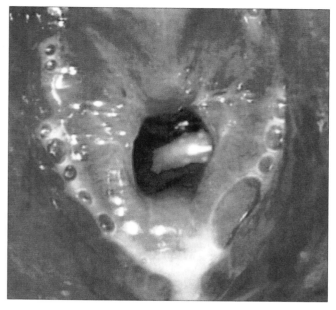

Figure 5-1. *Vaginal discharge in a prepubertal child.*

Cell culture confirmed by other tests remains the gold standard for evaluation of gonoccoal disease in children with suspected sexual abuse and the only evidence allowed in forensic cases. NAA tests are not reliable enough to be used in a group of patients where the prevalence is low, such as in prepubertal children. Bacterial strains with cultural characteristics and cell morphology similar to gonococci may be misidentified as *N. gonorrhoeae*. Therefore all positive cultures must be confirmed by at least two confirmatory bacteriologic tests.

A broad-spectrum (third-generation) cephalosporin is recommended as the initial treatment of gonococcal infection. Children with presumed or confirmed gonorrhea should also undergo testing for other STDs, such as *Chlamydia* infection, hepatitis B, HIV infection, and syphilis.

HUMAN IMMUNODEFICIENCY VIRUS

HIV is an RNA retrovirus that causes acquired immunodeficiency syndrome (AIDS). The two types of HIV are type 1 and type 2, the latter being extremely uncommon in the United States.

The clinical manifestations of HIV infection in children are varied and include failure to thrive, generalized lymphadenopathy, hepatomegaly, splenomegaly, diarrhea, or oral candidiasis. Other manifestations include central nervous system disease, cardiomyopathy, hepatitis, or recurrent invasive infections. Opportunistic infections are also common in HIV infection and can include *Pneumocystis carinii* pneumonia, *Mycobacterium* infection, *Cytomegalovirus* infection, *Cryptosporidium* infection, or candidiasis. The full spectrum of clinical manifestations and opportunistic infections associated with HIV infection are protean and beyond the scope of this chapter (American Academy of Pediatrics, 2000c).

Transmission of HIV to children can occur by one of four means: vertical transmission, breastfeeding, percutaneous or mucous membrane exposure to infected blood or body fluids, and sexual contact. The incidence of HIV infection acquired by pediatric victims of sexual abuse from HIV-infected perpetrators is unknown but is believed to be low. The question often arises of when to consider testing sexually abused children for HIV. A list of guidelines that may be useful for

Key Point:

HIV can be transmitted to children through vertically transmission, breastfeeding, exposure of percutaneous or mucous membranes to infected blood or body fluids, or sexual contact.

the clinician to consider has been proposed. *Consider testing sexually abused children or adolescents for HIV if:*

1. The perpetrator has:
    — known HIV infection
    — known risk factors for HIV infection:
        IV drug use
        multiple sexual partners
        bisexual or homosexual practices
2. The child or adolescent has:
    — had multiple assailants
    — another STD
    — history of vaginal or rectal penetration
    — known risk factors for HIV infection (see above)

3. The child/adolescent or parent requests testing

Before testing is done, pretest counseling must be performed, and posttest counseling must also be arranged. If the abuse was recent, seroconversion may not have occurred and may produce a false-negative result. Because of this, all patients should have repeat testing ideally at 6 weeks and at 3 and 6 months after the initial test.

Testing for HIV is done first with an enzyme immunoassay (EIA), which serves as a screening test. If this is positive, Western blot or immunofluorescent antibody tests should be used for confirmation.

If a child is discovered to have HIV, further investigation is needed to determine whether acquisition was via sexual abuse or other means. The child's mother should be tested for HIV to rule out vertical transmission. Other risk factors (as listed above) should be assessed for the probable source of the infection.

Treatment of HIV infection falls into three categories: postexposure prophylaxis, treatment of HIV infection, and treatment of opportunistic infections. Postexposure prophylaxis for HIV infection has recently been recommended in adults. However, data are lacking regarding its efficacy, especially in children. If postexposure prophylaxis is being considered for a child sexual abuse victim, consultation with a pediatric HIV specialist is recommended to choose the appropriate treatment regimen.

Antiretroviral therapy is indicated for most HIV-infected children. Because this form of treatment is a rapidly expanding and changing area, consultation with a pediatric HIV specialist is suggested to choose a treatment regimen. Early diagnosis and aggressive treatment of opportunistic infections is also important. Again, consulting with a pediatric HIV specialist should be considered (AAP, 2000c).

SYPHILIS

Syphilis is caused by a thin mobile spirochete, *Treponema pallidum.* The incidence of syphilis had dropped with the introduction of penicillin in the 1940s, but has increased dramatically in the United States during the late 1980s and early 1990s. Syphilis incidence in neonates and children closely parallels adult trends.

Key Point:

T. pallidum *infection (syphilis) is spread in utero or via intimate contact. In its congenital form, transmission occurs during pregnancy or birth and can occur at any stage of disease in the mother. Acquired syphilis in children resembles that seen in adults.*

Children can be infected with *T. pallidum* either in utero (congenital syphilis) or through intimate contact (acquired syphilis). Congenital syphilis occurs via transplacental transmission at any time during pregnancy or at birth; it can be transmitted at any stage of maternal disease. At the time of birth, infected infants may or may not have any signs of disease and may not show any signs for up to 2 years. The presentation of congenital syphilis may include hepatosplenomegaly, snuffles, lymphadenopathy, rash, or hemolytic anemia. Connors et al. (1998) diagnosed a case in a 6-month-old who had periosteal reaction in a long bone initially felt to be a fracture caused by abuse. If untreated, late manifestations of syphilis can develop, usually after age 2 years, and involve the central nervous system, bones, teeth, skin, and eyes. Late manifestations are found in approximately 40% of untreated patients (Starling, 1994).

Acquired syphilis in children is similar to the presentation seen in adults. It can be divided into the following three stages.

— Stage 1, or primary syphilis, appears as one or multiple indurated painless ulcers, or chancres. These occur at the site of inoculation and can last for 1 to 5 weeks.
— From 1 to 2 months later the secondary phase begins with a generalized maculopapular rash that classically involves the palms and soles. Condyloma lata, which are flat, gray-white coalescent papular lesions seen around the vulva or anus, can also present at this time **(Figure 5-2)**. It is important not to confuse this lesion with the more common condyloma acuminata, caused by human papillomavirus. Condyloma acuminata lesions are skin-colored and usually have a cauliflower-like surface.
— A variable latent period follows, and some patients then progress to the tertiary stage, which consists of dermal and cardiovascular manifestations.

Acquired syphilis is transmitted through infected oral or genital lesions (Neinstein et al., 1984). Because *T. pallidum* is fragile and survives only briefly outside the host, intimate contact is required for transmission (Starling, 1994). The evaluation of syphilis in the younger child may be confounded by an inability to obtain a history and to determine the potential for congenital infection. When syphilis is diagnosed outside the neonatal period, birth records should be scrutinized for evidence of congenital syphilis. Any case of noncongenital syphilis in children is considered to be caused by sexual abuse until proven otherwise.

The diagnosis of syphilis is usually made with serologic testing, although spirochete identification by microscopic darkfield examination gives a definitive diagnosis. Serologic confirmation of syphilis requires both a positive nontreponemal test and a treponemal test (to exclude false-positive results). Nontreponemal tests include the VDRL slide test, the rapid plasma reagin (RPR), and the automated reagin test (ART). These tests measure antibody directed against antigen from *T. pallidum*, antibody interaction with host tissues, or both. If high concentrations of antibody against *T. pallidum* are present, the nontreponemal tests can be falsely negative, called the ***prozone phenomenon***. These tests can also be falsely negative in early primary syphilis, latent acquired syphilis, and late congenital syphilis. Viral infections, connective tissue diseases, pregnancy, or Wharton's jelly contamination of cord blood can cause false-positive results.

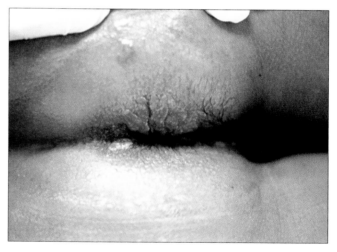

Figure 5-2. *Perianal condylomata lata lesion.*

To exclude false-positive results, any reactive nontreponemal test must be confirmed by a treponemal test. The tests that are currently used are the fluorescent treponemal antibody absorption (FTA-ABS) test and the microhemagglutination test for *T. pallidum* (MHA-TP). Positive treponemal tests usually remain that way for life.

Recommendations for serologic testing for syphilis in children who have been sexually abused have not reached consensus. Because the incidence of syphilis in sexually abused children is low, there is probably no benefit in screening every child. *The following are some criteria to determine which patients to screen for syphilis (Bays & Chadwick, 1993):*

Key Point:
Because the incidence of syphilis in sexually abused children is low, not every child requires screening.

— Children with evidence of other sexually transmitted diseases
— Adolescents
— Children with a family member, parent, or perpetrator with syphilis
— Children living in areas with a high incidence of syphilis

Serologic tests should be obtained 12 weeks after the alleged sexual contact or should be drawn and then repeated in 12 weeks to allow antibodies to develop (Sirotnak, 1994). Treatment of syphilis is with parenteral penicillin G. Recommendations for type of penicillin G and duration of therapy vary depending on stage of disease and clinical manifestions.

HERPES SIMPLEX

Herpes simplex viruses (HSVs) are double-stranded DNA viruses. The two types are HSV-1, usually involving the face and skin above the waist, and HSV-2 infection, usually involving the genitalia and skin below the waist. Either type of virus can be found in either site, depending on the source of infection.

HSV infection can be transmitted to an infant during birth through an infected maternal genital tract or by ascending infection. The majority of neonatal infections are caused by HSV-2. HSV infection can also be transmitted to a neonate (postnatal transmission) from a caregiver; these are often from nongenital sites. In newborns, HSV infection can manifest in one of three ways: (1) localized central nervous system disease, (2) disseminated disease, or (3) localized disease of the skin, eyes, and mouth. Initial symptoms of neonatal HSV infection can occur anytime in the first month of life.

Children and infants beyond the neonatal period can also become infected with HSV. Infection with HSV-1 usually results from contact with infected lesions. Infection with HSV-2 usually results from direct contact with infected genital secretions or lesions through sexual activity. Genital infections with HSV-1 can result from autoinoculation or heteroinoculation from oral lesions and can be the result of nonsexual contact. However, sexual abuse with oral-genital contact can be responsible for some genital HSV-1 infections. Whether the infection is with HSV-1 or HSV-2 does not confirm or disprove sexual abuse. Therefore determination of sexual abuse must rely on historical and other clinical information as well.

Genital herpes is characterized by tender vesicular or ulcerative lesions of the genitalia, perineum, or both. Systemic symptoms such as fever and malaise are often associated with the primary infection (Gardner & Jones, 1984). Tender inguinal adenopathy can also be seen.

The diagnosis of HSV infection is often made by visual inspection of lesions. The diagnosis can be confirmed with cell culture. Specimens should be of vesicle scrapings. Methods for culture confirmation include fluorescent antibody staining and enzyme immunoassays. Tzanck preparation, which is a histologic examination of lesions, has low sensitivity and is no longer recommended as a diagnostic test.

The differential diagnosis of genital herpes infection includes varicella-zoster infection (primary disease and reactivation), bullous impetigo, and contact dermatitis. It is not uncommon for children to have genital vesicular lesions from chickenpox (Simon & Steele, 1995). A Tzank smear will not differentiate between varicella-zoster (a herpes virus) and HSV.

TRICHOMONAS

Trichomonas vaginalis is a flagellated protozoan and is a common sexually transmitted organism in adolescents and adults. Infection is thought to be uncommon in prepubertal girls beyond the first few weeks of life because the prepubertal vaginal environment, which lacks glycogen and has a relatively high pH, is not conducive to the growth of trichomonads. As prepubertal girls approach menarche and the vaginal environment becomes more similar to that of an adult, *Trichomonas* infection becomes more of a potential.

T. vaginalis can be acquired during birth and causes a vaginal discharge in the first few weeks of life. Adolescent and adult females usually present with a pale yellow or

Key Point:
HSV infection can be transmitted through an infected maternal genital tract or by ascending infection, or it can come from a caregiver (usually nongenital transmission). After the neonatal period, children can acquire HSV infection through contact with an infected genital lesion, sexual activity, or direct contact with an oral lesion.

Key Point:
T. vaginalis *infection is more likely once the vaginal environment becomes more like that of an adult. Usually acquired through sexual contact, the presence of* T. vaginalis *raises a strong suspicion for sexual abuse.*

green vaginal discharge and vulvovaginal itching. They can also have dysuria and abdominal pain. Infected males can present with urethritis, epididymitis, or prostatitis. *Trichomonas* infection can also be asymptomatic. Prepubertal girls can present with vaginitis (Jones et al., 1985).

T. vaginalis is thought to be transmitted predominantly by sexual contact in adults. Although some studies have demonstrated the survival of *T. vaginalis* on toilet seats, no studies have confirmed that nonsexual transmission of *Trichomonas* infection occurs in either adults or children beyond the neonatal period (Jones et al., 1985). Therefore the identification of *Trichomonas* infection in children beyond the neonatal period should raise strong suspicion for sexual abuse.

The diagnosis of *T. vaginalis* is usually made by examination of a wet mount preparation of discharge. However, wet mount examination only detects organisms in 40% to 80% of infected individuals. If a wet mount is negative, a culture for *T. vaginalis* should be considered.

Treatment of *Trichomonas* infection is with metronidazole. Individuals infected with *T. vaginalis* should be tested for other STDs. In addition, children outside of the neonatal period should be evaluated for possible sexual abuse with a forensic interview and examination.

HUMAN PAPILLOMAVIRUS

Human papillomavirus (HPV) causes anogenital warts in both adults and children (condylomata acuminata). HPV is a nonenveloped, isosahedral, double-stranded DNA virus. Almost 70 virus types have been identified. Types 6 and 11 are found most often in condylomata acuminata, but types 16, 18, 31, 33, and 35 can also infect the genital tract. Cutaneous warts are most often caused by virus types 1 to 4, most notably by type 2.

HPV infection is almost exclusively an STD in the adult population. However, in children other modes of transmission do occur. Because of this, controversy often arises regarding the manner in which children acquire anogenital warts. There are four possible ways in which HPV lesions can be transmitted to a child: vertical or perinatal transmission; digital autoinoculation or heteroinoculation; fomite or casual contact; and sexual abuse.

Key Point:
Infection with HPV occurs almost exclusively as an STD in adults, but in children routes of transmission other than sexual abuse are possible: vertical or perinatal transmission; digital autoinoculation or heteroinoculation; or fomite or casual contact.

Evidence shows that each type of transmission occurs in childhood HPV infection. Perinatal infection occurs in utero or during passage through an HPV-infected birth canal. HPV has been isolated from the nasopharynx of neonates (Sedlacek et al., 1989). Both conjunctival papillomas containing HPV types 6 and 11 and juvenile laryngeal papillomatosis have been reported in children born to mothers with anogenital warts (Armstrong & Handley, 1997). The latency period between perinatally acquired HPV infection and the clinical appearance of lesions has not been well defined but is thought to range from weeks to possibly to as much as 5 years (Siegfried et al., 1998; Stevens-Simon et al., 2000).

Autoinoculation of HPV from nongenital warts most commonly occurs from hand warts via scratching. Heteroinoculation refers to transmission of HPV from a caretaker to a child by nonsexual contact, as may occur during diaper changes or bathing. There are reports of anogenital warts with HPV type 2 to support these types of transmissions (Gutman et al., 1993). Similarly, studies have documented that parents of children with anogenital HPV have cutaneous warts (Handley et al., 1997).

Fomite or casual transmission has been proposed to occur from infected secretions coming in contact with a child through sharing towels, underwear, or other fomites. There is no direct evidence to confirm that such a mechanism results in HPV infection in children.

Transmission of HPV infection via sexual abuse occurs by genital-genital contact, genital-anal contact, abusive digital fondling, or digital-anal or digital-vaginal contact. There is much disagreement in the literature regarding the prevalence of sexual abuse in children who present with anogenital warts. Some of the discrepancy comes from the different methods used to screen for warts and the variability in time of follow-up. Studies have been performed to assess the prevalence of genital HPV infections between sexually abused and nonabused preadolescent girls. Stevens-Simon et al. (2000) studied 40 preadolescent girls; HPV was detected in 5 (16%) of the 31 girls with confirmed or suspected sexual abuse and in none of the non abused girls.

Key Point:
In addition to a complete forensic interview and physical examination of the child to rule out sexual abuse, the history of a child with genital warts should include the answers to the following questions:
— Does a caregiver have a history of cutaneous warts?
— Does the mother have a history of cutaneous warts or abnormal Pap smears?

Important historical information to obtain when evaluating a child with genital warts includes a history of cutaneous warts in caregivers, maternal history of genital warts or abnormal Papanicolaou (Pap) smears, and a complete forensic interview and physical examination of the child for the evaluation of sexual abuse. This information may help to determine whether an HPV infection in a child is from sexual or nonsexual contact.

It has been proposed to use HPV subtype determination to indicate the source of HPV acquisition. However, isolation of subtypes 6 and 11 will not distinguish between sexual abuse and perinatal transmission. Similarly, isolation of subtype 2 will not distinguish between abusive genital fondling and innocent heteroinoculation or autoinoculation. Therefore historical, clinical, and social information must be considered to identify the mode of transmission when a child presents with anogenital warts.

The clinical manifestations of anogenital infection range from clinically inapparent infection to condylomata acuminata, described earlier (**See Figures 5-3, 5-4 and 5-5**). In males, lesions can be found on the shaft of the penis, the urethral meatus, the scrotum, or the perianal area. In females, lesions are seen on the labia and perianal area, and less commonly in the vagina and on the cervix. Most warts are asymptomatic, but they can cause itching, burning with urination, pain, and bleeding.

Often, the diagnosis of condylomata acuminata is made on the physical appearance alone. Acetic acid often turns mucosal lesions white and may be helpful during an evaluation. Confirmation of lesions is made with tissue biopsy, but biopsy should be reserved for cases in which the diagnosis is in doubt (Frasier, 1994). Newer techniques include polymerase chain reaction (PCR) to test for the presence of HPV DNA. This technique involves a superficial swab of the lesion, so it is noninvasive, but it has not yet been completely tested in the pediatric population (Siegfried et al., 1998; Stevens-Simon et al., 2000).

The differential diagnosis of condylomata acuminata includes condyloma lata, molluscum contagiosum, neurofibromatosis, histocytosis X, chronic benign pemphigus, and other neoplasms. The clinical differences in the lesion's appearance often make the diagnosis clear.

Children with anogenital warts should be referred to a dermatologist for regular follow-up and to discuss treatment options. One option is an initial period of observation because a proportion of cases spontaneously resolve. Topical treatments include liquid nitrogen, trichloroacetic acid, or podophyllin. These sometimes require multiple applications and are often irritating and painful to children. Condylomata acuminata can also be ablated by carbon dioxide laser or electrocautery, procedures that require general anesthesia. Ablation should be reserved for lesions that are too extensive to treat topically or those causing discomfort or other symptoms.

In adults, there is strong evidence of the association between anogenital HPV infection and anogenital neoplasm, particularly cervical carcinoma. HPV types 16, 18, 31, and 33 have been reported as high-risk oncogenic subtypes. At the present time, no data are available to assess the risk of subsequent anogenital neoplasm in children who have anogenital warts. Because of this unknown risk, regular follow-up on a long-term basis is recommended.

BACTERIAL VAGINOSIS

Bacterial vaginosis is an abnormal condition of the vagina characterized by a shift in the vaginal flora from the normally predominant Lactobacillus to an overgrowth of *Gardnerella vaginalis, Mycoplasma hominis,* and anaerobic bacteria.

Bacterial vaginosis is characterized by a vaginal discharge that is nonviscous, homogenous, white and has a malodorous fishy smell. It is usually not associated with abdominal pain, dysuria, or significant pruritus. Bacterial vaginosis may also be asymptomatic (Nyirjesy, 1999).

One of the controversies regarding bacterial vaginosis in the pediatric population concerns its mode of transmission. Some researchers feel that it is an STD, whereas others have questioned this association. Prepubertal girls with a history of sexual abuse were more likely to grow *G. vaginalis* from a vaginal culture (14.6%) than prepubertal girls in the control group who had no known history of sexual abuse (4.2%) (Bartley et al., 1987). Contrary to this study, Bump and Buesching (1988) found no statistically significant difference in the prevalence of bacterial vaginosis between sexually active and virginal adolescent girls.

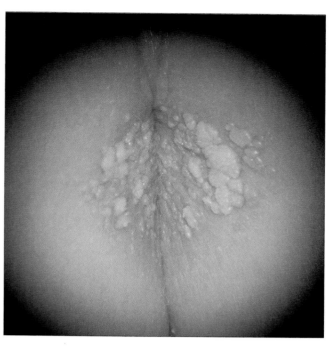

Figure 5-3. *Perianal warts (human papilomavirus).*

Whether the presence of bacterial vaginosis in a pediatric patient reflects disease acquired from sexual contact has important ramifications with respect to sexual abuse. If a child is found to have bacterial vaginosis, she should undergo a forensic interview as well as a forensic examination to determine if sexual abuse occurred. The child should also be tested for other sexually transmitted pathogens, such as *N. gonorrhoeae* and *C. trachomatis.* Culture for *G. vaginalis* is not recommended because this organism may be found in individuals without bacterial vaginosis.

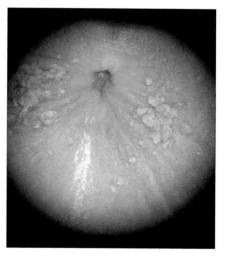

Figure 5-4. *Perianal warts (human papilomavirus).*

Key Point:
Some researchers classify bacterial vaginosis in children as an STD, but some do not. If the child has bacterial vaginosis, a forensic interview and forensic examination are required to determine if there has been sexual abuse.

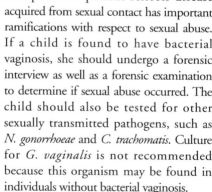

The diagnosis of bacterial vaginosis is made on clinical grounds. *The clinical diagnosis requires the presence of three out of four of the following symptoms or signs (Amsel's criteria) (AAP, 2000a):*

1. Homogeneous gray or white discharge on examination
2. Vaginal fluid pH >4.5
3. Positive amine test: mixing vaginal fluid with 10% potassium hydroxide results in a fishy odor
4. Presence of "clue cells": vaginal epithelial cells that appear "moth-eaten" or massively coated with coccobacilli on gram stain

The differential diagnosis of bacterial vaginosis includes other causes of vulvovaginitis in children, specifically the following: bacterial infections such as *N. gonorrhoeae, C. trachomatis, Streptococcus* species, *Hemophilus influenzae,* or

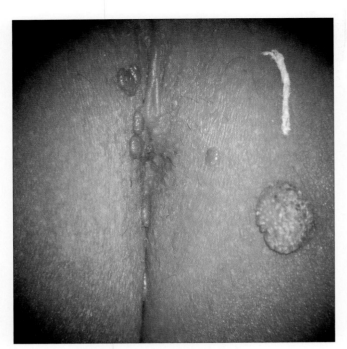

Figure 5-5. *Perianal flat warts (human papilomavirus).*

Key Point:
Transmission of HBV is via blood or body fluids. The mother can transmit HBV to her infant perinatally, or young children may transmit the virus horizontally when the prevalence of HBV is high. Those living in the same house as an HBV carrier are at an increased risk for infection.

Bacteroides species. Noninfectious causes of vulvovaginitis include foreign bodies, poor hygiene, and chemical and mechanical irritation (**Table 5-6**).

Treatment of bacterial vaginosis is with metronidazole. Patients with an allergy to metronidazole can be treated with clindamycin.

HEPATITIS B

Hepatitis B virus (HBV) is a DNA-containing hepadenovirus. HBV is transmitted through blood or body fluids, including semen, cervical secretions, and saliva. Modes of transmission include infusion of blood or blood products, percutaneous or mucous membrane exposure to blood or body fluids, and sexual activity. Transmission from mother to infant during the perinatal period occurs to infants born to hepatitis B-infected mothers. Horizontal transmission during early childhood occurs where the prevalence of HBV is high. Household contacts of HBV carriers are at increased risk for infection.

HBV infection can cause a wide range of symptoms. Individuals can be asymptomatic, have nonspecific symptoms such as anorexia or malaise, or have clinical hepatitis with jaundice. Acute infection leads to chronic infection in approximately 10% of individuals and greatly increases the risk for developing chronic liver disease or primary hepatocellular carcinoma later in life (AAP, 2000b).

Serologic antigen tests exist to detect the important components of the HBV, namely, hepatitis B surface antigen (HbsAg), hepatitis B core antigen (HbcAg), and hepatitis B e antigen (HbeAg). Hepatitis B surface antigen is detectable during acute infection. Anti-HBs identifies individuals who have had infection with HBV and also determines immunity after vaccination. Anti-HBc identifies individuals with acute or past HBV infection but is not present after immunization. The incubation period of acute hepatitis B infection is approximately 45 to 120 days; therefore for individuals with potential exposure to HBV, testing should be done at the initial presentation, at 3 months postexposure, and at 6 months postexposure (Crowe et al., 1996).

Table 5-6. Causes of Vulvovaginitis in Prepubertal Girls	
INFECTIOUS CAUSES	NON-INFECTIOUS CAUSES
Gonorrhea	Foreign body
C. trachomatis	Poor hygiene
Bacterial vaginosis	Chemical irritation
Streptococcus species	Mechanical irritation
Staphylococcus species	Allergy
Enterococcus	Rectovaginal fistula
Shigella species	Lichen sclerosis
H. Influenzae	
Bacteroides species	
Candida albicans	
T. vaginalis	
Helmenthic infections	
Enterobius vermicularis (pinworms)	
Varicella	

HBV is also transmitted through sexual activity. Therefore, if a child outside of the perinatal period is discovered to have acute hepatitis B infection, sexual abuse should be suspected. Vertical transmission is still possible if the infection is not clearly acute, and in this case the mother should be tested as well. If a child is sexually abused by a person with known HBV infection, that child is at increased risk of contracting HBV and should receive postexposure prophylaxis with one dose of hepatitis B immune globulin. In addition, vaccination with the hepatitis B vaccine should be initiated or revaccination given, unless the child is known to be allergic to the hepatitis B vaccine (AAP, 2000b).

Key Point:
When acute HBV infection is found in children older than the perinatal period, sexual abuse should be suspected even though other possibilities exist.

There is no treatment for acute HBV infection. Preexposure immunization with hepatitis B vaccine is the most effective means to prevent HBV transmission. Hepatitis B vaccination is recommended for all infants as part of the routine childhood immunization schedule. Children who have not been previously vaccinated should be immunized by age 11 or 12 years.

REFERENCES

American Academy of Pediatrics (AAP). Bacterial Vaginosis. In: Pickering LK, ed. *2000 Red Book: Report of the Committee on Infectious Diseases*. 25th ed. Elk Grove Village, Ill: American Academy of Pediatrics; 2000a:149-150.

American Academy of Pediatrics (AAP). Hepatitis B. In: Pickering LK, ed. *2000 Red Book: Report of the Committee on Infectious Diseases*. 25th ed. Elk Grove Village, Ill: American Academy of Pediatrics; 2000b:289-302.

American Academy of Pediatrics (AAP). Human immunodeficiency virus infection. In: Pickering LK, ed. *2000 Red Book: Report of the Committee on Infectious Diseases*. 25th ed. Elk Grove Village, Ill: American Academy of Pediatrics; 2000c:325-350.

Armstrong DKB, Handley JM. Anogenital warts in prepubertal children: pathogenesis, HPV typing and management. *Int J STD AIDS*. 1997;8:78-81.

Bartley DL, Morgan L, Rimsza ME. Gardnerella vaginalis in prepubertal girls. *Am J Dis Child*. 1987;141:1014-1017.

Bays J, Chadwick D. Medical diagnosis of the sexually abused child. *Child Abuse Negl*. 1993;17:91-110.

Bell TA, Stamm WE, Wang SP, et al. Chronic Chlamydia trachomatis infections in infants. *JAMA*. 1992;267:400-402.

Black CM. Current methods of laboratory diagnosis of Chlamydia trachomatis infection. *Clin Microbiol Rev*. 1997;10:160-184.

Branch G, Paxton R. A study of gonococcal infections among infants and children. *Public Health Rep*. 1965;80:347-352.

Bump RC, Buesching WJ. Bacterial vaginosis in virginal and sexually active adolescent females: evidence against exclusive sexually transmission. *Am J Obstet Gynecol*. 1988;158:935-939.

Connors JM, Schubert C, Shapiro R. Syphilis or abuse: making the diagnosis and understanding the implications. *Pediatr Emerg Care*. 1998;14:139-142.

Crowe C, Forster GE, Dinsmore WW, Maw RD. A case of acute hepatitis B occurring four months after multiple rape. *Int J STD AIDS*. 1996;7:133-134.

DeJong AR, Emmett GA, Hervada AA. Epidemiologic factors in sexual abuse of boys. *Am J Dis Child*. 1982;136:990-993.

Farrell MK, Billmire E, Sharmroy JA, et al. Prepubertal gonorrhea: a multidisciplinary approach. *Pediatrics*. 1981;67:151-153.

Frasier LD. Human papillomavirus infection in children. *Pediatr Ann*. 1994;23:354-360.

Gardner M, Jones JG. Genital herpes acquired by sexual abuse of children. *J Pediatr*. 1984;104:243-244.

Gilbaugh JH, Fuchs PC. The gonococcus and the toilet seat. *N Engl J Med*. 1979;301:91-93.

Girardet RG, McClain N, Lahoti S, et al. Comparison of the urine-based ligase chain reaction test to culture for detection of Chlamydia trachomatis and Neisseria gonorrhoeae in pediatric sexual abuse victims. *Pediatr Infect Dis J*. 2001;20:144-147.

Groth AN, Burgess AW. Sexual dysfunction during rape. *New Engl J Med*. 1977;297:764-766.

Gutman LT, Herman-Giddens ME, Phelps WC. Transmission of human genital papillomavirus disease: comparison of data from adults and children. *Pediatrics*. 1993;91:31-38.

Hammerschlag MR. Chlamydia trachomatis in children. *Pediatr Ann*. 1994;23:349-353.

Hammerschlag MR. Sexually transmitted diseases in sexually abused children: medical and legal implications. *Sex Transm Infect*. 1998;74:167-174.

Handley J, Hanks E, Armstrong K, et al. Common association of HPV 2 with anogenital warts in prepubertal children. *Pediatr Dermatol*. 1997;14:339-343.

Ingram DL, Everett D, Lyna PR, White ST, Rockwell LA. Epidemiology of adult sexually transmitted disease agents in children being evaluated for sexual abuse. *Pediatr Infect Dis J*. 1992;11:945-950.

Jenny C. Sexually transmitted diseases and child abuse. *Pediatr Ann*. 1992;21:497-503.

Jones JG, Yamauchi T, Lambert B. Trichomonas vaginalis infestation in sexually abused girls. *Am J Dis Child*. 1985;139:846-847.

Nair P, Glazer-Semmel E, Gould C, Ruff E. Neisseria gonorrhoeae in asymptomatic prepubertal household contacts of children with gonoccal infections. *Clin Pediatr*. 1986;25:160-163.

Neinstein LS, Goldenring J, Carpenter S. Nonsexual transmission of sexually transmitted diseases: an infrequent occurrence. *Pediatrics*. 1984;74:67-76.

Nyirjesy P. Vaginitis in the adolescent patient. *Pediatr Clin North Am*. 1999;46:733-745.

Schwarcz SK, Whittington WL. Sexual assault and sexually transmitted diseases: detection and management in adults and children. *Rev Infect Dis*. 1990;12:s682-s690.

Sedlacek TV, Lindheim S, Elder C, et al. Mechanisms for human papillomavirus transmission at birth. *Am J Obstet Gynecol*. 1989;161:55-59.

Shapiro RA, Schubert CJ, Myers PA. Vaginal discharge as an indicator of gonorrhea and Chlamydia infection in girls under 12 years old. *Pediatr Emerg Care*. 1993;9:341-345.

Sicoli RA, Losek JD, Hudlett JM, Smith D. Indications for Neisseria gonorrhoeae cultures in children with suspected sexual abuse. *Arch Pediatr Adolesc Med*. 1995;149:86-89.

Siegel RM, Schubert CJ, Myers PA, Shapiro RA. The prevalence of sexually transmitted diseases in children and adolescents evaluated for sexual abuse in Cincinnati: rationale of limited STD testing in prepubertal girls. *Pediatrics*. 1995;96:1090-1094.

Siegfried E, Rasnick-Conley J, Cook S, et al. Human papillomavirus screening in pediatric victims of sexual abuse. *Pediatrics*. 1998;101:41-47.

Simon HK, Steele DW. Varicella: pediatric genital/rectal vesicular lesions of unclear origin. *Ann Emerg Med*. 1995;25:111-114.

Sirotnak AP. Testing sexually abused children for sexually transmitted diseases: who to test, when to test and why. *Pediatr Ann.* 1994;23:370-374.

Starling SP. Syphilis in infants and young children. *Pediatr Ann.* 1994;23:334-340.

Stevens-Simon C, Nelligan D, Breese P, et al. The prevalence of genital human papillomavirus infections in abused and nonabused preadolescent girls. *Pediatrics.* 2000;106:645-649.

DIFFERENTIAL DIAGNOSIS

Philip Scribano, DO, MSCE

The evaluation of suspected child sexual abuse must include the possibility that the examination findings may result from a variation in the normal anatomy of a prepubertal child. In addition, several nonabusive traumatic injuries must be considered when evaluating the possibility of an abusive anogenital injury. Medical conditions that may appear to be traumatic abusive injuries must also be considered in the differential diagnosis of child sexual abuse.

Paramount to the protection of children from further abusive acts is early identification and a thorough understanding of the patterns and types of injuries sustained in child sexual abuse. However, the clinician must also evaluate and recognize conditions that may mimic child sexual abuse. This is of critical importance to avoid a mistaken diagnosis that can have significant negative consequences for the child, family, and falsely accused perpetrator.

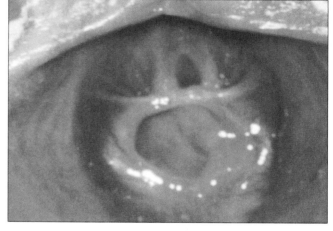

Figure 6-1. *Vestibular bands. (Courtesy of Dr. Lori Frasier, Salt Lake City, Utah)*

VARIATIONS OF NORMAL ANATOMY

GENITALIA

Variations of normal genital anatomy have been described. ***Vestibular bands*** (**Figure 6-1**), which are supporting structures of the urethra and superior hymen, have been confused as scarring of the genitalia. These linear structures are lateral to the urethra and hymen, are usually symmetrical, and connect to the lateral wall of the vestibule. Skin tags (**Figure 6-2**), septa, notches and clefts of the hymen, and congenital absence of the upper portion of the hymen have also been identified in normal, nonabused prepubertal girls and have been mistakenly reported as the traumatic injuries of sexual abuse. Superficial notches on the inferior half of the hymen have been observed in nonabused girls (Berenson et al., 2000); however, notches extending through more than 50% of the membrane were seen only in abused children. In the nonabused female, hymenal tags have been identified in more than 20% of girls (McCann et al., 1990). Vaginal columns, also normal, can protrude and cause an irregularity in the hymenal contour.

An important examination technique to adequately visualize the hymen and determine the presence of any irregularity in the rim is to place the child in the knee-chest position. Irregularities of hymenal tissue usually disappear because of the weight of the vaginal column. This will enable the hymenal rim to "smooth" out and resolve the irregularity seen previously.

Hymenal clefts are likely to be a congenital variant if they are a shallow concavity with smooth border and located in the anterior or anterolateral portions of the hymen. Clefts that are deep and angular and are located on the posterior aspect of the hymen must be evaluated further for sexual abuse (Bays, 2001). Congenital absence of the upper portion of the hymen has also been reported (Bays & Jenny, 1990).

Some normal findings can mimic old scarring of the genitalia. The ***linea vestibularis*** is a midline, linear structure extending from the posterior hymen to

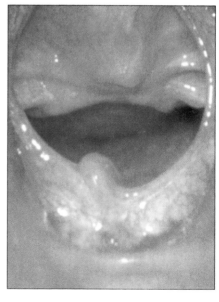

Figure 6-2. *Hymenal skin tag. (Courtesy of Dr. Lori Frasier, Salt Lake City, Utah)*

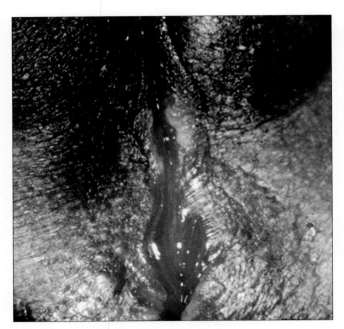

Figure 6-3. *Failure of midline fusion. (Courtesy of Dr. Frederick Berren, Hartford, Conn)*

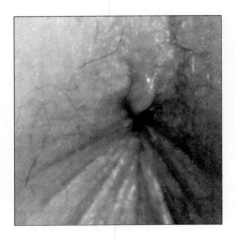

Figure 6-4. *Anal skin tag. (Courtesy of Dr. Lori Frasier, Salt Lake City, Utah)*

Key Point:
Clinicians need to be able to recognize both the patterns and types of injuries sustained during child sexual abuse and the conditions that may mimic abusive findings.

the posterior fourchette (Kellogg & Parra, 1991). The *median raphe* is a midline structure from the posterior fourchette along the perineum to the anal verge. The median raphe is less often confused with scarring in boys because it originates, uninterrupted from the ventral aspect of the penis, over the scrotal sac, through the perineum to the anal verge. These congenital structures are formed by fusion at the midline, and a ridge can develop as a result of that fusion. A failure of the midline fusion (**Figure 6-3**) mimics acute trauma. Follow-up examinations that reveal an unchanged, unhealed area suggest this structural abnormality is a congenital issue.

ANUS

Similar to the skin tags found on the hymen, anal skin tags (**Figure 6-4**) are also variations of normal physical structures. Much debate has centered around the concern that skin tags may be manifestations of prior anal trauma. However, more recent consensus with the evaluation of children who were not victims of abuse has identified anal skin tags in the general population. Specifically, if an anal skin tag is midline, it is likely to be a normal variant (Bays, 2001). Lateral skin tags should be regarded with some concern, and a detailed history of trauma should be ascertained before identifying these findings as normal.

Other anal findings mistakenly regarded as anal scarring include a smooth, midline external sphincter with a fan-shaped area in the posterior midline (McCann et al., 1989). Perianal erythema is a nonspecific finding that can result from infectious causes such as group A streptococcal disease or infectious colitis causing venous congestion; inflammatory processes such as Crohn's disease; or dermatologic conditions such as lichen sclerosus. (A more detailed description of each entity is reported elsewhere in this chapter.)

The degree of anal dilation has been of concern regarding repeated anal abuse, yet consensus regarding this finding is still lacking. A recent classification system provides one possible interpretation of anal dilation as a nonspecific finding for dilation of any size, with or without stool present in the rectal vault, or, if the child is examined in the knee-chest position for 30 seconds or greater (Adams, 2001). Often, significant dilation of the anus can occur because of retained stool and conditions such as chronic constipation and neurogenic patulous anus (Agnarsson et al., 1990). Post-mortem dilation is another nonabuse cause of anal dilation (McCann et al., 1996).

NONABUSIVE TRAUMA

The evaluation of anogenital trauma in the prepubertal child requires some understanding of the mechanisms by which these injuries occur. Most commonly, accidental genital injuries have been described as caused by a straddling of an object such as a bicycle or during climbing and falling onto an object (**Figure 6-5**). The child strikes the object, causing injury to the urogenital structures. The injuries sustained are the result of compression of the soft tissues against the bony margins of the pelvic outlet, specifically the pubic symphysis, rami, or adductor longus tendon. The most common mechanism of urogenital straddle injuries is a fall on a bicycle crossbar (25% to 39%), followed by a fall on furniture (23% to 36%), a fall on miscellaneous objects without climbing (11%), a fall while climbing on playground equipment (10% to 25%), a fall on the back of a shoe or ice skate (4%), running into an object (3%), and other miscellaneous falls (13%) (Bond et al., 1995; Dowd et al., 1994). Straddle injuries should be considered an extremely unlikely mechanism of injury in children under age 9 months, given their developmental limitations in ambulation (Dowd et al., 1994). As with any trauma evaluation, a determination of how the injury occurred should be ascertained from the child and/or caregiver if the child is nonverbal. Any inconsistencies with the history provided or no history provided should prompt concerns for maltreatment.

Most nonpenetrating injuries involve the upper structures of the vulva such as the mons pubis, clitoris, and labia. However, one study identified as many as 34% of injuries posterior to the hymen (Bond et al., 1995). Penetrating injuries may occur because of falls onto pointed objects and may produce laceration injuries to the posterior fourchette, hymen, vagina, or rectum. These injuries must be thoroughly evaluated for the exact details of the mechanism of injury before attributing an accidental means to this type of trauma.

Because of the rich blood supply of the external genitalia, a relatively minor injury can manifest with excessive bleeding, especially when the unestrogenized vagina, hymen, or adjacent structures are involved (Merritt, 1998). Often the challenge of accurately assessing the location of bleeding requires sedation or general anesthesia because of the pain and anxiety associated with examination.

Vulvar hematomas, commonly the result of straddle injuries, can be very painful and may prevent the child from urinating because of the pain and swelling of the urogenital structures. Vaginal injuries should be regarded as very unusual accidental injuries unless the history and associated findings are consistent with an accidental, penetrating mechanism. Unusual hymenal or vaginal accidental penetrating injuries include impalement

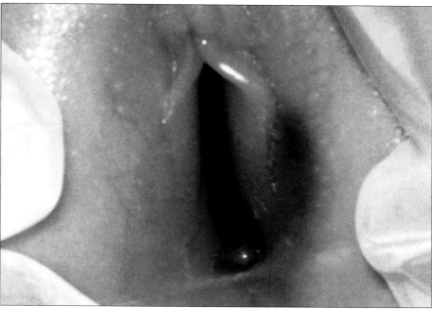

Figure 6-5. *Straddle injury. (Courtesy of Dr. Lori Frasier, Salt Lake City, Utah)*

from a sharp object, or high-pressure water that insufflates the vagina causing laceration (Merritt, 1998). Most of these injuries, however, are probably the result of sexual assault.

Nonabusive traumatic urogenital injuries are most common in females (over two thirds of cases). However, males are apt to present with scrotal trauma (36% to 57% of male injuries), which were mostly lacerations caused by straddle mechanisms, followed by penile ecchymoses and/or laceration (25% to 43%) (Dowd et al., 1994; Kadish et al., 1998). With regard to anal trauma in males, isolated anal trauma or trauma localized to the 10 to 2 o'clock and/or the 5 to 7 o'clock positions should cause concern for abuse, whereas isolated genital trauma may be more indicative of an accidental mechanism (Kadish et al., 1998).

Other nonabusive anogenital injuries include zipper entrapment, and these should be easily identified by history and localized external injury. Children involved in motor vehicle crashes may sustain a pelvic fracture caused by a crush injury. Sharp bony fragments can penetrate the vagina and lower urinary tract. Fissures of the posterior fourchette or anus can be iatrogenically introduced during an examination that includes traction of the labia or buttocks (Bays, 2001). An ingested, sharp foreign body that traverses the gastrointestinal tract may, on passage from the anus, cause trauma; however, this is a rare possibility. Although foreign bodies are coated with mucus and fecal matter to make even passage of a sharp pin unlikely to cause trauma, a lacerated rectal mucosa caused by a swallowed fishbone has been reported (Black et al., 1982). Typical child masturbation should not cause genital injury, although concern as to the nonabusive nature of minor abrasions and contusions as a result of masturbation reported in mentally retarded girls is still under debate. Sexual abuse must be considered in this at-risk population or a preverbal child before attributing the cause of the minor genital trauma to masturbation (Hyman et al., 1990).

Key Point:
Nonabusive trauma may occur, but the history and physical findings in these accidental cases should be consistent with the mechanism of injury.

Injury to the perineum with perianal bruising, rectal prolapse, or evisceration of the bowel have been reportedly caused by children sitting on suction drain vents in swimming pools (Cain et al., 1983; Centers for Disease Control [CDC], 1992).

DERMATOLOGIC DISORDERS

Lichen sclerosus et atrophicus is a chronic, benign inflammatory skin disorder characterized by white, shiny macules and papules that coalesce to form a confluent, hypopigmented, atrophic plaque (**Figure 6-6**). Typically, the vulvar and perianal areas are involved in an hourglass or "figure eight" pattern. The hymen is not involved. Hemorrhagic, bullous lesions, fissures, and ulcers can lead to confusion with the traumatic injuries (acute or chronic) of a sexual assault (Powell & Wojnarowska, 2000; Wood & Bevan, 1999). Although males can also be affected with phimosis as the most common problem, lichen sclerosus et atrophicus affects females to males in a ratio of 10:1 (Loening-Baucke, 1991). It most commonly occurs in adulthood, but up to 15% of cases occur in children, many of which are in the preschool age. Other parts of the body can be affected, including the upper part of the trunk, forearm, neck, and face (Loening-Baucke, 1991).

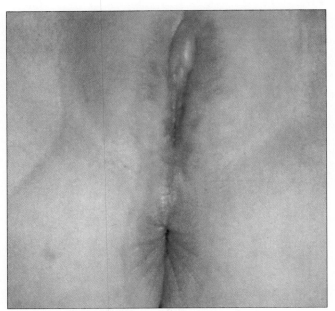

Figure 6-6. *Lichen sclerosus et atrohicus.*
(Courtesy of Dr. Lori Frasier, Salt Lake City, Utah)

Typical symptoms include anogenital itching, pain, and bleeding. Chronic, unremitting disease predisposes the development of labial adhesions or phimosis. Diagnosis is most often made clinically; however, biopsy can confirm the characteristic findings of lichen sclerosus et atrophicus.

A uniformly effective treatment has not been described, although treatment with hydrocortisone cream (1%) twice daily until symptoms abate and subsequently when symptoms recur appears to be effective (Bracco et al., 1993; Dalziel & Wojnarowska, 1993). Two thirds of premenarchal girls have improvement or resolution of their lesions before menarche (Loening-Baucke, 1991).

Seborrheic dermatitis is a common diaper rash in infants presenting similarly to lesions more commonly occurring on the face and scalp. The lesions are slightly greasy and yellow with an erythematous base, and the mucosa is spared. It is not usually pruritic. Most notable is the postinflammatory hypopigmentation and possible fissures that may develop in severe cases (Siegfried & Frasier, 1997).

Allergic reactions causing contact dermatitis can occur on any region of the body, including the anogenital region. Contact dermatitis results from irritation caused by the use of potentially irritating cleaning products and lotions or simply from infrequent or irregular hygiene practices. Erythema, scaling, blistering, and edema may be present.

Hanks & Venters (1992) describe an interesting complication of bedwetting. The use of a bedwetting alarm introduced a genital rash that was vesicular over the labia and inner thigh, prompting a child protection service evaluation. One month later, the child's twin sister developed a similar rash. On further questioning, the history was provided that both children had been using a bedwetting alarm that was nickel plated. After a dermatologic evaluation, nickels were taped to the inner arms of both children, and they developed a vesicular eruption similar to the prior episode. The importance of a detailed history of any and all products that may come in contact with the anogenital area cannot be overemphasized.

Psoriasis of the diaper area (erythematous, thick, silvery, scale-like lesions) may occur in infants. Examination of the nails and other skin areas may assist in the proper diagnosis (Dodds, 1997).

If irritated, cavernous or strawberry hemangiomas (**Figure 6-7**), the most common benign vascular tumors of infancy, can be difficult to identify and misdiagnosed as acute sexual abuse (Levin & Selbst, 1988). Lesions can be present on the hymen, vulva, vagina, or perineum and can bleed or ulcerate, which occurs in about 5% of cases. Present at birth, these tumors grow in proportion to the growing infant and appear as small, red masses with an irregular border (Bays, 2001; Hurwitz, 1993c; Siegfried & Frasier, 1997).

Pemphigus disorders are characterized as severe, chronic bullae that develop on normal-appearing skin and mucous membranes. Rare in children, bullous pemphigoid can present as large, tense bullae on normal-appearing or erythematous skin. Associated bullae may be observed in the mouth as well as lower abdomen and thigh regions. Symptoms include mild pruritus, pain, and occasionally bleeding. ***Pemphigus vulgaris*** is an autoimmune disorder characterized by flaccid vesiculobullous lesions of 1 to 3 cm in size with persistent erosions. Commonly affected areas include the face, scalp, neck, and anogenital regions, as well as "pressure areas" of the feet, back, and mouth. A Tzanck smear may identify acantholytic epidermal cells, in contrast to multinucleated giant cells seen in herpesvirus infections (Hurwitz, 1993a).

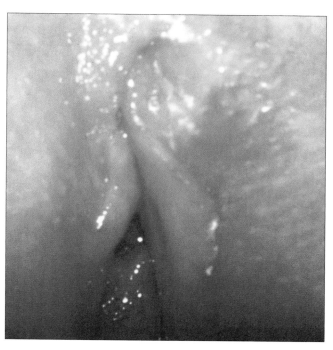

Figure 6-7. *Strawberry hemangioma. (Courtesy of Dr. Lori Frasier, Salt Lake City, Utah).*

INFECTIOUS DISORDERS

Vulvovaginitis is a common inflammatory problem in prepubertal girls caused by a less prominent labia majora protecting the thinner structures of the vulva, low estrogen presence (which increases susceptibility of the vaginal mucosa to irritation and infection), and a neutral pH of the vagina providing an optimal growth milieu for bacteria (Jaquiery et al., 1999). Other factors leading to inflammation include children's hygiene habits, which increase the chance of chronic irritation or bacterial contamination.

Although the majority of prepubertal girls with vulvovaginitis do not have an infectious etiology, let alone a sexually transmitted infection, one should consider bacterial diseases in the differential diagnosis if there is a visible vaginal discharge on examination along with moderate to severe inflammation (Jaquiery et al., 1999). Bacterial culprits include *Staphylococcus aureus* (which may also present with impetigo in the anogenital region), group *A Streptococcus*, *Enterococcus*, and *Shigella*. Even if there are no identified risk factors and no disclosure of sexual abuse, one should consider *Neisseria gonorrhea* in the differential diagnostic evaluation if

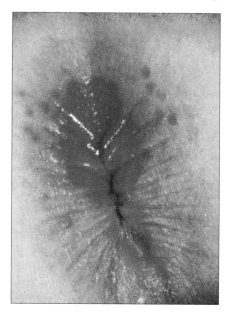

Figure 6-8. *Perianal erythema due to group A streptococcus. (Courtesy of Dr. Lori Frasier, Salt Lake City, Utah)*

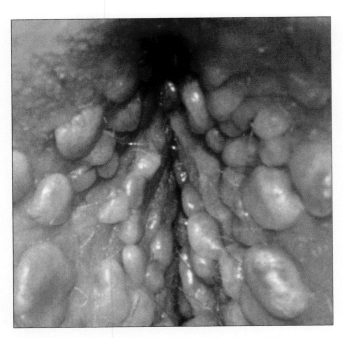

Figure 6-9. *Human papillomavirus: anal. (Courtesy of Dr. Lori Frasier, Salt Lake City, Utah)*

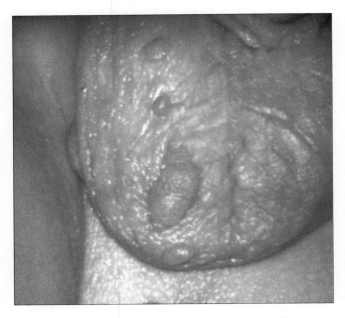

Figure 6-10. *Human papillomavirus: scrotal. (Courtesy of Dr. Lori Frasier, Salt Lake City, Utah)*

evaluating for bacterial vaginitis. Depending on specific laboratory processing, evaluation of *N. gonorrhea* and group *A Streptococcus* may require additional swabs for specific organisms because of the different growth media required.

Group A streptococcal infection can also manifest as intense perianal erythema (**Figure 6-8**) or, in males, balanitis. This is primarily a disease of early childhood, and its incidence is similar to that of streptococcal impetigo, but its age distribution is very different from the age distribution of streptococcal pharyngitis. However, in a series of 23 children with perineal group A streptococcal infection, 92% of affected children had group A streptococcal pharyngitis identified by throat culture (Mogielnicki et al., 2000).

In adults, vulvar or anal human papillomavirus (HPV) warts are felt to be acquired by sexual transmission. However, perinatal acquisition, autoinoculation, heteroinoculation from hand contact and diapering, and fomite transmission with shared bath towels or swimsuits have been reported with HPV infection in children (Bays, 2001). These warts are typically soft, are less than 0.5 mm, and may have a papular or more verrucous shape (**Figure 6-9**). They often coalesce along skin folds in a symmetric, mirror distribution and usually spare the anal verge (Siegfried & Frasier, 1997). In males the scrotal region may be the predominant site of infection (**Figure 6-10**). Usually, children are asymptomatic but may complain of itching or bleeding. An association of recent varicella infection and subsequent, rapid progression of anogenital HPV infection has been reported in three children under age 3 years in whom child protection investigations ruled out sexual abuse (Persaud & Squires, 1997).

Because of the extremely high prevalence in adults (10% to 80% of asymptomatic, sexually active young women), the increasing prevalence of HPV infection identified in children is predictable; however, concern for sexual transmission should still exist (Siegfried & Frasier, 1997). With the benefit of DNA typing, the source of HPV infection can sometimes be identified by comparing the type-specific infection in the child and mother, thus increasing the probability of vertical transmission. Anogenital condyloma accuminata is often the result of HPV types 6 and 11, but types 16, 18, 31, 33, 34, 35, 45, and 56 have been isolated in asymptomatic patients (Siegfried & Frasier, 1997). Subtypes 13 and 32 have been isolated to the oral mucosa exclusively (Muram & Stewart, 2000). A detailed history should include prior evidence of maternal infection and/or abnormal Papanicolaou smear and other wart infections in the mother as well as other family members. Given the difficulty in accurately estimating the true latency of onset of disease from initial exposure, a child protection investigation for sexual abuse should be undertaken in children older than age 3 to 4 years in whom no perinatal acquisition can be easily explained (American Academy of Pediatrics, 1999; McCune et al., 1993; Stevens-Simon et al., 2000).

It is important to consider varicella infection in the differential diagnosis of vesicular lesions in the perineum or vulva. A report of a 6-year-old girl described isolated, 3 to 4 mm vesicular lesions with an erythematous base located over the labia majora and a few other tender, erythematous areas noted around the clitoris without any other skin involvement (Boyd & Jordan, 1987). These lesions were present for 2 days before further involvement of the skin confirmed the diagnosis of varicella. A Tzanck smear is not sufficient to make the diagnosis, and viral culture should be performed when question arises as to whether herpes simplex or varicella virus is the infectious agent. Another herpesvirus, Epstein-Barr infection, has also been associated with genital ulcers and can be identified by genital swabs for polymerase chain reaction testing for the Epstein-Barr virus DNA or by serologic tests (IgM to Epstein-Barr viral antigen) (Taylor et al., 1998).

If herpes simplex virus (HSV) is isolated, it is important to evaluate the possibility of autoinoculation, either from oral lesions with gingivostomatitis, or with an intermediate autoinoculation from infection of the digit (herpetic whitlow). The subtype (HSV1, HSV2) alone is not sufficient to determine the source of original herpes simplex infection in a child, although type 1 is more common in the mouth and type 2 in the genital mucosa (Corey, 1983). With this caveat, however, a child presenting with genital herpes necessitates a child protection investigation in most circumstances to determine if the infection was sexually transmitted. Viral culture is the gold standard for identification, although polymerase chain reaction has been used to identify herpesvirus infection. It does not differentiate the herpes simplex virus subtypes (Beards, 1998; Muram & Stewart, 2000).

Molluscum contagiousum (**Figure 6-11**), a common poxvirus infection producing characteristic, pale, umbilicated papules, is self-limiting. Infectivity occurs with contact with an infected person or contaminated objects, and epidermal injury is not a necessary prerequisite for inoculation of the virus (Highet, 1992). Although any area of skin may be affected, it is rare on palms, soles, and mucous membranes. It can be localized to the inner thighs and perineum, causing some concern for sexual abuse. Although this infection is not regarded as a sexually transmitted disease in children, the CDC does categorize molluscum as a sexually transmitted disease in adults. Because of the self-limiting nature of the disease, curettage or cryotherapy is rarely indicated.

Schistosomiasis is another nonsexually transmitted cause of anogenital wart-like lesions. Evidence of infection was recovered in a 12-year-old female with multiple vulvar and perineal warts and a purulent vaginal discharge as well as from a 14-year-old female with a single vulvar wart (Onuigbo et al., 1999). Surgical excision of the warts in both children revealed granulomas containing the terminally spined ova of the worm *Schistosoma haematobium*. Both children were treated with antifungal agents with resolution of their infestations.

Pinworm infestation *(Enterobius vermicularis)* can also be a cause of vulvar bleeding or vulvar and/or anal itching, and can be diagnosed by the characteristic small, white adult worms easily visualized on examination. Symptoms are usually greatest at night when the worms are most active. Alternatively, transparent tape may be applied to the anus to collect any eggs present. The eggs can be visualized on a glass slide by using a low-power light microscope. A similar nuisance infestation is scabies, which may be localized to the anogenital region in addition to the more common areas of

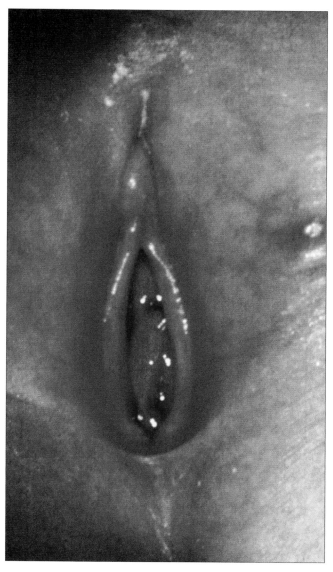
Figure 6-11. *Molluscum contagiousum. (Courtesy of Dr. Lori Frasier, Salt Lake City, Utah)*

the web spaces of fingers, wrists, elbows, axillae, abdomen, and waist. It is characterized by a pruritic, erythematous, papular rash, usually worst during the nighttime hours when the adult female mites are most active.

A retained foreign body, most commonly toilet tissue, is not an uncommon occurrence in children. It is crucial to obtain an optimal examination, which includes visualization into the vagina to rule out the presence of a foreign body, especially when a foul-smelling discharge is observed. Recurrent urinary tract infection should also prompt suspicion of a retained foreign body, as was the case in a 4-year-old girl who had suprapubic pain, dysuria, and urinary frequency. There was no history of foul-smelling discharge or bleeding. A plastic suppository shell, which caused chronic irritation to the bladder, was removed from the posterior vaginal wall (Yu, 1997).

Candidal diaper dermatitis is a common fungal infection in infants with erythema of the vulva and perineum and satellite lesions at the outer aspects of the involved skin. However, candidal vaginitis in the prepubertal child should prompt further evaluation of recent antibiotic use, diabetes mellitus, or altered immune function, because this condition is very unusual in the prepubertal girl (Farrington, 1997).

Key Point:
A broad range of dermatologic and infectious conditions may cause physical findings that mimic findings possible in cases of child sexual abuse. A careful history, a detailed physical examination, and appropriate laboratory/diagnostic testing will help clarify the presence or absence of these conditions.

INFLAMMATORY DISORDERS

Perianal lesions of Crohn's disease have been mistakenly diagnosed as sexual abuse (Stratakis et al., 1994). Skin tags, fissures, thickened perianal skin, fistulas and abscesses, and scarring caused by complications of Crohn's disease can be easily confused with other entities, including sexually transmitted diseases. Anal involvement of Crohn's disease is present in 21% to 72% of affected children (Stratakis et al., 1994). Intestinal manifestations of Crohn's disease may be absent, and vulvar lesions such as erythema, edema, and ulceration may be the first presentation of the disease in children (Schroeder, 2000).

Kawasaki syndrome (mucocutaneous lymph node syndrome) is a vasculitis characterized by fever for 5 or more days and several distinct clinical findings: cervical adenopathy; bilateral conjunctival infection; changes to the mucus membrane such as dry, cracked lips and strawberry anal skin; and changes to the extremities such as edema, erythema, and desquamation. An erythematous rash of the perineum that progresses to desquamation of the region can precede the onset of the more diagnostic findings of Kawasaki syndrome (Hurwitz, 1993b). Given the significance of early diagnosis to avoid the complication of coronary artery aneurysm, prompt treatment is important.

The triad of oral aphthous stomatitis, ulcers of the external genitalia, and inflammatory disease of the eye structures (uveitis, iritis, iridocyclitis) characterizes Behçet's syndrome (Hurwitz, 1993b). Genital ulcers occur in 10% of patients. The ulcers are often painless and may heal with scarring on resolution by 7 to 14 days. Recurrence is common. Often the differential diagnosis includes herpes simplex and syphilis, causing this syndrome to be confused with sexual abuse.

MISCELLANEOUS DISORDERS

Idiopathic calcinosis cutis is a complication of excessive calcium deposition caused by medical conditions, such as collagen vascular diseases or endocrinologic disorders that create an increased calcium state, or occurring idiopathically. The appearance of these lesions (firm, white papules approximately 3 to 10 mm in size) can mimic molluscum contagiosum or genital warts, thus causing concern about the possibility of transmission of a sexually transmitted disease (Bernardo et al., 1999).

Treatment is directed at the underlying cause. If the cause is idiopathic, surgical excision is the recommended treatment. However, spontaneous resolution has been reported.

Disorders of the skin that can be mistakenly attributed to bruising as a result of child maltreatment include erythema multiforme, idiopathic thrombocytopenic purpura and other bleeding diatheses, Henoch-Schönlein purpura, and mongolian spots.

Some conditions may cause urethral bleeding or abnormalities of the urethra, including hemangioma, polyp, ureterocele, and prolapse of the urethra, which can be mistaken for acute trauma. Urethral prolapse (**Figure 6-12**), seen most commonly in prepubertal African-American girls, is often associated with a history of increased intra-abdominal pressure (crying, straining with defecation), which predisposes to the development of prolapse (Bays & Jenny, 1990; Bays, 2001).

Rectal prolapse can be confused with anal trauma and sexual abuse. Predisposing medical conditions include cystic fibrosis, myelomeningocele, prune belly syndrome, or other conditions requiring straining, such as chronic constipation or excessive cough.

Hair tourniquet syndrome, constrictive injuries of the appendages caused by an inconspicuous strand of human hair, is more common on fingers and toes. However, similar injuries can occur on the penis or clitoris, causing significant pain, erythema, and occasional bleeding at the structures, thus raising undue suspicion of child abuse (Rich & Keating, 1999). Because of the inflammation and potential ischemia resulting from the constriction, it is important to remove the encircling strand of hair before any further injury occurs.

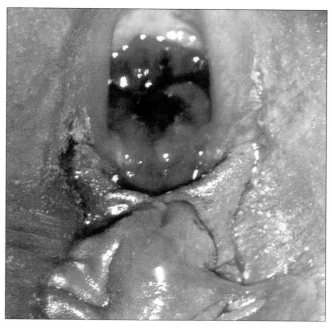

Figure 6-12. Urethral prolapse. (Courtesy of Dr. Mary J. Spencer, Escondido, Calif)

Labial agglutination or fusion of the labia minora is a common problem seen in the infant resulting from any inflammatory condition of the vulvar region, including diaper dermatitis, vulvovaginitis, and urinary tract infection. The denuded labial epithelium becomes agglutinated as the labia closely appose in the diapered child (**Figure 6-13**) (Gibbon et al., 1999). With a peak incidence of approximately 3% in 1-to-2-year-olds, the presence of labial agglutination in the diapered infant is not cause for concern over sexual abuse in this age-group (Leung et al., 1993). In the older school-aged child, however, this phenomenon has been associated with sexual abuse, especially in the Caucasian girl (Berenson et al., 2000), and a focused evaluation should be undertaken in this population.

CONCLUSION

Given the vast array of conditions that may be mistaken for child sexual abuse, it is important to be aware of the differential diagnosis of anogenital conditions mimicking trauma from sexual abuse. An understanding of variations to the normal anogenital anatomy in children is crucial for understanding what is abnormal. The manifestations of nonabusive trauma; dermatologic, infectious, and inflammatory conditions; and other, less common disorders must be considered by the clinician who is evaluating a child for sexual abuse.

REFERENCES

Adams JA. Evolution of a classification scale: medical evaluation of suspected child sexual abuse. *Child Maltreat.* 2001;6:31-36.

Agnarsson U, Warde C, McCarthy G, Evans N. Perianal appearances associated with constipation. *Arch Dis Child.* 1990;65:1231-1234.

American Academy of Pediatrics: Committee on Child Abuse and Neglect. Guidelines for the evaluation of sexual abuse of children. *Pediatrics.* 1999;103:186-191.

Bays J. Conditions mistaken for child sexual abuse. In: Reece M, ed. *Child Abuse: Medical Diagnosis and Management.* 2nd ed. Philadelphia, Pa: Lippincott Williams & Wilkins, 2001:287-306.

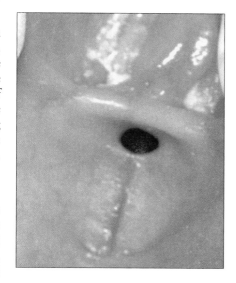

Figure 6-13. Labial agglutination. (Courtesy of Dr. Lori Frasier, Salt Lake City, Utah)

Key Point:
Because genital findings may represent a serious underlying medical condition, it is important to complete a careful differential diagnostic process, considering all possibilities.

Bays J, Jenny C. Genital and anal conditions confused with child sexual abuse trauma. *Am J Dis Child.* 1990;144:1319-1322.

Beards G, Graham C, Pillay D. Investigation of vesicular rashes for HSV and VZV by PCR. *J Med Virol.* 1998;54:155-157.

Berenson AB, Chacko MR, Wiemann CM, Mishaw CO, Friedrich WN, Grady JJ. A case-control study of anatomic changes resulting from sexual abuse. *Am J Obstet Gynecol.* 2000;182:820-834.

Bernardo BD, Huettner PC, Merritt DF, Ratts VS. Idiopathic calcinosis cutis presenting as labial lesions in children: report of two cases with literature review. *J Pediatr Adolesc Gynecol.* 1999;12:157-160.

Black CT, Pokorny WJ, McGill CW, et al. Ano-rectal trauma in children. *J Pediatr Surg.* 1982;17(5):501-504.

Bond GR, Dowd MD, Landsman I, Rimsza M. Unintentional perineal injury in prepubescent girls: a multicenter, prospective report of 56 girls. *Pediatrics.* 1995;95:628-631.

Boyd M, Jordan SW. Unusual presentation of varicella suggestive of sexual abuse. *Am J Dis Child.* 1987;141:940.

Bracco GL, Carli P, Sonni L, et al. Clinical and histologic effects of topical treatments for vulvar lichen sclerosus. *J Reprod Med.* 1993;38:37-40.

Cain WS, Howell CG, Ziegler MM, Finley AJ, Asch MJ, Grant JP. Rectosigmoid perforation and intestinal evisceration from transanal suction. *J Pediatr Surg.* 1983;18:10-13.

Centers for Disease Control. Suction drain injury in a public wading pool—North Carolina, 1991. *MMWR.* 1992;41:333.

Corey L, Adams HG, Brown ZA, et al. Genital herpes simplex virus infections: clinical manifestations, course, and complications. *Ann Intern Med.* 1983;98:973-983.

Dalziel KL, Wojnarowska F. Long term control of vulvar lichen sclerosus after treatment with a potent topical steroid cream. *J Reprod Med.* 1993;38:25-27.

Dodds ML. Vulvar disorders of the infant and young child. *Clin Obstet Gynecol.* 1997;40:141-152.

Dowd MD, Fitzmaurice L, Knapp JF, Mooney D. The interpretation of urogenital findings in children with straddle injuries. *J Pediatr Surg.* 1994;29:7-10.

Farrington PF. Pediatric vulvo-vaginitis. *Clin Obstetr Gynecol.* 1997;40:135-140.

Gibbon KL, Bewley AP, Salisbury JA. Labial fusion in children: a presenting feature of genital lichen sclerosus? *Pediatr Dermatol.* 1999;16:388-391.

Hanks JW, Venters WJ. Nickel allergy from a bed-wetting alarm confused with herpes genitalis and child abuse. *Pediatrics.* 1992;90:458-456.

Highet AS. Molluscum contagiosum. *Arch Dis Child.* 1992;67:1248-1249.

Hurwitz S. Bullous disorders of childhood. In: Hurwitz S, ed. *Clinical Pediatric Dermatology: A Textbook of Skin Disorders of Childhood and Adolescence.* 2nd ed. Philadelphia, Pa: WB Saunders Co; 1993a:446-447.

Hurwitz S. Vasculitic disorders. In: Hurwitz S, ed. *Clinical Pediatric Dermatology: A Textbook of Skin Disorders of Childhood and Adolescence.* 2nd ed. Philadelphia, Pa: WB Saunders Co; 1993b:543-554.

Hurwitz S. Vascular disorders of infancy. In: Hurwitz S, ed. *Clinical Pediatric Dermatology: A Textbook of Skin Disorders of Childhood and Adolescence.* 2nd ed. Philadelphia, Pa: WB Saunders Co; 1993c:243-247.

Hyman SL, Fisher W, Mercugliano M, Cataldo MF. Children with self-injurious behavior. *Pediatrics.* 1990;85:437-441.

Jaquiery A, Stylianopoulos A, Hogg G, Grover S. Vulvovaginitis: clinical features, aetiology, and microbiology of the genital tract. *Arch Dis Child.* 1999;81:64-67.

Kadish HW, Schunk JE, Britton H. Pediatric male rectal and genital trauma: accidental and nonaccidental injuries. *Pediatr Emerg Care.* 1998;14:95-98.

Kellogg ND, Parra JM. Linea vestibularis: a previously undescribed normal genital structure in female neonates. *Pediatrics.* 1991;87:926-929.

Leung AKC, Robson WLM, Tay-Uyboco J. The incidence of labial fusion in children. *J Paediatr Child Health.* 1993;29:235-236.

Levin AV, Selbst SM. Vulvar hemangioma simulating child abuse. *Clin Pediatr.* 1988;27:213-215.

Loening-Baucke V. Lichen sclerosus et atrophicus in children. *Am J Dis Child* 1991;145:1058-1061.

McCann J, Reay D, Siebert J, Stephens BG, Wirtz S. Postmortem perianal findings in children. *Am J Forensic Med Pathol.* 1996;17:289-298.

McCann J, Voris J, Simon M, Wells R. Perianal findings in prepubertal children selected for non-abuse: a descriptive study. *Child Abuse Negl.* 1989;13:179-193.

McCann J, Wells R, Simon, Voris J. Genital findings in prepubertal girls selected for nonabuse: a descriptive study. *Pediatrics.* 1990;86:428-439.

McCune KK, Horbach N, Dattel BJ. Incidence and clinical correlates of human papillomavirus disease in a pediatric population referred for evaluation of sexual abuse. *Adolesc Pediatr Gynecol.* 1993;6:20-24.

Merritt DF. Evaluation of vaginal bleeding in the preadolescent girl. *Pediatr Surg.* 1998;7:35-42.

Mogielnicki NP, Schwartzman JD, Elliott JA. Perineal group A streptococcal disease in a pediatric practice. *Pediatrics.* 2000;106:276-281.

Muram D, Stewart D. Sexually transmitted diseases. In: Heger A, Emans SJ, Muram D, eds. *Evaluation of the Sexually Abused Child.* 2nd ed. New York, NY: Oxford Press; 2000:187-223.

Onuigbo WIB, Anyaeze CM, Ozumba BC. Sexual abuse simulated by schistosomiasis. *Child Abuse Negl.* 1999;23:947-949.

Persaud DI, Squires J. Genital papillomavirus infection: clinical progression after varicella infection. *Pediatrics.* 1997;100:408-412.

Powell J, Wojnarowska F. Childhood lichen sclerosus and sexual abuse are not mutually exclusive diagnoses. *BMJ.* 2000;320:311.

Rich MA, Keating MA. Hair tourniquet syndrome of the clitoris. *J Urol.* 1999;162:190-191.

Schroeder B. Vulvar disorders in adolescents. *Obsetr Gynecol Clin North Am.* 2000;27:35-48.

Siegfried EC, Frasier LD. Anogenital skin diseases of childhood. *Pediatr Ann.* 1997;26:322-331.

Stevens-Simon C, Nelligan D, Breese P, Jenny C, Douglas JM. The prevalence of genital human papillomavirus infections in abused and nonabused preadolescent girls. *Pediatrics.* 2000;106:645-649.

Stratakis CA, Graham W, DiPalma J, Leibowitz I. Misdiagnosis of perianal manifestations of Crohn's disease. *Clin Pediatr.* 1994;33:631-633.

Taylor S, Drake SM, Dedicoat M, Wood MJ. Genital ulcers associated with acute Epstein-Barr virus infection. *Sex Transm Infect.* 1998;74:296-297.

Wood PL, Bevan T. Lesson of the week: child sexual abuse enquiries and unrecognised vulval lichen sclerosus et atrophicus. *BMJ.* 1999;319:899-890.

Yu TJ. Urinary tract infection with a neglected vaginal foreign body. *J Urol.* 1997;157:1475-1476.

Chapter 7

Screening for and Treatment of Sexual Abuse Histories in Boys and Male Adolescents

William C. Holmes, MD, MSCE

Introduction

The sexual abuse of boys and male adolescents is not uncommon, yet the discourse surrounding childhood sexual abuse often addresses males in a separate chapter, a paragraph of disclaimer, a footnote, or not at all. This marginalization of male sexual abuse minimizes the clinical problem in a way that does not reflect reality, an unfortunate process readily perceived by abused boys. Clinicians who are part of this pervasive dynamic become, often through no fault of their own, complicit in the silence of abused boys. Silence begets silence, a cycle fed by ignorance as well as fears about male victimhood and male sexuality. This chapter specifically focuses on the problem of male sexual abuse and the clinician's role in identifying histories of sexual abuse in young male patients, as well as the information needed when responding to disclosure and when referring patients for treatment.

The Problem

To roughly estimate how underrepresented male sexual abuse is, publications on sexual abuse cited in OVID-MEDLINE from 1995 to 2000 were identified using the search term "sexual abuse," and limited to English language and age less than 19 years. The search was further restricted by placing "male" and "female" limits on results. A total of 749 citations were found after limiting the set with "male," compared with 1190 citations found after limiting the set with "female," indicating that, at best, 6 publications about sexual abuse of young boys and adolescent males exist for every 10 publications about sexual abuse of young girls and adolescent females. The actual ratio is considerably less. Many publications identified with the search term "sexual abuse" and limited by the term "male" report on the sexual abuse of females perpetrated by males. Many also report findings about small subsamples of males subsumed within much larger subsamples of females, making the unique characteristics surrounding sexual abuse of males unidentifiable. A review of the literature in 1998 that surveyed research from the preceding 15 years identified only 166 publications that reported on 149 samples that included at least 20 males and reported results for males separately (Holmes & Slap, 1998). This number is considerably less than the 749 citations found in the Internet search noted above. A relative paucity of information, then, is a major challenge inherent in alerting clinicians to unique aspects of male sexual abuse. Added to this is the larger challenge of cultural pressures surrounding masculine gender socialization.

Understanding the cultural norms of masculine gender socialization is the first task to pursue when examining the issues surrounding sexually abused boys and male adolescents. These cultural norms are often at their peak influence when abuse occurs in boys' lives, determining not only how the boys respond to the abuse they have experienced, but also how family, friends, clinicians, and law enforcement personnel respond to the abuse history when it is disclosed or, more often, when feeling threatened with its imminent disclosure. Discomfort and sometimes outright silencing of young males who seek disclosure are routine. These responses emanate from fear regarding open discussions of male sexuality, lack of knowledge about the actuality of male victimization, and disorientation resulting from disruptions of beliefs about normative behavior operating within the central tenets of masculine identity.

Key Point:
Understanding the cultural norms of masculine gender socialization is the first task in examining issues concerning sexually abused boys and male adolescents. One of the core moves in male gender socialization is the movement away from the feminine.

At its core, the process of male gender socialization requires the boy to move away from the feminine, an act that moves the boy away from mother, female caregiver, and the ubiquitous presence of female teacher (48 of 49 teachers in primary schools are women, and after-school programs to which many children go are staffed primarily by women). Since at least half of children grow up in fatherless homes, and fewer than 15% of children who grow up in homes with a father present receive any amount of primary caregiving from their fathers, the person(s) and role model(s) to whom boys turn when they move away from the feminine are absent (Jolliff & Horne, 1999; Smith, 2000).

Disregard of the feminine and absent masculine role modeling leads to boys' maturational progress being heavily guided by surrounding cultural phenomena. Reports by the national child advocacy organization, Children Now, describe how television, a substantial presence in the lives of children, helps to define masculinity (Heintz-Knowles et al., 1999; Massna et al., 1999). In a national poll, three fourths of children aged 10 to 17 years described males on television as violent. More than two-thirds described them as angry. Children did not think that "sensitive" was a word that could be used to describe television's male characters. In a sampling of the shows these children reported watching, some level of violence appeared in over half of the television shows and movies most popular among adolescent boys. Three fourths of males in the programs and movies sampled performed antisocial behaviors such as ridiculing, lying, and engaging in aggressive or defiant acts. Sports commentators consistently used the language of war, martial arts, and weaponry to describe sports action. Traditionally masculine images of speed, danger, and aggression were often used in the commercials shown during programs boys watched. Regardless of circumstances, men did not cry.

Pollack (1998) calls the male gender socialization process propagated by cultural representations, absent fathers, and rejection of the feminine the "Boy Code." Pollack describes four injunctions of this code: the "sturdy oak" injunction; the "give 'em hell" injunction; the "big wheel" injunction; and the "no sissy stuff" injunction. The sturdy oak is stoic, stable, and independent. Boys are not to share pain or grieve openly. They are to be confident when they feel afraid, certain when uncertain, and independent when desperate for love, attention, and support. Meanwhile, they should "give 'em hell." They should be macho, high-energy, and violent supermen, all while being strikingly cool, presenting the front of a "big wheel." Everything is going all right, everything is under control, even if it isn't. If these injunctions have not provided enough structure for maintaining the Code, the final straitjacket is the prohibition against expressing feelings or urges seen as "feminine" —no sissy stuff. No dependence, no warmth, no empathy. Those who break this final injunction are met with ridicule, taunts, and shame-inducing epithets. They are "girls" and/or "faggots." Combined, these injunctions often push boys to live in painful silence, full of repression, denial, and limitation, pursuing only what the culture expects of and for them.

This is the case for those boys unchallenged by other, external forces. What happens when an act of sexual abuse occurs? If the abuse is at the hands of a male perpetrator, how is the boy to disclose having participated in a homosexual act when avoidance of homosexuality at any cost is an overriding concern of one who is living inside the Code? How does he explain to himself the fear response of his own body that resulted in an erection during the abuse episode? How does he talk about the pain of anal rape? He is not to feel pain, and if he does, he is not to express it. He is not to identify himself to others as being allied in any way with the feminine, and worse, certainly not in any way that would be perversely misidentified within the frame of abuse as a male lover of males. If the abuse is at the hands of a female perpetrator, how is the boy to disclose pained expressions of confusion, ambivalence, or distress? When the successful culmination of the Code is sex with a woman, how does a boy configure abuse by a woman as victimizing, particularly if the abuser physically pleasured the boy, engendering a sense of complicity clouded by desire? Unlike the female child/adolescent in such a situation, we accord greater importance to the response and actions of the male body than to the cognitive level of development of the male child and adolescent. The Code says that the male body supercedes his mind. The mind attached to the body is further restricted from identifying as victim by the culture ascribing solely to femininity the role of the victim. And, how, if the female perpetrator is the boy's mother, does he report her when she is his primary caregiver and his father is absent?

This is the lived position of most boys and male adolescents who are survivors of sexual abuse. This is the boy or male adolescent who sits across from the clinician in the examination room. He is hiding truth, protecting himself and the clinician from the tumult of upending cultural constructions of the masculine. He desperately wants someone to help him, to protect him, to heal him, but he desperately fears disclosing to the healthcare provider how flawed he is. Many clinicians might suspect his secret, but also seek the comfort of hiding (Holmes & Offen, 1996). Clinicians are, after all, equal participants in the culture and perpetuators of the Code.

The literature does not support an assumption of male invulnerability. Studies of boys and male adolescents, most of which were completed in junior to high school samples, report sexual abuse history rates of 4% to 16% (Bagley et al., 1995; Boney-McCoy & Finkelhor, 1995a; Harrison et al., 1997; Hernandez et al., 1993; Hibbard et al., 1990; Kohan et al., 1987; Lodico et al., 1996; Nagy et al., 1994; Nelson et al., 1994; Risin & Koss, 1987; Siegel et al., 1987). Nelson et al. (1994) report a rate of abuse occurring in the prior week of 2% in 9th to 12th grade boys. One large-scale, nationally representative study of the incidence of sexual abuse in boys and male adolescents was completed in 1986 and found an incidence rate of one (SE, 0.31) per 1000 (Cappelleri et al., 1993). Studies of adult men from the general population confirm that rates in the upper half of the range reported above are most likely. Large, random-sample, US and Canadian studies (the first completed by telephone, the second house-to-house) report rates of childhood sexual abuse histories in adult men to be 7% (Canada) to 16% (United States) (Finkelhor et al., 1990; MacMillan et al., 1997). These results not only can be considered to be representative of general populations of adult men, they also can be considered to be referable to general populations of boys and male adolescents (who are living through the time period for which historical information was gathered from adult men in the noted studies). As many as 1 in 6 boys coming to a pediatrician's office, then, may have had some type of sexual abuse experience; 1 in 50 male adolescents may have been abused in just the previous week.

Sexual abuse experienced by boys and male adolescents includes both non-contact and contact interactions. Non-contact interactions can occur in many forms. Exhibitionism includes someone exposing himself/herself to the boy; engaging in some sort of sexual activity, from masturbation to intercourse, in front of the boy; asking or forcing the boy to expose himself; asking or forcing the boy to engage in some sort of sexual activity in front of the perpetrator(s) or a camera; or some

Key Point:
Non contact interactions can vary from exhibitionism to verbally or visually stimulating the boy sexually via a pornographic medium. Contact abuse does not necessarily mean direct physical touching. Non-contact interactions can culminate in touching of the boy's genitals or other eroticized body parts through clothing. Eroticized or frankly sexualized body-to-body contact with clothing on is also contact abuse.

combination of these activities. Non-contact interactions may involve verbally or visually stimulating the boy sexually via a pornographic medium (ie, reading pornographic materials to him, showing him pornographic pictures or video). Contact abuse does not necessarily require actual touching of the skin. Non-contact interactions described above (i.e., visual stimulation) that culminate with the perpetrator touching the boy's genitals or other eroticized body parts through clothing are contact abuse. Eroticized or frankly sexualized body to body contact, with clothing on, is contact abuse. Other contact abuse includes a range of activities: deep kissing; prolonged, eroticized, or frankly sexualized touch; manual-genital contact of or by the perpetrator; orogenital contact of or by the perpetrator; oroanal contact of or by the perpetrator; anal penetration of the victim or perpetrator; and vaginal penetration of the perpetrator. Penetration of the boy can include entry by another's penis into the boy's mouth or anus. However, penetration also can be accomplished using fingers or other objects, and thus can occur with a female perpetrator, indicating that questions about penetrative activity should be asked regardless of the sex of the perpetrator.

Male victims report that three or more types of the aforementioned sexually abusive acts occur during a "typical" abusive experience (Pierce & Pierce, 1985). Fondling by and of the perpetrator is the most frequently reported act (55% to 91% of cases) (Ellason et al., 1996; Finkelhor et al., 1990; Kendall-Tackett & Simon, 1992; Lenderking et al., 1997; McClellan et al., 1997; Moisan et al., 1997; Schulte et al., 1995).

Anal penetration is the next most frequently reported act (37% to 70% of cases in a majority of reports) (Cupoli & Sewell, 1988; Doll et al., 1992; Ellason et al., 1996; Finkelhor et al., 1990; Fromuth & Burkhart, 1987; Holmes, 1997; Hunter, 1991; Huston et al., 1995; Hutchings & Dutton, 1993; Kendall-Tackett & Simon, 1992; Lenderking et al., 1997; McClellan et al., 1997; McCormack et al., 1992; Moisan et al., 1997; Reinhart, 1987; Risin & Koss, 1987; Roane, 1992; Robin et al., 1997b; Sarwer et al., 1997; Whiffen & Clark, 1997).

Orogenital contact occurs at rates (12% to 55%) somewhat lower than those for penetration: 15% to 38% of victims report being fellated, and 12% to 35% of victims report being forced to perform fellatio or cunnilingus (Cupoli & Sewell, 1988; Doll et al., 1992; Ellason et al., 1996; Fromuth & Burkhart, 1987; Holmes, 1997; Huston et al., 1995; Kendall-Tackett & Simon, 1992; McClellan et al., 1997; Moisan et al., 1997; Pierce & Pierce, 1985; Reinhart, 1987; Roane, 1992; Schulte et al., 1995).

Knowing this information and being able to discuss it frankly with boys and male adolescents who have experienced such activity is important. Understanding of the types of acts that can happen to a boy, rather than discomforting confusion about what a boy is trying to explain in his less cognitively adept language, is critical. Armed with knowledge, the physician, nurse, or other healthcare provider can play the crucial roles of listening attentively, understanding disclosures, helping boys to break their gnawing silence, and shepherding them into care.

THE SOLUTION

Because spontaneous disclosure and discovery of sexual abuse is uncommon in boys, the mode of presentation assumed in the type of evaluation described in Chapter 3 will be infrequent in boys, especially in older boys. Thus a screening strategy is very important if abuse histories are to be identified and appropriately managed clinically.

The healthcare provider's office is the place where boys are most likely to be seen, usually at least yearly, and where questions frequently are asked, answers anticipated, and examinations performed. Acute, chronic, and preventive care occur at the healthcare office. Much of the standardized preventive care that occurs during routine healthcare visits do not focus on problems that affect up to 1 in 6 children. This provides the first argument for considering routine screening of abuse and violence in the life of boys. If any question remains, consider the fact that in an average year, approximately 400,000 boys under age 18 years are victims of physical abuse or neglect, 80,000 boys are arrested for having run away from home, 4500 boys commit suicide, and 3000 boys are murdered (Kiselica & Horne, 1990). Abuse and violence screening in boys and male adolescents should be standard operating procedure.

How Should Providers Do This?

The provider must begin by creating an environment that demonstrates willingness to consider male sexual abuse as a common reality. This more indirect method can set the stage for conversations that may not even require active, verbal screening on the part of the provider. One of the best routes for doing this is to have reading material in the waiting room. A number of books present male characters as potential or actual victims of sexual abuse. A provider should include these books in the waiting room in addition to books that have female characters. Three examples of books that span pediatric age groups are:

— *Stranger Safety* (ages 3 to 5 years; Roo Publications, St. Petersburg, Fla; $4.95)
— *The Right Touch* (ages 6 to 9 years; Illumination Arts Publishing Company, Bellevue, Wash; $15.95)
— *The Paper Knife* (ages 10 to 18; iUniverse.com, Inc., Lincoln, Neb; $14.95)

Direct, verbal screening is the next step. This questioning should take place within the safety of a private, clinical interaction, not only on a paper screening form completed by the patient or his parent in the waiting room. Although using forms to screen for abuse histories is another way to help create an environment that is conducive to detection of unidentified abuse, direct questioning in the clinical interaction is critical because some individuals would not be comfortable acknowledging abuse histories on a form that could be seen by many individuals other than the provider. As the developmental status of the boy allows, direct questioning should occur with the boy or male adolescent alone. These expectations should be made clear to the parent/caregiver and the child at the outset of the interview: "The way I work with my patients is to speak with them and their parents first, and then, to take some time when just the two of us — the child and I — sit and talk, about their health, about their life." The nervous parent/caregiver can be provided a seat right outside the closed door if necessary, but a time for private conversation, during which direct screening can occur, usually is crucial. It tells the boy that he has independent agency, creating an environment that empowers him to disclose sensitive information from which he may be protecting his parent/caregiver (or his parent/caregiver may be seeking to keep private).

Whenever the provider asks abuse- and/or violence-related screening questions, it is often helpful to provide an explanatory and normalizing introduction. For example, he or she might say, "I'm finding out that boys experience abuse and violence in their lives more than I thought, so I've begun to ask all the boys in my practice about these kinds of experiences. Some boys tell me that bad things do happen to them. They might have been beaten up badly by someone, just once or more regularly. Someone might have touched their body in a sexual way or done some other sort of sexual thing to them, sometimes by force, that they didn't want to have happen. Has this ever happened to you?" Sitting quietly while waiting for a response is often the best tactic. Despite the fact that tension may build and be uncomfortable, distraction with jokes and/or other humorous asides is strongly discouraged. The provider must remain outside the confines of what the Boy Code requires.

The provider should anticipate an immediate "no" response from most boys. This does not mean, however, that the nay-saying boy or male adolescent has not experienced any of these types of events. The provider's response, then, should not be to say, "good," or any other emphatic, rewarding-of-silence judgment on a "no" answer. This is not to suggest that the provider should be disappointed the boy has not been abused or that he or she should encourage the manufacturing of histories when none exist. Rather, this recommendation highlights the need to recognize that both boys and the practitioner may prefer silence to the discomfort of disclosure. In response to a "no" answer, then, the provider should project an "open door" policy. For example, he or she might say, "if anything like this has ever happened to you, and you're just not ready to tell me, or if it were to happen to you in the future, I want you to know that you can talk to me about it at any time. In fact, I'm asking you to talk with me about it. That would be one sure way to begin working through all the feelings and challenges that an experience like that causes for kids your age. This is true for your friends as well. If you know another boy who has been abused in some way, encourage him to talk to his doctor about it." This is not leading or encouraging the boy to admit to abuse that did not happen; rather, it seeks to counteract the tendency of boys to deny, defer, dissuade, distract, and deligitimize when confronted by their own histories.

The screening questions should be asked at each visit. Boys in particular need this; their reluctance to disclose victimizing experiences requires vigilant, sensitive inquiry that communicates to them that someone cares, someone will listen, and someone will take action on their behalf. This subtle education can even be lighthearted and become direct in the process; for example, a provider might say, "Here's that annoying part of the visit when I always ask about abuse and violence. You know why I always ask about this don't you? Abuse happens to boys, too, but they often are too embarrassed to talk about it . . . so, I like to make sure that the boys I take care of know that they never need to be worried about that with me. They should not be embarrassed to talk with me about bad things that have happened to them." With this diligent, sensitive, caring inquiry, the abused boy finally may disclose. However, it should be remembered that boys who have finally decided to disclose still may do so initially with indirect, imprecise language, referring generically, for example, to "a lot of family stress" (Froning & Mayman, 1990). The provider must listen carefully to boys' answers. As important as the answers may be for what they say, the answers may be equally important for what they do not say.

If a boy and/or male adolescent discloses an abusive history in response to screening, a nonjudgmental, validating, empowering, and advocating comment (or series of comments) should be the provider's first response. A number of possible comments are applicable in this situation:

1. "I think you are a brave person to have told me what you did. It's like what a superhero would do, and I'm particularly glad you did because I can help you."
2. "I'm sorry this happened to you."
3. "It was not your fault."
4. "I'm here to help you."
5. "It's my job, along with your family member [family member's name], to make sure you are safe from now on."

These initial comments are important in response to disclosure: they affirm the boy's decision to tell and the provider's willingness to help. They also provide a supportive environment during a time when the boy may not remember many of the specifics of what is said in response to his disclosure, unless, of course, the comments are in some way pejorative or make him feel sorry he has disclosed. Unfortunately, the boy will always remember negative comments or words that discourage further disclosure. The immediate aftermath of disclosure is often full of ambivalence: fear, regret, exhilaration, anticipation, worry, loss, relief, happiness that someone finally knows, anxiety about what the future holds, and so forth. These feelings may be coupled with bodily symptoms, such as tachycardia, sweating, dizziness, or blushing, that may require a few minutes to resolve before continuing with additional history taking and examination. The provider might, again, be kindly forthright with the boy, stating, "I see that this is very upsetting for you to talk about. I admire how strong you have been in deciding to tell me. I would like to ask you some additional questions about what you have just told me, but I was wondering if you would like me to ask you some questions about other things first, then talk about the abuse in a few minutes?"

If the boy prefers, the provider should proceed with simple questioning about other topics such as school, friends, home life, family relationships, and so forth. Although these clearly are not difficult descriptions of the abusive experience, they all are areas that can be affected in the aftermath of abuse. They are important, although less challenging, aspects of the history. The provider should be carefully attuned to detecting reported changes in these areas of the boy's life. The provider also might ask about more health-related issues even if he or she has already done so. These could focus on risky activities, such as drug and alcohol use, sexual behavior with peers, perpetration of violence on others, gang participation, or other types of risky activities. Boys and male adolescents who have been sexually abused report much higher rates of these types of potential abuse-related outcomes.

An association between sexual abuse and substance use, for example, has been consistently reported (Bartholow et al., 1994; Dembo et al., 1987; Dembo et al., 1989, 1990; Embree & DeWit, 1997; Hernandez et al., 1993; Hibbard et al., 1990; Hussey et al., 1992; Nagy et al., 1994; Nelson et al., 1994; Robin et al., 1997a, 1997b; Schulte et al., 1995; Simpson et al., 1994; Windle et al., 1995). Sixth grade boys who were either sexually abused or both physically and sexually abused report rates of multi-substance abuse that are 12 and 44 times higher than non-abused boys ($p<0.0000005$); twelfth grade boys from the same groupings report rates that are 3 and 10 times higher ($p<0.0000005$) (Harrison et al., 1997). Nagy et al. (1994) concur, documenting that sexually abused high school boys are two times more likely than non-abused high school boys to use alcohol currently and five times more likely to use drugs currently ($p<0.05$). Nelson et al. (1994) indicate current use of alcohol, marijuana, and cocaine by abused versus non-abused boys are two, four, and ten times higher ($p<0.001$), respectively. The rate of injection drug use may be higher in abused versus non-abused boys as well, and its use appears to begin in adolescence for boys who have been sexually abused (Bartholow et al., 1994; Holmes, 1998; Zierler et al., 1991).

Proportionally more abused than non-abused males also report difficulty controlling sexual feelings and are more likely to perpetrate coercive sexual acts against others (Becker & Stein, 1991; Burgess et al., 1988; Freund et al., 1990; Fromuth et al., 1991; Hernandez et al., 1993; Hussey et al., 1992; Janus et al., 1987; Langevin et al., 1989; Lodico et al., 1996; McClellan et al., 1997; McCormack et al., 1992; Roane, 1992; Rubinstein et al., 1993; Sansonnet-Hayden et al., 1987; Stevenson & Gajarsky, 1991; Violato & Genuis, 1993; Worling, 1995a, 1995b). Abused males also note engaging more frequently in high-risk sexual behaviors such as prostitution and unprotected anal intercourse (Bartholow et al., 1994; Burgess et al., 1987; Carballo-Dieguez & Dolezal, 1995; Lenderking et al., 1997; Zierler et al., 1991). They have more lifetime sexual partners, use condoms less frequently, and have higher rates of sexually transmitted diseases and unintended pregnancy in their partner(s) (Bartholow et al., 1994; Lenderking et al., 1997; Nagy et al., 1994; Nelson et al., 1994; Resnick & Blum, 1994; Weber et al., 1992; Zierler et al., 1991). These difficulties may be present soon after abuse begins; however, they can be latent for an extended time, and may begin, recrudesce, or become worse during puberty, even in boys who were abused years before entry into adolescence.

Key Point:

If the boy is uncomfortable, proceed with simple questions concerning other topics, such as school, friends, home life, family relationships, etc. During this questioning, be aware that relationships have been found between sexual abuse and substance use, difficulty controlling sexual feelings, coercive behavior, PTSD, major depression, anxiety disorders, borderline personality disorder, antisocial personality disorder, paranoia, dissociation, somatization, bulimia, anger, aggressive behavior, poor self-image, poor school performance, running away from home, self-destructive tendencies, and legal problems. If these arise during further questioning, consider them red flags.

Outcomes also are thought to include more frequent problems with coercive behavior, posttraumatic stress disorder (PTSD), major depression, anxiety disorders, borderline personality disorder, antisocial personality disorder, paranoia, dissociation, somatization, bulimia, anger, aggressive behavior, poor self-image, poor school performance, running away from home, and legal trouble (Bagley et al., 1995; Bartholow et al., 1994; Boney-McCoy & Finkelhor, 1995b; Briere et al., 1988; Brown et al., 1997; Burgess et al., 1987; Friedrich & Schafer, 1995; Gibby-Smith, 1995; Harrison et al., 1990; Hernandez et al., 1993; Hibbard & Hartman, 1992; Hibbard et al., 1990; Hunter, 1991; Hussey et al., 1992; Janus et al., 1987; Langevin et al., 1989; Moisan et al., 1997; Nagy et al., 1994; Nelson et al., 1994; Paris et al., 1994; Remafedi et al., 1991; Resnick & Blum, 1994; Robin et al., 1997b; Roesler & McKenzie, 1994; Rosen & Martin, 1996; Schulte et al., 1995; Whiffen & Clark, 1997; Windle et al., 1995; Wolfe et al., 1994). Self-destructive tendencies may be best indicated by a rate of suicide attempts that is 1.5 to 14 times higher in sexually abused than non-abused males (Bagley et al., 1995; Bartholow et al., 1994; Boudewyn & Liem, 1995; Briere et al., 1988; Brown & Anderson, 1991; Deykin & Buka, 1994; Harrison et al., 1990; Hernandez et al., 1993; Langevin et al., 1989; Nagy et al., 1994; Nelson et al., 1994; Remafedi et al., 1991; Resnick & Blum, 1994; Windle et al., 1995).

Although simple questions about things other than the abuse experience(s) are intended to be momentarily diversionary for the boy by highlighting friendly conversation and building trust, a potential foundation of information can begin to be built. The information may reveal many areas for concern. Counsel about this concern may best be delayed until future clinical encounters occur unless the behavior is life threatening. Whenever counseling does occur, however, the provider should avoid shame-based approaches to risk-prevention. Abused boys' shame is substantial enough without adding to it.

As the conversation or time dictates, the provider will need to reintroduce the subject of the abuse. The boy's feelings should be acknowledged when doing this: "I'm going to bring us back to the subject of the abuse. I know this may not be easy for you. When I have talked to other patients of mine about the abuse they experienced, it was not uncommon for them to feel a little embarrassed about it. Just as I assured them, I will assure you now, that I'm comfortable with whatever you feel you are able to tell me. I may ask you some questions about things that you may not be ready to talk about. If you would rather not talk about it now, I would like for you to say that rather than tell me something that isn't true. We can talk about that particularly embarrassing thing at some future visit. If you think you can manage to tell me the answer to my question, however, even though you're scared and nervous and embarrassed, I promise I will respect your feelings to go slow or take a break if you need that. Okay? . . . How do you feel, so far, about talking about this with me?" Acknowledging the boy's possible discomfort while being direct about what the provider is going to talk about next and assuring the boy that the provider is comfortable talking about the subject of sexual abuse may help to initiate a sense of trust. Counteracting what the boy has learned from the Code, these kind of statements will tell him that his feelings are important and that the provider is not only interested in but also able to handle feelings the boy may find frighteningly powerful. The Code is robust, however; one should assume that counteracting it, while maintaining trust, will require an ongoing process.

The next step is to establish a common ground with regard to use of names for different body parts. Boys and male adolescents should not be expected to use formal words for body parts (Levitt, 1990). As with the other items on the agenda so far, this issue is broached in a direct way. The provider might begin by saying, "Different people have different names for body parts and I'm okay with that.

Because I'm a doctor, I tend to use words like 'penis' when I'm talking about a 'penis,' but other people sometimes use other words. Some kids I see here have talked about their 'dick' instead of using the fancy word 'penis.' The same is true for other body parts, whether they're boys' and men's or girls' and women's—body parts, and for words about things people do with their body parts, such as sexual things. I want you to know I'm comfortable with whatever words you use for anything . . . but I also want you to know that I might need to ask sometimes what a particular word means. Okay?" Another suggestion is to show the boy anatomical dolls or to draw pictures, using these guides to ask the boy for his preferred words for different body parts. Boys too shy to use anatomical words may point to the pictures as they describe what happened with parts of the body (Levitt, 1990). These approaches indicate to the child that his agency, in the context of discussing these highly charged events, is paramount.

As one progresses to the details of who did what to whom when, the provider must remember that the process of disclosure may occur in stages, with only a scant structure of the story originally disclosed. The clinician should be empathic when necessary, but should not be visibly, overly emotive in response to the specifics of disclosure, especially during the initial stages of disclosure. The boy's own emotions may be overwhelming enough for him without his feeling some sense of responsibility for someone else's emotions. The focus should be on acknowledging the boy's experience: "That must have been scary for you." Furthermore, when asking follow-up questions or reflecting back to the boy what the provider has heard, the provider should be careful about labeling sexual acts, because any signs of discomfort or potentially pejorative labeling of interactions (i.e., "homosexual") may interfere with the process of disclosure. For example, instead of saying, "Did he perform homosexual acts on you?" a physician might provide a descriptive prompt, "Did he put his penis into the place where your bowel movements come out?"

Key Point:
The focus should remain on acknowledging the boy's experience.

References to male perpetrators in some of the prior examples is not meant to imply that most sexual abuse of boys and male adolescents is at the hands of other males. This is not known with certainty. Large-sample studies report that anywhere from 53% to 94% of perpetrators are male. Some studies suggest that a large number of female perpetrators may exist, some of whom appear to be adolescent-aged baby-sitters (Doll et al., 1992; Finkelhor et al., 1990; Risin & Koss, 1987; Ryan et al., 1996). Some smaller-sample studies of older adolescents and young adults report ranges with even lower rates of male perpetrator abuse (22% to 73%), indicating rates of female perpetrator abuse that are as high as 78% (Formuth & Burkhart, 1987; Johnson & Shrier, 1987; Moisan et al., 1997; Rubinstein et al., 1993; Violato & Genuis, 1993). Adult sample studies, however, often report higher male perpetrator rates, ranging from 63% to 90% (Carballo-Dieguez & Dolezal, 1995; Holmes, 1997; Hunter, 1991; Hutchings & Dutton, 1993; Nuttall & Jackson, 1994; Okami, 1991; Roesler & McKenzie, 1994). These data may indicate that boys and male adolescents may revise their perceptions of abuse as they age.

Representations of sexual interactions operating within power structures that would be considered abusive if the sexes of the perpetrator and abused were switched not only exist within the culture, they are thought to be dramatically compelling or, alternatively, funny. Gartner (1999) illustrates this cultural trend with a New Yorker cartoon published in August 25, 1997. In the cartoon, a boy about 10 or 11 years old lies in bed with an older woman, at least in her twenties, and both are smoking. The boy says, "I want you to know that I've always felt that you were more to me than just a babysitter." Such representations of male sexual abuse teach boys that what they may have perceived to be abuse is desirable behavior, especially when committed by a woman. Comparable depictions of sexual abuse of girls by men are more likely to be considered offensive or even pornographic. Although a boy's experience may have been traumatizing to him, he is encouraged to be proud about the interaction or to see it as funny, interesting, or some other variation of a compelling life event, certainly not as illegal. All of this adds to the confusion that he may be experiencing as a result of event-related arousal and even pleasure. Abusive sexual experiences with female perpetrators often may become defined, concurrently or retrospectively, then, as normative rather than abusive.

It is also uncertain whether most individuals who sexually abuse males come from within or outside the family. Most large-sample studies report that over half of perpetrators are extra-familial and that perhaps well under half of these are not known to victims (Doll et al., 1992; Finkelhor et al., 1990; Hernandez et al., 1993; Lodico et al., 1996; Risin & Koss, 1987; Siegel et al., 1987). So, the majority of perpetrators, then, appear to be located outside the family, and to be known by the boy. The age of the boy appears to be a factor in whether or not the perpetrator has a prior relationship to the boy. Young boys under the age of 6 years are at comparatively greater risk for abuse by family members and acquaintances, whereas older boys over 12 years old are at comparatively greater risk for abuse by someone outside the family, particularly by strangers (Doll et al., 1992; Faller, 1989; Gordon, 1990).

Key Point:
Do not assume the sex of the perpetrator or the identity during questioning of the boy.

Consequently, in their questioning, healthcare providers should assume neither the sex nor the identity of the perpetrator. They should do their best not to perpetuate the misperceptions of boys who have been sexually abused by female perpetrators, perhaps stressing in their educational comments about abuse and violence that perpetrators can be anyone: male or female; a person who looks the same as the child or different; an individual who is known or unknown; or someone from inside or outside the family. This caution goes beyond concerns related to screening and follow-up questioning in the event of disclosure because notes from a clinical encounter can be useful in legal proceedings, and pejorative questioning may be particularly unhelpful in this regard.

A physician's testimony in court may be allowed as evidence, which is an exception to the usual hearsay rule (Levitt, 1990). Testimony is more likely to be admissible if discussions are not leading in any way, and are documented with extreme specificity and precision. Readable notes are very helpful in this regard, and audio- and/or videotaping of the interview may also be useful. The boy's willingness to fully disclose may be hampered by audio- or videotaping, however, so their potential effect should be considered fully. Taking notes during the midst of a particularly difficult disclosure might even be a substantial interference. However, legal concerns make taking notes appropriate. Therefore, thorough explanation should be provided to the boy as to why documentation is necessary, as well as to what precautions will be taken to ensure confidentiality. If note taking becomes too intrusive, giving the boy uninterrupted attention during disclosure and affirming his care and safety are paramount. Whether notes are written during or soon after disclosure, they should document the child's demeanor throughout the clinical encounter. They also should document what things were disclosed spontaneously. The provider should note what questions were asked by whom and whether answers were spontaneous, hesitant, or completely not forthcoming. It is necessary to identify who else was present in the room and any role they played in asking questions or retrieving and/or formulating answers.

At some point in the discussion following disclosure, the provider should make it clear that he or she is required by law to report known sexual abuse of a minor. Mandated reporting laws differ by state, but "minor" is usually defined as someone less than age 18 years. This is a particularly challenging issue for boys and male adolescents who have finally managed to resolve their embarrassment, shame, and fear enough to allow themselves to disclose to a trusted provider. They may be disturbed that their "secret" must now be reported to a bureaucratic structure that may initiate further proceedings with the potential for disclosing what they have kept hidden to the very people they least want to know that they have broken the silence. There are contingencies that surround mandated reporting that can be discussed and resolved with the boy and/or his protective caregiver. Any plan for reporting the abuse must ensure the safety of the boy and that no further abuse will occur, and must be documented by the provider. When the boy was last abused, by whom, where the perpetrator currently resides, and what protective structures are in place to avoid future abuse are all questions that must be answered as part of this discussion.

These questions can also be a nice entry into discussion about overprotection, a threat to independence that sometimes results from disclosure of abuse. Fear of overprotection and further loss of independence may act as a deterrent to continuing discussion of what happened and the ongoing emotional and psychologic consequences.

In addition to the patient who has made a spontaneous disclosure, there are some other scenarios that may occur in a pediatrician's office that should be mentioned. Some providers may be asked to assess a boy who has already made a disclosure to the police or to a social service agency. The provider should review any records (such as social work or social agency reports) about the event(s) of abuse before seeing the boy. The provider should be familiar with as many details of the allegations as possible (Levitt, 1990). The provider should meet briefly with the parent(s) alone. The provider should find out what the parent(s) know(s). Because the parent(s) may not know about the disclosures, it is best to not volunteer this information. The provider should find out what their concerns are and ask for their perception of why they are there. Similar to the spontaneous disclosure scenario described above, it is appropriate to speak next to the boy or male adolescent alone. The interviewer can start the same way, by asking him for his perception of why he is there. Otherwise, recommendations about how to proceed with discussions of abuse experiences that are spontaneously disclosed should be followed, although they should be altered in accordance with the contingencies of the event(s) being discussed (i.e., recency of abuse, identity of perpetrator, who has requested provider's involvement, and why). If referral to the current provider has been made, for example, to clarify allegations or to document the consistency of the description of experiences across providers, comparison between what the child or adolescent tells you and what the reports say would be instructive. Again, depending on the reason for the referral, these inconsistencies may or may not be noted and further inquiries made. (Chapter 3 details more fully with what parents and children should be asked.)

An examination is important to any evaluation of sexual abuse. These details have been covered exhaustively in other sections of this book (see Chapters 3 and 14). There are some additional, particular details to consider, however, with regard to boys or male adolescents. For the examination, and perhaps even for the detailed interview before it, boys may benefit from having both male and female providers available from which to choose. If the perpetrator was a man, the boy may feel safer having a female physician do the examination; if the perpetrator was a woman, he may feel safer having a male physician do the examination. If the provider does not have skills with or specific knowledge about forensic-level examinations should that be necessary, he or she should refer the patient to a site that does have expertise. (See Chapters 4 and 15, which describe when examinations of this type are needed.)

If the provider must refer the boy, the boy should be assured that he can and should continue to see the provider after he receives care at the other site. Also, it is good to broadly describe for the boy what he will experience at the specialty site, and to note that the individuals who will complete the examination there are experts. Briefly, the boy can anticipate (McEvoy et al., 1999):

— A physical examination while fully naked (to document presence/absence of lacerations, bite marks, abrasions, bruising, redness, and swelling; and to allow swabbing of any secretions)

Key Point:
It is essential to make it clear that the you are mandated by law to report known sexual abuse of a minor in accordance with state laws. This may be challenging with a boy or male adolescent who is finally acknowledging his secret, which must now be reported to a bureaucratic structure that may initiate proceedings where the secret is disclosed to the very people from whom he has been hiding it.

Key Point:
An examination is an important component of the evaluation of sexual abuse. Certain aspects particular to males should be considered:

— Have both male and female of providers available from which the victim may choose.

— If you are not prepared to complete this part of the assessment, refer the patient to a site that has the needed expertise.

— Broadly describe for the boy what he will experience at the specialty site.

— Keep available a sexual assault examination kit.

— Refer the boy to a therapist with expertise in treating sexually abused boys, not just girls.

— Insertion of a sigmoidoscope into the rectum
— Urethral orifice swabbing
— Pictures taken of his genital and perineal region
— Combing of his pubic hair (if present)
— Swabbing of his throat
— Combing of his facial hair (if present)
— Blood tests for presence of drugs

If a sexual abuse specialty clinic or provider does not exist near the clinical location of the scenarios described above, that provider should have a sexual assault examination kit available. (See http://www.tritechusa.com/Crime/sexual-victim.htm for an example of a commercial site that sells kits of this type.)

Referral to a therapist with expertise specifically in treating sexually abused boys is a crucial step in the "assessment and plan" phase. The therapist can be a psychologist or clinical social worker, but he or she should have access to a psychiatrist in the event the boy requires psychopharmacological treatment. Experience and expertise with boys are critical, yet not always easy to find. Lack of experience with boys can be detrimental to a successful outcome. Sending a boy to a therapist with expertise in the treatment of girls can lead to care that focuses on the wrong areas, misses other issues entirely, and can emphasize the marginalization the boy may already feel. Attending a site that is primarily for girls may highlight his own concerns that he is a rarity, that he is feminized, or that there are no other boys like him. The provider should spend some time identifying an individual or group of individuals to whom referral is appropriate by checking personal references or contacting national organizations such as the National Organization on Male Sexual Victimization, at www.nomsv.org, that might have referral networks. Listening to patients' feedback about those therapists who have been particularly helpful or unhelpful enables the provider to make effective referrals.

In some circumstances, the necessary expertise with boys may need to be superceded by expertise in early childhood development. Treatment of preschool males, for example, requires skills beyond facility with sex and gender specifications surrounding treatment of the abused child (Hewitt, 1990). In early childhood, comprehensive knowledge about cognitive, social, emotional, and sexual development of very small children is required, with an eye toward the norms and pathologies of the current stage of development, and where the child is headed to in the next stage. Also, there must be an ability and desire to work with small children and their parents, with specific expertise in clinical approaches such as play therapy. It would be ideal, however, were these skills to be coupled with expertise in the particular needs of boys.

Key Point:
No matter how old the victim is, the pediatrician should send a letter to the therapist to whom the referral has been made stating what is known about prenatal, birth, infancy, and childhood history; substantial medical problems; primary caregiver history; past and current descriptions of growth and cognitive/emotional development; and an account of what has happened with regard to abuse history (how and whether disclosure occurred, details of abuse events, perpetrator identity, parent/family response, legal involvement); and the child's response.

No matter how old the boy is, however, the pediatrician should send a letter to the therapist to whom he or she has referred the boy. In the letter, the provider should include what he or she knows about prenatal, birth, infancy, and childhood history; substantial medical problems; primary caregiver history (separations, changes, limitations of caregiver, etc.); past and current descriptions of growth and cognitive/emotional development; and the account of what has happened with regard to abuse history (how/whether disclosure occurred, details of abuse events, perpetrator identity, parent/family response, legal involvement); and how child has responded to all of this (Hewitt, 1990).

Froning and Mayman (1990) suggest that boys older than preschool ages be involved in therapeutic experiences that include group and family therapy. Group therapy with other boys counteracts the pervasive sense that many abused boys have that they are alone. It provides dialogue with others who, quite surprisingly to the boy, often have gone through just what he has gone through. The process can build trust, and it may limit distortions of the male self. Family therapy may help to address the enormous pressures that exist or develop in families after disclosures of abuse and can serve to educate the family about the numerous nuances of recovery for boys. Whether in these settings or in personal therapy, issues that should be addressed include a feeling by some boys that they are "damaged goods"; guilt; fear; depression; low self-esteem and poor social skills; repressed anger and hostility; impaired ability to trust; blurred role boundaries and role confusion; pseudo-mature behavior with a concomitant failure to accomplish developmental tasks; and self-mastery and control (Cabe, 1999; Sgroi, 1982). This basic knowledge of some of the suggested therapeutic options as well as some of the issues that usually must be addressed should give the healthcare provider a knowledge and language base from which to keep abreast of where the boy and his family are in the process of treatment.

Some families will not pursue treatment after disclosure has occurred. For those who do not, it is the responsibility of the provider to continue supportive care to the boy (even though this may need to be done in the guise of medical care as an explanation to parents and/or for insurance-related reasons). Frequent visits to the primary care provider should be scheduled for the boy, particularly in the time period immediately after disclosure. While any necessary physical and laboratory evaluations will be required at these interactions, the most important activity will be asking the boy about how he is doing, providing positive feedback on the progress he is making, and continuing to advocate counseling to the boy's caregiver, especially if he is not doing well.

For these boys and male adolescents in particular, but also for boys who have been referred for psychological care successfully, some recommendations about specific needs within clinical interactions are important to follow (Cabe, 1999). Limits and boundaries in the relationship must be clear and consistent. Clinical interactions should begin and end on time — even if it means that other patients' scheduled care is rearranged. Extreme caution should be taken with touch of any kind without the patient's permission. Other individuals should be invited into a clinical interaction only with the child's permission. The child must feel free to discuss with the provider intimate parts of his life without fear of unnecessary disclosure to others. Only threats of suicide, other self-injury, and/or injury to others should be reported, and the patient should be warned of this exception to confidentiality at the beginning of and during the clinical relationship. It is important to try to give the boy as much control as possible within the clinical interaction. While he may not control what things must be covered during the clinical interaction, he may be presented with controlling the order in which these items are addressed; the order of questions to be asked; when, how, and with whom the examination is to be completed; and so forth (Froning & Mayman, 1990).

Healthcare providers may be particularly helpful in reducing the shame of abuse that boys experience, especially because healthcare providers are viewed as "experts" on the body. Boys may be particularly troubled by and ashamed about erectile responses and pleasure experiences during their abuse. The provider can educate the boy about physiology and in doing so can normalize the boy's response. For example, a provider can say, "If someone pokes you in the eye, it will probably tear up. If someone tickles you, you'll probably laugh. If someone touches your private parts, it will probably feel good" (Froning & Mayman, 1990). This type of assurance alone can be invaluable.

Engagement with the family of the boy is invaluable as well (see **Table 7-1** for some basic counsel for families). Often, providers miss this opportunity, either because they underestimate their own contribution to others' lives or because they just do not know what would be helpful. At the very least, listening carefully, answering questions when possible, educating when the opportunity arises, and acknowledging and empathizing with the immense amount of fear, anger, and sadness present in the boy's and family's lives can go a long way toward helping to

---

Table 7-1. Recommendations for Parents/Family Members of Sexually Abused Boys

Do <u>Not</u>	Do
1. Pry into physically intimate details of experiences, but be fully accepting of these details should victim choose to divulge them.	1. Allow victim to talk about details he would like to talk about.
2. Ask questions that begin with "Why?" These can easily be misconstrued as blaming questions.	2. Reassure him that he isn't responsible for what happened, you don't blame him, and you don't think that he is weak. At the same time, encourage discussion of self-blaming beliefs and other self-doubts.
3. Minimize the gravity of what has happened, such as by making jokes about abuse events.	3. Be careful about attempts to reduce tension (humor that reflects one's own discomfort is inappropriate).
4. Encourage threats of revenge against perpetrator. Victim may worry about the the safety of those exacting revenge, and threats may affect legal remedies.	4. Respect victim's wishes with regard to disclosure. He should determine, when possible, who is and is not told, how, when, why, and so forth.
5. Seek the "remedy" of distraction, or "taking his mind off it." The victim should be the one to request distraction. However, distraction should not be the primary mode of resolving abuse history.	5. Remind family and friends to be careful in comments they make that could be understood, misunderstood, or purposely meant to imply blame.
6. Assume that because the victim is quiet, stoic, and seemingly unharmed by the abuse that he is not upset, angry, hurt, confused, and in other ways harmed by the abused.	6. Remind family/friends that the victim has privacy needs. At the same time, don't isolate the victim because this can confirm beliefs he is damaged.
7. Take personally increased concerns by the male victim surrounding communication about either the event, the confusion after the event, or even generalizing this to all things in the relationship. He may be establishing boundaries.	7. Be careful about how the victim is "protected." Disclosure can be regretted if it leads to restrictive rules having more to do with fears than real threats. Encourage him to resume his normal life.
8. Become demeaning if school performance declines. Inform school personnel on a "need to know" basis, and then, only with discussion about this with victim.	8. Be aware of behavioral change, such as loss of appetite, withdrawal, sleep disturbance, fears of being alone or being touched, excessive crying, bedwetting, sexual preoccupations, or alcohol and drug use, that may indicate difficulties victim is unable to articulate.

From *McEvoy AW, Rollo D, Brookings JB*. If He Is Raped: A Guidebook for Parents, Partners, Spouses, and Friends. *Holmes Beach, Fla: Learning Publications, Inc.; 1999.*

set a steadier course for those who are buffeted by the sometimes chaotic aftermath of sexual abuse. Abused boys in particular often endure an all-encompassing, self-consuming suffering. Providers can meet this "with an accurate and child-focused empathy, . . . [I]f we recoil at his disclosures . . . he will not disclose . . . if we do not feel his pain, he will [continue to] endure it alone" (Cabe, 1999).

CONCLUSION

Over time, after the immediate issues that surround disclosure of sexual abuse are resolved, boys who disclose sexual abuse histories should engage the medical system in much the same way any other boy or teenager would. He is likely to have numerous issues, however, that his peers do not have. New and recrudescent concerns often appear as he traverses new developmental milestones. These should be expected and respected. Continually encouraging psychological care whenever circumstances warrant is recommended. Such care should be normalized for him so that he anticipates that mental health care may be routine for him throughout his life, at least when the outcomes of sexual abuse are characteristically prevalent (i.e., adolescence, marriage, birth of a child, confrontations with the perpetrator).

With regard to his routine medical care, the American Medical Association Guidelines for Adolescent Preventive Services (GAPS) (1997) recommends that each adolescent should have three complete physical examinations (once in the years 11 to 14, years 15 to 17, and years 18 to 21). Also, adolescents should be asked annually about sexual behaviors, and sexually active teenagers should be screened for sexually transmitted diseases (STDs). This aspect of adolescent health care can make a teenager embarrassed, nervous, and/or upset. Adolescents who have been sexually abused should be kept informed of what future care will entail, perhaps via a set of guidelines charted by age level, and they should be maximally prepared for what to expect during the current as well as the next visit. A genital examination in a boy whose perpetrator fondled and then raped him, for example, may be a focus of great concern and agitation for this male patient. Providers must expect and respect these concerns.

Most importantly, the healthcare provider can remain informed enough to know the unique features of male sexual abuse, the cultural nervousness surrounding it, and the resulting internal challenges for abused boys in maintaining silence in the midst of great personal pain, upheaval, confusion, anger, and sadness. The informed, sensitive provider can have the distinct honor of being able to help an entire patient subpopulation that otherwise tends to remain hidden, hurting, and sometimes hurtful. The rewards for such awareness are immeasurable.

REFERENCES

American Medical Association (AMA). Department of Adolescent Health. *Guidelines for Adolescent Preventive Services (GAPS)*. 1997. Available at: http://www.ama-assn.org/ama/upload/mm/39/gapsmono.pdf. Accessed February 26, 2002.

Bagley C, Bolitho F, Bertrand L. Mental health profiles, suicidal behavior, and community sexual assault in 2112 Canadian adolescents. *Crisis*. 1995;16:126-131.

Bartholow BN, Doll LS, Joy D, et al. Emotional, behavioral, and HIV risks associated with sexual abuse among adult homosexual and bisexual men. *Child Abuse Negl*. 1994;18:747-761.

Becker J, Stein RM. Is sexual erotica associated with sexual deviance in adolescent males? *Int J Law Psychiatry*. 1991;14:85-95.

Boney-McCoy S, Finkelhor D. Prior victimization: a risk factor for child sexual abuse and for PTSD-related symptomatology among sexually abused youth. *Child Abuse Negl*. 1995a;19:1401-1421.

Boney-McCoy S, Finkelhor D. Psychosocial sequelae of violent victimization in a national youth sample. *J of Consult Clin Psychol*. 1995b;63:726-736.

Boudewyn AC, Liem JH. Childhood sexual abuse as a precursor to depression and self-destructive behavior in adulthood. *J Trauma Stress*. 1995;8:445-459.

Briere J, Evans D, Runtz M, et al. Symptomatology in men who were molested as children: a comparison study. *Am J Orthopsychiatry*. 1988;58:457-461.

Brown GR, Anderson B. Psychiatric morbidity in adult inpatients with childhood histories of sexual and physical abuse. *Am J Psychiatry*. 1991;148:55-61.

Brown LK, Kessel SM, Lourie KJ, et al. Influence of sexual abuse on HIV-related attitudes and behaviors in adolescent psychiatric inpatients. *J Am Acad Child Adolesc Psychiatry*. 1997;36:316-322.

Burgess AW, Hartman CR, McCormack A. Abused to abuser: antecedents of socially deviant behaviors. *Am J Psychiatry*. 1987;144:1431-1436.

Burgess AW, Hazelwood RR, Rokous FE, et al. Serial rapists and their victims: reenactment and repetition. *Ann N Y Acad Sci*. 1988;528:277-295.

Cabe N. Abused boys and adolescents: Out of the shadows. In: Horne AM, Kiselica MS, eds. *Handbook of Counseling Boys and Adolescent Males: A Practitioner's Guide*. Thousand Oaks, Calif: Sage Publications, Inc; 1999:199-215.

Cappelleri JC, Eckenrode J, Powers JL. The epidemiology of child abuse: findings from the Second National Incidence and Prevalence Study of Child Abuse and Neglect. *Am J Public Health*. 1993;83:1622-1624.

Carballo-Dieguez A, Dolezal C. Association between history of childhood sexual abuse and adult HIV-risk sexual behavior in Puerto Rican men who have sex with men. *Child Abuse & Neglect*. 1995;19(5):595-605.

Cupoli JM, Sewell PM. One thousand fifty-nine children with a chief complaint of sexual abuse. *Child Abuse Negl*. 1988;12:151-162.

Dembo R, Dertke M, La Voie L, et al. Physical abuse, sexual victimization and illicit drug use: a structural analysis among high risk adolescents. *J Adolesc*. 1987;10:13-33.

Dembo R, Williams L, La Voie L, et al. Physical abuse, sexual victimization and illicit drug use: replication of a structural analysis among a new sample of high-risk youths. *Violence Vict*. 1989;4:121-138.

Dembo R, Williams L, La Voie L, et al. A longitudinal study of the relationships among alcohol use, marijuana/hashish use, cocaine use, and emotional/psychological functioning problems in a cohort of high-risk youths. *Int J Addictions*. 1990;25:1341-1382.

Deykin EY, Buka SL. Suicidal ideation and attempts among chemically dependent adolescents. *Am J Public Health*. 1994;84:634-639.

Doll LS, Joy D, Bartholow BN, et al. Self-reported childhood and adolescent sexual abuse among adult homosexual and bisexual men. *Child Abuse Negl*. 1992;16:855-864.

Ellason JW, Ross CA, Sainton K, et al. Axis I and II comorbidity and childhood trauma history in chemical dependency. *Bull Menninger Clin*. 1996;60:39-51.

Embree BG, DeWit ML. Family background characteristics and relationship satisfaction in a native community in Canada. *Soc Biol*. 1997;44:42-54.

Faller KC. Characteristics of a clinical sample of sexually abused children: how boy and girl victims differ. *Child Abuse Negl*. 1989;13:281-291.

Finkelhor D, Hotaling G, Lewis IA, et al. Sexual abuse in a national survey of adult men and women: prevalence, characteristics, and risk factors. *Child Abuse Negl*. 1990;14:19-28.

Freund K, Watson R, Dickey R. Does sexual abuse in childhood cause pedophilia: an exploratory study. *Arch Sex Behav*. 1990;19:557-568.

Friedrich WN, Schafer LC. Somatic symptoms in sexually abused children. *J Pediatr Psychol.* 1995;20:661-670.

Fromuth ME, Burkhart BR. Childhood sexual victimization among college men: definitional and methodological issues. *Violence Vict.* 1987;2:241-253.

Fromuth ME, Burkhart BR, Jones CW. Hidden child molestation: an investigation of adolescent perpetrators in a nonclinical sample. *J Interpersonal Violence.* 1991;6:376-384.

Froning ML, Mayman SB. Identification and treatment of child and adolescent male victims of sexual abuse. In: Hunter M, ed. *The Sexually Abused Male.* Vol 2. New York, NY: Lexington Books; 1990:199-224.

Gartner RB. *Betrayed as Boys: Psychodynamic Treatment of Sexually Abused Men.* New York, NY: Guilford Press; 1999:356.

Gibby-Smith BM. Correlations of grade point averages at a rural college with reports of abuse in rural families. *Psychological Rep.* 1995;77:619-622.

Gordon M. Males and females as victims of childhood sexual abuse: an examination of the gender effect. *J Fam Violence.* 1990;5:321-332.

Harrison PA, Edwall GE, Hoffman NG, et al. Correlates of sexual abuse among boys in treatment for chemical dependency. *J Adolec Chem Dependency.* 1990;1:53-67.

Harrison PA, Fulkerson JA, Beebe TJ. Multiple substance use among adolescent physical and sexual abuse victims. *Child Abuse Negl.* 1997;21:529-539.

Heintz-Knowles K, Li-Vollmer M, Chen P, et al. *Boys to Men: Entertainment Media Messages about Masculinity.* Oakland, Calif: Children Now; 1999.

Hernandez JT, Lodico M, DiClemente RJ. The effects of child abuse and race on risk-taking in male adolescents. *J Nat Med Assoc.* 1993;85:593-597.

Hewitt S. The treatment of sexually abused preschool boys. In: Hunter M, ed. *The Sexually Abused Male.* Vol 2. New York, NY: Lexington Books; 1990:225-248.

Hibbard RA, Hartman GL. Behavioral problems in alleged sexual abuse victims. *Child Abuse Negl.* 1992;16:755-762.

Hibbard RA, Ingersoll GM, Orr DP. Behavioral risk, emotional risk, and child abuse among adolescents in a nonclinical setting. *Pediatrics.* 1990;86:896-901.

Holmes G, Offen L. Clinicians' hypotheses regarding clients' problems: are they less likely to hypothesize sexual abuse in male compared to female clients? *Child Abuse Negl.* 1996;20:493-501.

Holmes WC. Association between a history of childhood sexual abuse and subsequent, adolescent psychoactive substance use disorder in a sample of HIV seropositive men. *J Adolesc Health.* 1997;20:414-419.

Holmes WC, Slap GB. Sexual abuse of boys: definition, prevalence, correlates, sequelae, and management. *JAMA.* 1998;280:1855-1862.

Hunter JA. A comparison of the psychosocial maladjustment of adult males and females sexually molested as children. *J Interpersonal Violence.* 1991;6:205-217.

Hussey DL, Strom G, Singer M. Male victims of sexual abuse: an analysis of adolescent psychiatric inpatients. *Child Adolesc Soc Work J.* 1992;9:491-503.

Huston RL, Parra JM, Prihoda TJ, et al. Characteristics of childhood sexual abuse in a predominantly Mexican-American population. *Child Abuse Negl.* 1995;19:165-176.

Hutchings PS, Dutton MA. Sexual assault history in a community mental health center clinical population. *Comm Ment Health J.* 1993;29:59-63.

Janus M, Burgess AW, McCormack A. Histories of sexual abuse in adolescent male runaways. *Adolescence.* 1987;22:405-417.

Johnson RL, Shrier D. Past sexual victimization by females of male patients in an adolescent medicine clinic population. *Am J Psychiatry.* 1987;144:650-652.

Jolliff D, Horne AM. Growing up male: the development of mature masculinity. In: Horne AM, Kiselica MS, eds. *Handbook of Counseling Boys and Adolescent Males: A Practitioner's Guide.* Thousand Oaks, Calif: Sage Publications, Inc; 1999:3-23.

Kendall-Tackett KA, Simon AF. A comparison of the abuse experiences of male and female adults molested as children. *J Fam Violence.* 1992;7:57-62.

Kiselica MS, Horne AM. Preface: For the sake of our nation's sons. In: Horne AM, Kiselica MS, eds. *Handbook of Counseling Boys and Adolescent Males: A Practitioner's Guide.* Thousand Oaks, Calif: Sage Publications, Inc; 1990:xv-xx.

Kohan MJ, Pothier P, Norbeck JS. Hospitalized children with history of sexual abuse: incidence and care issues. *Am J Orthopsychiatry.* 1987;57:258-264.

Langevin R, Wright P, Handy L. Characteristics of sex offenders who were sexually victimized as children. *Ann Sex Res.* 1989;2:227-253.

Lenderking WR, Wold C, Mayer KH, et al. Childhood sexual abuse among homosexual men: prevalence and association with unsafe sex. *J Gen Intern Med.* 1997;12:250-253.

Levitt CJ. Sexual abuse of boys: A medical perspective. In: Hunter M, ed. *The Sexually Abused Male.* Vol 1. Lexington, Mass: Lexington Books; 1990:227-240.

Lodico MA, Gruber E, DiClemente RJ. Childhood sexual abuse and coercive sex among school-based adolescents in a midwestern state. *J Adolesc Health.* 1996;18:211-217.

MacMillan HL, Fleming JE, Trocme N, et al. Prevalence of child physical and sexual abuse in the community: results from the Ontario Health Supplement. *JAMA.* 1997;278:131-135.

McClellan J, McCurry C, Ronnei M, et al. Relationship between sexual abuse, gender, and sexually inappropriate behaviors in seriously mentally ill youths. *J Am Acad Child Adolesc Psychiatry.* 1997;36:959-965.

McCormack A, Rokous FE, Hazelwood RR, et al. An exploration of incest in the childhood development of serial rapists. *J Family Violence.* 1992;7:219-228.

McEvoy AW, Rollo D, Brookings JB. *If He Is Raped: A Guidebook for Parents, Partners, Spouses, and Friends.* Holmes Beach, Fla: Learning Publications, Inc; 1999:112.

Messner M, Hunt D, Dunbar M, et al. *Boys to Men: Sports Media Messages about Masculinity.* Oakland, Calif: Children Now; 1999.

Moisan PA, Sanders-Phillips K, Moisan PM. Ethnic differences in circumstances of abuse and symptoms of depression and anger among sexually abused black and Latino boys. *Child Abuse Negl.* 1997;21:473-488.

Nagy S, Adcock AG, Nagy MC. A comparison of risky health behaviors of sexually active, sexually abused, and abstaining adolescents. *Pediatrics.* 1994;93:570-575.

Nelson DE, Higginson GK, Grant-Worley JA. Using the youth risk behavior survey to estimate prevalence of sexual abuse among Oregon high school students. *J School Health.* 1994;64:413-416.

Nuttall R, Jackson H. Personal history of childhood abuse among clinicians. *Child Abuse Negl.* 1994;18:455-472.

Okami P. Self-reports of "positive" childhood and adolescent sexual contacts with older persons: an exploratory study. *Arch Sex Behav.* 1991;20:437-457.

Paris J, Zweig-Frank H, Guzder J. Risk factors for borderline personality in male outpatients. *J Nerv Ment Dis.* 1994;182:375-380.

Pierce R, Pierce LH. The sexually abused child: a comparison of male and female victims. *Child Abuse Negl.* 1985;9:191-199.

Pollack W. *Real Boys: Rescuing Our Sons from the Myths of Boyhood.* New York, NY: Random House; 1998.

Reinhart MA. Sexually abused boys. *Child Abuse Negl.* 1987;11:229-235.

Remafedi G, Farrow JA, Deisher RW. Risk factors for attempted suicide in gay and bisexual youth. *Pediatrics.* 1991;87:869-875.

Resnick MD, Blum RW. The association of consensual sexual intercourse during childhood with adolescent health risk and behaviors. *Pediatrics.* 1994;94:907-913.

Risin LI, Koss MP. The sexual abuse of boys: prevalence and descriptive characteristics of childhood victimizations. *J Interpersonal Violence.* 1987;2:309-323.

Roane TH. Male victims of sexual abuse: a case review within a child protective team. *Child Welfare.* 1992;71:231-239.

Robin RW, Chester B, Rasmussen JK, et al. Factors influencing utilization of mental health and substance abuse services by American Indian men and women. *Psychiatr Serv.* 1997a;48:826-832.

Robin RW, Chester B, Rasmussen JK, et al. Prevalence, characteristics, and impact of childhood sexual abuse in a Southwestern American Indian tribe. *Child Abuse Negl.* 1997b;21:769-787.

Roesler TA, McKenzie N. Effects of childhood trauma on psychological functioning in adults sexually abused as children. *J Nerv Ment Dis.* 1994;182:145-150.

Rosen LN, Martin L. The measurement of childhood trauma among male and female soldiers in the U.S. Army. *Milit Med.* 1996;161:342-345.

Rubinstein M, Yeager CA, Goodstein C, et al. Sexually assaultive male juveniles: a follow-up. *Am J Psychiatry.* 1993;150:262-265.

Ryan G, Miyoshi TJ, Metzner JL, et al. Trends in a national sample of sexually abusive youths. *J Am Acad Child Adolesc Psychiatry.* 1996;35:17-25.

Sansonnet-Hayden H, Haley G, Marriage K, et al. Sexual abuse and psychopathology in hospitalized adolescents. *J Am Acad Child Adolesc Psychiatry.* 1987;26:753-757.

Sarwer DB, Crawford I, Durlak JA. The relationship between childhood sexual abuse and adult male sexual dysfunction. *Child Abuse Negl.* 1997;21:649-655.

Schulte JG, Dinwiddie SH, Pribor EF, et al. Psychiatric diagnoses of adult male victims of childhood sexual abuse. *J Nerv Ment Dis.* 1995;183:111-113.

Sgroi SM. *Handbook of Clinical Intervention in Child Sexual Abuse.* Lexington, Mass: Lexington Books; 1982:387.

Siegel JM, Sorenson SB, Golding JM, et al. The prevalence of childhood sexual assault: The Los Angeles Epidemiologic Catchment Area Project. *Am J Epidemiol.* 1987;126:1141-1153.

Simpson TL, Westerberg VS, Little LM, et al. Screening for childhood physical and sexual abuse among outpatient substance abusers. *J Substance Abuse Treatment.* 1994;11:347-358.

Smith K. *Who's Minding the Kids? Child Care Arrangements*: Fall 1995. Washington, DC: US Census Bureau; 2000. Current Population Reports, P70-70:27.

Stevenson MR, Gajarsky WM. Unwanted childhood sexual experiences relate to later revictimization and male perpetration. *J Psychol Human Sexuality.* 1991;4:57-70.

Violato C, Genuis M. Factors which differentiate sexually abused from nonabused males: an exploratory study. *Psychological Rep.* 1993;72:767-770.

Weber FT, Gearing J, Davis A, et al. Prepubertal initiation of sexual experiences and older first partner predict promiscuous sexual behavior of delinquent adolescent males: unrecognized child abuse? *J Adolesc Health.* 1992;13:600-605.

Whiffen VE, Clark SE. Does victimization account for sex differences in depressive symptoms? *Br J Clin Psychol.* 1997;36:185-193.

Windle M, Windle RC, Scheidt DM, et al. Physical and sexual abuse and associated mental disorders among alcoholic inpatients. *Am J Psychiatry.* 1995;152:1322-1328.

Wolfe DA, Sas L, Wekerle C. Factors associated with the development of posttraumatic stress disorder among child victims of sexual abuse. *Child Abuse Negl.* 1994;18:37-50.

Worling JR. Adolescent sibling-incest offenders: differences in family and individual functioning when compared to adolescent nonsibling sex offenders. *Child Abuse Negl.* 1995a;19:633-643.

Worling JR. Sexual abuse histories of adolescent male sex offenders: differences on the basis of the age and gender of their victims. *J Abnorm Psychol.* 1995b;104:610-613.

Zierler S, Feingold L, Laufer D, et al. Adult survivors of childhood sexual abuse and subsequent risk of HIV infection. *Am J Public Health.* 1991;81:572-575.

DISABILITY AND SEXUAL VIOLENCE

Sharon W. Cooper, MD, FAAP

Sexual assault knows no boundaries. Victims of assault may be children or adults, male or female, healthy or ill, and able or disabled. In light of this fact, it is imperative that healthcare providers, social service members, and the legal and law enforcement communities gain a better understanding of the universal nature of this type of abuse.

On occasion, acute sexual assault may occur within the context of chronic sexual abuse. The victim may have been a willing or unwilling partner, but on a specific occasion abuse occurs with force, without consent, or with coercion. In the circumstance of a child, consent is not an issue if the assailant is an individual who is either an adult or older by 4 years or more (age differences vary from state to state). The use of force makes the episode more traumatic and the long-term effects more significant. When chronic sexual abuse has been present and the most recent event has been within 72 hours, a full medical evaluation including a rape kit is indicated. The actual type of assault need not be genital penetration, but may constitute any number of sexual acts that leave the victim traumatized, ashamed, or with the feeling of helplessness and fear.

Approximately 54 million Americans report some level of disability, and 26 million describe their disability as severe (Holmes, 1999). Between 4% and 5% of Americans have a developmental disability, including mental retardation, autism, cerebral palsy, and severe learning disabilities (LaPlante & Carlson, 1996). The child or adult with a disability is a special patient when sexual assault is the concern. Often the disclosure of the event may be delayed, or, in the circumstance of a nonverbal individual or someone with minimal communication skills, may be expressed behaviorally or with physical evidence such as bruises or bleeding. As is the case in victims without disabilities, the most likely offender will be known to the victim.

In the case of an individual with a physical disability, there is an additional phenomenon associated with sexual and physical abuse referred to as disability-related abuse, in which perpetrators withhold needed equipment and assistance to coerce sexual contact. Orthotic equipment such as wheelchairs, walkers, or braces; medications; transportation; assistance with getting out of bed or hygienic care; or therapy are all necessary services that may be withheld. This type of disability-related abuse is more common when the sexual assault is perpetrated by an aide or a healthcare provider. This also may occur within the independent living center scenario. Sexual assault has an impact upon victims with disabilities that is similar to that experienced by other patients, with the added caveat that reporting is less likely to be believed or investigated. In addition, the presence of a disability increases the risk of sexual exploitation whereby abusers encourage or coerce sexual contact between individuals with disabilities who otherwise might not be at all attracted to each other.

Case Study

A.G. presented to the Emergency Room because of a disclosure of sexual assault to her mother. This child was 10 years old and had been diagnosed with severe spastic diplegia with speech and language delay associated with mild dysarthria secondary to periventricular leukomalacia. She was the product of a 30-week gestation with respiratory distress syndrome and an intraventricular hemorrhage that resulted in subsequent cerebral palsy. Her motor delays were so significant that she was nonambulatory and used a manual wheelchair. She had moderate impairment of her fine motor skills and upper extremity strength. Her cognition was low normal. Her speech and language delay problems were manifested by dysarthria with prolonged and deliberate pronunciations and numerous articulation defects, so that her degree of intelligibility was about 75%. Nevertheless, she had keen command of pragmatics in her language and was easily determined to be a competent historian. She described the fact that while at her place of out-of-home after school care, an adult uncle had repetitively urged his 16-year-old nephew to, "Start out with this one!" A.G. recounted her verbal protestations, which went unheeded, and the painful experience of having her legs pulled apart despite the spastic hip adductor contractures for which she received physical therapy on a regular basis. She was able to recall each of the verbal instructions of the adult, which were sprinkled with laughter and profanity. This had happened on one occasion, and she subsequently developed anxiety, fearfulness of all men, recurrent nightmares, insomnia, episodes of crying, and withdrawn behaviors. Her mother initially was skeptical of her report, but brought her to medical care. Her physical examination revealed bruising on her inner thighs, edema and redness of the hymen, and fresh tears noted on the posterior fourchette. Law enforcement was initially planning to forgo a full investigation, assuming that this child would not be seen as a credible witness.

INCIDENCE OF ABUSE

The incidence of abuse and assault among persons with disabilities is significantly higher than in the general population. Although sexual victimization occurs in at least 20% of females and 5% to 10% of males in the United States, it is estimated that as high as 90% of people with developmental disabilities will experience sexual abuse or assault at some point in their lives. Forty-nine percent will experience 10 or more abusive events (Valenti-Hein & Schwartz, 1995). Additional studies reveal that the likelihood of rape is very great: 15,000 to 19,000 people per year in the disabled population (Sobsey, 1994).

Concern for sexual assault in association with general maltreatment brought to light by Crosse et al. in the 1993 study conducted by the National Center on Child Abuse and Neglect (NCCAN), entitled *A Report on the Maltreatment of Children with Disabilities*. This research was prepared in response to the Child Abuse Prevention, Adoption, and Family Services Act of 1988. This law focused on abuse of children with physical, intellectual, or emotional disabilities. Data were collected from a sample of 35 child protective services agencies from across the country, which provided information on all cases of substantiated maltreatment of children over a 6-week period in 1991. A total of 1834 children had substantiated abuse during the study period and the study found the following:

— An estimated 23 out of 100 children per year are maltreated in the United States.

— Of those children who were abused, 17.2% had disabilities, and of all the children who were sexually abused, 15.2% had disabilities.

— Abused children with disabilities were more likely to be male and typically older than children without disabilities who were abused.

— The incidence of maltreatment (e.g., number of children maltreated annually per 1000 children) among children with disabilities was 1.7 times higher than the incidence of maltreatment for children without disabilities. When this fact was dissected further, it was noted that children with disabilities had higher rates of all types of abuse: Children with a disability were 2.1 times more likely to be physically abused than children without disabilities, 1.8 times more likely to be sexually abused, and 1.6 times more likely to be neglected.

— The disability itself directly led to or contributed to child abuse in 47% of maltreated children with disabilities. The most common disabilities noted were emotional, learning disabilities, physical disabilities, and speech or language delay or impairments (Crosse et al., 1993).

The overrepresentation of children with disabilities on the rolls of child protective service cases bears further discussion. Superficially, it is thought that these children are at higher risk because of the increased burden of care associated with their conditions. Care providers who have marginal coping mechanisms would certainly be more likely to neglect and physically abuse such individuals because of frustration, a sense of being overwhelmed, and a possible lack of attachment to the child who has not fulfilled their parental expectation. These theories, however, do not explain the matter of sexual abuse in this population. The dynamics of sexual assault, often associated with violence, and a need for power and control, might better describe the circumstances of sexual abuse in children with significant disabilities.

HATE CRIMES AGAINST PERSONS WITH DISABILITIES

Disability bias takes many forms, including hate crimes. Laws such as the Fair Housing Amendments Act of 1988, the Americans with Disabilities Act of 1990, and the Rehabilitation Act of 1973 are designed to protect people with disabilities from this type of prejudice.

The presence of a physical or mental disability is a recognized risk for victimization from a hate crime. Such a travesty would include physical and/or sexual assault based solely on one's race, religion, gender, disability, or sexual orientation. The presence of a disability as a category for the cause of a hate crime has been included in 21 state statutes, although it is not as yet included in the federal law, the Hate Crimes Prevention Act of 1999. Despite that fact, persons with disabilities are included in the Summary of Hate Crime Statistics, 2000 published in the Federal Bureau of Investigation (FBI) Uniform Crime Reports (FBI, 2000). This report cited 36 incidents of hate crimes based on disability that were reported to the federal authorities. It is thought that this number is a significant underestimation of the incidence of the crime because many jurisdictions do not have a special category for assault and battery based on the presence of a disability. Perpetrators of such crimes have included gangs, youth offenders, and adults who are generally outside of the caregiving role. Victims may be of any age or sex, and in most cases, their disability is apparent.

In 1990 Sobsey and Mansell outlined 5 "cultural myths" that contribute to the erroneous thinking about persons with disabilities. The acceptance of the following myths further propagates the development of psychological justification of a hate crime mentality.

Key Point:
The myths that can propagate the development of psychological justification of a hate crime include the following:
— the "Dehumanization" myth
— he "Damaged Merchandize" myth
— the "Feeling No Pain" myth
— the "Disabled Menace" myth
— the "Helpless" myth

— The "Dehumanization" Myth: Labels such as "vegetative state" suggest that a person with a disability is something less than a full member of society and serves to dehumanize the individual. Perpetrators may rationalize their abusive behavior as not really injuring another person.

— The "Damaged Merchandise" Myth: Similar to dehumanization, this myth asserts that the life of the individual with a disability is "worthless" and that he or she has nothing to lose. Such a philosophy can lead to the justification of cessation of minimal support (such as providing food, water, or medication) to a person who is otherwise relatively functional, especially after a catastrophic event such as a traumatic brain injury. This thinking is aligned with advocates for euthanasia of children with severe disabilities, who rationalize that such killing is in the best interest of the child. An example was a well-publicized case in Canada, argued in the courts in 1997, which involved a father's so-called "compassionate homicide" of his 13-year-old daughter with cerebral palsy.

— The "Feeling No Pain" Myth: People with disabilities are thought of as having no feelings or as being immune to pain and suffering. There is no basis for this myth and, in fact, individuals with disabilities experience the same range of emotions found in any person.

— The "Disabled Menace" Myth: Perceived as different, individuals with disabilities are often considered unpredictable and dangerous, whether or not there is any foundation for the fear. Classical literature such as Steinbeck's *Of Mice and Men* (1937) or Hugo's *Notre Dame de Paris* (1917) has promoted the stereotype in which men with mental or physical impairments were seen as a menace to the small community in which they lived. Adherence to this myth may motivate people to prevent community facilities, such as group homes for adults with mental retardation, from being developed in their neighborhoods.

— The "Helpless" Myth: Beliefs or perceptions that individuals with disabilities are helpless and unable to take care of themselves undermine their self-esteem and ability to take on decisions related to daily life. This in turn makes the individual more vulnerable to abuse and manipulation (Sobsey & Mansell, 1990).

The prevalence of these myths with respect to hate crimes is unknown. However, in-depth case analysis of crimes against disabled people might direct prevention strategies targeting misconceptions that exist in the general population. Exaggerations of these misconceptions may contribute to the development of high-risk behavior patterns that tend to lead to the commission of a crime.

Nursing Home and Group Home Residents

A recent report of the General Accounting Office (GAO) to the United States Congress in March 2002 revealed that the federal and state governments provide oversight for almost 17,000 nursing homes in the nation. Investigations noted that inadequate state procedures allowed extensive delays in the investigation of serious allegations of elder abuse (General Accounting Office [GAO], 1999). In addition, state surveys identified serious deficiencies that caused harm to residents and a risk for serious injury or death in more than 25% of nursing homes in the nation (GAO, 1999). The most recent data reveals that even though guidelines are now in place, investigations are not taking place within the 10 working days of their receipt (GAO, 2000). Three states were intensively reviewed for physical abuse and sexual abuse occurrences in nursing homes: Georgia, Illinois, and Pennsylvania. It was determined that sexual abuse and physical abuse allegations were not reported promptly and that law enforcement was rarely summoned to investigate. Criminal background checks of personnel working in the nursing homes were incomplete, and when allegations were substantiated, there was minimal disciplinary action. Criminal prosecutions were extremely rare, despite severe abuse.

Studies conducted regarding the severe impact of sexual assault and abuse in the nursing home and elderly population point out that there are serious problems with potentially devastating consequences (Burgess et al., 2000). Factors such as forced dependence, poor communication with relatives, and failure to recognize multiple victim assault scenarios contribute to the incidence of abuse of individuals who reside in nursing homes in America (Payne & Cikovic, 1995).

Cases of untreated sexually transmitted diseases, severe posttraumatic stress disorder in patients with emerging dementia, and associated physical abuse consistent with sadistic sexual assault have been reported and reviewed. Problems of delayed medical care and investigations with subsequent compromised evidence have contributed to the inability of law enforcement to respond appropriately to this form of sexual assault. In the states reviewed, more than 60% of complaints were submitted more than 2 days after an event had occurred. Although federal statutes are in place, poor enforcement has led to a sense of apathy and a free range for sex offenders, who escape offender registries in these circumstances despite disclosures by victims. This problem exists in part because nursing home employees create an environment of fear of retribution against residents making complaints regarding a care provider.

Often, other personnel employed by the facility witnessed the sexual assault and failed to report it. In other circumstances, residents informed a family member who did not take the matter further. Family support was intermittent because of the fear that the resident would be asked to leave the facility and the prospect of finding a new place for the resident to live was daunting. Residents who informed a staff member would be admonished to keep the information to themselves, so that there would be no disruption in the day-to-day management of the facility. Occasionally, visual evidence of injury detected by concerned staff members would be the primary indication that a resident had been assaulted. Failure to disclose by the victim was either due to the suppressive milieu or the nature of the victim's disability. These issues and others make the medical evaluation and further investigation of sexual assaults in nursing home residents more difficult.

Examination of a nursing home resident may be difficult because of joint contractures, resistance of the victim owing to the pain of the assault itself, or difficulty in communicating with patients suffering from dementia and cognitive impairments. Careful documentation of any physical findings is essential and the examination should be conducted in the same way as with a nonverbal victim, with documentation of all behavioral changes noted by reliable historians. A rape kit is indicated, because the GAO report of 1999 revealed delays in criminal background checks of nursing home personnel hid a significant number of employees with prior histories of abuse complaints.

It is also important to note that nursing home residents are often immunocompromised and may have had minimal sexual experiences. The onset of symptoms such as fever, malaise, changes in blood pressure, or skin rashes in a resident who has either disclosed or been deemed to have been sexually assaulted require a thorough medical assessment looking for sexually transmitted diseases that may be attacking vital organs such as the myocardium. Failure to recognize the occasional systemic presentation or failure to seek medical care in a timely manner for such residents could cause undue harm or death.

Evaluation of the Child or Adult with a Disability

Several actions should be taken in the evaluation of a child or adult with a disability for a sexual assault. Initially, the patient presents for healthcare either because of a verbal or behavioral disclosure of assault, or because there were suspicious circumstances leading to an evaluation, particularly in a nonverbal individual. In the first situation, the method of disclosure is very important. If a victim with a disability comes for healthcare with evidence of severe physical bodily harm as well as genital trauma, the practitioner must provide a concise but extremely detailed account of the history both as given by the victim and as given by any other reliable observer. It is extremely important to be able to speak with someone familiar with the victim. Unlike a patient with no developmental problems, those who have mental illness or developmental delay may be unable to communicate to a stranger in a meaningful manner. Consider the person whose primary form of communication is sign language. If a sign language interpreter is not available within the acute care setting, the medical record should cite that such is the case, and as soon as is feasible, a history should be taken with a certified interpreter. The record should not indicate that a history could not be obtained.

With nonverbal individuals who have been found, for example, with their clothing awry, stains in their underwear or diaper, or highly suspicious bruising in or around the genitals, collateral interviews must be obtained to assess the opportunity for

Key Point:

If a victim with a disability comes for health care with evidence of severe physical bodily harm and genital trauma, the practitioner must provide a concise but extremely detailed account of both the history as related by the victim and that offered by any other reliable observer.

assault. Typically, the history is provided by a nonoffending care provider who, upon discovery of such findings, seeks medical care immediately for the victim. This person may well have no knowledge of potential perpetrators, but may be able to list possible persons who have been with the child or adult within a certain time frame. Documentation of the last time that the individual was seen as normal is very important in investigating these types of circumstances. The development of behaviors may not have occurred at this point, so the behavioral history may not be helpful unless this event constitutes one of several episodes. In the latter situation the history of change in behavior may well represent the sentinal event, which yields clues to a successful investigation.

In the circumstance of an individual who is in residential care, interviews of multiple caregivers will be necessary to better discern if the change in behaviors points more toward a fearfulness of bodily harm (such as always covering the genitalia in a protective manner during hygiene care) or anxiety regarding a target person. Such information must be obtained through careful questioning of a uniform nature of all care providers who have come into contact with the victim. Additional history should be obtained from other residents who may have witnessed the sexual assault and are afraid to disclose or who have been victims themselves of the same perpetrator.

When a child or youth is brought to medical care from a group home or residential treatment facility, factors that make the child more vulnerable to abuse must be considered. Experts cite that the nature of a caregiver-resident relationship is inherently unequal because the caregiver ultimately has power and control. The caregiver has a position of authority. Victims may feel powerless to resist the propositions of a caregiver for fear of losing their affection, fear of retaliation, or because they have been conditioned to be compliant (Furey, 1994). Caregivers can withhold normal daily items that assist in making the living environment pleasant. Removal of toys or sentimental keepsakes represents unspoken threats of retaliation. A caregiver may isolate the victim for fabricated actions, thus reinforcing to the child that it is wiser to acquiesce to the requests for sexual favors than to resist. The child will often feel that there is no resource for help because the specific caregiver has such a position of authority. This is also relevant to the child for whom mental illness is the cause of residential care.

Key Point:
Whenever a child is being brought for medical care for a possible sexual assault within a home or extended care facility, a call should be made immediately to law enforcement to attempt to secure the crime scene before intentional or unintentional tampering of evidence takes place.

Whenever a child is brought medical care due to a possible sexual assault within a home or extended care facility, a call should be made immediately to law enforcement to attempt to secure the crime scene before intentional or unintentional tampering of evidence takes place. Jurisdiction for child protective services depends on licensing practices, the definition of the roles of the specific Child Protective Service employees (e.g., investigative workers vs. treatment workers) and state guidelines. It is possible that certain situations will not fall within the purview of a social service agency. A victim with developmental delay may require photographs of various rooms in the facility to be able to describe better the actual scene of the assault. The acute medical care setting may not have pictures of the residential facility available, but should obtain them as soon as possible to facilitate gathering the most accurate history.

Key Point:
It is important to remember that one of the purposes of the medical history is to obtain verbal evidence. A careful behavioral history is also needed, because family members or care providers who know the child well can attest to any changes in the normal routines.

It is important to remember that one of the purposes of the medical history is to obtain verbal evidence. The hearsay exception, therefore, allows for far more leading questions than would be allowed in a psychological forensic interview. In addition, speech and language delay may be such that a person with a disability can respond only to "yes" and "no" questions, although this approach should be a last resort for obtaining information. Assistance from a family member or other person familiar with the disabled victim is invaluable in learning the range of language present in that individual. Free association conversation may not be a meaningful option with this type of patient, and nonverbal responses such as facial expressions, smiles, eye contact, and changes in affect may be very important when discussing various caregivers.

A careful behavioral history is also of paramount importance, because family members or care providers who know the child well can attest to any changes in their normal routines. Defensive startle behaviors such as covering of the eyes or ears, extreme reluctance to accept assistance with toileting, recent onset of sleeping in a fetal position, or withdrawn behaviors with self-imposed isolation are some behavior changes that should cause concern. Emotional lability, easy agitation, and fearfulness during bathing or toileting form another group of signs that should be documented in the process of evaluating visually impaired children. Children with sight may demonstrate similar behaviors but these may be restricted to those times when a perpetrator is in their vicinity. These children may not know their assailants well enough to be able to name them, or they may know them well and be hesitant to disclose their identity because of threats. Threats are often communicated to silence children who do not have disabilities in cases of child sexual assault and sexual exploitation.

DISCLOSURE

In documenting a history of sexual assault or child sexual abuse, a careful understanding of the method and content of disclosure is crucial. If a patient has a developmental level within the very early childhood range, a disclosure might simply be blurted out within the context of toileting or bathing. Often children who are cognitively less than age 5 years will not have learned the concept of a "secret" and feel comfortable in revealing very intimate information without reservations. Some examiners may choose to discount such a disclosure as if it constitutes simple environmental contamination and seemingly has no validity. However, if the patient has not demonstrated sexually reactive behaviors in the past and has not had a habit of verbalizing in a sexually explicit manner, there is no reason to disbelieve the factual nature of the information any more than one would disbelieve other statements that the child is making (Gil & Johnson, 1993).

Disclosure may be incomplete because of the child's poor understanding of the specific events that took place. For example, a statement given by a 4-year-old while walking with her mother in an otherwise innocuous situation was, "Patrick licks me too hard!" Further exploration by the mother revealed that this child was referring to being the victim of recurrent assault by a 26-year-old male who was performing cunnilingus upon her. Although an individual with developmental delay may not understand the concept of unacceptable physical boundary violation, he would still be able to describe the incident within the context of its sensation. Verbalized sensory memory is very important to document, because this strongly infers experiential learning. If a child or an adult with developmental delay has been told a story about being platonically kissed by a care provider, it is not likely that they would be able to describe the sensation of having their lips and mouth penetrated by another's tongue and exactly how that felt without the strong probability that they had indeed experienced this sensation. This would, therefore, negate the probability of a suggested memory for a child with developmental delay. Research regarding suggested memory has primarily assessed children who have normal development, speech, and language (Ceci et al., 1992). One cannot extrapolate that this research has merit in the disabled population. In addition, a history of a painful experience involving the genitalia, anus, or breasts should hold significant merit in the absence of any normal physical explanation (e.g., candidal vaginitis or severe constipation).

Key Point:
Verbalized sensory memory is very important to document, because this strongly infers experiential learning.

At times, disabled children disclose extremely sexually explicit information, such as forced fellatio or anal penetration. Indications of such forms of abuse may be frankly stated or demonstrated through gesture language, generally in response to direct questioning. Such utterances or mimes are well outside the normal range of psychosexual development and knowledge. Consequently, they should be documented verbatim or as descriptively as possible and considered as unlikely to have been suggested. The exception to this rule is present when a child may have been exploited through exposure to a significant amount of pornography as a method of grooming for future abuse. This form of exploitation may have definite impact on a child's sexual knowledge and a history of such exposure is important to elicit. Typically, video pornography would more likely be the source of the visual memory of a very sexually explicit encounter. It is important to remember that this form of desensitization by an assailant does not negate the reality of a true sexual assault. It may merely explain a delay in disclosure or a feeling in the victim that their sexual behavior constitutes "What big girls do," a frequently described justification offered to them by a perpetrator.

Sensory information such as tastes, smells, sounds made by the perpetrator, or tactile descriptions such as wet, hard, or soft are all very relevant within the context of a sexual assault history and should be carefully documented. This information is not generally within the realm of fantasy and in all probability represents objective history about the event.

As is the case with children and youths without disabilities, coercion to fabricate may occur. Fortunately, research has revealed that disclosures under these circumstances are rare and are not necessarily associated with divorce and custody. There may well exist a good faith concern on the part of a parent to ensure that nothing has happened to the child during a visitation event. Clinicians who have experience in evaluating children for sexual abuse readily recognize the risk of a false disclosure when there has been a parental threat such as: "I'm going to take you downtown for a lie detector test, and if you don't tell me everything, someone will really get hurt!" Individuals with disabilities are at risk to behave in a more compliant manner than those who are not disabled, in attempts to ensure that they will be liked and included by others. This learned compliance is often carefully instilled in them by their parents, to facilitate their social acceptability. Consequently, the risk for such a victim's acquiescence to pressure for a disclosure of details, which may not be accurate, is greater. If possible, it is imperative for the clinician to carefully explore and document the method of disclosure, before beginning the victim interview.

HEARING-IMPAIRED VICTIM

If the victim is hearing impaired and a parent or care provider is fluent in sign language, it is possible to obtain a cursory history before having access to a certified sign language interpreter. The same set of standards regarding obtaining a history from an individual alone should be used as much as is feasible within the limitations of availability of services within an acute care setting. The common feelings of self-blame also exist in the disabled victim and will require reassurance from a familiar person or supportive hospital personnel. The hearing-impaired victim may be very traumatized because of an inability to anticipate an attack or difficulty in communicating with the assailant. It is essential to remember that most assailants of persons with disabilities are known to the victim and may be in a caregiving role. This betrayal of trust may cause increased anxiety whenever the victim is away from what is perceived to be a safe place.

Actual interviewing techniques with a hearing-impaired victim should include careful eye contact despite the fact that questions may be interpreted by a sign language expert. The clinician should follow the standard method of interviewing to include rapport building and free association conversation before embarking on the sexual assault history. Setting the victim at ease is an important part of the medical evaluation, because use of threats by the perpetrator may cause the victim to be fearful of giving a full disclosure. Reassurance that the encounter is of a medical nature is also important, particularly in those healthcare facilities that have

Key Point:
The clinician should follow a standard method of interviewing, including rapport building and free-association conversation before embarking on the sexual assault history. Reassurance that the encounter is of a medical nature is also important, particularly in health care facilities that have a separate sexual assault evaluation area.

a separate sexual assault evaluation area. The young victim must understand that even though the examination room may be decorated in a childlike manner, this is indeed a "check-up," and it is important to tell the truth so that the examiner can assure that "the child's body will be alright." Because of the conduit of information through the sign language interpreter, the medical provider should tell the victim that he or she will repeat what the provider believes the victim communicated to ensure complete understanding of the history as given. Reassurance should be stated that this effort is to confirm that the medical care provider truly understands the details the victim is communicating.

Review of the behaviors of the hearing-impaired victim should be discussed both with a supportive family member or care provider and with the victim. Often care providers are unaware of sleep dysfunction, situational anxieties, specific fearfulness, or intrusive thoughts. Consequently, because of the high association of post-traumatic stress disorder after either a single incident of sexual assault or multiple occurrences, these specific symptoms should be discussed during the discussion of history and behaviors with a hearing-impaired victim.

VISUALLY IMPAIRED VICTIM

Obtaining a history from a visually impaired victim requires empathy and the realization that data will include primarily nonvisual sensory information. If the individual is an adult who has lost vision during the adult years, the ability to describe what was experienced and link this to known visual imagery will be both intact and revealing. Such individuals often have a significant amount of anxiety because of the loss of an extremely important ability. The presence of acute traumatic stress may cause the process of obtaining a medical history to be difficult and prolonged. Reassurance that whatever information can be given will be helpful often allows the victim to carefully reconstruct the total experience.

Details such as the time of day or place of assault must be explained in more depth, based on the victim's normal means of making these determinations. For example, if the victim speaks of having returned from a place of work to the home and that the bus takes 1 hour to reach that point, he or she may be able to establish an approximate time when the assault occurred despite the inability to see a clock.

Careful questioning in a step-by-step fashion may provide important information, such as the smell of alcohol on the breath of the assailant, the sensation of facial hair as might be present in a person with a beard, or the recognition of a regional accent in the assailant's verbal demands. If a weapon was used, the victim may recall exactly where a knife barely penetrated her skin, for example, and the examiner might be able to document the presence of a skin reaction at that site in the physical examination. This is particularly important if the assailant is known to the victim and the defense of a consensual sexual encounter arises.

Children and adolescents, who have lost their sight either from birth or very early in life, often have language delay as well. It is theorized that lack of visual stimulus to reciprocally communicate in response to visual cues is the likely cause. This lack of visual stimulus also contributes to the associated motor delays frequently noted in visually impaired infants and toddlers since the stimulus to reach and procure, and the subsequent associated verbal communication is absent. Victims of sexual assault who are visually impaired are often able to describe auditory and olfactory details, which may have limited value in the resultant identification of an assailant. However, because the perpetrator is most likely to be known to the victim, questions during the medical encounter might include the reasons that convince the victim of the identity of the assailant.

When visual impairment accompanies other disabilities such as a cognitive delay or hearing loss, the victim may demonstrate tactile defensiveness after a sexual assault. This is manifested as combativeness and might lead investigators to believe that no sexual assault could have occurred. It is also important to assure law enforcement that disabled victims may be assaulted regardless of their apparent "attractiveness" or lack thereof. Sexual assault is rarely romantically motivated, and the presence of bias on the part of an investigator should be addressed to ensure the highest motivation of the investigative process (Sorensen, 1997).

Although a child who is only visually impaired can speak and hear, it is common for mild speech and language delays to exist once the child has surpassed age 18 to 24 months. These delays stem from a lack of visual stimulus, which is a natural incentive for enhanced vocabulary acquisition. Children who lose their vision after age 5 years have a higher incidence of independence and better language development. One language parameter noted to be problematic is the incorrect use of personal and possessive pronouns, such as confusing "his" and "their." This has impact on the ability of such a victim to give a thorough history of a sexual assault. Consequently, it is wise to screen language concepts in a visually impaired child or adult sexual assault victim and assure that the child is responding reliably, consistently, and with expressive understanding. Identification of body parts might need to be done with tactile reinforcement, so that the examiner will be assured of understanding what the victim is trying to communicate. Words such as "down there" are often used for the genitalia, and the medical record should reflect gesture language to ensure the accuracy of communication intent.

Review of behaviors and feelings should be conducted in a manner similar to that of the hearing-impaired victim, with intentional verbal redundancy to assure that the examiner has a clear understanding of the information being communicated by the assaulted individual.

COGNITIVELY OR BEHAVIORALLY IMPAIRED VICTIM

In considering the medical evaluation for sexual assault of a victim with a disability of a cognitive and behavioral nature, nonverbal documentation may constitute the essence of the history. For this reason, it is important that a care provider familiar with the habits and behaviors of the victim be included in the evaluation. From the behavioral perspective, a change in behavior is the most important time line event. An acute sexual assault may represent only a point amidst numerous sexual encounters with the same or other assailants. It is therefore imperative to seek a very careful behavioral history of a victim with a disability. Although instruments have been devised to assess sexualized behaviors in normally developing children in the United States between age 2 and 12 years, no such studies have been devised for children with various forms of disabling conditions. Non-abused children without disabilities have more sexualized behaviors (e.g., overt masturbation) at younger ages and as they become older, fewer behaviors are seen. It is important to recognize the actual developmental age or age equivalence of the disabled child when determining if sexualized behaviors may be age appropriate. This realization of cognitive age equivalence is also important in discerning the method of interviewing in the acute care setting as well as the expectations of the examiner for some degree of cooperation.

Behavior changes that might be acutely present in a sexually assaulted developmentally delayed child or adult would include the following:

— Irrational fearfulness of a person, place, or object

— Emotional lability

— Problems with arousal such as hypersomnolence or insomnia

— Changes in activity level (e.g., hyperactive or withdrawn)

— Distractibility

— Anger outbursts

Key Point:
It is wise to screen the language concepts of a visually impaired child or adult sexual assault victim and ensure that the child is responding reliably, consistently, and with expressive understanding.

Key Point:
It is imperative to seek a very careful behavioral history for victims with disabilities.

— Separation anxiety behaviors

— Increased masturbation

— Sexualized behaviors

These behaviors are essentially the same as those seen in a sexually assaulted child with normal development. However, sexualized behaviors are often expressed along a continuum, with normal sexual exploration representing one end of the bell-shaped curve and sexually molesting behaviors at the other end of the curve. Points between may be differentiated by including self-imposed behaviors (e.g., masturbation or inserting objects into themselves) as compared to children who demonstrate extensive mutual sexual behaviors (Gil & Johnson, 1993). Although research has not been done to affirm this theory in the developmentally delayed population, it is probable that the frequency of sexualized behaviors in the assault victim would increase with cognitive age. Acute traumatic stress symptoms can be seen in developmentally delayed children who have been victims of sexual assault, and compassionate, understanding care helps to reassure a frustrated and often guilt-ridden non-offending parent.

Because the most common perpetrator of sexual assault and abuse is someone of at least an acquaintance relationship, the developmentally delayed victim demonstrates the same degree of confusion as is seen in young children. Unfortunately, children with mental retardation, for example, are taught to be compliant with authority figures and to seek assistance. Consequently, they may not perceive that anyone has "hurt" them or "touched them in a bad way." Gaining information presents problems if questions are presented in a "yes-no" format. In addition, for cognitively or developmentally impaired victims who have been assaulted by non-painful means, reporting may be delayed as the person struggles with the meaning of the experience.

MOTOR-IMPAIRED VICTIM

The victim of sexual assault who has a motor impairment presents special considerations in the medical evaluation. Motor delays may be from the central nervous system to the distant muscle fiber.

Patients with gross and fine motor delays may be classified as shown in **Table 8-1**. Depending on the etiology of these motor delays, cognition may be spared. Cerebral palsy is a category of static motor dysfunction that is most often present at or shortly after birth. The exception is the traumatic brain injury victim, who often has significant gaps in motor, cognitive, and behavioral function. Other forms of cerebral palsy, such as spastic diplegia, are frequently the result of prematurity or may be secondary to perinatal asphyxia. Eighty-five percent of individuals with hemiplegia have both normal intelligence and the capability of complete independent living. Those persons with athetosis also have a higher incidence of near normal intelligence, although dysarthria may lead to poor speech intelligibility and the impression that the patient is not cognitively intact. Receptive language in such patients is often age appropriate. Keeping this in mind is important when determining a patient's ability to respond to questions regarding a sexual assault. In this instance, questions should be framed so that close to monosyllabic responses could suffice for information. A family member or other individual who is accustomed to the victim's communication style is invaluable to assist the examiner in understanding what is being communicated. Corroborative information from family members or others who are frequently with the victim should be obtained to better enhance the victim's credibility. Such corroboration would include the weather on the day of the assault, who was present in the house or facility, what time of day the assault may have taken place, to whom the victim may have made a disclosure, and the overall tendency to tell the truth that the familiar observer could affirm from experience.

Key Point:

Eighty-five percent of individuals with hemiplegia have both normal intelligence and are capable of completely independent living. Receptive language in patients with athetosis is often age appropriate, which should be borne in mind when determining the patient's ability to respond to questions concerning a sexual assault.

Table 8-1. Examples of Neurological Causes of Motor Delay

Central Nervous System	Hypoxic ischemic injury to the brain	Cerebral palsy, possible mental retardation
	Neuronal migration anomaly	Cerebal palsy and mental retardation
Spinal Cord Disorder	Spina bifida	Paraplegia with or without hydrocephalus
	Spinal cord injury	Paraplegia/quadriplegia
Anterior Horn Cell Disease	Spinal muscular atrophy	Hypotonia/areflexia
Neuropathies	Metachromatic leukodystrophy	Degenerative hypotonia with extreme weakness
Neuromuscular disorders	Myasthenia gravis	Ptosis, respiratory and generalized weakness, fatigue
Myopathies	Muscular dystrophy	Progressive proximal muscle weakness

Other causes of motor delay might include physiologic system dysfunctions such as those seen in patients with skeletal dysplasias, severe short stature with obesity, and compromised respiratory function.

INTERVIEW TECHNIQUES

It is helpful to frame questions within a certain topic once rapport has been established, so that the individual can focus on specific facts. For example, when discussing where the sexual assault occurred, the examiner should seek descriptions from the victim of the entire place, such as a home or school. Identifying normal rooms, such as a classroom or a lunchroom, assists the victim in thinking about the whole day and placing the event within the context of a school day.

Once the individual has been able to describe various locations in or around the scene of the crime, the examiner should verbally define that he or she wishes to talk about "the place where you got hurt, at school." This allows the individual with a disability to begin to recall how he or she came to be at the scene and chronologically what happened next. Children and adults with disabilities have a more difficult time shifting from topic to topic mentally and consequently should be assisted as much as possible in making such transitions. If an event occurred outside, for example, asking about weather conditions will help in corroboration of the event. One can confirm from weather reports easily if the conditions described by the victim were true on that day.

Redundancy in questioning for children and adults with disabilities increases the chance that both the examiner and the victim will be talking consistently about the same thing at the same time. Rephrasing questions allows one to ask the individual in several ways about the same information. When a victim is unchanged in the response, the examiner can feel more assured that there is no confusion regarding the facts. In addition, talking slowly is very helpful for such patients, because

Key Point:
Children and adults with disabilities have a more difficult time shifting from topic to topic mentally and should be assisted as much as possible in making these transitions.

complex sentences and sentences that run together in content and meaning can confuse a victim significantly. Recognizing that the receptive language age equivalent may be far less than chronological age will assist the examiner in having realistic expectations of question structure (Walker, 1999).

Words should be chosen with care when questioning persons with disabilities regarding what specifically happened. Terms such as "hurt" or "touch" may not reflect their recollection of the event. "Touch" may mean something that one does to a microwave oven. In the sexual assault scenario, "hurt" may or may not be appropriate. When a victim has been assaulted in an oral manner, for example, pain may not be the sensation that was experienced. Instead, words such as "put" or "placed" should be considered in the medical interview. "Did he put his hand right here?" If the victim does not have a consistent term for the genitalia or other anatomic areas, the examiner should point to the victim's body, not his or her own. Alternative choices are to use simple picture board symbols or to allow the victim to draw what happened. In questioning the victim, knowing what terms are used for anatomic parts of the body is helpful. Establishing if the assault has occurred once or more often is important in both interpretations of the physical findings and in discerning reasons for delayed disclosure.

In a residential facility where there are multiple care providers a victim may not be able to identify or name a specific perpetrator, unless the individual is very familiar with the names of caregivers. The ability to describe the individual is hampered by limitations in language, but the victim may be able to describe the person's normal duties with respect to care-providing responsibilities. For example, a disabled individual may give the history that "it was the man who always takes us to the lunchroom." The examiner should seek as much information as possible for the record so that investigators will have probable cause to put together a photographic line-up of employees within the institution. Most residential homes should have photographic identification badges for their employees, which are helpful as long as they are not so outdated that workers no longer resemble their photos. In this scenario, circumstantial information is also helpful, such as other staff observations of a specific individual who may have been seen exiting the victim's room. The timing of the assault may be established best by physical findings and collaborative history from others in the residential facility. This is important because of the difficulty with date and time definitions in a person who is cognitively delayed.

When taking a medical history from the victim, it is important to consider a gradual approach to seeking information. In some states and jurisdictions, the hearsay exception associated with a medical history must also meet the test that the victim understands that he or she is in a medical encounter. Consequently, it is important for the examiner to introduce herself as a physician, and that the individual is at a hospital or a special clinic, "to help people who may have been hurt or are sick." Establishing the fact that the encounter is for a medical diagnosis or treatment is essential, and it is even more important in the child or adult with a disability. Once this relationship has been made clear, any facts that are subsequently gathered are more likely to be acceptable within a court of law.

A brief test of mental status and short-term memory is helpful. This facilitates one's gauge of the victim's ability to observe, remember, and communicate. The presence of some degree of language delay should not be surprising. In a study of young children ages 4 to 7 years whose development was otherwise normal but who had been maltreated, all had a 12- to 18-month delay in both expressive and receptive language (Lyon & Saywitz, 1999). The most common disability in children is speech and language delay, which may compound cognitive, motor, and behavioral abnormalities. The examiner must assess if the victim is able to state his or her name and age, and where the examination is taking place. If the victim is unable to spontaneously give his or her whole name, the examiner should ask, "Do you have more names?" Questions regarding family members should be included if the victim resides with the family or sees them often. However, if the individual is in residential care, he or she may be unable to respond competently to questions about family members.

If the victim is accompanied by a parent, it is important to ask what the victim calls the parent before asking further questions about the family. Information regarding residence and time spent there assists in knowing if questions about the family residence are appropriate. The individual may not know his or her age if birthdays are events that go unacknowledged in that residence. It is important to know this information before asking the victim. Typically, children and adolescents are taught their ages and this concept is reinforced throughout the year. However, as they become older and more dependent on the care provider, actual age may become a less important detail. Asking if birthdays are times of celebrations in the environment in which this person lives will establish that the individual understands what a birthday is, although he or she may not remember his or her own birthday or age.

Questions about daily routines, such as, "What do you do when you get up in the morning?" encourage free association conversation in the rapport-building phase of the medical history. They also establish the victim's ability to recall normal activities of daily living. Prompts such as, "What happens after that?" are helpful in affording the examiner the opportunity to evaluate spontaneous language content and the ability of the victim to speak in terms of concrete actions versus more abstract feelings. Questions such as, "Do you stay home all day?" can assist the victim in expressing place and person concepts. They may also allow him or her to speak of an alleged perpetrator in an indirect fashion, so that the examiner might learn the terminology used in reference to this person and use those same terms. Using questions regarding yesterday, today, and tomorrow help to establish that the child has an understanding of time.

PHYSICAL EXAMINATION

Examinations in such settings may be very difficult and require sedation to complete evidence collection. Particularly if there is obvious evidence of genital trauma, sedation and pain management are indicated. Examination under anesthesia is also an option.

Several barriers limit access to a normal physical examination experience for a victim with a disability in the clinic and hospital setting. For adults and youths with disabilities, inaccessible parking and lack of ramps and curb cuts make reaching the healthcare facility problematic. On reaching the facility, interior and exterior doors that are wide enough and easy enough to open are important when a victim arrives with minimal assistance. When a woman or man arrives who is using a mobility device, the route through the facility should be such that maneuvering is optimal. If the waiting area for sexual assault victims is separate from the mainstream emergency room waiting area, space should be adequate to accommodate victims in wheelchairs without their having to be in the direct line of traffic to examination rooms. Other physical barriers to patients with disabilities include countertops and sign-in areas that are not low enough for a seated patient. Chairs should be provided for those who cannot stand while waiting to complete necessary paperwork. Examination tables should have motorized adjustable height and head supports. This will facilitate the patient's ability to transfer to a table from a wheelchair, for example, with minimal need for assistance, which reinforces independence. Toilets also should be accessible and dressing rooms large enough for a person using a wheelchair to navigate.

One of the most significant consequences of access barriers to patients with disabilities is the fact that disabled women are less likely to have regular pelvic examinations than other women (Nosek et al., 1995). Providing for dignified and independent access for disabled sexual assault victims ensures that neither the patient nor a staff member will be injured during a transfer onto the examination table. Asking each woman what would make the examination more comfortable should be a part of the examination process. Patients who are able to respond to this question understand their personal circumstances far better than an unfamiliar aide. Their direction helps maintain a patient-centered care system. In women or men with cerebral palsy, osteoporosis may have caused the sexual assault to be associated with an occult fracture. If the patient seems to be in pain and unable to tolerate simple manipulation, pelvic, hip, and lower extremity films should be obtained before the examination to assure that no fracture has occurred.

Positioning of the patient's legs for an adequate and complete pelvic examination for women with range of motion restrictions secondary to spasticity of the lower extremities is a most important consideration. Restricted range of motion may be encountered with women or children who have had a stroke, spina bifida, cerebral palsy, multiple sclerosis, or orthopedic injuries. Patients who have knee flexion or extension contractures may have to be examined with the legs lifted upward rather than using stirrups. Maximum abduction is best accomplished by as much knee flexion as is possible in the spastic patient.

The temperature of the room and table can cause a victim with lower extremity spasticity to become far more rigid and unable to relax, particularly if either is too cold. Occasionally, pulmonary compromise is another consideration, particularly in patients with a tracheostomy. Maintaining the table in a 45-degree angle may present some difficulty for the examiner but facilitates the patient's tolerance of the examination. Administration of oxygen should be considered in the patient whose disability is associated with shortness of breath or where scoliosis makes the examination more difficult with respect to positioning. It may be necessary to examine the patient in a bed rather than on a firm examination table because the latter may cause far more discomfort for the victim.

It is necessary that extra personnel be on hand to assist with the examination for such tasks as stabilizing the lower extremities. Involuntary leg movements are not uncommon in women who are having this type of examination. However, in women with neurological conditions affecting the lower extremities, spasticity is often more pronounced. This can be managed by gentle stretching of the lower extremities during positioning as well as application of a 2% lidocaine gel to the perineum. Any rapid movements can result in both pain and increased spasticity, and should be avoided.

When the examination entails a woman with a spinal cord injury above the level of T-6, there is a potential for the development of autonomic dysreflexia. Autonomic dysreflexia (also known as autonomic hyperreflexia, paroxysmal hypertension in spinal cord injury, hypertensive autonomic crisis, and paroxysmal neurogenic hypertension) is the reaction of the autonomic nervous system to discomfort in visceral organs such as the cervix, uterus, bladder, or rectum, all of which are manipulated during the pelvic examination (Welner, 1988). There is a paroxysmal reflex sympathetic discharge as a result of this noxious stimulation of the autonomic nervous system. These patients may already have this complication because of the sexual assault. Signs and symptoms may include an increase or decrease in heart rate, irregular pulse, labile hypertension, facial flushing, headache, nasal congestion, nausea, pupillary dilation, muscle spasms, and diaphoresis (**Table 8-2**).

Management of autonomic dysreflexia during a sexual assault examination should include placing the patient in a semi-upright position if he or she is supine, loosening of the clothing or constrictive devices such as a spinal brace, administration of a rapid acting antihypertensive agent, pain control, immediate bladder catheterization, and treating infection. Further intervention may require

Key Point:
Dignified and independent access to the examination ensures that neither a victim nor a staff member is injured during transfer onto the examination table. Asking each woman what would make the examination more comfortable should be a part of the examination process. Patients who are able to respond to this question understand their personal circumstances far better than an unfamiliar aide, and allowing their direction is very helpful in maintaining a patient-centered care system.

Key Point:
Factors that are helpful in providing a more comfortable examination experience include the following:
— *Positioning of the patient's legs*
— *Warming the temperature of the room and table*
— *Positioning of the table in a 45-degree angle to avoid pulmonary compromise*
— *Administration of oxygen*
— *Examining the patient on a bed rather than a firm examination table if more comfortable for the patient*
— *Employing extra personnel to assist with the examination*

assistance from an anesthesiologist. The patient may not be able to verbalize symptoms, therefore monitoring blood pressure would be a minimum precaution for any spinal cord injured patient requiring a pelvic examination.

Another group of patients who will require careful management when being examined for sexual assault are spina bifida patients. These patients have a high incidence of latex allergy, which can lead to anaphylaxis in extreme cases. Consequently, the examiner must be careful to use latex-free gloves during the examination. If a clean intermittent catheterization is to be done before or after the examination either to empty the bladder or to collect evidence, a latex-free catheter must be used.

A rape kit should be used to collect evidence. The possibility of having acquired a sexually transmitted disease should be considered and discussed. Certain disabilities are associated with poor immune response, and the disabled victim may be at greater risk than other victims. Pregnancy prophylaxis should be considered as well as appropriate counseling of the victim and family so that actions that are in the best interest of the patient may be expedited.

In a sexual assault case, there are two crime scenes: the victim and the site where the crime occurred. Both "scenes" deserve meticulous attention to ensure the integrity of results. Evidence collection is extremely important at the crime scene as well as when the child or youth is brought to the health care facility owing to the possibility that the perpetrator of sexual assault of a disabled person is a serial offender. Evidence from the present crime may indicate a modus operandus similar to other crimes. Furthermore, the commission of these crimes may lack careful efforts to disguise the identity of the assailant. If an ambulance has been dispatched, the sexual assault examiner should carefully review Emergency Medical Service

Table 8-2. Autonomic Dysreflexia (or Hyperreflexia)	
Etiology	Painful stimuli of visceral organs that result in the activation of the autonomic nervous system receptors leading to paroxysmal sympathetic discharges. Bladder and bowel distension are the most common causes.
Target vessels	Aorta, large vessels of the brain
Manifestations	Diffuse muscle spasms, usually in the lower extremities
Trigger organs	Visceral organs such as the bladder, cervix, rectum, and uterus
Potential gynecologic triggers	Pelvic, rectal, or urologic examinations; severe menstrual cramps; pelvic pain; ruptured ovarian cyst; UTIs; perineal pain as is seen in fecal impaction; decubitus ulcers
Treatment	Semi-supine positioning, loosening of clothing and other constrictive devices, rapid-acting antihypertensive agent, pain control, immediate bladder catheterization, and treating infection. Possible anesthesia consultation.
Complications	Seizures, intracranial hemorrhage, coma
Risk of death	Significant

(EMS) records. Often, fictitious histories change from the time that the EMS personnel arrive at the scene to the time that a more careful story is provided in the emergency room setting. Inconsistencies in the perpetrator history is the rule rather than the exception in all forms of abuse. Any forensic clues to the potential identity of the perpetrator should be documented carefully, stored in the sexual assault kit, and communicated with the law enforcement response team. Careful studies have shown the greatest yield for positive forensic evidence in the prepubertal child sexual assault victim is from the clothing gathered and submitted with the rape kit (Christian et al., 2000). The DNA evidence present in this material was found to be more reliable than those fluids found on the victim's body. Realization of this fact requires a mandatory, careful retrieval of any and all articles of clothing the child was known to have been wearing at the probable time of the crime. From a crime scene perspective, this includes discarded diapers or wipe cloths that might be present at the scene.

DNA laboratory analysis involves examination of a DNA strand at 13 specific locations. The DNA profile evidence can be compared to a known source, such as profiles maintained in a databank of convicted sex offenders. The most comprehensive databank has been established by the Federal Bureau of Investigation and is called the Combined DNA Index System (CODIS), which includes both known perpetrator DNA evidence as well as DNA samples taken from crime scenes where no suspect is known. This affords law enforcement the opportunity to identify a suspect or link serial crime scenes. This is particularly important when the victim is disabled, because suspect identification might be marginal or less than the level of proof required in a court of law.

A DNA result may fall into one of three categories: inclusion, exclusion, or inconclusive. Inclusion refers to the circumstance when the DNA profile of a known individual matches the DNA profile from the crime scene. The strength of this inclusion depends in part, however, on the number of DNA locations examined and the statistics reflecting how often the general profile would be found in the general population. Rare DNA patterns will have a stronger case for the suspect to have been at the scene of the crime. However, if the DNA pattern is very common, such as might be seen in 1 in 2000 people, the biological evidence is less assured. Increasing the number of DNA locations tested generally results in more powerful statistics.

Key Point:
A DNA result may fall into one of three categories:
— Inclusion
— Exclusion
— Inconclusive

When there is no DNA match between the suspect and the crime scene, the profile is referenced as "excluded." Exclusion does not necessarily mean that a suspect is innocent. It is possible that no body fluids may have passed between the victim and the assailant even though a sexual assault took place.

Inconclusive results indicate that DNA testing did not produce information that would allow an individual to be either included or excluded as the source of the biological evidence. There may be several reasons for an inconclusive result. Even with the ability to reclaim DNA from minute sources, there may have been insufficient quantity or quality of DNA to produce definitive typing results. Another example of inconclusive DNA results might occur when the evidentiary sample contains a mixture of DNA from several individuals, as might occur in a gang rape scenario. Even if the suspect's DNA is found in this source, the presence of DNA from other sources may prohibit the establishment of an inclusive or exclusive result (Turman, 2001).

Violence associated with sexual assault, although uncommon in the disabled child and youth, requires close surveillance for head and neck injury, facial trauma, and other bodily injuries. If the victim's disabilities include communication difficulties, the clinicians must be very thorough, as if examining a very young child, to be assured of discovering every affected site. Defensive wounds, which usually occur to the upper extremities when the victim assumes a defensive posture, should be carefully noted. Injuries that result from defending against the assailant's hand or weapon can be seen on the upper outer arms, shoulders, or palms of the hands.

Case Study

John M. was a 21-year-old male with Down syndrome and autistic behaviors. He lived with his mother during the weekends and was in a residential facility during the week. Mrs. M. had recently terminated a 3-year relationship with George, a man who admitted the need for a gay partner. Even though he had established residence with his friend, he continued to visit Mrs. M. and to take John for overnight visits on the weekends. Mrs. M. did not note any change in John's behavior until one evening as she was assisting him with bathing after he had spent the weekend with George. Mrs. M., who was a school nurse, noticed that John's anal area was red and tender. She told John to stand in the tub, and asked what had happened. John's only response was to point toward his anus and say, "George." She immediately brought him to the emergency room.

The emergency room evaluation was difficult and inconclusive. John had to wait for 2 hours before being seen and was very anxious in such an unfamiliar environment. No attempts were made to question John or to establish rapport with him. When the examiner was unable to convince John to let him remove his clothing or to take a prone knee-chest position on the examination table to be examined, the evaluation came to a rapid conclusion. It was deemed inappropriate to consider sedation to complete the examination. Mrs. M. was very distressed both by the process and by the frustration of being unable to confirm or dismiss the disclosure that John had made. He was referred to a subspecialty clinic for child sexual abuse.

At the specialty clinic, John's history was obtained from his mother and copies of his most recent complete psychometric evaluation were reviewed. The clinician discussed with Mrs. M. the best ways to get John to cooperate with the examination and learned that he would be most willing if his mother was not only in the room, but also a participant in the examination process. Mrs. M. described behavior changes in John, which had not been present before his weekend with George. These changes included separation anxiety, increased perseveration, poor sleeping noted at his residential facility, and markedly increased masturbation. Using her guidance, John spent some time with the examiner alone while a better understanding of his communication level was established.

John's 2-year-old psychometric evaluation revealed that he was functioning at the 4-year level cognitively. This was important information that allowed the examiner to better phrase her questions to John, because most of his responses were in one- and two-word sentences. When presented a picture of an Asian American boy, John became excited, pointed at the picture and said, "John, John!" John was able to identify receptively all body parts on both the drawing and himself. When asked if he was hurting today, John expressed understanding and shook his head, "No." As the examiner talked about each of his body parts asking again about hurting, John's response was consistently negative until the examiner used his word for buttocks. This caused John to immediately become sad and have downcast eyes, accompanied by the response, "Yes." When pointing to the buttocks on the drawing, John quickly stated, "George, George." The examiner used other tasks to distract John from his body parts for a short time and then returned to a new drawing of an Asian American boy. Again, when the examiner indicated the buttocks on the drawing, John responded quickly, "George!"

Later when brought to the examination room, John was very cooperative with the examiner. His mother was in the room and facilitated his removal of his clothes. He understood her instruction to "bend over" without problems, and the examiner could look at John's anus with a colposcope more easily and completely. John again pointed to his anus and said, "George, George." The anal examination was normal.

Discussion

John made unsupervised overnight visits with George for several months. He had no behavioral changes, according to his mother, although she was not with John most of the week. In addition, despite the fact that Mrs. M.'s boyfriend had admitted to a preference for male partners, she saw her own son as "still a child" and felt no qualms about allowing him to spend nights at the home of George.

At the specialty clinic, background information essential to evaluating this patient included a general health and medical history from his mother, and further information regarding his cognition and communication. The examiner needed to know that John was primarily monosyllabic in his communication skills in order to interview him in the best manner. Information regarding memory, perseveration, compulsions, and social skills was important in interpreting John's disclosure. The degree of autism needed to be fully discussed before the examiner interviewed John in order to avoid triggers that might cause John to lapse into auto-stimulatory behaviors. It was important to learn if John was able to respond to such questions as "who" or "what," which may be too abstract for a person with autistic behaviors. In addition, it was helpful to know whether care provider communication was augmented with sign language and whether phrases were limited to one- or two-word sentences. This information was obtained from the nonoffending care provider who sought medical care. A careful pre-interview, therefore, was valuable in preparing to talk with John. Separation issues also were explored so that the interview method could be adapted so as to avoid increasing John's agitation due to his inability or unwillingness to separate from his mother.

In the emergency room setting, attempts were made to examine John, but his anxiety became too great and, in a hysterical frenzy, he became combative. He was discharged with recommendations to follow up with his primary care physician in 24 to 48 hours. A rape kit was unsuccessfully attempted. The primary care physician made a referral to a child sexual abuse clinic.

Sexual assault associated with exploitation is even more difficult to address in light of the fact that photography that may have been done may have been completed while the child was chemically influenced and could not recall any details of the episode.

Exploitation involving production of child pornography has been well documented in evidence analysis of criminal cases. Treatment of children who are sexually assaulted in conjunction with photo documentation may be obviously delayed. Physical disabilities are often more evident in these types of cases, and in the rare circumstance that a child is brought for medical care after such victimization, there is often a scenario of multiple perpetrators of sexual assault.

SEXUAL ASSAULT AND HOMICIDE

When sexual assault has resulted in a homicide of a disabled child or youth, the cause of death is usually strangulation, often associated with blunt trauma to the head and/or stabbing. Frequently, two of these three causes are present and occasionally all three (DiMaio & Dana, 1998). The child victim is frequently severely torn through the vagina or rectum or through both. This is especially the case when the child is quite small because of the size of the vagina and rectum. When the victim is a youth, genital trauma is often less severe, although not invariably so. When present, there may be abrasions, superficial lacerations, or contusions at the introitus of the vagina, most commonly at the 6 o'clock position. Bruising to the inner thighs is not uncommon, and there also may be bite marks noted on the breasts in female children and youths.

Anal injuries in the sexual assault homicide case may be minor and, if present, are at the anal verge, scattered around the circumference in a random fashion (DiMaio & Dana, 1998). Examination of the perineum, the perianal area, and the thighs using an ultraviolet light may reveal seminal deposits, which fluoresce, although this is nonspecific. Swabs of all of these areas should be done for further analysis.

In the homicide victim who is disabled, preexisting medical problems may contribute to death. For example, many children with congenital syndromes have significant underlying heart disease. Adolescents with Williams syndrome may have undiagnosed critical supravalvular aortic stenosis, pulmonic valvular stenosis, hypoplasia of the aorta, or other arterial anomalies (Buyse, 1990). Forty percent of children and youths with Down syndrome have endocardial cushion defects, ventricular septal defects, or patent ductus arteriosus. Depending on the availability of medical care for these children, there may or may not be evidence of prior open-heart surgery. The presence of such conditions as these may complicate their ability to tolerate a violent assault.

Vertebral anomalies, particularly of the cervical spine, may predispose a child or youth with a disability to death during a sexual assault. Individuals with Down syndrome have a 12% incidence of atlantoaxial instability, a condition that usually requires physical education modifications in school and with certain sports. Attempted strangulation or hyperflexion and extension of the neck of such patients, as can occur with severe shaking or facial blunt trauma, might cause cervical spine dislocation with spinal cord injury and possibly death. Patients with severe scoliosis associated with neuromuscular disease will also be at higher risk for skeletal injury. Spastic quadriplegia, spinal muscular atrophy type II, and spina bifida are examples of motor problems that contribute to such complications. Nonambulatory individuals often have significant osteoporosis, causing ease of fractures. Visually impaired victims may be killed without the perpetrator realizing that identification would be very difficult. However, the motive for homicide in the sexual assault victim may not be only to hide potential evidence and discovery. A perpetrator may attempt to disguise the crime by burning or burying the body, hoping to destroy evidence of the sexual nature of the original act.

MULTIDISCIPLINARY CONSIDERATIONS

Even in the Emergency Room setting, a team decision making process is indicated particularly when the victim has a disability. Many communities have established a sexual assault response team (SART). The expertise of specially trained sexual assault investigators, in conjunction with a sexual assault nurse examiner (SANE) and possibly a prosecutor with advanced training in sexual assault cases is invaluable. In the circumstance of a disabled victim, physical evidence of an acute sexual assault is self-explanatory. However, in the circumstance of a non/verbal child victim, who may have been assaulted more than 24 hours before, and who may have no physical evidence whatsoever of a sexual encounter, review of custody or other extenuating concerns that might support either a coerced or spontaneous false allegation should at least be considered. When a team documents that there has been attention to this possibility and discerns that enough evidence exists to discount this hypothesis, the credibility of the final decision is increased. Such documentation may be included in the medical record, dependent upon jurisdictional considerations.

In the institutional setting, contamination of caregiver histories may occur even without a specific motive to suppress information. Law enforcement questioning will be important in determining what is rumor and what acts actually have been observed. The sexual assault may have been witnessed, or the victim may have been discovered very shortly after the event occurred. If a child with mental retardation, for example, is brought from a residential care center, the person who made the original complaint should be interviewed rather than others who initially deny any knowledge of the assault. On occasion, a victim may not present as an emotionally traumatized person, but instead with sexually reactive behaviors that might indicate abuse of a chronic nature.

When a sexual assault victim survives and is brought for medical care with or without the assistance of EMS, 3 other components are necessary to document for legal considerations:

1. The child's method and content of disclosure

2. A history of changes in the behavior of the child victim

3. Physical examination findings, which would include the child's behavior during the examination

Key Point:
Recognizing that acute sexual assault in the child or youth is often a single event within a context of chronic sexual abuse leads the examiner to revise the typical medical interview.

Recognizing that acute sexual assault in the child and youth is often a single event within a context of chronic sexual abuse requires that the examiner revise the typical medical interview. This is also the case when a disability is present. It is essential in some jurisdictions to establish with the victim the understanding that the examiner is a healthcare professional and that this encounter is, indeed, a "check-up." This is to make it clear that the history that is being obtained is for the purpose of establishing a medical diagnosis and to render treatment. Due to the forensic nature of the sexual assault examination, it is a legal ploy that evidence so collected be excluded, because the patient did not understand the medical nature of the examination. In light of the fact that a disabled patient might have impaired cognition, it is even more important to document that the patient expresses an understanding that they are "here to see the doctor and to make sure that their body will be all right." Although acute sexual assault evaluations are typically in a hospital setting, there are many facilities that have special areas for rape and assault victims to be interviewed and examined separate from the frenzy of a busy emergency room. Failure to inform the victim with a disability of this fact as well as documenting the victim's understanding may, depending on various state statutes, lead to a successful suppression of the medical history, which usually meets the hearsay exception.

Establishing that a victim is competent to give a medical history should be feasible if the person's cognitive developmental level is at least age 4 years. If the person is an adult with mental retardation but is capable of self-care and has mastered activities of daily living, it is probable that mental competence can be established for clinical purposes. Gathering information from a familiar care provider regarding the child's or youth's short- and long-term memory, reliability to recount normal facts, and expressive and receptive language abilities is very important. Although a disabled individual may not be able to read, he or she may be able to consistently recall incidents that have had a major impact on his or her memory. It is helpful to access information regarding the patient's performance on standardized instruments of cognitive abilities, including verbal and performance skills, such as are noted on the Wechsler Intelligence Scale for Children (Wechsler, 1992). Adaptive abilities measured by tests such as the Vineland Adaptive Behavior Scale or the Adaptive Behavior Rating Scale indicate social maturity and levels of self-help skills (Vineland Adaptive Behavior Scale, 1984; Hawthorne Adaptive Behavior Rating Scale, 1987). Often individuals who have cognitive impairments score in a much more functional range than would be reflected in intelligence tests. These instruments facilitate a description of the person's ability to function in society and to achieve normal living, despite an IQ score. It is important to remember that although patients may have multiple disabilities, they may have extreme capabilities to recount recent events.

Sexually explicit knowledge is not along the normal psychosexual developmental continuum of children or youths with or without significant disabilities. Consequently, individuals who use sexually explicit language in describing events that have happened to them must have acquired the vocabulary from either environmental exposure of a chronic nature or through sexual experiences that have been explained in this manner. Access to and use of pornography, for example, is not usually seen in this group unless it has been intentionally provided for the purpose of victim grooming or to facilitate exploitation. It is possible that a disabled adult might purchase significant amounts of pornography, but children and youths are generally still supervised in such a manner that exposure would be rare.

At times, inference of the abuse site may occur through the patient's subsequent behavior. There may be what appears to be an irrational fear of or an aversion to a specific room or area in the home or facility. This behavior is not different from what is sometimes noted in children and adolescents who have no developmental problems and constitutes another historical component regarding the site of assault. This information is often provided in the situation of chronic sexual abuse, and it is important to note that the acute sexual assault victim often comes for medical care after the most recent event within the context of recurrent episodes.

Other behaviors that may be seen in a sexually abused developmentally delayed child or adolescent depend on the victim's experience with the sexual assault and/or prior abuse. If the sexual experience was not painful, the victim may present with recurrent autostimulatory behaviors and masturbation. When force, coercion, and painful assaultive events have occurred, the child often has signs of acute traumatic stress and extreme fearfulness. Many behaviors consistent with chronic child sexual abuse may exist, and obtaining a careful history regarding those types of manifestations is indicated. Sexual offending behaviors or recurrent mutual sexual behaviors may be difficult to eradicate in this population and will require a careful and consistent behavioral modification plan so that the victim may return to a lifestyle that is as normal as possible and be accepted socially in the least restrictive environment.

The issue of consent must also be addressed with the child or adolescent with a disability (Lumley & Miltenberger, 1997). It is not uncommon for a sexual assault victim who is nonverbal to be reported as a consensual partner with a similar aged sibling or other person with a disability. Sibling abuse either represents parental or caretaker neglect, or a convenient fabrication of the etiology of a sexual assault. The focus of the issue of consent is not volition alone but includes the victim's ability to understand the nature of the sexual act and its consequences as well as his or her ability to understand and use actual volition (Parker & Abramson, 1995). An adolescent who is developmentally disabled usually lacks an adequate foundation for understanding a consensual sexual relationship. Such a person has typically lacked experience in dating or formal sex education. Without confirmation of an understanding of sex education, this individual would not satisfy the legal criteria for distinguishing between a consensual sex act and sexual abuse (Parker & Abramson, 1995).

Key Point::
An adolescent who is developmentally disabled typically lacks experience in dating or formal sex education. Without confirmation of an understanding of sex education, this individual would not satisfy the legal criteria for distinguishing between consensual sex acts and sexual abuse.

In the emergency room setting the role of the social worker becomes immensely important, because information regarding the victim's functional levels and language comprehension will assist the practitioner in crafting appropriate questions. In addition, family information, past reports to child protective services or law enforcement, and assistance regarding who might represent an uninformed but nonoffending parent or care provider are invaluable adjuncts to the ultimate disposition for the victim. For example, should there be prior reports to CPS of neglect or sexual abuse, the decision at the time of this new medical encounter may be made for out-of-home placement, until a more in depth investigation could take place. Information regarding an uninformed but non/offending care provider would assist as well in determining if the patient would be at risk for coercion to recant. The hospital social worker can also assist in victim advocacy options should other factors such as domestic violence, substance abuse, or an abusive therapist/patient relationship play a role in the victimization of the child or disabled adult. It is important to remember that 48.1% of perpetrators of sexual abuse against people with disabilities gained access to their victims through disability services (Sobsey, 1994).

Another aspect of sexual assault in conjunction with sexual exploitation is the mentally impaired child who is being prostituted by a family member (Tharinger et al., 1990). This places the child at risk for physical and emotional abuse, in addition to sexual assault. Fifty-two percent of victims involved in prostitution suffer from posttraumatic stress disorder during the time that they are working as prostitutes. Children who are marketed by family members are at high risk for sexually transmitted diseases, more severe genital trauma, and exposure to HIV and AIDS. The underlying mental impairment and a conditioned compliance to authority figures causes these children to be difficult to rescue. They constitute a profit-making venture for their relatives. Data collected from research regarding sexual exploitation of juveniles estimated the number of sexually exploited children living in their own homes between the ages of 10 and 17 years in the general populations to be approximately 73,000, a much higher number than previously assumed. Victim interviews pointed strongly to the nuclear family as the catalyst for this form of exploitation (Aarji, 1997; Estes & Weiner, 2001; O'Brien, 1991).

Competence to testify in court has legal ramifications and includes 4 factors:

1. A present understanding of the difference between a truth and a lie as well as an indication that the person feels compelled to speak the truth

2. The mental capacity at the time of the occurrence of the event to observe or receive accurate impressions of the event

3. Memory sufficient to retain an independent recollection of the observations

4. The capacity to communicate into words that memory and to understand questions about the event (Melton, 1981)

In the child or youth with a disability, establishing that there is an understanding between a truth and a lie rests on information from a care provider familiar with the individual. Children and youths may certainly participate in pretend play, but this normal developmental behavior does not preclude their ability to understand truths and lies and to be reliable historians. It is also important to resist the temptation to stereotype children and youths with disabilities as unreliable witnesses. For example, children with certain types of cerebral palsy, such as choreoathetosis and hemiplegia, have a high incidence of normal intelligence, although verbal dysarthria may make their oral communication difficult for the layperson to understand. For this reason, use of a family member may be necessary in the history component of the evaluation, to ensure that the examiner fully comprehends the meaning of what the victim is expressing. This is one indication for an interview with a parent or familiar care provider present. Some adolescents with choreoathetosis are almost completely nonverbal, but may be able to type their communications accurately. Exploration of this form of communication will be important for the examiner of the sexual assault victim. Many such youths use laptop assistive communication devices and may be able to express more fully the details of their assault through this manner.

SUMMARY

Children and adults with a disability are at higher risk for all forms of abuse. Sexual assault may occur within the context of many problems, including a hate crime, elder abuse, or disability related abuse, in which perpetrators withhold needed interventions, such as wheelchairs, medications, transportation or other necessary assistance. Although sexual victimization occurs in at least 20% of females and 5% to 10% of males in the Unites States, it is estimated that more than 90% of people with disabilities will experience sexual abuse or assault in their lifetime. Numerous myths exist that contribute to the perception that persons with disabilities are in some manner "immune" to the physical and emotional impact of sexual assault. A significant number of disabled children and adults are sexually assaulted by a provider of a therapeutic service. Obtaining a medical history, being aware of behavioral changes, and following similar procedures for obtaining forensic evidence in the physical examination is very important in the evaluation of these types of cases. It is important to modify one's approach to the interview and the physical examination as one makes accommodations for the existing disability. Recognizing specific medical conditions which may become life threatening due to the assault or the examination is imperative. Disabled individuals who are assaulted with resultant death may have medical conditions which contribute more to the death than the trauma of the assault itself. Implementation of a team approach even in the Emergency Room setting provides the most ideal manner of decision making regarding the investigative process. Inclusion of consideration of sexual exploitation by family members is another important point for clinicians who find disabled sexual assault victims who appear to be involved in prostitution. It is imperative to keep an open mind and be vigilant in attention to detail for the evaluation of these types of victims, as careful clinical assessment will yield a court-worthy case.

APPENDIX: DIRECTORY OF SERVICE PROVIDERS

(First Response to Victims of Crime Who Have a Disability. Washington DC: US Department of Justice; Office of Justice Programs; Office for Victims of Crime; October 2002.)

Alzheimer's Disease

Alzheimer's Association
(800) 272-3900; (312) 335-8882, TTY
www.alz.org

Alzheimer's Association's *Safe Return Program*
Crisis Line: (800) 572-1122; (314) 647-5959, TTY
Nonemergency Line: (888) 572-8566; (888) 500-5759, TTY
www.alz.org/caregiver/programs/safereturn.htm

Americans with Disabilities Act of 1990 and Section 504 of the Rehabilitation Act of 1973

Americans with Disabilities Act Information Line
(800) 514-0301; (800) 514-0383, TTY
www.usdoj.gov/crt/ada/adahom1.htm

Office of Justice Programs
US Department of Justice
(202) 307-0690; (202) 307-2027, TTY

Blindness or Visual Impairment

American Council of the Blind
(800) 424-8666
www.acb.org

American Foundation for the Blind
(800) 232-5463; (212) 502-7662, TTY
www.afb.org

Deafness or Hard of Hearing

National Association of the Deaf
(301) 587-1788; (301) 587-1789, TTY
www.nad.org

National Institute on Deafness and Other Communication Disorders
(800) 241-1044; (800) 241-1055, TTY
www.nidcd.nih.gov

Registry of Interpreters for the Deaf
(703) 838-0030; (703) 838-0459, TTY
www.rid.org

Mental Illness

National Alliance for the Mentally Ill
(800) 950-6264; (703) 516-7227, TTY
www.nami.org

National Depressive and Manic-Depressive Association
(800) 826-3632
www.ndmda.org

Treatment Advocacy Center
(703) 294-6001
www.psychlaws.org

Mental Retardation

American Association on Mental Retardation
(800) 424-3688
www.aamr.org

National Down Syndrome Congress
(800) 232-6372
www.ndsccenter.org

The Arc of the United States
(800) 433-5255
www.thearc.org

Other National Victim Resources

Battered Women's Justice Project
(800) 903-0111
www.bwjp.org

Childhelp USA/Forrester National Child Abuse Hotline
(800) 422-4453; (800) 222-4453, TTY
www.childhelpusa.org

Family Violence Department's Resource Center on Domestic Violence:
Child Protection and Custody
(800) 527-3223
http://nationalcouncilfvd.org

Family Violence Prevention Fund/Health Resource Center
(888) 792-2873; (800) 595-4889
www.endabuse.org

Mothers Against Drunk Driving
(800) 438-6233
www.madd.org

National Center for Missing and Exploited Children
(800) 843-5678; (800) 826-7653, TTY
www.ncmec.org

National Center for Victims of Crime
(800) 394-2255; (800) 211-7996, TTY
www.ncvc.org

National Children's Alliance
(800) 239-9950
www.nca-online.org

National Clearinghouse for Alcohol and Drug Information
(800) 729-6686; (800) 487-4889, TTY; (800) 735-2258, TTY Relay Service
www.health.org

National Clearinghouse on Child Abuse and Neglect Information
(800) 394-3366
www.calib.com/nccanch

National Coalition Against Domestic Violence
(800) 537-2238; (800) 553-2508, TTY
www.ncadv.org

National Criminal Justice Reference Service
(800) 851-3420; (877) 712-9279, TTY
www.ncjrs.org

National Domestic Violence Hotline
(800) 799-7233; (800) 787-3224, TTY
www.ndvh.org

National Fraud Information Center
(800) 876-7060
www.fraud.org

National Organization for Victim Assistance
(800) 879-6682
www.try-nova.org

Office for Victims of Crime Resource Center
(800) 627-6872; (877) 712-9279, TTY
www.ojp.usdoj.gov/ovc/ovcres

Parents of Murdered Children
(888) 818-7662
www.pomc.org

Rape, Abuse & Incest National Network
(800) 656-4673
www.rainn.org

REFERENCES

Aarji SK. *Sexually Aggressive Children: Coming to Understand Them.* Thousand Oaks, Calif: Sage Publishing; 1997.

Americans with Disabilities Act of 1990.

Burgess A, Dowdell E, Prentky R. Sexual abuse in nursing home residents. *J Psychosoc Nurs.* 2000;38(6):10-18, 48-49.

Buyse ML. *Birth Defects Encyclopedia.* Dover, Mass: Blackwell Scientific Publications; 1990.

Ceci S, Leichtman M, Putnick M, eds. *Cognitive and Social Factors in Early Deception.* Hillsdale, NJ: Erlbaum; 1992.

Child Abuse Prevention, Adoption, and Family Services Act of 1988. Pub L No. 100-294, Sec. 101 [42 U.S.C. 5101].

Christian CW, Lavelle JM, De Jong A, Loiselle J, Brenner L, Joffe M. Forensic evidence findings in prepubertal victims of sexual assault. *Pediatrics.* 2000;106:100-107.

Crosse S, Kaye E, Ratnofsky A, et al. *A Report on the Maltreatment of Children with Disabilities.* Washington, DC: US Department of Health; Administration for Children and Families; Administration of Child, Youth, and Families; National Center on Child Abuse and Neglect; 1993.

DiMaio VJM, Dana S. *Handbook of Forensic Pathology.* Austin, Tex: Landes Bioscience; 1998.

Estes RJ, Weiner NA. *The Commercial Sexual Exploitation of Children in the U.S., Canada and Mexico.* Philadelphia, Pa: University of Pennsylvania; 2001:59.

Fair Housing Amendment Act of 1988.

Federal Bureau of Investigation (FBI). *Summary of Hate Crime Statistics.* Washington, DC: Federal Bureau of Investigation; 2000.

Furey EM. Sexual abuse of adults with mental retardation: who and where. *Ment Retard.* 1994;32:173.

General Accounting Office (GAO). *Additional Steps Needed to Strengthen Enforcement of Federal Quality Standards.* Washington, DC: US General Accounting Office; 1999. Publication GAO/HEHS-99-46.

General Accounting Office. *Nursing Homes: Complaint Investigation Processes Often Inadequate to Protect Resident.* Washington, DC: US General Accounting Office; 1999. Publication GAO/HEHS-99-80.

General Accounting Office. *Nursing Homes: Sustained Efforts Are Essential to Realize Potential of the Quality Initiatives.* Washington, DC: US General Accounting Office; 2000. Publication GAO/HEHS-00-197.

Gil E, Johnson TC. *Sexualized Children Assessment and Treatment of Sexualized Children and Children Who Molest.* Rockville, Md: Launch Press; 1993.

Hate Crimes Prevention Act of 1999.

Hawthorne Adaptive Behavior Rating Scale. Columbia, Mo: Hawthorne Educational Services, Inc; 1987.

Holmes JF. US population: a profile of America's diversity—the view from the Census Bureau, 1998. *The World Almanac and Book of Facts.* Mahwah, NJ: Primedia Reference; 1999.

Hugo V. *Notre Dame de Paris.* New York, NY: PF Collier & Son; 1917.

LaPlante M, Carlson D. *Disability in the US: Prevalence and Causes, 1992.* US Department of Education; National Institute on Disability and Rehabilitation Research; 1996. Disability Statistics Report 7.

Lumley VA, Miltenberger RG. Sexual abuse prevention for persons with mental retardation. *Am J Ment Retard.* 1997;101:459.

Lyon T, Saywitz K. Young maltreated children's competence to take the oath. *Appl Dev Sci.* 1999;3:16-27.

Melton G. Procedural reforms to protect child victim: witnesses in sex offense proceedings. In: Bulkley J, ed. *Child Sexual Abuse and the Law.* Washington, DC: American Bar Association National Legal Resource Center for Child Advocacy and Protection; 1981.

Nosek MA, Young ME, Rintala D, Howland C, Clubb F, Bennett J. Barriers to reproductive health maintenance among women with physical disabilities. *J Women's Health.* 1995;45:505-518.

O'Brien M. *Taking Sibling Incest Seriously.* Newbury Park, Calif: Sage Publishing; 1991.

Parker T, Abramson PR. The law hath not been dead: protecting adults with mental retardation from sexual abuse and violation of their sexual freedom. *Ment Retard.* 1995;33:257-258, 261-262.

Payne B, Cikovic R. An empirical examination of the characteristics, consequences, and causes of elder abuse in nursing homes. *J Elder Abuse Negl.* 1995; 7(4):61-74.

Rehabilitation Act of 1973. Amendment Section 508; 1998.

Sobsey D. *Violence and Abuse in the Lives of People with Disabilities: The End of Silent Acceptance?* Baltimore, Md: Paul H. Brookes; 1994.

Sobsey D, Mansell S. The prevention of sexual abuse of people with developmental disabilities. *Dev Disabilities Bull.* 1990;18:55-66.

Sorensen DD. The invisible victims. *Impact.* Minneapolis, Minn: University of Minnesota, Institute on Community Integration (UAP)/Research and Training Center on Community Living; 1997.

Steinbeck J. *Of Mice and Men*. Salinas, Calif: Covici-Friede; 1937.

Tharinger D, Horton B, Millea S. Sexual abuse and exploitation of children and adults with mental retardation. *Child Abuse Negl.* 1990;14:371-383.

Turman K. *Understanding DNA Evidence: A Guide for Victim Service Providers.* Washington, DC: Office for Victims of Crime; 2001:1-11.

Valenti-Hein DC, Schwartz LD. *The Sexual Abuse Interview for Those with Developmental Disabilities.* Santa Barbara, Calif: James Stanfield Co; 1995.

Vineland Adaptive Behavior Scale. Circle Pines, Minn: American Guidance Service; 1984.

Handbook on Questioning Children: A Linguistic Perspective. Washington, DC: American Bar Association Center on Children and the Law; 1999.

Wechsler D. Wechsler Intelligence Scale for Children. 3rd ed. San Antonio, Tex: Harcourt Brace Educational Measurement; 1992.

Welner SL. *Caring for the Woman with a Disability*. Philadelphia, Pa: Lippincott-Raven; 1988.

MULTIDISCIPLINARY TEAMWORK ISSUES RELATED TO CHILD SEXUAL ABUSE

Angelo P. Giardino, MD, PhD
Eileen R. Giardino, PhD, RN, CRNP

Child sexual abuse is a multifaceted problem that is best dealt with using an interdisciplinary approach to care and services. Ideally, various disciplines participate jointly in a clinical process that is team-oriented, collaborative, and focused on providing the child and family with the best care possible (Schmitt, 1978; Wilson, 1992). This chapter describes the clinical teamwork needed to work with children and families dealing with sexual maltreatment. It also addresses broader teamwork required among agencies to best serve children and families. The specific agencies and clinical services discussed are child protective services (CPS), the mental health system, health care professionals, and the court system. This chapter specifically addresses the mandated reporting responsibility, participation in the joint investigation process, interactions with the mental health system, and court-related responsibilities of professionals who serve children and families who have experienced abuse.

TEAM APPROACH

Many details are needed to complete the medical evaluation for child sexual abuse. The healthcare practitioner who conducts the evaluation is responsible for identifying and reporting suspected child sexual abuse and for completing an accurate medical evaluation, including history, physical examination, and collection of laboratory specimens (Hibbard, 1998; Sgroi, 1982). Throughout the process, the practitioner must collaborate with various disciplines and agencies represented on the multidisciplinary team. Collaboration is necessary to provide medical treatment and to make appropriate referrals for the child and family for services such as mental health counseling or social services (Jenny, 1996a, 1996b, 2002). Meticulous documentation of the medical evaluation is essential because of possible court proceedings involving the cooperation of health care practitioners cooperate (Dubowitz & Bross, 1992; Myers, 1996).

Ludwig (1977) describes the interdisciplinary approach to child maltreatment as a series of individuals with different backgrounds coming from different disciplines and traditions that contribute to the solution of the same problem. "When a child is . . . sexually abused, the ideal set of events is that doctors treat injuries, therapists counsel the child, social services works with the family, police arrest the offender, and attorneys prosecute the case" (Hammond et al., 1997, p.1). Achieving the ideal interdisciplinary approach requires that the health care provider effectively interact with a number of disciplines and agencies. The benefits of teamwork in addressing child maltreatment are many and include improved information sharing among clinicians, joint decision making and planning among team members, collaborative educational approaches, and mutual support among team members (Ludwig, 1981; Siegler & Whitney, 1994; Wilson, 1992).

Considering the individual child and the community level of response to child maltreatment, many prominent national organizations and governmental agencies have called for an interdisciplinary model to address the needs of the child and family (Bross et al., 1988; DePanfilis & Salus, 1992b; Dinsmore, 1993; Ells, 1998; Helfer & Schmidt, 1976; Schmitt, 1978). In practical terms, a child suspected of being a victim of abuse must tell his or her story to many different people in health care, CPS, and law enforcement. Teamwork helps to enhance communication among agencies and disciplines and allows for a more unified approach to the interviews that are conducted by participating agencies and disciplines. The possibility of joint interviews and fact-gathering efforts among professionals and agencies may occur when there are common goals, mutual understanding of professional roles and responsibilities, and an atmosphere characterized by open communication (Pence & Wilson, 1994).

There are excellent rationales for a coordinated response to child maltreatment. Foremost is a reduction in the number of the interviews the already traumatized child must endure. Coordination also minimizes the number of people involved in the case while potentially providing a better quality of evidence uncovered for both criminal prosecution and civil litigation. Coordination of services helps provide essential information to the investigating and treating service organizations while decreasing the potential for conflicts between and among various involved agencies (Dinsmore, 1993).

Key Point:

The interdisciplinary team shares the responsibility for collecting and processing the components of a sensitive and thorough assessment and works directly with the child and family. Formal protocols should guide the work of the team so that agencies and disciplines adhere to the same standards.

The interdisciplinary team shares the responsibility of collecting and processing the components of a sensitive, thorough evaluation of the child and family (DePanfilis & Salus, 1992a; Ludwig, 1981). Many authorities agree that a team's work should be guided by formal protocols that minimize the chance for failure to adhere to agreed upon standards of thoroughness and excellence (DePanfilis & Salus, 1992a, 1992b; Dinsmore, 1993; Pence & Wilson, 1994; Schmitt, 1978). Formal protocols at the state, local, or organizational level are most helpful when they address specific details of shared responsibilities and how these are to be carried out. Important aspects of joint interdisciplinary collaboration include clarity with regard to the roles and responsibilities of each of the involved agencies, and delineation of the steps that must be accomplished at each stage of the process or intervention. Explicit declaration of time frames essential for completion of each step and assignment of responsibility for carrying out each step of the protocol. Finally, joint protocols should contain practical advice for handling both routine and special circumstances that may arise during the investigation and treatment phases of a case (DePanfilis & Salus, 1992b).

Conflict among individuals and agencies is inevitable in a teamwork environment. However, experience has demonstrated that team success is measured by the effectiveness with which conflict is resolved rather than by the amount of conflict generated (Ells, 1998; Sands et al., 1990). Team members need not agree on every point of a case, but they must resolve differences in a manner that does not compromise the core objectives of the team and the underlying goal of serving children and families who are dealing with maltreatment issues. Conflicts related to fundamental issues of the team's work need constructive attention and time to build consensus. The team should quickly address less important, peripheral issues and move rapidly onward to focus its attention on the more important, central issues that require discussion and resolution (Baglow, 1990; Fargason et al., 1994). In interdisciplinary work related to child maltreatment, conflict frequently revolves around the tension and emotion that may be associated with decision making, interpersonal relationships, competition, territorialism, and perceived lack of cooperation (DePanfilis & Salus, 1992b).

Ells (1998) suggests ways that teams can deal with conflict constructively. The first important step toward constructive conflict resolution is for interdisciplinary teams to keep sight of their purpose outlined in the group's mission statement. The following is Ells' outline for dealing with team conflict:

— Look forward to opportunity, not backward to blame.

— Be respectful. Consider each person's point of view. Listen to one another. Be sure each position is understood. Restate the other's position in your own words.

— Clarify the opposing point of view. Find something positive in each view. Avoid defending your own point of view until you understand the opposing view.

— Voice opposing points of view.

— State your position clearly and firmly, but without excessive emotion.

— Once you have been heard, do not continue to restate your position.

— Avoid personalizing your position and stay focused on the issue.

— Offer suggestions rather than mere criticism of other points of view.

— Remember that conflict with a team is natural and work toward a mutually agreeable resolution.

— Base resolutions on consensus, not abdication of responsibility or integrity.

— Keep focused on the team's agreed-upon purpose and refer to your protocol for guidance.

REPORTING

It is the responsibility of healthcare providers to report all cases of suspected sexual abuse. This is known as mandated reporting. Legislation exists in every state that requires specific healthcare professionals to report suspected cases of maltreatment to the designated CPS agency (Zellman & Faller, 1996). Healthcare providers are mandated reporters of maltreatment because they are likely to come in contact with abused children in the course of their work. Although states vary in the list of professionals who are required to report, physicians and nurses are mandated in every state (Myers, 1998).

Although reporting is mandated, there are barriers that keep people from reporting some suspected cases. Recognizing the problems healthcare professionals face in reporting, state laws generally include provisions designed to remove barriers from the duty to report (Zellman & Faller, 1996). These provisions include the following:

— Immunity for good faith reporting (a person can still be sued in civil court but can claim immunity under this statute in the case)

— Standards to guide reasonable suspicion (concern of possible maltreatment need not be absolutely diagnosed prior to reporting)

— Rules regarding anonymity of the reporter

— Relaxation of privileged communication rights, such as the doctor/patient privilege, that would apply in a setting other than child maltreatment

— Procedures for reporting and how the information is processed

— Guidelines regarding protective custody for the child if deemed necessary for the child's safety

— Penalties for failure to report (Goldner et al., 1996; Zellman & Faller, 1996)

Mandated reporters must report situations that reach the level of suspicion for abuse. Such reporters are not afforded professional judgment or flexibility in such cases and do not have discretion in this matter (Myers, 1998). The triggering level for reporting may be a difficult issue for healthcare professionals depending on the case. Different state statutes use various wordings to describe the level of suspicion that requires reporting, including such phrases as cause to believe, reasonable cause to believe, known or suspected abuse, reason to suspect, and observation or examination that discloses evidence of abuse (Myers, 1998).

Even though the phrases describing levels of suspicion for abuse vary, the overarching intent remains to ensure that healthcare professionals report suspicions of possible maltreatment when clinical interactions would lead a competent professional to consider child abuse or neglect as a reasonably likely diagnosis or cause to explain the case before them (Myers, 1998). However, uniform compliance with mandated reporting laws by healthcare providers remains a concern. Data from National Incidence Studies (NIS) conducted by the federal government reveal a discrepancy between the number of cases recognized by a wide range of professionals compared to the number of cases reported specifically to the CPS agency (Sedlak & Broadhurst, 1996). Even after considering possible data collection reasons, there are recognized cases that are not receiving CPS investigation. Fortunately, the majority of mandated reporters do comply routinely with mandated reporting responsibility, but occasionally, professionals do fail to report cases that certainly meet reporting standards. Failure to report cases of suspected child maltreatment is serious and may have serious consequences for the child as well as for the provider who fails to report, including possible civil or criminal action and penalties (Myers, 1998).

Many reasons motivate professionals to report suspected maltreatment (Zellman & Faller, 1996). The primary motivation is to stop further maltreatment and to get help for the family (Kempe, 1978). It is also important to help the family see the seriousness of the problem. There is great incentive to comply with the mandated reporter law/workplace policies and procedures because failure to do so has serious consequences on professional practice. Another reason to report is to bring CPS expertise into the case (Zellman & Faller, 1996).

COLLABORATIVE INVESTIGATION AND INTERVENTION

When dealing with child sexual abuse, the child, family, and healthcare team often becomes involved with a variety of community and governmental agencies. Among these organizations are those providing social services and supports, the police who investigate crimes, mental healthcare providers who provide psychologic and psychiatric treatment, and the court system that oversees civil and criminal actions that result from the case.

Key Point:
The state or county CPS agency generally serves as the responsible governmental entity because of legal mandate. In any alleged child sexual abuse, the CPS agency plays a central role in reporting, investigation, and treatment, working closely with other parts of the team.

The state or county CPS agency is usually designated as the responsible governmental entity because of legal mandate. The CPS agency is central to reporting, investigation, and treatment related to alleged child sexual abuse. Depending on the circumstances of the case and the locality where the alleged abuse occurred, the police department or law enforcement personnel, and in some cases, the district attorney's office or prosecutors may also become involved.

CHILD PROTECTIVE SERVICES

CPS agencies (both state and county) are responsible for receiving reports and investigating cases of child abuse. Several states also include law enforcement personnel in this stage of the process. CPS is also the lead agency in the assessment of child and family social service needs, the development of an intervention strategy that includes treatment for the child and family, and ongoing follow-up and monitoring of cases of child maltreatment until they closed. CPS often works closely with law enforcement to investigate cases of suspected maltreatment. CPS also works with the courts to determine issues involving custody and parental rights (Dubowitz & DePanfilis, 2000).

LAW ENFORCEMENT AGENCIES

Police or other law enforcement agencies become involved because sexual abuse is a crime (Lanning, 2002; Lanning & Walsh, 1996). Law enforcement personnel are responsible for the criminal investigation and are specially trained in conducting interviews, collecting crime scene evidence, and interrogating suspects (Cage & Pence, 1997). CPS and the police often call upon the healthcare providers to interpret information uncovered during the investigation. Various mental healthcare providers, such as psychiatrists, psychologists, mental health social workers, and counselors, may be included in the investigation.

The Police Foundation and the American Public Welfare Association collaborated on a joint project identifying models that best characterized the kinds of joint investigation programs between law enforcement and CPS Agencies (Sheppard & Zangrillo, 1996). The models vary in the amount of formal collaboration that occurs between law enforcement and CPS agencies. CPS agencies report that approximately 20% of CPS investigations of child maltreatment are jointly conducted, whereas law enforcement agencies report that 80% to 95% of police investigations are jointly conducted with CPS (Sheppard & Zangrillo, 1996). This disparity is due to joint investigations occurring more often in severe cases, which inevitably require police involvement. Approximately 42% of cases jointly investigated are substantiated (Sheppard & Zangrillo, 1996). The highest number of joint investigations between CPS and police occur in child maltreatment cases where sexual abuse is alleged (Sheppard & Zangrillo, 1996). Please see **Table 9-1** for a schematic detailing joint investigations of child sexual abuse.

In general, the typical CPS process consists of six stages: intake, initial assessment/ investigation, family assessment, case planning, service provision, and evaluation of family progress and case closure (DePanfilis & Salus, 1992a). Each CPS process stage is highlighted in **Table 9-2**.

The typical law enforcement investigation of child maltreatment revolves around criminal aspects of child abuse and neglect. Police officers play key roles in the investigative process because, in addition to reporting and investigating cases of child maltreatment, they collect and preserve evidence for criminal prosecution in these cases (Pence & Wilson, 1994). The criminal investigative role consists of a series of interviews with multiple people who may be able to shed light on details related to the abuse situation. These people include the child, nonoffending caregivers, siblings and other potential victims, relatives and friends of the victim, and the actual suspected perpetrator(s) (Lanning, 2002; Lanning & Walsh, 1996). Law enforcement also gathers physical evidence and searches the crime scene when indicated. Ideally, the criminal investigation uses a collaborative team approach with the other agencies involved.

Law enforcement officers also support child protective services because they may accompany CPS caseworkers to isolated, potentially dangerous locations (Pence & Wilson, 1994). Police can provide immediate response to emergency situations through their availability 24 hours a day, 7 days per week. They can enforce standing court orders and may assist in removing children from the home when danger is imminent. Police also arrest suspects if they have reason to believe that the person or persons may seek to flee the jurisdiction.

MENTAL HEALTH PROFESSIONALS

Mental health professionals are vital components of the interdisciplinary team evaluating and treating child sexual abuse. Their role is to help the child deal with the short- and long-term impact of maltreatment. Psychiatrists, psychologists, and other mental health professionals assist in the initial evaluation and provide treatment after the assessment. Within the context of a forensic evaluation, mental healthcare providers may also be asked to assess the risk to the child of further abuse (Bond, 1978; DePanfilis & Salus, 1992b; Sgroi, 1982; Stern, 1978).

Key Point:
The six stages of the CPS process are:
1. *Intake*
2. *Initial assessment/investigation*
3. *Family assessment*
4. *Case planning*
5. *Service provision*
6. *Evaluation of family progress and case closure*

Table 9-1. Typical Case Progression in Joint Investigations

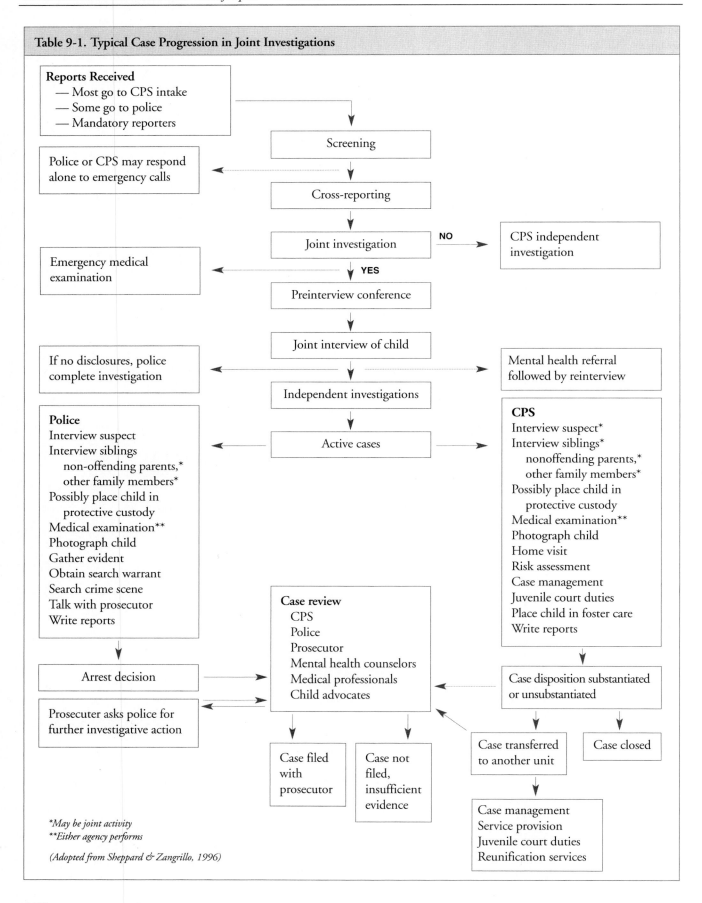

Reports Received
— Most go to CPS intake
— Some go to police
— Mandatory reporters

Police or CPS may respond alone to emergency calls

Emergency medical examination

If no disclosures, police complete investigation

Police
Interview suspect
Interview siblings
    non-offending parents,*
    other family members*
Possibly place child in
    protective custody
Medical examination**
Photograph child
Gather evident
Obtain search warrant
Search crime scene
Talk with prosecutor
Write reports

Arrest decision

Prosecuter asks police for further investigative action

Screening

Cross-reporting

Joint investigation   **NO** →   CPS independent investigation

↓ **YES**

Preinterview conference

Joint interview of child

Independent investigations

Active cases

Mental health referral followed by reinterview

CPS
Interview suspect*
Interview siblings*
    nonoffending parents,*
    other family members*
Possibly place child in
    protective custody
Medical examination**
Photograph child
Home visit
Risk assessment
Case management
Juvenile court duties
Place child in foster care
Write reports

Case disposition substantiated or unsubstantiated

Case review
    CPS
    Police
    Prosecutor
    Mental health counselors
    Medical professionals
    Child advocates

Case filed with prosecutor

Case not filed, insufficient evidence

Case transferred to another unit

Case closed

Case management
Service provision
Juvenile court duties
Reunification services

*May be joint activity
**Either agency performs

(Adopted from Sheppard & Zangrillo, 1996)

Table 9-2. Child Protective Services Process

Phase	Description
Intake	— Receive reports of suspected child sexual abuse — Evaluate reports against statutory and agency guidelines — Determine urgency of response — Educate reporters on state laws, agency guidelines, and CPS functions
Initial assesment investigation	Gather sufficient information to decide: — If child sexual abuse has occured — Level of risk for future maltreatment — If child is safe at home — Types of services needed to reduce risk
Family assesment	— Obtain information about nature, extent, and causes of risk — Gain deeper understanding of how abuse occured — Analyze personal and environmental factors that conributed to abuse
Case planning	— Determine strategies to change conditions and behaviors that resulted in child sexual abuse — Collaborative planning is best when possible — Court often involved
Service provision	— Care plans implemented — CPS arranges, provides, and/or coordinates the delivery of services to child and family

Adapted from DePanfilis D, Salus MK. Child protective services: A guide for caseworkers. Washington, DC: US Department of Health and Human Services, National Center on Child Abuse and Neglect; 1992a.

Services provided in the home are another level of intervention for the abused child. A treatment plan developed by mental health care providers outlines supports beneficial to the positive long-term outcome of child abuse. Home services include in-home supports, services in the child's own home, wrap-around mental health services, and even placement in substitute care (e.g., foster care and kinship care settings). Collaboration with the education system encourages the development of service plans that may include early intervention, special education, after-school activities, and recreational enrichment activities. Care and services are ideally rendered in a manner that empowers the family and incorporates any strengths and abilities the family may bring to the situation (Dubowitz & DePanfilis, 2000).

COURTS AND JUDICIAL PROCEEDINGS

Court appearances are stressful events for both the child and the healthcare provider involved in cases of child sexual abuse. The effect of court proceedings on the child is of concern to the healthcare provider because court is an adult-oriented environment that uses adversarial proceedings to solve problems that may be confusing and overwhelming to a child (American Academy of Pediatrics [AAP], 1999). Studies on the emotional effects of testimony on sexually abused children show varying results of positive and negative effects (Runyan & Toth, 1991). Related to providing testimony, children tend to have high levels of anxiety preceding court appearance. It appears that the presence of maternal support for the child contributes to improved emotional health (Wolraich et al., 1999). Healthcare providers can be of great assistance to the child and family through support, care, and advocacy. Often, mental health referrals to therapists with legal expertise may help the child through a difficult time (Wolraich et al., 1999).

Children become involved with the court system for various reasons. Some include concerns regarding possible maltreatment, contested custody arrangements within divorce proceedings, and adoption issues. Other reasons involve suspected offenses the child committed (often called delinquency offenses) and traffic offenses (Goldner et al., 1996; Katner & Plum, 2002). Regardless of whether proceedings are in juvenile or family court, children enter a formal adult setting designed to resolve contentious adult disputes in an adversarial, rule-driven manner. Court proceedings are generally anxiety-producing situations for children because of the adversarial nature of the process and the formal rules that govern the discussion (AAP, 1999; Bulkley et al.,1996).

It is rare that a child is called as a witness in a nonabuse-related criminal or civil case. Child maltreatment and divorce-related custody disputes account for the majority of child court appearances (Wolraich et al., 1999). Fortunately courts recognize the need to handle children differently from adults, owing mainly to a child's dependence on adults and the child's varying understanding about the proceedings (Wolraich et al., 1999). Judges can modify the court environment to make it more child sensitive through aspects such as complexity of language used, size of furniture, and orientation of judge to child witness (Runyan & Toth, 1991).

Juvenile Courts

Juvenile or family court is governed by state laws and typically separated from adult court. The structure of juvenile court varies from state to state. Some states separate juvenile court from adult courts, whereas other states hear child protection cases in juvenile sessions of regular courts that handle all types of cases. When a child protection case is heard in a court with a general civil and criminal docket (schedule), it is more common for the case to be delayed because of the issues that arise when dealing with other types of cases. Also, general jurisdiction trial court judges may be less familiar with child welfare issues (Feller et al., 1992).

Juvenile court exercises power over minors brought into the system because of all forms of child abuse, neglect, abandonment, unwillingness to submit to parental control (incorrigibility), and delinquency (committing criminal offenses). Juvenile court may ask a child witness to provide factual information that may result in taking the child into state custody (Wolraich et al., 1999). Currently two legal doctrines underlie the role of the juvenile court in child maltreatment cases (Bulkley et al., 1996). The doctrines, *parens patriae* and best interests of the child, are described as follows:

Key Point:
Whether in juvenile or family court, children enter a formal adult setting designed to resolve contentious adult disputes in an adversarial, rule-driven format. For children, court proceedings usually produce anxiety because of the adversarial environment and the formal rules.

— *Parens patriae*: the government has the authority to step in and limit the parents' authority over their children when the court perceives a danger to the children's physical or mental health.

— *Best interests of the child*: the government must consider what is reasonably in the child's best interest when deciding if the child should be removed from the care of the parents or be allowed to remain in the care of the parents.

In the current court system, families have a right to autonomy over decisions they make, privacy for their deliberations and actions, and the ability to stay whole or together as they choose (Bulkley et al., 1996). These rights are not absolute, however, and the government may step in if there is a compelling reason to protect the children from harm. The purpose of juvenile court relative to child maltreatment is to do the following:

— Protect the child from further maltreatment and harm

— Provide services and treatment to the child and family

— Terminate parental rights

— Provide permanent placement for the maltreated child

—Order mental health evaluation of children and parents when needed (Bulkley et al., 1996)

Juvenile court developed alongside the movement toward professional social work and the increased use of social services to support families and protect children (Goldner et al., 1996). The juvenile court exercises state authority to intervene in a family over the objection of a parent to protect a child. The juvenile court system is unique in that it may rely on the input of nonlegal professionals to make informed decisions for the welfare of the child. Judges welcome information from CPS caseworkers, psychiatrists, private agency social workers, physiologists, and physicians. Juvenile courts recognize that their decisions, which profoundly affect the safety and well being of a child, are only as good as the input they receive (Feller et al., 1992).

Key Point:
Judges in juvenile court usually welcome information from CPS caseworkers, psychiatrists, private agency social workers, physiologists, and physicians because their decisions can only be as good as the information at their disposal.

The juvenile court has broad discretion in addressing issues and invokes judicial authority to facilitate the social welfare system's goal of rehabilitating and treating the abusive family when possible. Guiding principles that underlie juvenile court authority include:

— Children are presumed to lack the mental competency and maturity possessed by adults

— The child's caregivers must be shown to be unfit, unable, unwilling, or unavailable to care adequately for the child before the court intervenes

— Court intervention may be taken to promote the best interests of the child (Goldner et al, 1996)

In general, the CPS agency files a petition with the juvenile court asking for the court's involvement to protect the child. The initial hearing determines whether the child should be removed from the family's home in order to keep him or her safe from further abuse or injury. From here, trial preparation begins in which evidence will be presented to the judge from both sides that will determine if maltreatment has occurred. If the judge decides that abuse or neglect has occurred, then the case moves on to a deposition hearing in which the judge will decide who will have custody of the child and what protection is necessary. Options include:

Key Point:
The two roles that a health professional may be asked to assume in the court process are (1) providing direct knowledge of information pertinent to the specific case at hand or (2) providing the court with an interpretation of the information that has been offered (expert witness).

— Protective supervision order: offers a wide range of structure

— Temporary removal of child: foster care, kinship care

— Permanent removal of child: with termination of parental rights

Criminal Court

Child abuse is a crime in all states. Through state penal codes and criminal laws, each state defines specifics about sexual abuse, physical abuse, emotional abuse, and neglect (Myers, 1998). Because states vary in their definitions, healthcare providers must become familiar with the specifics that govern practice in their states (NCCANI, 2000).

Although many people advocate full prosecution of all cases of child maltreatment, this ideal has not been achieved. A number of reasons underlie why full prosecution is not possible. First, juvenile courts were traditionally viewed as the ideal place for handling the child abuse and neglect cases because of their focus on the family needs and the provisions of services to the child and family. Second, it is very difficult to "prove" child maltreatment in criminal court because of constitutional rights concerning evidence afforded defendants in criminal court; for example, rules of evidence, search and seizure, standards for guilt (beyond a reasonable doubt, the right to confront witness and examine and cross-examine) (Bulkley et al., 1996). Third, criminal court is seen as especially threatening and potentially damaging to children secondary to (1) multiple interviews, (2) inevitable delays that extend over years, (3) insensitive questioning, and (4) defendant's right to face-to-face confrontation in court (Goldner et al., 1996; Katner & Plum, 2002). The family may also be damaged during criminal proceedings, especially when the offender is a parent.

Court proceedings may lead to consequences that affect the home, caregivers, and the child. Consequences include (1) loss of employment, (2) loss of income, (3) disruption or dissolution of the family, (4) incarceration of a parent and potential feeling of guilt on the part of the child, and (5) if there is an acquittal, designation of the child by family as disruptive and diminishment the child's value within the family.

There are many reasons for prosecuting perpetrators of child sexual abuse (Bulkley et al., 1996). The process may clearly establish the perpetrator as solely responsible for the maltreatment. Prosecution may help to vindicate the victim and establish a sense of fairness while recognizing the innocence of the victim. In addition, finding a perpetrator guilty should reduce the risk for further episodes of maltreatment and create a criminal record for offender. Prosecution may also ensure that the offender is treated, although the availability of effective offender treatment is often inadequate.

Expert Versus Fact Testimony

The healthcare provider's contribution to the court process involving child sexual abuse typically includes sharing the record of the medical evaluation and providing interpretation of the findings to the court. Healthcare providers may be asked to participate in two different roles. One is to provide direct knowledge of information surrounding the specific case at hand, referred to as being a fact witness (Finkel & Ricci, 1997). The other role is to provide the court with interpretation of the information being discussed, referred to as being an expert witness. Expert testimony is permitted in court proceedings when the expert is felt to have a broad base of knowledge and expertise in the details concerning child sexual abuse situations (Myers, 1996).

Healthcare providers who prepare for either expert witness or fact testimony should familiarize themselves with all details of the case (Myers, 1996, 1998). It is necessary to obtain copies of the medical records to avoid relying on memory (these cases may go to trial many months or years after the date of the evaluation) and to meet with the attorneys involved to understand the types of questions that might be posed.

Support for the Child During Court Proceedings

Supports are available to children to help prepare them for the experience of court proceedings. Child advocacy centers as well as healthcare providers can help the child work through what to expect in court and how to deal with the questioning process required in the courtroom. Court preparation helps ensure that the child has a supportive person to accompany the child to court and explains to all involved what to expect in the courtroom. Preparation also includes clarifying that the child is not judged by performance in the courtroom (Wolraich et al., 1999). Court schools help the child deal with fears of what to expect in court by role-playing types of questions and appropriate answers (Runyan & Toth, 1991). In New York, for example, children under age 10 years cannot testify unless they know the difference between opinion and fact. Court school helps prepare younger children to understand the meaning of an oath and to distinguish between the opinion and fact (Christian, 2000).

After the court appearance date, it is important to schedule a follow-up visit with the healthcare provider to identify how the child is dealing with the stress and anxiety surrounding court preparation and appearance. Evaluation is made for acute stress manifestations, adjustment problems, and the child's daily functional status, such as school performance or social functioning (Wolraich et al., 1999). Referral to mental health services is recommended when necessary.

IMPACT ON THE CHILD

There is no universal set of responses or uniform impact from the experience of sexual abuse on a child or adolescent (Kendall-Tackett et al., 1993). Individual differences in response to the trauma of childhood abusive events have been attributed to the nature of the abuse experience and individual psychologic adaptation (McCann et al., 1988). Physical and mental health disorders are found in evaluating the long-term impact of sexual abuse on adults with a history of sexual assault (Golding, 2000). For example, adult women survivors of sexual assault were more likely to have medically unexplained physical symptoms (Golding, 2000).

The impact on physical health of child sexual abuse is generally limited and, once identified, is treated with standard medical therapies (Jenny, 1996a, 1996b, 2002). Using an organ system approach, Berkowitz (1998) summarizes the more commonly recognized medical effects of child sexual abuse. A number of physical effects can be plausibly attributed to the impact of sexual abuse. These are in addition to immediate injuries and possible sexually transmitted diseases that may be identified during the initial medical evaluation.

Commonly identified physical effects include various gastrointestinal disorders. These are thought to be secondary to stressful events that may cause subsequent acid secretion and intestinal motility. Disorders associated with sexual abuse are frequently termed "functional," because they tend to show no structural, infectious, or metabolic basis. Included among these are irritable bowel syndrome, nonulcer dyspepsia, and chronic abdominal pain (Berkowitz, 1998).

Gynecologic and urologic disorders may be seen as potentially related to the inappropriate focus on the child's genital region that occurs in the context of sexual activity. In general, survivors with long-term gynecologic symptomotology associated with child sexual abuse tend to have no organic etiology identified. Common symptoms include chronic pelvic pain, dysmenorrhea, and menstrual irregularities (Berkowitz, 1998).

Somatization may be seen in sexual abuse cases when there is a preoccupation with bodily processes. Conflicting research in this area makes firm statements difficult, but some clinical population studies suggest that somatization may account for increased complaints of chronic headache and backache as well as other functional neurologic complaints in children and adults who have been sexually abused (Berkowitz, 1998).

The mental health impact of child sexual abuse is related to the fundamental harm inflicted upon the child by the imposition of developmentally inappropriate sexual behavior (Berliner & Elliott, 1996, 2002). The perpetrator's actions place the psychologic foundation of the child's sense of self-worth, normal development, and normal adjustment mechanisms at risk (Sgroi, 1975; Summit, 1983).

Several continua of mental health symptoms exist, including the following:

1. A symptom severity continuum ranging from mild to severe

2. A course of effects ranging from relatively short-term effects to those that are long-term, sometimes even lifelong

3. Internalization versus externalization of symptom pattern ranging from those who respond to stress by internalization, manifested in depression and withdrawal, to those who respond by externalization, manifested by aggression and disruptive behaviors

Each child faces abusive experiences with a personal set of coping behaviors and environmental realities that moderate the severity, acuity, and expression of responses to sexual abuse. Possible impacts on mental health have been described that include the following (Berliner & Elliott, 1996, 2002):

Behavioral problems: clinically significant increases in problematic behavioral problems have been identified when children who have been abused are compared with children who have not been abused. This includes generic behavioral problems as well as increased sexual behaviors.

Posttraumatic stress disorder (PTSD) symptoms: related to the child's response to the anxiety around the sexual abuse. Although many children do not meet the full criteria for a formal PTSD diagnosis, many demonstrate symptoms characteristically associated with PTSD.

Interpersonal difficulties: associated with the child's view of himself or herself after the abuse and his or her ability to establish trusting relationships.

Cognitive and emotional distortions: conflicting evidence makes clear statements difficult in this realm, but complex and multidetermined symptom patterns have been observed clinically. School performance and emotional functioning seem most at risk.

Adult survivors of child sexual abuse often have problems in functioning that are related to early damaging sexual experiences (Sgroi & Bunk, 1988). Research has described a link between sexual abuse and a host of emotional and behavioral dysfunctions. Among these problems are depression, low self-esteem, suicide attempts, multiple personality disorder, school failure, regressive behavior, post-traumatic stress disorder, drug and alcohol abuse, running away, sexual promiscuity, prostitution, and delinquent behavior (Bachmann et al., 1988; Jenny et al., 1986; Whitman & Munkel, 1991).

CONCLUSION

There are many benefits attending coordinated, collaborative team approaches to the investigation and treatment of child sexual abuse. An interdisciplinary approach helps to address the issues involved in the complicated process of identification, evaluation, and investigation of the child's situation. It is ideal when the various disciplines jointly participate in a process focused on providing the child and family with the best possible care (Schmitt, 1978; Wilson, 1992). The members of an effective interdisciplinary team understand the importance of the input of the other team members. Healthcare providers collaborate with CPS, law enforcement officers, and mental health providers as the case unfolds. The child's best interests are served when this multidisciplinary teamwork occurs in an open environment that fosters collaboration and information sharing. Each part of the team must prioritize the needs of the child at all times.

REFERENCES

American Academy of Pediatrics (AAP). Guidelines for the evaluation of sexual abuse of children: subject review (RE9819). *Pediatrics.* 1999;103:1-9.

Bachmann GA, Moeller TP, Benett J. Childhood sexual abuse and the consequences in adult women. *Obstet Gynecol.* 1988;71:631-642.

Baglow LJ. A multidimensional model for treatment of child abuse: a framework for cooperation. *Child Abuse Negl.* 1990;14:387-395.

Berkowitz CD. Medical consequences of child sexual abuse. *Child Abuse Negl.* 1998;22:541-550.

Berliner L, Elliott DM. Sexual abuse of children. In: Briere J, Berliner L, Bulkley JA, Jenny C, Reid T, eds. *The APSAC Handbook on Child Maltreatment.* Thousand Oaks, Calif: Sage Publications; 1996:51-71.

Berliner L, Elliott DM. Sexual abuse of children. In: Myers JEB, Berliner L, Briere J, Hendrix CT, Jenny C, Reid TA, eds. *The APSAC Handbook on Child Maltreatment.* 2nd ed. Thousand Oaks, Calif: SAGE Publications; 2002:55-78.

Bond JR. The psychologist's evaluation. In: Schmitt BD, ed. *The Child Protection Team Handbook.* New York, NY: Garland Publishing, Inc; 1978:121-133.

Bross DC, Krugman RD, Lenherr MR, Rosenberg DA, Schmitt BD, eds. *The New Child Protection Team Handbook.* New York, NY: Garland Publishing Inc; 1988.

Bulkley JA, Feller JN, Stern P, Roe R. Child abuse and neglect: Laws and legal proceedings. In: Briere J, Berliner L, Bulkley JA, Jenny C, Reid T, eds. *APSAC Handbook on Child Maltreatment.* Thousand Oaks, Calif: Sage Publications; 1996:271-296.

Cage RL, Pence DM. Criminal investigation of child sexual abuse. *Portable Guide to Investigating Child Abuse.* Washington, DC: US Department of Justice; 1997.

Christian NM. Teaching young victims how to survive in court. *The New York Times,* October 29, 2000.

DePanfilis D, Salus MK. *Child Protective Services: A Guide for Caseworkers.* Washington, DC: US Department of Health and Human Services, National Center on Child Abuse and Neglect; 1992a.

DePanfilis D, Salus MK. *A Coordinated Response to Child Abuse and Neglect: A Basic Manual.* Washington, DC: US Department of Health and Human Services, National Center on Child Abuse and Neglect; 1992b.

Dinsmore J. *Joint Investigations of Child Abuse: Report of a Symposium.* Washington, DC: US Department of Health and Human Services, National Center on Child Abuse and Neglect; 1993.

Dubowitz H, Bross DC. The pediatrician's documentation of child maltreatment. *Pediatr Leg Med.* 1992;146:596-599.

Dubowitz H, DePanfilis D, eds. *Handbook for Child Protection Practice.* Thousand Oaks, Calif: Sage Publications Inc; 2000.

Ells M. *Forming a Multidisciplinary Team to Investigate Child Abuse: Portable Guide to Investigating Child Abuse.* Washington, DC: US Department of Justice; 1998.

Fargason CA, Barnes D, Schneider D, Galloway BW. Enhancing multi-agency collaboration in the management of child sexual abuse. *Child Abuse Negl.* 1994;18:859-869.

Feller JN, Davidson HA, Hardin M, Horowitz RM. *Working with the Courts in Child Protection.* Washington, DC: US Department of Health and Human Services, National Center on Child Abuse and Neglect; 1992.

Finkel MA, Ricci LR. Documentation and preservation of visual evidence in child abuse. *Child Maltreat.* 1997;2:322-330.

Golding J. Long term physical health problems associated with sexual assault history. *The APSAC Advisor.* 2000;13:16-20.

Goldner JA, Dolgin CK, Manske SH. Legal issues. In: Monteleone J, ed. *Recognition of Child Abuse for the Mandated Reporter.* 2nd ed. St. Louis, Mo: GW Medical Inc; 1996:191-210.

Hammond CB, Lanning KV, Promisel W, Shepherd JR, Walsh B. Law enforcement response to child abuse. *Portable Guide to Investigating Child Abuse.* Washington, DC: US Department of Justice; 1997.

Helfer RE, Schmidt R. The community-based child abuse and neglect program. In: Helfer RE, Kempe CH, eds. *Child Abuse and Neglect: The Family and the Community.* Cambridge, Mass: Ballinger Publishing Co; 1976:229-265.

Hibbard RA. Triage and referrals for child sexual abuse medical examinations from the sociolegal system. *Child Abuse Negl.* 1998;22:503-513.

Jenny C. *Medical Evaluation of Physically And Sexually Abused Children: The APSAC Study Guide 3.* Thousand Oaks, Calif: SAGE Publications; 1996a.

Jenny C. Medical issues in sexual abuse. In: Briere J, Berliner L, Bulkley JA, Jenny C, Reid T, eds. *The APSAC Handbook on Child Maltreatment.* Thousand Oaks, Calif: Sage Publications; 1996b:195-226.

Jenny C. Medical issues in sexual abuse. In: Myers JEB, Berliner L, Briere J, Hendrix CT, Jenny C, Reid TA, eds. *The APSAC Handbook on Child Maltreatment.* 2nd ed. Thousand Oaks, Calif: SAGE Publications; 2002:235-247.

Jenny C, Sutherland SE, Sandahl BB. Developmental approach to preventing the sexual abuse of children. *Pediatrics.* 1986;78:1034-1038.

Katner D, Plum HJ. Legal issues. In: Giardino AP, ed. *Recognition of Child Abuse for the Mandated Reporter.* 3rd ed. St. Louis, Mo: GW Medical Inc; 2002:309-350.

Kempe CH. Sexual abuse, another hidden pediatric problem: the 1977 C. Anderson Aldrich Lecture. *Pediatrics.* 1978;62:382-389.

Kendall-Tackett KA, Williams LM, Finkelhor D. Impact of sexual abuse on children: a review and synthesis of recent empirical studies. *Psychol Bull.* 1993;113:164-180.

Lanning KV. Criminal investigation of sexual victimization of children. In: Myers JEB, Berliner L, Briere J, Hendrix CT, Jenny C, Reid TA, eds. *The APSAC Handbook on Child Maltreatment.* 2nd ed. Thousand Oaks, Calif: SAGE Publications; 2002:329-347.

Lanning KV, Walsh B. Criminal investigation of suspected child abuse. In: Briere J, Berliner L, Bulkley JA, Jenny C, Reid T, eds. *The APSAC Handbook on Child Maltreatment.* Thousand Oaks, Calif: Sage Publications; 1996:246-270.

Ludwig S. Team teaching of the multidisciplinary approach. *Child Abuse Negl.* 1977;1:381-386.

Ludwig S. A multidisciplinary approach to child abuse. *Nurs Clin North Am.* 1981;16:161-165.

McCann J, Pearlman LA, Sakheim DK, Abrahamson DJ. Assessment and treatment of the adult survivor of childhood sexual abuse within a schema framework. In: Sgroi SM, ed. *Vulnerable Populations: Evaluation and Treatment of Sexually Abused Children and Adult Survivors.* Vol 1. Lexington, Mass: Lexington Books; 1988:77-101.

Myers JEB. Expert testimony. In: Briere J, Berliner L, Bulkley JA, Jenny C, Reid T, eds. *The APSAC Handbook on Child Maltreatment.* Thousand Oaks, Calif: Sage Publications; 1996.

Myers JEB. *Legal Issues in Child Abuse and Neglect Practice.* 2nd ed. Thousand Oaks, Calif: Sage Publications; 1998.

National Clearinghouse on Child Abuse and Neglect Information (NCCANI). *Statutes-at-a-Glance: Definitions of Child Abuse and Neglect.* Washington, DC: NCCANI; 2000:1-7.

Pence D, Wilson C. *Team Investigation of Child Sexual Abuse: The Uneasy Alliance.* Thousand Oaks, Calif: Sage Publications; 1994.

Runyan DK, Toth PA. Child sexual abuse. In: Krugman RD, Leventhal JM, eds. *Report of the Twenty-Second Ross Roundtable on Critical Approaches to Common Pediatric Problems.* Columbus, Ohio: Ross Laboratories; 1991.

Sands RG, Stafford J, McClelland M. "I beg to differ:" conflict in the interdisciplinary team. *Soc Work Health Care.* 1990;14:55-72.

Schmitt BD, ed. *The Child Protection Team Handbook.* New York, NY: Garland Publishing Inc; 1978.

Sedlak AJ, Broadhurst DD. *Third National Incidence Study of Child Abuse and Neglect (NIS-3 Final Report).* Washington, DC: US Department of Health and Human Services; 1996. Contract #105-94-1840.

Sgroi SM. Sexual molestation of children: the last frontier in child abuse. *Child Today.* 1975;4:18-21, 44.

Sgroi SM, ed. *Handbook of Clinical Intervention in Child Sexual Abuse.* Lexington, Mass: Lexington; 1982.

Sgroi SM, Bunk BS. A clinical approach to adult survivors of child sexual abuse. In: Sgroi SM, ed. *Vulnerable Populations.* Vol 1. Lexington, Mass: Lexington; 1988:137-186.

Sheppard DI, Zangrillo PA. Coordinating investigations of child abuse. *Public Welfare.* 1996;54:21-31.

Siegler EL, Whitney FW, eds. *Nurse-Physician Collaboration.* New York, NY: Springer Publishing Co; 1994.

Stern HC. The psychiatrist's evaluation of the parents. In: Schmitt BD, ed. *The Child Protection Team Handbook.* New York, NY: Garland Publishing Inc; 1978:109-120.

Summit RC. The child sexual abuse accommodation syndrome. *Child Abuse Negl.* 1983;7:177-192.

Whitman BY, Munkel W. Multiple personality disorder: a risk indicator, diagnostic marker and psychiatric outcome for severe child abuse. *Clin Pediatr.* 1991;30:422-428.

Wilson EP. Multidisciplinary approach to child protection. In: Ludwig S, Kornberg AE, eds. *Child Abuse: A Medical Reference.* 2nd ed. New York, NY: Churchill Livingstone; 1992:79-84.

Wolraich ML, Aceves J, Feldman HM et al. American Academy of Pediatrics. Committee on psychosocial aspects of child and family health. The child in court. *Pediatrics*. 1999;104(5:1):1145-1148.

Zellman GL, Faller KC. Reporting of child maltreatment. In: Briere J, Berliner L, Bulkley JA, Jenny C, Reid T. eds. *The APSAC Handbook on Child Maltreatment*. Thousand Oaks, Calif: Sage Publications; 1996.

Chapter 10

Documentation and Report Formulation: The Backbone of the Medical Record

Martin A. Finkel, DO, FACOP, FAAP

The medical record functions as the vehicle to reflect and articulate the clinical encounter between the health care providers, the child and/or adolescent patient, and the caregiver. The medical record for children suspected of experiencing inappropriate sexual contact shares most of the core elements of the standard medical record/consultation format found in either office- or hospital-based practice. Acceptable medical practice dictates that clinicians follow the standard set of assessment parameters used in the evaluation of any medical condition. The constructs under which a medical diagnosis is formulated begin with the clinician understanding the "disease" entity and its clinical expression. When a patient comes to the physician, a medical history is obtained along with a review of the patient's past medical history, including a detailed review of systems and appropriate developmental and social history.

In suspected sexual abuse examinations, the examiner should presume that there is a significant probability that child protective services (CPS), law enforcement, and defense counsel will review the record. In contrast, most office records are only reviewed in the context of a peer review or in a malpractice action. The medical record documenting suspected sexual abuse must be constructed with exacting attention to detail in anticipation of legal scrutiny. It must be legible, well constructed, and educational, and the conclusions must be defensible (Myers, 1997, 1998). The medical history and any visual findings should be carefully documented. The clinician also must articulate a diagnosis and treatment recommendations (Finkel & Ricci, 1997). The credibility of the diagnostic assessment will come into question if the record is incomplete and/or poorly formulated (Boyce et al., 1996; Parra et al., 1997). These basic principles also apply to any aspect of medical practice and should not be unique to the evaluation of child sexual abuse.

This chapter will describe core elements of the information to be obtained, how to obtain the information, and how to document the medical history and physical examination. In addition, legal concepts that have general application to patient medical records but take on special significance in suspected sexual abuse will be discussed. The latter part of this chapter provides suggestions on how to tie all the pieces together to formulate a clear, defensible diagnosis.

Documenting the Clinical Evaluation

Clinicians document their interactions with their patients in various ways. Documentation runs the gamut from very precise language reflecting historical details of the medical history to a synthesis of the information gathered.

For example, in most busy practices the clinician may ask a series of questions, listen to the patient's responses, and at some time either after the history or examination, summarize the interaction and record salient points. Although a style that synthesizes and organizes information while deleting irrelevant points may be acceptable for general medical practice, it is not acceptable for documenting the medical history in suspected child sexual abuse. When obtaining a medical history, the clinician must record verbatim the questions asked and the responses provided by the child and/or caregiver. It is precisely the idiosyncratic statements of children and their responses to questions that illustrate an age-inappropriate understanding of sexual activities and/or knowledge of symptom-specific complaints temporally related to events that provide the greatest insight into what a child may have experienced. Therefore it is critically important that the medical record reflect the exact details of the history obtained. This is accomplished by recording the questions asked and the responses provided at the time of the interview. This will require the clinician to set the pace of questioning in concert with his or her ability to record the responses given.

The clinician also must learn to craft questions that are developmentally appropriate and that are not leading or suggestive. There is a clear continuum regarding leading, suggestive, and coercive questioning. Questions that do not imply a particular response and are open ended tend to provide the clearest understanding of what a child may have experienced.

THE MEDICAL RECORD

The medical record crystallizes the information gathering process that leads to the formulation of a diagnosis. For allegations of child sexual abuse, it is best to envision a puzzle in which several disciplines other than medicine can and will provide valuable information not readily accessible to the medical care provider. In some cases the medical piece of this puzzle may be sufficient to stand on its own, whereas in other cases it is the collective observations and information gathered that provide an understanding of what a child may have experienced. The medical record not only serves as the vehicle to formalize a diagnostic assessment for the clinician but also serves as a tool to inform caseworkers, law enforcement, and the courts that will have access to the medical record. The medical record is generally reviewed in the context of case management discussions in a multidisciplinary team review.

PURPOSE OF THE MEDICAL EXAMINATION

Children suspected of experiencing age-inappropriate sexual activities are at risk for incurring both anogenital and extragenital trauma as well as sexually transmitted diseases. In addition, children and adolescents may express significant concerns about their sense of body intactness that can be addressed only in the context of a complete medical examination. The medical examination is an essential component of the complete assessment of any child suspected of being sexually abused and is critical in addressing the health concerns of the child and the caregiver.

In the evaluation of a child suspected of being abused, clinicians need to work in a collaborative fashion with professionals from CPS, mental health, and law enforcement. This is due to statutorily mandated reporting of child abuse and concerns for the investigation. Although the examination and the medical report may have investigative value, the clinician must make it clear to child protection and law enforcement that the purpose for examining a child suspected of being abused is to diagnose and treat any residual consequences of the alleged sexual contact that may be found. The medical professional's primary concern is the patient's well being, therefore all aspects of the examination are conducted in a manner therapeutic to the child, whether through reassurance, treatment for acute injuries, or care of sexually transmitted diseases.

The clinician's diagnosis and recommendations not only serve the child's needs directly but also help nonmedical colleagues understand the child's specific treatment needs and facilitate the child receiving appropriate care.

When the examination is seen to serve the purposes of diagnosing and treating both abnormality (residual to concerns) and normality, all children suspected of being abused deserve the benefit of an examination. For many children and parents the issue of normality will be equal in importance to abnormality. Physicians treat patients either through the direct provision of medicine or the time-honored benefit of reassuring the patient and addressing both rational and at times unrealistic concerns. The health benefit of reassurance by a clinician that the child's body is not injured and that there will be no long-term adverse health consequences can be enormously beneficial.

ESTABLISHING THE DIAGNOSING AND TREATING PHYSICIAN RELATIONSHIP

A child or adolescent comes to a medical provider either because he or she personally has recognized a need for healthcare, a guardian has recognized a need for medical attention, or a CPS and/or law enforcement professional who understands the potential medical consequences of sexual contact has referred the child. It is important to explain in a developmentally appropriate way that the examination is for the purpose of diagnosis and treatment. Explaining the purpose of the examination and documenting that the child understood that he or she was being seen for diagnosis and treatment enhances the potential admissibility of the child's medical history under the diagnosing and treating physician's exception to hearsay. The admissibility of out-of-court statements is important because it allows the clinician to explain fully the basis on which the diagnostic assessment was formulated. Many medical conditions are diagnosed without confirmatory laboratory tests or specific examination findings, but rather are based on a constellation of presenting symptoms and signs.

The purpose of the examination can be explained in variety of ways, depending on the child's age. For example, the clinician might begin with an introductory comment such as, "You know that when you have gone to the doctor in the past and not felt well the doctor asks you all kinds of questions like, 'Does your tummy hurt? Do you have a headache? Have you had a fever?' The reason the doctor asks questions is simply to understand what may have been bothering you so the doctor can decide what parts of your body to look at and decide whether you will need any special tests or medicines to get better. I will be asking you some questions about what happened. The questions I am going to ask are not to embarrass you or make you uncomfortable but simply to help me understand what happened. If I understand what happened, I can do a better job of taking care of you and decide whether you need special tests or medicines to get you better." It is important to allow the child to express any special concerns. Once it is clear that the child understands the purpose of taking the medical history, it is important to encourage the child to tell the doctor the truth. The child usually agrees to do so. It is necessary to follow any response by asking the child to explain why it is important to tell the truth. The child might respond by saying; "That way the doctor can help me get better." A natural transitional question would be to inquire whether the child has any worries or concerns that he or she would like to share.

Children may appreciate the need to see a physician if they have been injured but would not be expected to understand fully the potential consequences of sexual interactions. Parents also may not fully appreciate the potential consequences of the sexual interactions and should receive guidance in seeking diagnostic and treatment services. Thus, it is incumbent on medical professionals to educate parents, colleagues in child protection, mental health professionals, and law enforcement

Key Point:
The clinician's diagnosis and recommendations serve the child's needs directly, help nonmedical colleagues understand the child's specific treatment requirements, and facilitate the child receiving appropriate care.

personnel regarding the potential medical consequences of sexual abuse and the need to make referrals to diagnostic and treatment services for children suspected of being sexually abused.

MEDICAL HISTORY DOCUMENTATION

The old maxim that if it is not in the record, it wasn't done or considered applies as much to the medical record as it would to any other type of documentation. The clinician cannot rely on an independent recollection of an interaction with a patient with limited notations when assessing children for possible maltreatment. The medical record must reflect accurately the evaluation and stand on its own. A well-structured and comprehensive record is a testament to the thoroughness with which the clinician obtained the medical history, conducted the examination, and formulated a diagnosis.

Information regarding the presenting concerns is obtained from a variety of sources, each of which must be weighed regarding relevance. When individuals other than the child offer information, it is generally considered hearsay and therefore should not be used in formulating the clinical diagnosis. The clinician's diagnosis will rely on the interpretation and integration of the following:

— The medical history
— Physical examination findings
— Laboratory test results

When obtaining a medical history from the child and/or caregiver, all information is recorded verbatim. It is inadequate to simply provide a summary note. Documentation should reflect all introductory comments along with the exact questions asked and the child's verbatim response. In part, the basis for the hearsay treatment exception is the presumption that when a patient goes to the physician, he or she will tell the truth because it is in the patient's best interest to do so. It is logical to conclude that if the patient tells the truth to the physician, the physician can make the diagnosis and get the patient better quickly. The treatment exception, therefore, allows for admissibility of the child's description of symptoms, sensations, or pain associated with the presenting concern. In addition, the child's description of the cause of the injury or "illness" may provide idiosyncratic details that it would be difficult to explain if the child had not experienced a specific causal event. If the child states that the injury or contact was at the hands of a particular individual, it is necessary to explain why the identity of that individual would be important to the diagnosis at hand (Myers, 1998). If children are either to young to verbalize their experience or emotionally unavailable to do so, then the examiner observes and records behavioral changes and emotional state.

Information provided by CPS, law enforcement personnel, or a nonoffending parent regarding the presenting concerns is important but should not be relied on as the sole information when formulating a diagnosis. Background information from sources other than the child is often helpful in understanding the context in which an alleged event occurred, but does not negate the need to speak to the child independently.

In some communities, clinicians have been discouraged from speaking to the child about the alleged experience. The basis for this is the presumption that the retelling will be traumatic to the child and/or the concern that there may be discrepancies between the new information and the initial disclosure. In regard to the first issue, children may find retelling the event to an understanding medical professional to be therapeutic and an opportunity to express personal worries or concerns. One child said, "I can tell you because you're a doctor." In regard to the issue of potential discrepancies in details from subsequent histories, the clinician should not compromise the ability to conduct a complete and thorough assessment including a medical history from the child. If discrepancies arise, they should be addressed. Many questions asked by the clinician for medical diagnostic purposes would not be expected to have been addressed by nonmedical professionals, and the history obtained by the clinician has the potential to enhance the understanding of what a child might have experienced.

COMPONENTS OF THE MEDICAL RECORD

The medical record in sexual abuse cases is similar to the traditional medical record. In most pediatric assessment settings, basic information regarding the child's medical history is appropriately obtained from a parent, usually the mother. The same is the case in suspected sexual abuse cases. The clinician may begin with a review of the child's past medical history, including a detailed review of systems. If the child is present in the room when the past medical history is being reviewed, it is best not to discuss any of the details of the child's alleged experiences but to reassure the child that he or she will be spoken to independently and will have an opportunity to share any worries or concerns before the examination. Children can be asked to think about any worries or concerns they might have while mom is being asked all these boring questions. After the medical history is obtained the child should be asked to leave the room, and the nonoffending parent or caregiver should then provide an understanding of the presenting concern he or she either observed personally or heard through a third party. The information obtained from the caregiver is important to frame the issue but generally should not be used in formulating a diagnosis because it will be considered hearsay. When hearsay is used in formulating a diagnosis, the use of such information should be qualified and appropriately noted. The "chief complaint" or history of the alleged contact is obtained whenever possible from the child independent of the caregiver.

Components of the medical history should include the following:

1. Birth history
2. Family history
3. Social history
4. Developmental history
5. Hospitalizations/emergency room visits
6. Surgery
7. Medications/allergies
8. Review of body systems with particular attention to genitourinary and gastrointestinal systems
9. History obtained from the caregiver regarding the presenting concern
10. History obtained from the child

When the child's caregiver is unavailable to provide the medical history, the referring agency should be asked to try to obtain medical records for review. The history obtained from the caregiver should be structured to obtain the best possible chronology of events and/or observations. For example, if the child made a statement to a caregiver in a manner that was spontaneous and idiosyncratic, it would be important to understand the circumstances under which the statement was made. The caregiver should be asked to provide as exact a recollection of the child's disclosure or observed behavior as possible and the caregiver's reaction to the disclosure. Questions to the child should be asked in a way that encourages the child to provide contextual detail to observations and statements.

REVIEW OF SYSTEMS

All body systems should be included in the medical history; however, the genitourinary (GU) and gastrointestinal (GI) review of systems take on special importance. The GU and GI systems can provide information that may have special relevance to the issue of sexual contact. The importance of the review of systems stems in part from the need to identify any current or preexisting medical conditions that should be considered when assessing GU or GI complaints possibly associated with sexual contact. Routine medical practice requires consideration of a differential diagnosis whenever signs and symptoms that may have a variety of etiologies are present. If the child has had either GI or GU symptoms for reasons unrelated to the alleged sexual contact, knowledge of such symptoms can be used in legal proceedings to undermine the conclusion that the presence of the same symptoms results from sexual contact.

When children experience genital fondling, vulvar coitus, or coitus, they may be able to provide important historical details of post-fondling dysuria, post-vulvar coital dysuria, or "honeymoon cystitis" that can confirm with medical certainty that they have experienced genital trauma. Dysuria results from rubbing and resultant superficial trauma to the periurethral and/or vestibular structures. The injuries incurred from fondling or vulvar coitus are generally superficial and heal very quickly without residual evidence (Finkel, 1989).

When the child's review of systems reveals a history of urinary tract infections and the child experienced associated dysuria, it should be anticipated that someone may attempt to suggest that knowledge of this symptom is the result of a prior infection and not of inappropriate contact. The clinician can address these challenges by conducting a thorough review of systems. When considering preexisting conditions, the clinician must evaluate carefully the temporal relationship between a set of symptoms and the child's complaint(s) referable to the contact. GU questions should include the following:

— History of urinary tract infections, vaginal discharges, vaginal odor, vaginal bleeding, diaper dermatitis, or urinary incontinence
— Use of bubble baths
— Treatment for any sexually transmitted diseases
— Menstrual history
— Use of tampons
— Abortions
— Accidental genital injuries
— Vaginal foreign bodies
— Prior examinations of the genitalia for any reason other than routine health care
— Self-exploratory activities/masturbation

The review of GI systems should include the following:

— Age of toilet training and whether there were any difficulties
— Use of rectal suppositories, enemas, or medications for inducing bowel movements
— History of constipation or painful bowel movements
— Frequency and character of stools
— History of recurrent vomiting, diarrhea, bloody stools, hemorrhoids, fecal incontinence, rectal itching, or pin worm infestation

Myers (1997, 1998) has identified a number of issues that, if addressed, will result in a more thorough and defensible medical record. Key steps in compiling a legally defensible medical record are as follows:

1. Document the child's age at the time of the statement.
2. Note the duration of elapsed time between the suspected abuse and the child's statements.
3. Specify who was present when the child made the statement, where the statement was made, and to whom it was made.
4. Document whether specific statements are made in response to questions or are spontaneous.
5. Note whether the child's responses are made to leading or nonleading questions.
6. Note if the child's statement was made at the first opportunity that the child felt safe to talk.

7. Document the emotional state of the child. Note if the child was excited or distressed at the time of the statement and, if so, what signs or symptoms of excitement or distress were observed.
8. Document whether the child was calm, placid, or sleeping before making the statement, or soon thereafter.
9. Use the exact words that the child used to describe the characteristics of the event.
10. Document the child's physical condition at the time of the statement.
11. Note any suspected incentives for the child to fabricate or distort the truth.

RECORDING THE PHYSICAL EXAMINATION FINDINGS

Anyone who reviews the documentation of an examination of a child suspected to have been sexually abused should be able to see from the manner in which the record is structured and the details provided that a complete and thorough assessment was conducted and that the documentation reflects such. Introductory statements should reflect the purpose for which the examination was conducted and background information regarding how the child came for an examination. The record should include the overall medical condition of the child, offer the general physical examination findings, and describe in meticulous detail the appearance of all genital and anal structures and any relevant extragenital findings. A detailed report demonstrates that the examiner understands the importance of being thorough and has reflected such in recording the examination findings in a precise manner. Any physical findings interpreted to be either diagnostic or supportive of the diagnosis should have visual documentation to augment the written record. Photographic and/or video documentation eliminates the opportunity for an adversary to request that a child undergo a repeat examination if a second opinion is sought. This author believes that all examinations should include objective documentation of the genital and anal structures whether diagnostic findings are present or not. This is justified because children can remain at risk for something of an inappropriate nature to occur in the future. If so, the baseline documentation of an initial examination may prove to be a useful reference if there is a concern in the future. Baseline documentation can be of particular value in circumstances when a child comes in the context of a custody dispute or the allegations are unsubstantiated but are of concern. Photographic, colposcopic, and videocolposcopy methods of visual documentation have become routine and the standard of care in evaluating suspected sexual abuse (Finkel & Ricci, 1997).

DESCRIBING THE PHYSICAL EXAMINATION

The description of the physical examination begins with a general assessment of the child's health, including vital signs and appropriate measurements. The examination generally proceeds in a head-to-toe fashion, and the record should note findings relevant to the concerns at hand as well as any medical conditions that need attention. Children should not have only an anogenital examination without attention to their general well-being. Children who experience sexual abuse may experience physical abuse and neglect and have findings on examination that must be addressed in concert with the disclosure of sexual abuse.

The appearance of the genitalia and anus and any extragenital findings germane to the concern should be described in detail and further documented by photographs. In the absence of acute or chronic signs of trauma, it is not appropriate to simply conclude that there is no evidence of sexual abuse or that the examination is "normal." Rather than using truncated summary words such as "normal examination" or "no evidence of sexual abuse," the clinician should provide a clear description of the examination findings and account for the absence of acute or chronic residual evidence when historical details support the concern that the child experienced something of a sexually inappropriate nature. Conclusions such as "the examination neither confirms nor denies the history provided" or that an examination without diagnostic residual is "consistent with the history of sexual

Key Point:
A detailed report demonstrates that the examiner understands the importance of being thorough and has reflected such in recording the examination findings precisely. Any physical findings interpreted to be either diagnostic or supportive of the diagnosis should have visual documentation to augment the written record. Photographic and/or video documentation eliminates the opportunity for an adversary to request that a child undergo a repeat examination if a second opinion is sought.

abuse" are equally inadequate. Ambiguous conclusions are best avoided. The diagnostic assessment should integrate the physical examination findings, laboratory results, and medical history in a manner that is clear and descriptive.

Reliance on a preformed checklist that designates findings as either normal or abnormal should be avoided. The excerpt from a complete report in Table 10-1 illustrates an alternative way of describing genital and anal examination findings. The example is limited to illustrating the description of the anogenital aspects of the physical examination.

PUTTING IT ALL TOGETHER: FORMULATING A DIAGNOSIS

The following section provides examples showing how to of integrate anogenital examination findings and the medical history in various clinical scenarios into a consultative report.

The medical record is the sum and substance of the medical evaluation. The diagnosis must be formulated in a manner that is clear and defensible. The clinician must consider and incorporate salient aspects of each of the following when formulating a diagnosis:

1. Historical details and behavioral indicators reflective of the contact
2. Symptoms that can be directly associated with the contact
3. Acute and healed genital/anal injuries

Table 10-1. Description of an Anogenital Examination When Diagnostic Findings Are Not Present

The child was examined in both the supine frog-leg and knee-chest positions. The examination was conducted with the use of videocolposcopy at 4, 6, 10, and 16 magnifications with white and red free light and recorded. The child was Tanner Stage 1 for both breast and pubic hair development and Huffman Stage 1 for estrogenization of external genitalia. The clitoral hood, labia majora, and labia minora were well formed without acute or chronic signs of trauma. After separation of the labia majora and minora, the structures of the vaginal vestibule were examined. There was no abnormal degree of redness, vaginal discharge, or malodor. There was some redundancy to the tissue surrounding the urethral meatus. The hymenal membrane orifice had a crescentic configuration with an uninterrupted thin velamentous border along its edge from 2 to 10 o'clock with the child supine. The transverse hymenal orifice diameter measured between 3 and 5 mm, depending on the degree of labial separation, traction, and relaxation. The external surface of the hymenal membrane, fossa navicularis, and posterior fourchette did not demonstrate any acute or chronic signs of injury. There was a fine, lacy vascular pattern to vestibular mucosa. The appearance of the hymenal membrane orifice was unchanged in the knee-chest position. There were no stigmata of sexually transmitted disease. The external anal verge tissues and perineum were examined in the supine knee-chest position with the legs flexed onto the abdomen. There was a symmetrical rugal pattern, normal sphincter tone, and a constrictive response to separation of the buttocks. There were no postinflammatory hypopigmentary or hyperpigmentary changes. Slight venous pooling was evident during the latter part of the examination and disappeared with anal constriction. There were no acute or chronic signs of trauma to the external anal verge tissues, the distal portion of the anal rectal canal, or the perineum.

---

4. Extragenital trauma
5. Forensic evidence
6. Sexually transmitted diseases

An important purpose of the medical record is to educate all who review issues such as the following:

1. Why there may be discrepancies between a child's perception of the experience and what actually happened
2. Why children who provide clear histories of injuries as a result of the contact may not have diagnostic residual findings
3. The types of symptoms secondary to trauma that might be anticipated when a child experiences genital fondling, genital-to-genital contact, or anal trauma

Throughout the diagnostic and treatment process and report writing clinicians must be objective, know the limitations of their clinical observations, incorporate differential considerations, and formulate a diagnosis in a manner that is unbiased.

The following examples reflect common clinical scenarios that require the formulation of very different diagnostic assessments:

1. Inappropriate sexual contact by history and/or behaviors is described; however, there is no diagnostic residual evidence on examination.
2. Diagnostic findings are present that reflect inappropriate contact, such as trauma, sexually transmitted diseases, and/or seminal products, and are supported by descriptive history and/or behavior.
3. Diagnostic findings reflect inappropriate contact, such as trauma, sexually transmitted diseases, and/or seminal products, without descriptive history and/or behavior.
4. Inappropriate sexual contact that can be confirmed with medical certainty without healed residua.
5. Insufficient historical or behavioral details exist to support a concern of inappropriate sexual contact with a nondiagnostic physical examination.

CASE STUDIES

The constellation of historical, behavioral, and examination findings will vary from case to case. Each of the following scenarios illustrates how one diagnostic assessment could be formulated:

1. *Inappropriate sexual contact by history/behavior is described; however, there is no diagnostic residual evidence on examination.* The medical history presented by this 8-year-old girl reflects progression of a variety of inappropriate sexual activities over time, initially represented to her in a caring and loving context. Although the initial interactions were described as playful, the activities progressed with correspondingly escalating threats to maintain secrecy. The young girl did not complain of experiencing any physical discomfort after the genital fondling or the stroking of her uncle's genitalia. During the medical history, she asked what that icky stuff was that came out of his pee pee and explained that she had to wipe it from her peach using a tissue. In addition, she said that she was worried that people could tell just by the way that they looked at her that she had to do those disgusting things. In light of the history regarding contact with genital secretions, she is at risk for contracting a sexually transmitted disease. I have evaluated this young lady for sexually transmitted diseases. Treatment and follow-up will be initiated should any of the test results be positive. Her physical examination does not demonstrate any acute or chronic residua to the sexual contact nor would it be anticipated in light of her denial of discomfort associated with the contact. Her body image concern is common among children who experience sexual abuse. I do not believe there is any alternative explanation for this child's history of progressive engagement in sexual activities,

threats to maintain secrecy, detailed description of a variety of sexually explicit interactions, and concerns about body image other than from experiencing such. The most significant impact of her inappropriate sexual experiences is psychologic. She needs to be evaluated by a clinical child psychologist to assess the impact of her inappropriate experiences, develop a therapeutic plan, and provide anticipatory guidance regarding body safety.

2. *Diagnostic findings are present that are reflective of inappropriate contact, such as trauma, sexually transmitted diseases, and/or seminal products, and are supported by descriptive history and/or behavior.* This 7-year-old girl provided a clear and detailed medical history reflecting her experiencing genital-to-genital contact and being coerced into placing her mouth onto her father's genitalia.

She perceived the genital-to-genital contact to involve penetration into her vagina. She provided a history of bleeding and pain after the genital-to-genital contact. Although her disclosure occurred 1 month after the last stated contact, her physical examination demonstrates diagnostic residua to such. On physical examination, there is well-defined healed transsection of the posterior portion of her hymen extending to the base of its attachment on the posterior vaginal wall. This finding is diagnostic of blunt force penetrating trauma and reflects the introduction of a foreign body through the structures of the vaginal vestibule, through the hymenal orifice, and into the vagina. She did not complain of physical discomfort associated with the history of oral genital contact, although she stated that her father peed in her mouth. Contact with ejaculate places her at risk for a sexually transmitted disease. She has been evaluated for sexually transmitted diseases. Should any of the tests be positive, treatment and follow up will be initiated.

3. *Diagnostic findings reflect inappropriate contact, such as trauma, sexually transmitted diseases, and/or seminal products, without descriptive history and/or behavior.*

This 10-year-old girl was unable to provide adequate details by history to fully understand the scope of sexually inappropriate activities for which there has been a concern. Although seminal products were found on her underwear, none were found on examination nor would it be anticipated in light of the fact that the last suspected contact was 2 weeks prior. This child's disclosure to her best friend regarding sexual interactions with a family "uncle" resulted in an investigation and the request for an examination to diagnose and treat any residua to the suspected sexual abuse. When an attempt was made to obtain the medical history, this young lady appeared very withdrawn, would not make eye contact, nor would she engage in meaningful conversation. During the examination, she demonstrated a degree of "cooperativeness" that was disturbing. Throughout the examination, she appeared as if she was dissociating from the examination process.

Her genital examination did not demonstrate any acute or chronic signs of trauma or stigmata of sexually transmitted diseases. The anorectal examination demonstrated a well-defined linear scar at 5 o'clock in the knee-chest position. With anoscopy the scar was observed to extend from the external anal verge tissues across the anoderm and to the pectinate line. The appearance of the scar was enhanced with the use of a red free filter and recorded on 35 mm film and through videocolposcopy.

Although this young lady appeared emotionally unavailable to provide historical details regarding inappropriate sexual activities, the recovery of seminal products in her underwear and the presence of a healed laceration of the anal tissues confirms with medical certainty that she experienced blunt force penetrating trauma. This young lady would benefit from being seen by a child psychiatrist to assess the emotional impact of her experience, provide appropriate medication, and develop a treatment plan.

4. *Inappropriate sexual contact that can be confirmed with medical certainty without healed residua.* This 9-year-old girl provided a detailed history of various sexually inappropriate interactions with her stepfather spanning a 6-month time frame. The initial activities were represented to her as a special game in a loving context. The most recent event, 10 days prior to the disclosure, involved her stepfather placing his "stuff" into her "coochie." When asked to explain what she meant by "inside," with the use of an anatomic model of the female genitalia, she demonstrated that she thought his "stuff" was placed inside in the adult sense of penetration. On physical examination, there were no acute or chronic signs of trauma or sexually transmitted diseases. The edge of the hymenal membrane was without interruption. The orifice diameter was 5 mm with traction and insufficient to have allowed introduction of a foreign body such as a penis into the vagina. Although this young girl perceived the genital-to-genital contact to involve penetration into the vagina, penetration was limited to the structures of the vaginal vestibule.

When asked if any of the touching hurt, she provided a history of discomfort that followed the rubbing of his genitalia on hers but denied seeing anything that made her know she was hurt. When asked in what way it hurt, she stated that it hurt her after her stepfather stopped touching her and she went to go "pee pee." When asked to describe the discomfort, she stated that it stung. The discomfort with urination only lasted a day, and she denied ever having felt anything like that before. Her review of systems was negative for any alternative explanation for the history of dysuria. The symptom of dysuria temporally related to the genital-to-genital contact reflects trauma to the periurethral area as a result of rubbing. The only way this young girl could know about the symptom of dysuria temporally related to the genital-to-genital contact is by experiencing such. This confirms with medical certainty that she experienced penetration into the vaginal vestibule. The trauma incurred to the distal urethra/ vestibular mucosa was superficial and has since healed without residua, as anticipated.

5. *Insufficient historical or behavioral details exist to support a concern of inappropriate sexual contact with a nondiagnostic physical examination.* This 2-year-old boy was examined to address the concern that he may have been touched in a sexually inappropriate manner. This concern arose because of a diaper rash, intermittent self-stimulatory behaviors, and some resistance to having his diaper changed. Mom raised the question as to whether her son may have been touched in a sexually inappropriate manner to account for the genital irritation, increased genital touching, and resistance to having his diaper changed. Mom stated that she had been sexually abused by her father as a child and wanted to protect her son from the same. The maternal grandparents occasionally baby sit for her son. His physical examination is positive for diaper dermatitis caused by *Candida albicans* with secondary impetiginous lesions. The historical and behavioral details that have been provided are insufficient to confirm with medical certainty that this boy has experienced anything of a sexually inappropriate nature. The constellation of behavioral changes can be attributed to his diaper dermatitis and was not the result of any sexually inappropriate contact. This child, as all children, should receive anticipatory guidance regarding body safety in a developmentally appropriate manner. I obtained baseline documentation of the appearance of his anogenital anatomy that will serve as a reference should there be any concerns in the future. The present concerns afford an opportunity for this child's mother to address any unresolved issues concerning her own experience and exercise caution in leaving her child in the care of any individual about whom she has concern.

Less frequent clinical presentation scenarios may include the following:

1. Identification of a healed injury on examination with no prior suspicion of abuse in the absence of historical or behavioral indicators.

2. A child presenting with a concern by a caregiver without clear historical or behavioral details to support the concern.

3. A sexually transmitted disease is diagnosed in a young child for whom no explanation for how the child contracted the disease is available following a complete investigation.

4. Fabricated or misinterpreted behaviors and/or history alleging sexual abuse generally in a young child.

The diagnostic assessments presented as case studies in this chapter represent a few ways in which the clinician can articulate findings and interpret them to those who will need to reference the consultative report. A clear and detailed medical record will reduce the likelihood that the clinician will need to appear in court to explain the record. The medical report should make appropriate recommendations for any follow-up medical care and mental health services.

CONCLUSION

When children are suspected to have experienced sexually inappropriate activities the health care professional plays a very important role. The health care provider's primary focus is the diagnosis and treatment of residual consequences to alleged sexual abuse. As discussed earlier the examination is for both the detection and treatment of "abnormality" and the determination of "normality," and as such should be conducted for both purposes (Finkel & Giardino, 2001).

The clinician has a responsibility to gather information necessary to formulate a diagnosis in an objective manner. The responsibility also extends to the formulation of a clear, descriptive report that states the basis on which the clinical diagnosis was made and can be supported. The manner in which the consultative report is constructed and supported by appropriate documentation speaks to the level of skill of the clinician. The clinician's assessment should be informative for colleagues in child protection and law enforcement who must interpret the medical evaluation and who must consider the information within the context of a multidisciplinary perspective.

A clearly written and defensible report will serve clinicians well in any legal proceedings for which they may be required to testify. Detailed consultative reports can reduce the chances of appearing in court as the record can stand on its own.

REFERENCES

Boyce MC, Melhorn KJ, Vargo G. Pediatric trauma documentation: adequacy for assessment of child abuse. *Arch Pediatr Adolesc Med.* 1996;150:730-732.

Finkel MA. Anogenital trauma in sexually abused children. *Pediatrics.* 1989; 84:317-322.

Finkel MA, Giardino AP. *Medical Evaluation of Child Sexual Abuse: A Practical Guide.* Newbury Park, Calif: Sage Publications; 2001.

Finkel MA, Ricci LR. Documentation and preservation of visual evidence in child abuse. *Child Maltreat.* 1997;2:322-330.

Myers JEB. *Evidence in Child Abuse and Neglect Cases.* 3rd ed. New York, NY: John Wiley; 1997.

Myers JEB. *Legal Issues in Child Abuse and Neglect Practice.* 2nd ed. Thousand Oaks, Calif: Sage Publications; 1998.

Parra JM, Huston RL, Foulds DM. Resident documentation of diagnostic impression in child sexual abuse evaluations. *Clin Pediatr.* 1997:36:691-694.

Chapter 11

NETWORKS AND TECHNOLOGIES

Randell Alexander, MD, PhD
J. M. Whitworth, MD

NETWORKS

Sexual abuse examinations require a level of sophistication that is akin to cardiac catheterization, electroencephalographic (EEG) analysis, and other complex interpretive procedures. Learning how to conduct, document, interpret, and communicate about these examinations requires considerable training and experience.

In the past, many examiners have been self-taught or had short training opportunities. What has made this relatively inadequate education acceptable for so many years has been the ongoing supplementation by attendance at child abuse conferences, consultation with colleagues, and years of experience. However, this approach is haphazard and results in outcomes of variable quality. Although part of the solution to the development of state-of-the-art expertise is the establishment of forensic pediatric fellowship training, it is also necessary to establish networks that enable physicians to communicate regularly.

Formal networks link child abuse physicians (e.g., forensic pediatricians) to other advanced medical care providers (e.g., nurse practitioners). Networks accomplish a variety of functions, including the following:

1. Enhancing the education of practitioners regarding child abuse and process issues such as reporting, investigation, and court procedures

2. Creating peer review mechanisms, thereby

    a. improving accuracy and increasing uniformity of conclusions

    b. avoiding "conclusion creep" (a gradual change in how findings are interpreted when not periodically contrasted against the interpretations of others)

    c. ensuring quality assurance

    d. lending additional weight to the solidity of conclusions as they are perceived by others (e.g., judges)

3. Incorporating interdisciplinary decision making more regularly

4. Providing greater consultation opportunities between members of the network and professionals in the community

5. Improving the opportunities for research by creating a larger database than individual practitioners or clinics could maintain alone

6. Establishing a larger, more organized coalition for child abuse advocacy

7. Allowing an opportunity for reduction of professional stress by providing professional and personal support for practitioners

The structure of networks varies considerably, ranging from small, loose coalitions to large, highly detailed organizations. This chapter describes more organized and detailed systems. Such systems increasingly employ sophisticated equipment for child abuse identification, computer documentation, and telemedicine applications. To support such an infrastructure, not only is a traditional interdisciplinary team of professionals important, but also nontraditional members such as information technologists and electronic technicians. Research and development administrators are needed to support the technologies, capabilities, and fiscal realities of these new enterprises.

Ultimately, building a network is not about creating more elaborate organizations, but about protecting children. Success of these networks is determined by how professionally children are cared for, how accurately sexual abuse is detected and identified, and how well this information is communicated to others.

DESIGNING A TELEMEDICINE SYSTEM THAT PROTECTS CHILDREN

Because of new technology, the distance over which information can be shared is almost unlimited. Electronic information, including patient records, photographs, real-time images, video, and databases, is almost instantaneously available to anyone with access to commercially available hardware and software. The equipment for virtual assessment is available to everyone with the financial resources. This is a far cry from the days when the distance of the examiner from a patient was limited by the length of stethoscope tubing. As we learn about this technology, our enthusiasm drives a desire to expand services to new patient populations and improve our communications with colleagues doing the same work. Information technology specialists provide electronic vistas for collaborations beyond our wildest dreams a short time ago.

In general, pediatricians have been slow to embrace virtual assessment because of the importance of the interaction between the physician and the parent/child dyad. This focus is appropriate and should be the driving force behind system design.

Electronic system design is easily accomplished by any qualified engineer, but if primary clinical considerations are not addressed, the equipment sits unused at the evaluation site, a constant reminder of a waste of precious resources that could have gone toward the care of children. Although technology is important in supporting clinical activities, the clinical activities must be central to the planning, implementation, and operation of a system. It is easy to become enthralled with the technology and be willing to bend the clinical activity to meet the capability of the equipment, rather than demanding modifications in the equipment to meet the clinical need.

Key Point:
A successful telemedicine program begins with a detailed needs assessment that focuses early on profiling the target consumer for the program. It also cannot be assumed that professional personnel in the field will find the equipment as exciting as the designer, especially if they feel it is intimidating or intrusive. In brief, the concept of "If you build it, they will come" does not work.

A successful telemedicine program begins with a detailed needs assessment that focuses early on profiling the target consumer for the program. If the people surrounding the target consumer are unwilling or unable to use the electronic equipment or service, the service will languish. Even if the program is designed for professional quality assurance, the actual and potential impact on the patient still must be considered. It cannot be assumed that families and children, by definition, would rather not travel to a center to be evaluated, or that the child will find a virtual experience equal to an in-person encounter. It also cannot be assumed that professional personnel in the field will find the equipment as exciting as the designer, especially if practitioners find it intimidating or believe it to be intrusive. In brief, the concept of "If you build it, they will come" does not work (Whitworth, 2001a).

The use of telemedicine in child abuse cases is not new. There are several programs in which "store and forward" technology has been used for consultation with centers of excellence and for quality assurance and peer review. The use of telemedicine technology for real-time evaluations, however, is new and offers challenges as well as significant rewards for clinicians and children. In short, it is an effective tool to extend expertise to rural communities, increase the accuracy of diagnosis, reduce unnecessary investigations, and extend the range of multidisciplinary teams. Several years of experience with virtual assessment in child abuse has convinced us of the effectiveness of this tool in many assessment activities, but has also emphasized the need for careful pre-planning.

The design of a child-centered telemedicine program for abuse begins with a careful analysis of the status of children's examinations in the focus community. The needs assessment must answer several questions, as follows:

1. Do the individuals and agencies perceive a problem with quality or access to examinations?

   a. If neither is true, the program is doomed.

2. Who will be working directly with the patient at the distant location?

   a. If there is a sensitive, committed professional who can be trained in all aspects of crisis intervention, and in communicating subtle examination findings effectively, and in using the equipment, a telemedicine program may succeed.

3. Is there an adequate patient population to maintain examiners' skills?

   a. An examiner who sees one patient a month will not maintain adequate skills.

4. Are those responsible for investigation willing to use the facilities and be convinced the results are accurate?

   a. The users of the service must see the results from a telemedicine examination as providing something that improves their ability to do their job.

5. Is the technology available adequate to accurately diagnose the problems likely to be present at the distant site?

   a. Technology for evaluation depends on adequate transmission speeds. In some locations, the use of real-time evaluations is impossible.

6. Who is going to assume the long-term costs and personnel commitments for the program?

   a. A program in which transmission of records for consultation is the norm and consultation is done at leisure requires a small long-term commitment. Real-time assessment, on the other hand, requires a huge time and personnel commitment with the associated commitment to financial support. Reimbursement issues must be addressed creatively.

In the deployment of a new telemedicine program, there are two critical elements. First, the community must know about the program in detail, and key players in abuse evaluations must have a sense of participation or partial ownership. Second, all users must receive detailed training and support from the center to develop and maintain a sense of partnership in doing good things for abused children.

STATE NETWORKS

The Child Protection Team Program of the State of Florida, Department of Health, Children's Medical Services Telnet Initiative provides real-time evaluations of children alleged to be abused in two hub (expert) sites and 15 peripheral sites. The hubs provide 24-hour-a-day coverage for emergency and scheduled evaluations in rural areas with challenging geographic and service delivery problems. Connections between the hubs and peripheral sites are provided by either ISDN (three bonded lines providing 384 kb/sec) or 1/4 T-1 lines. Peripheral sites are provided with telemedicine transmission equipment and a variety of peripherals to accomplish all standard evaluations of abuse allegations. The peripheral sites are operated by registered nurses recruited and trained specifically for the program, and the hub sites are operated by board-certified pediatricians or pediatric Advanced Registered Nurse Practitioners (ARNP) recognized as experts in the evaluation of allegations of abuse.

The process for a distant examination is based on a written protocol, which is designed for each peripheral site. The investigator contacts the on-call nurse who, in

Key Point:
The community must know about the program in detail and key players in abuse evaluations must have a sense of participation or partial ownership. In addition, all users must receive detailed training and support from the center to develop and maintain a sense of partnership in doing good things for abused children.

turn, contacts the hub examiner on call. The suitability of a telemedicine examination is determined and the need for emergency local medical assessment is addressed. If a telemedicine examination is appropriate, the child and investigator travel to the peripheral site while the consultant travels to the hub site. This process usually takes 45 to 60 minutes. Before connection, the nurse speaks with the child, investigators, and family and explains the process, after which the connection is made. The hub examiner also speaks with the parents and the child, and reassurances are given about the examination. A medical history is gathered as well as a history related to the allegation. The parents are often asked to leave the room during the history of the allegation, but the nurse remains to provide support for the child. A standard pediatric health assessment is accomplished with the nurse acting as the hands of the hub examiner. This may include a colposcopic examination in sexual abuse cases. A record is created including photographs by the hub examiner. Evidence collection may be done by the nurse locally. The hub examiner speaks with the child, the family, and the investigator separately after the examination. The hub examiner maintains all photographs and records of the event and will share records with qualified investigators.

Our experience has convinced us of several things related to the use of telemedicine technology in child abuse evaluations:

1. Patient acceptance in all age-groups has been excellent. It is rare for a child to refuse to cooperate. Observation would lead us to believe that the telemedicine experience actually enhances patient comfort and cooperation in some cases.

2. The photographic product from telemedicine is equal to that produced on site and is adequate for peer review and quality assurance review. The distance between hub and peripheral site is immaterial.

3. Court challenges of data have been minimal and unsuccessful.

4. Evaluation of patients in the early stages of diagnosis has reduced the number of unnecessary investigations.

5. The need to travel long distances for evaluation has diminished for families and investigators.

6. Immediate feedback for investigators is available after each examination (Whitworth, 2001b).

It is clear that this technology is a reliable, cost-effective method of expanding the effective range of multidisciplinary teams in a statewide system. In addition, this technology has potential for use in interviewing and other assessment activities (Whitworth et al., 2002).

DISTANCE LEARNING

Distance learning refers to teaching beyond the range of one's voice. Perhaps the first widespread application of this concept was the development of the printing press, which allowed communication of ideas that transcended the immediate space and time of the speaker. In recent times, distance learning has come to mean use of television and/or computers as a means of education.

This process can be passive or interactive, a fixed system or one that uses the Internet. For example, a number of states (e.g., Georgia and Iowa) have developed statewide dedicated videoconferencing networks that can be adapted for patient examination, but are used primarily to connect fixed sites (typically classrooms).

In these arrangements, not only is the distance learning like a closed circuit television system, but also it is interactive in that students at a remote site can speak to (even interrupt) the presenter. These and similar systems are either hardwired or use satellite connections (Block, 2001). The initial costs of building such a system

Key Point:
Telemedicine technology is a reliable, cost-effective method of expanding the effective range of multidisciplinary teams in a statewide system.

Key Point:
Distance learning refers to teaching beyond the range of one's voice. Beginning with the printing press, methods to achieve distance learning include television, computers, "store and forward" technology using a network, and videoconferencing.

are very high, and scheduling of any education program must compete with other users. Use of such systems for child abuse education has been very limited.

Systems that are more specific for child abuse education have been part of larger telemedicine networks. This can be accomplished by "store and forward" technology that allows posting of an image to other members of the network, perhaps asking for an opinion or functioning as a test. The advantage of this approach is that users can log onto a secure website or respond to an e-mail at a time of their own convenience. If communication occurs over the Internet, it is highly desirable that additional encryption be made given the highly sensitive nature of the photographs in sexual abuse cases. This can be accomplished by proprietary software (e.g., ImageQuest, Second Opinion), or by off-the-rack encryption software (which tends to make it more difficult for the receiver unless he or she has the same software). Images sent digitally can be altered by each party to add arrows, question marks, and other notations to aid the learning process.

Another option is videoconferencing. Users are able to connect over the Internet with a video camera, monitor, computer, and sound system (e.g., the computer's speakers). The video camera can be fairly inexpensive if only speakers' faces are to be seen, but a much higher resolution (and more expensive) camera is necessary if images are to be transmitted. Some systems may piggyback on existing high-speed connections that may be more dedicated to child abuse networking (e.g., Florida). The overall affordability and flexibility (e.g., not having to share use with other parties) makes this a strong option for distance learning.

As technologies evolve even further, it should be possible to incorporate video streaming to view talks at national or state conferences so that the observer does not need to travel (Block, 2001). The financial implications of such an arrangement pose an opportunity for established conferences, but also open the way for copying or for unauthorized viewers.

The rapid development of distance learning technologies enables forensic pediatricians more timely access to other opinions, improves their knowledge base, and should improve the care of children.

FUNDING

The equipment necessary for effective electronic communications depends on the needs of the group wishing to use the technology. If, for example, there is only a need to establish peer review or consultative relationships between examiners, all that is needed is access to the Internet via a commercially available e-mail account. Text and photographs can be exchanged as often as desired. The only concern is that commercial e-mail is not secure, so patient information must be depersonalized or encrypted. For distribution to larger groups, a listserv can be employed with distribution to many recipients simultaneously. There are several commercial sources for development and maintenance of a listserv.

Larger network deployments require a much more ambitious investment and the recruitment of partners to accomplish the goals of the group. Federal funding sources for the deployment of telemedicine services are an attractive solution to purchasing expensive equipment and transmission lines, but do not offer long-term solutions to operational costs and should not be relied on to fund other than start-up costs. Planning should begin by assessing the existing networks using high-speed or broadband technology in your area. Few users employ their bandwidth on a full-time basis. These users might include your state information technology provider, state universities, statewide banks, power companies, telephone companies, Internet providers, or weather services. Any of these providers may have a "backbone" that might be shared to provide a service to abused children as a public service at a much lower cost than developing an independent network. It is also often true that some of these providers may have underutilized equipment that might be modified to the needs of a medical examination. It is generally accepted that the minimum transmission speed needed to do real-time medical evaluations for a child abuse application is 384 kilobytes/sec, whereas a slower speed is acceptable for teleconferencing.

The recruitment of partners for the project is essential for the utilization of the network as well as for survival. Law enforcement has a vested interest in supporting your proposed program. You can speed the process of providing medical information about allegations, reduce the travel distance and time for police officers, improve the quality of medical assessments, and provide a medical expert on call. For this, law enforcement is often willing to invest in your program. Similarly, prosecutors can expect an improvement in the quality of assessments and availability of experts for prosecutions. Local hospitals, other service providers, and county commissions find that their ability to provide a community service to abused children is improved and will often see the advantages of investing in the infrastructure or operations.

TECHNOLOGIES

Many nonmedical child abuse professionals, general pediatricians, and others have little appreciation of the strides in technology used for medical assessment of child abuse in the last 10 to 15 years (Alexander, 2001a). Forensic pediatricians also may have a variable appreciation for these advances, and many have significant funding constraints that preclude their use of available technologies.

Existing technologies for the medical assessment of sexual abuse exhibit a wide range of sophistication. However, the most important component in any technologic apparatus is the expertise of the examiner. When an examiner with expertise looks at a child's genitalia without any visual aid, this can be an excellent means to detect potential physical evidence. The prime disadvantage of this approach is the inability to provide visual documentation for later review or a second opinion. Although it is very uncommon that photographs are shown in juvenile or criminal court, a medical consultant for the defense sometimes reviews them. Drawings are sufficient for nearly all court purposes, but not as helpful for medical review.

Visual documentation is helpful for teaching purposes and as a means for peer review. Computer graphics applications are proving extremely useful in court and the classroom, especially with shaken baby syndrome (Lauridson & Parrish, 2001). They enable the student (or juror) to better understand the anatomy, physiology, and biomechanics of injury. Increased application of computer graphics to the field of sexual abuse should result in improved understanding of how genital injuries occur and how they heal (J. McCann, personal communication, 4/23/01).

Using technology that is available today, sexual abuse evaluations in the future will increasingly make use of improved imaging, links to remote locations, and teleconferencing to improve the response for children (Alexander, 2001b)

COLPOSCOPY: IMAGING SEXUAL ABUSE

Colposcopy in child abuse cases evolved as a means to better visualize the genitalia of young girls (Teixeira, 1981; Woodling & Heger, 1986). The colposcope is an instrument designed for gynecologists to evaluate and document lesions of the cervix in adult patients. The instrument is a low-power microscope to which a light source and camera are attached. It was found to be equally useful in evaluating the genitalia of children alleged to be sexually abused. Although colposcopy is not essential to perform an effective examination, it offers the capability of standardizing documentation, preserving evidence of what was seen by the examiner, and providing magnification of small lesions. Macrophotography can also be used when a colposcope is not available.

As better equipment became available and as expertise increased, there was a need to improve collection of photographic evidence and to create a more detailed information

Key Point:
The most important component in any technologic apparatus is the expertise of the examiner.

base. To accomplish this, the colposcope was linked to a computer with software to capture not only still photographs, but also digital images and video clips and to create medical records. Photography has become essential in all sexual abuse examinations for evidentiary and peer review purposes.

Photographic images should be collected based on a protocol that ensures that each part of the examination is captured. If a lesion is found, several views should be photographed to ensure a clear representation on at least one of the views. The mechanics of using the colposcopic eyepieces while capturing an image are difficult, but this problem can be partially solved by using the image on a computer screen for focus and capture *(Figures 11-1 to 11-3)*.

Evaluations

Store and forward evaluations are accomplished by an independent examiner in one location capturing images and a medical record, then transmitting those images electronically or physically to another independent examiner for consultation, interpretation, or review. The record must be stored by one examiner and then forwarded to another for review and comment (thus the term store and forward). The review by the distant examiner may be at any time after the transmission, and the quality of the review is totally dependent on the quality of the captured material at the originating site. For this reason, there are distinct limitations to the usefulness of store and forward communications, which include the following:

— Focus and clarity of photographs

— Selection of photographs for transmission

— Sometimes incomplete historical information

— Timeliness of feedback

While the completeness of photographic documentation can be improved using video clips, the size of typical clips makes transmission problematic.

Many examiners still use standard photographs to document examination findings, which requires photo processing, printing, and then scanning into a format suitable for transmission. This introduces inordinate delays in store and forward formats. Many facilities have replaced standard photographic equipment with digital imaging. Digital imaging offers many advantages in that photographs can be stored on a computer, can be printed at any time needed, can maintain original quality over time, and can be transmitted electronically as often as needed. Modern digital equipment can produce images equal to analog images. Although there is concern about the ability to alter digital images, in reality there are multiple ways to ensure the integrity of an image in court. These include software that precludes modification or alteration of an original, and/or the testimony of the examiner in court that the image depicts what was actually seen.

Synchronous (real-time) evaluation of children with allegations of abuse is a new application of an older

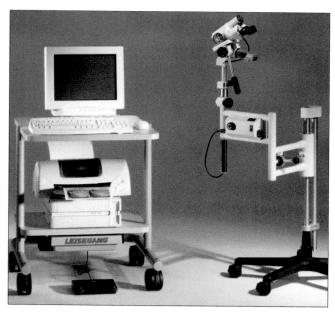

Figure 11-1. The ImageQUEST Colposcopy Image Documentation System with 3MTL colposcope and Balance-O-Matic arm.

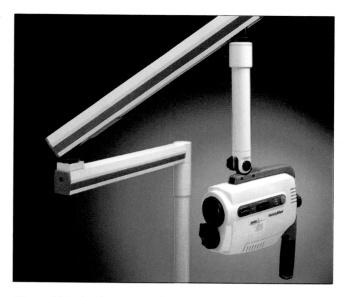

Figure 11-2. A colposcope with articulating arm.

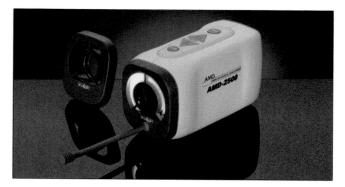

Figure 11-3. The AMD 2000 patient camera.

technology to address some of the difficult issues in accessibility of services. Florida has the luxury of having a multidisciplinary team system that is over 20 years old. The system supports 23 teams with a physical presence in 26 locations in the state. Despite this system, in many counties reasonable acute access to the experts at team sites is problematic for geographic reasons. In addition, the number of medical professionals willing to work in this stressful field is limited, with the recruitment of new providers roughly equaling the exit of experienced providers. The challenge therefore was to provide local services in a timely manner utilizing the experts in team centers more efficiently by recruiting a new cadre of medical extenders in the field and linking them electronically in real time. These extenders in the field are nurses. To evaluate the system, two team sites were selected as "hub" sites.

Each team (hub) site is responsible for providing expert levels of medical child abuse assessments to specific remote sites by using the communication infrastructure developed. To ensure around-the-clock coverage by medical experts, each remote site can be linked to the other hub site as well.

Each distant location is equipped with a rolling cart that allows use in multiple locations. A personal computer was integrated into the cart and was fitted with a video capture card and electronic medical record software for recording data and capturing digital still images. The equipment includes the following:

— Tandberg Health Care System III (hub sites) and Tandberg 8000 units (remote sites). Although these two models have different codecs that have different bandwidth upper ends and differing numbers of video/audio inputs/outputs, they are fully interoperable.

    * Leisegang colposcope model number 3DLSUL with LM2PR analogue camera

— AMD colposcope with articulating arm model number 7800

— AMD 2500 general examination camera, which uses a single 1/4 inch CCD with 1X and 50X lenses that snap on/off.

In designing the infrastructure, the engineering team decided to build a parallel network to compare T-1 lines with ISDN lines. This system has provided consistent high-quality transmission with markedly improved access to care by an expert and has made the expert available for many more examinations than ever before. The system has survived court challenges and is now ready for further deployment.

ELECTRONIC RECORD

Records of sexual abuse examinations can be kept in various formats:

— Paper hardcopy. This may consist of written descriptions perhaps supplemented by drawings. This is the traditional medical record. The advantage is that it is easy to read. Disadvantages are the considerable storage requirements and labor in copying a record.

— Conventional 35mm photographs or slides. These may be kept as part of the written record or in a separate file. Photographs may be dislodged from the rest of the written record. They have the same advantages and disadvantages already noted.

— Videotape of the forensic genital examination. This method provides more perceptual information than a photograph alone, but results in storage problems even if multiple examinations are captured on the same tape.

— Digital photographs or short digital video clips. Resolution of these images is increasingly more detailed, and most systems now take adequate images. Photographs use considerable memory, and video clips take very large amounts. If video clips are to be held in memory, several 10- to 15-second clips are sufficient to capture the examination without exhausting the computer's memory capacity. Although many images can be saved on the computer's hard drive, they should also be stored on a CD RW (rewriteable CD). These discs can hold numerous digital photographs and are small enough to be easily stored. In addition, computer images and video clips can be stored in a server, which has immense storage capacity.

In addition to images of the examination, the entire medical record can be electronic, reducing or eliminating the need for storage of a hardcopy record. Other advantages include the following:

— Ease of access

— Ability to combine text and photographs in a seamless record

— Ability to tailor specific formats for dissemination to others. For example, a copy could be sent to child protective services or police, but without the genital photographs or video clips. If certain information in the text is later deemed "inadmissible" (i.e., for a legal proceeding), an edited copy can be created with a few keystrokes.

As with images, the electronic record should be backed up. If this can be accomplished in another location, it increases the security that a disaster in one location will not erase a record of the child's medical evaluation.

SUMMARY

The evolution of networks and technologies is rapidly advancing. The end result will be to arm medical examiners with an array of tools and communication avenues that will increase their sophistication and improve the care of children. As this health component improves, better data will be available for child protective services, police, and the court to make wise decisions.

REFERENCES

Alexander R. Networks and technologies. *American Professional Society on the Abuse of Children (APSAC) Advisor.* 2001a;13:2.

Alexander R. Vision for the future. *American Professional Society on the Abuse of Children (APSAC) Advisor.* 2001b;13:3-5.

Block R. Telemedicine and distance learning in the child abuse intervention field. *American Professional Society on the Abuse of Children (APSAC) Advisor.* 2001;13:8-9.

Lauridson J, Parrish R. Computer graphics in child abuse and neglect. *American Professional Society on the Abuse of Children (APSAC) Advisor.* 2001;13:14-16.

Socolar R, Fredrickson D, Block R, Moore J, Tropez-Sims S, Whitworth J. State programs for medical diagnosis of child abuse and neglect: case studies of five established or fledgling programs. *Int J Child Abuse Negl.* 2001;25:441-456.

Teixeira WR. Hymenal colposcopic examination in sexual offenses. *Am J Forensic Med Pathol.* 1981;3:209-214.

Whitworth JM. How to design a telemedicine system that actually protects children. *American Professional Society on the Abuse of Children (APSAC) Advisor.* 2001a;13:6-7.

Whitworth JM. Synchronous evaluations of child abuse. *American Professional Society on the Abuse of Children (APSAC) Advisor.* 2001b;13:19.

Whitworth JM, Wood B, Morse K, Rogers H, Haney M. The Florida Child Protection Team Telemedicine Program. In: Oakley AMM, Woolten R, eds. *Teledermatology.* New Zealand: Royal Academy of Medicine, LTD; 2002:35-149.

Woodling BA, Heger A. The use of the colposcope in the diagnosis of sexual abuse in the pediatric age group. *Child Abuse Negl.* 1986;10:111-114.

OVERVIEW OF ADOLESCENT AND ADULT SEXUAL ASSAULT

Judith A. Linden, MD, FACEP, SANE
Janet S. Young, MD

Sexual assault is a crime of violence, often motivated by aggression and rage, with the assailant using sexual contact as a weapon for power and control. Rape is distressingly prevalent in the United States, with 1 out of every 6 women and 1 out of every 33 men experiencing an attempted or completed rape in his or her lifetime (Tjaden & Thoennes, 2000). The first modern definition of rape can be found in English common law in 1756. Rape was defined as carnal knowledge of a woman not one's wife by force, or against her will. In 1962 the United States Model Penal Code updated the definition of rape: "A man who has sexual intercourse with a female, not his wife, is guilty of rape…if he compels her to submit by force or threat of force or threat of imminent death, serious bodily injury, extreme pain, or kidnapping" (United States Model Penal Code, 1962, quoted in Epstein & Langenbahn, 1994). This definition was also vague and extremely limiting because it was gender specific, did not include intimate partner rape, and required a demonstration of the victim's resistance to sexual contact (severe injuries). In the 1970s, with influence from the feminist movement, many laws pertaining to rape were reformed throughout the United States. Although state laws vary somewhat as to the definition of rape, most state laws currently define rape more broadly using gender-neutral language. Most states define rape using three criteria: (1) any vaginal, anal, or oral penetration by a penis, object, or other body part; (2) lack of consent, communicated with verbal or physical signs of resistance, or if the victim is unable to consent by means of incapacitation because of age, disability, or drug or alcohol intoxication; and (3) threat of or actual use of force. Modern definitions of rape also include rape by taking advantage of incapacitated individuals, such as children, the disabled, and the elderly. A more recent revision increases the penalty for drug-facilitated rape, most commonly with gamma hydroxybutyrate (GHB) or Rohypnol (flunitrazepam). The Drug Induced Rape Prevention and Punishment Act of 1996 is a federal statute that provides a penalty of up to 20 years in prison for the intent to commit a crime of violence against an individual by distribution of a controlled substance to that individual without his or her knowledge. Some states, such as Massachusetts, further amended state law in 1998 to specifically include Rohypnol ("roofies," "roche," "Mexican valium"), GHB ("liquid X," "liquid E," "grievous bodily harm," "everclear," "liquid sex," "easy lay"), and ketamine ("special K").

Sexual assault is more broadly characterized as any unwanted sexual contact, thus encompassing a range of behaviors, including rape, incest, molestation, fondling or grabbing, or forced viewing of or involvement in pornography. Statutory rape includes the rape of any minor not able to give consent and often carries a more stringent punishment. The age of consent varies from 14 to 18 years, depending on the state of residence.

Rape has also been recognized as a weapon of war throughout the centuries, used to humiliate and undermine the enemy in conflict. However, it is also perpetrated by

Key Point:
Sexual assault is broadly defined as any unwanted sexual contact.

soldiers against their own people in wartime. The International Criminal Tribunal for the Former Yugoslavia recognized rape as a crime against humanity for the first time in 1996. In 1998 the International Tribunal for Rwanda found Jean-Paul Akayesu guilty of genocide and for the first time found rape to be an act of genocide (Ramsay, 1999).

EPIDEMIOLOGY

The scope of sexual assault in the United States cannot be fully understood by focusing on reported statistics. These figures, however, provide the only means of comprehending a rough estimate of the problem. Statistics reported by law enforcement agencies such as the Federal Bureau of Investigation Uniform Crime Reports (FBI UCR), which rely on police reports, are inaccurate because of extremely low reporting rates (FBI, 1999). The FBI UCR recorded 100,000 rapes in the United States in 1990. The 1992-1993 National Crime Victimization Survey (NCVS) included both reported and unreported, attempted and completed rapes, and estimated 550,000 rapes annually, five times as many rapes as the FBI UCR (Bachman & Saltzman, 1995). The 1990-1992 National Women's Study used a broader definition of rape as an event "which occurred without the woman's consent, involved the use of force or threat of use of force, and involved penetration of the victim's vagina, mouth or rectum" (Kilpatrick et al., 1992, introduction). This study estimated 680,000 rapes annually. A more recent survey, the National Violence Against Women Survey (1995-1996) (US Department of Justice, 1995; Tjaden & Thoennes, 1998) estimated 1 million rapes or attempted rapes annually in the United States: 876,000 in women and 111,000 in men. The average annual number of rapes per respondent was 2.9 for women and 1.7 for men. This figure is nine times higher than the FBI UCR statistics. This indicates that one out of every six women in the United States (or 18%), has been the victim of an attempted or completed rape in her lifetime (Tjaden & Thoennes, 2000).

Most rapes are never reported to the police or health care providers. Experts estimate that only between 16% and 30% of rapes are reported to law enforcement agencies (Bachman & Saltzman, 1995; Kilpatrick et al., 1992). Adolescents are even less likely to report (Kilpatrick & Saunders, 1997). A recent study in an urban emergency department found a 39% lifetime prevalence of sexual assault, with 46% having reported the crime to law enforcement officials and 43% seeking medical care (Feldhaus et al., 2000). However, this study reveals a higher lifetime prevalence and reporting rate than other studies.

Male victims are less likely to report rape unless serious injuries are present (Pino & Meier, 1999). Males are more likely than females to report physical injuries without reporting the accompanying sexual assault and are more likely to use denial as a coping mechanism (Kaufman et al., 1980). Explanations for lower reporting rates by males include the fear of being labeled as weak if they show emotional pain, fear of being labeled as homosexual, and shame of not being able to defend themselves. Contrary to popular rape mythology, the majority of males who rape males are not homosexual, and the majority of males who are raped are not homosexual.

Sexual assault is a "tragedy of youth," often affecting youths and adolescents disproportionately (Kilpatrick et al., 1992). The National Women's Study reported that 29% of all rapes occurred when the victim was less than age 11 years, while another 32% occurred between ages 11 and 17 years (Kilpatrick et al., 1992). This report also indicates that a perpetrator known or trusted by the victim most often commits the assault. According to the National Women's Study, only 22% of women were raped by strangers ("blitz" rapes). Twenty-nine percent of women were raped by acquaintances, 9% by ex-husbands, 11% by stepfathers, 10% by boyfriends, and 16% by other relatives (Kilpatrick et al., 1992). Victims with a known assailant are less likely to report the crime or receive medical care (Feldhaus et al., 2000; Koss et al., 1988).

Reasons for not reporting sexual assault are numerous. The most common reasons for not reporting include fear of family, friends, and others finding out (70%); fear of the assault being made public by the media (50%); fear of being blamed (68%); fear of retaliation; and perceived shame or actual stigma associated with being the victim of sexual assault (Kilpatrick et al., 1992). Victims are less likely to report the rape to police if they do not fit into the classic definition of rape victim as a woman raped by a stranger. These "silent victims" continue to have many of the mental health and physical sequelae of rape but often do not receive the crucial resources available.

Although rape is an act of violence, it is often also an act of opportunity. The one common link that identifies rape victims is that the rapist has access to the victim. This helps explain why a known assailant perpetrates 80% of rapes. Most victims and perpetrators are of the same race, supporting the theory that access is the most important risk factor (Sanford et al., 1979). Many rapists prey on vulnerable victims who may be seen as less likeable or credible, such as the homeless or substance abusers. Contrary to popular rape myths, more attractive, provocatively dressed individuals are not more likely to be victims of rape.

The classic rape victim, with whom providers easily empathize, is the victim of a "blitz rape," or random act of rape by a stranger. This is actually fairly uncommon.

"Confidence rape," in which the victim has had a previous nonviolent relationship with the assailant, occurs more often. Examples include a friend or acquaintance who uses deceit (such as offering a ride home), an assailant who controls the victim by age or rank, and an assailant who exploits someone unable to give consent. In the "stress-sex" situation the victim initially consents to contact, but the assailant then becomes abusive and violent, forcing further sexual activity without consent. This is a common scenario for date rape and prostitutes who are raped. Although many people are less likely to label this situation rape, the experience can be just as frightening and devastating as that of a blitz rape.

Key Point:
Victims often do not report rape or seek medical care, particularly if the assailant is known to them; the majority of attacks are by someone known to the victim, and thus are not reported.

PUBLIC HEALTH IMPLICATIONS

With an incidence of sexual assault between 680,000 and one million annually, or 1.3 to 2 forcible rapes per minute, the cost to US public health systems is enormous (Kilpatrick et al., 1992; Tjaden & Thoennes, 2000). Most cost calculations take into account only the short-term 'tangible' costs (e.g., property and productivity lost, medical bills). The National Institute of Justice (1996) calculated not only the tangible financial cost of sexual assault, but also the intangible costs (such as pain, suffering, risk of death, disability and long term emotional trauma), calculated using civil law damage suit methodology. From 1987 to 1990 the out-of-pocket (tangible) expense to society was calculated as $5100 per sexual assault, making rape the most costly crime in the United States, exceeding even murder. If the effect on the survivor's quality of life is quantified (intangible costs), this figure increases to $87,000 annually per assault (National Institute of Justice, 1996). Sexual assaults cost over $127 billion each year, amounting to over $425 for each man, woman, and child in the United States (National Institute of Justice, 1996).

The public health costs also encompass the long-term health effects of sexual victimization. Survivors of sexual assault are more likely to develop mental health problems when compared to women who had never been raped (Kilpatrick et al., 1992; Nadelson et al., 1982; Walker et al., 1995). The National Women's Study reported an eight-fold increase in major depression compared to women who had never been sexually victimized. An estimated 3.8 million adult American women have rape-related posttraumatic stress disorder (PTSD) (Kilpatrick et al., 1992). There is also considerable evidence that sexual assault victims demonstrate higher rates of alcohol and drug use (Kilpatrick et al., 1992).

The effects on the physical health of the survivor continue for years. Sexual assault survivors show an increased use of the health care system. In one study, nearly all women survivors visited a physician for problems unrelated to the sexual assault during the next 2 years and had outpatient costs that were 2.5 times greater than that of nonvictims. Physician visits by rape victims increased 56% (4.1 to 7.3 visits per year) in the year following the rape. This increase persisted for 2 years, until the end of the study (Koss et al., 1991). Somatic complaints that develop after an undisclosed assault, such as insomnia, gastrointestinal symptoms, or gynecologic or sexual dysfunction, often lead to costly medical evaluation (Walker et al., 1993).

Finally, unwanted pregnancy is a major public health concern, with 5% of rapes resulting in pregnancy. Based on current rape statistics, approximately 32,000 resultant pregnancies a year contribute significantly to the cost of treating survivors of sexual assault (Holmes et al., 1996). Unfortunately, many unwanted pregnancies resulting from rape occur in adolescent victims of incest who do not seek medical care immediately after the assault.

Sexual assault is a crime that has devastating consequences for the survivor and the family, causing loss of physical and emotional well-being, decreased productivity, and loss of life. The crime also contributes tremendous financial costs to society. Although perpetrators should be held responsible for sexual assault, it is difficult to prosecute and hold them accountable. It is even more difficult to predict who is likely to commit sexual assault in order to prevent the crime. It is therefore important to focus on identifying populations at increased risk of sexual victimization and to create effective strategies for prevention and early intervention.

POPULATIONS AT RISK

Although rape is pervasive in the United States, some populations may be at increased risk of sexual assault. The greatest risk factor for sexual assault is female gender, with approximately 70% to 90% of rape victims of the female gender and 10% to 23% male (Bachman & Saltzman, 1995; Tjaden & Thoennes, 2000).

The second greatest risk factor for sexual assault is young age (Bachman & Saltzman, 1995; Kilpatrick et al., 1992; Tjaden & Thoennes, 2000). In one large telephone survey, 61% of rape victims were younger than age 17 years at the time of the assault, and only 6% of the rapes occurred after age 29 years (Kilpatrick et al., 1992). In another study, 54% of rape victims were under age 15 years at first rape, and 83.4% were less than age 25 years (Tjaden & Thoennes, 2000). Adolescents and young adult women are most at risk for acquaintance and date rape. Some studies suggest that more than 75% of adolescent rapes are committed by an acquaintance (Kilpatrick et al., 1992; Kilpatrick & Saunders, 1997). Women attending college have a three times greater risk of rape compared to the general population, and are often raped by someone they know (Koss et al., 1987).

Past victimization is a strong risk factor for revictimization (Kilpatrick et al., 1992; Tjaden & Thoennes, 2000). Sexual assault in childhood is one of the most powerful risk factors for sexual assault as an adult (Acierno et al., 1999). Women with a history of rape or attempted rape as an adolescent are two to five times more likely to be revictimized than women without a history of sexual assault (Gidycz et al., 1993; Hanson & Gidycz, 1993; Kilpatrick et al., 1992). It is unclear whether this increased risk is related to ongoing environmental factors such as family violence, living in an unsafe neighborhood or home, homelessness, or high-risk behaviors. Women in physically and emotionally abusive relationships also experience higher rates of rape and sexual assault. They are more likely to experience repeated rapes and serious physical injuries and are less likely to report to health care providers and law enforcement agencies (Feldhaus et al., 2000; Koss et al., 1988).

The mentally incapacitated are at higher risk for sexual victimization. Possible explanations include a decreased ability to perceive dangerous situations. They are

Key Point:
The greatest risk factors for becoming a victim of sexual assault are female gender, adolescence, and young adulthood.

more likely to be targeted by predators because they appear to be vulnerable and less likely to be taken seriously (Acierno et al., 1997).

Women in the military and institutionalized women have reported sexual assault rates that are significantly higher than the general population (Sadler et al., 2000). The assailants are often in positions of power and relatively immune from repercussion or prosecution.

IMMEDIATE REACTIONS TO SEXUAL TRAUMA

The majority of rape victims do not seek immediate medical assistance: only 30% to 43% seek medical care after a rape (Feldhaus et al., 2000; Tjaden & Thoennes, 2000). The physical and emotional reactions associated with sexual victimization are as varied as the patients who experience them are. There is no "normal" or "abnormal" response. Immediate reactions may include shock and disbelief, shame and self-blame. The victim may experience anger directed toward the assailant, or toward health care workers, advocates, or law enforcement officials. Outward behavior can include anything from sobbing and crying to presenting a quiet, calm demeanor. The most intense fear during and immediately after a rape is often the fear of death. Although many victims may not suffer severe injuries, the fear of death during the assault can be extremely intense. Other initial concerns include fear of contracting a sexually transmitted disease (STD), fear of pregnancy, and fear of serious genital injuries that would affect sexual functioning. Transmission of human immunodeficiency virus (HIV) has emerged as one of the most intense fears among survivors. In addition to fear, a rape victim's emotional responses may include anxiety, helplessness, and guilt.

Burgess and Holmstrom (1974) first described the "rape trauma syndrome" in the 1970s after interviewing rape survivors at Boston City Hospital. They defined the rape trauma syndrome as a group of "behavioral, somatic, and psychological reactions, which are an acute stress reaction to a life-threatening situation" (Burgess & Holmstrom, 1974, p. 982, author's emphasis). They identified two phases of response to rape: the acute "disorganization phase" (lasting several weeks) and the "reorganization phase" (lasting from several weeks to years) (Burgess & Holmstrom, 1974). In the initial disorganization phase the survivor experiences somatic reactions to rape, such as pain from physical trauma, headaches and sleep disturbances, gastrointestinal symptoms, and genitourinary symptoms. Almost half of rape survivors have physical complaints at early follow-up, although the majority have a normal examination (Holmes et al., 1998). The survivor also continues to display some of the initial emotional reactions, such as fear, humiliation, self-blame, anger, and revenge. The recall of the event is often clouded by intense feelings of guilt, helplessness, and fear (Burgess & Holmstrom, 1974; Nadelson et al., 1982).

During the reorganization phase, the survivor often continues to experience somatic symptoms. Symptoms of nonspecific anxiety are usually manifest and can be associated with the development of phobias. Survivors may fear being indoors if they were raped inside, or fear crowds. During this phase, survivors often change addresses and phone numbers frequently.

DELAYED EFFECTS ON THE SURVIVOR

Survivors of sexual assault often experience increased rates of posttraumatic stress disorder (PTSD), depression, suicidal ideation, substance abuse, and physical complaints, such as pelvic pain, abdominal pain, and headaches. One study that evaluated women who came to a gastroenterology clinic found a significant increase in psychiatric disorders, medically unexplained symptoms, and physical abuse in sexual assault survivors compared to women who had never been sexually assaulted (Walker et al., 1995). One of the most debilitating after-effects of sexual assault is PTSD. The hallmarks of the disorder include persistent reliving of the event and behavioral changes to avoid stimuli associated with the trauma. Almost one third of sexual assault survivors develop PTSD at some time, almost six times the number of people who develop PTSD within the general population (Kilpatrick et al., 1992). In a prospective study of hospital-referred rape victims, 97% met PTSD criteria at initial assessment, and almost half still met the criteria 2 months later (Rothbaum et al., 1992). In one study, half of all survivors interviewed 2 to 3 years after the sexual assault reported continued feelings of intense terror, horror, or fear about the possibility of being killed by the rapist. Many remained suspicious of others, feared being alone, and experienced sexual dysfunction (Nadelson et al., 1982).

Major depression is extremely common in rape survivors, with almost 30% reporting at least one episode. Rape survivors are three times more likely to experience a major depressive episode at some time during their lives than are nonvictims. Increased rates of suicidal ideation and suicide attempts have also been noted in survivors of sexual assault, with one third reporting that they had contemplated suicide, a rate four times greater than among the general population, and 13% reporting an actual suicide attempt, a rate 13 times higher than among the general population (Kilpatrick et al., 1992).

Many survivors report increased use of alcohol and other drugs, as well as alcohol and drug-related problems (Kilpatrick et al., 1992). Increased use of alcohol and drugs may represent an attempt to self-medicate the painful emotions associated with sexual victimization. Ironically, the use of alcohol and drugs often places the survivor at increased risk for revictimization. One study found that rape survivors were 5 times more likely to have used prescription drugs nonmedically, 6 times more likely to have used cocaine, and 10 times more likely to have used hard drugs other than cocaine (e.g., heroin). This study also found that survivors were 13 times more likely to have had two or more alcohol-related problems (for example, trouble at work/at school/with police, health problems, difficulty with family/friends, auto accidents or accidents at home) than nonvictimized women and 26 times more likely to have had two or more serious drug abuse problems (Kilpatrick et al., 1992). Survivors with PTSD were even more likely to have drug- and alcohol-related problems.

Key Point :
The long-term effects of rape can be devastating and include physical and psychiatric disorders, including major depression, PTSD, and drug and alcohol abuse.

Survivors demonstrate increased medical visits in the first year after assault compared to nonvictimized women, even when visits for follow-up of assault related injuries and routine check-ups are excluded (Kimmerling & Calhoun, 1994). Physical symptoms such as chronic pain, headache, gastrointestinal symptoms, and gynecologic symptoms may be more common in women with a history of sexual assault. Proposed explanations include physical injury, posttraumatic increased autonomic arousal, effects of chronic stress on the immune system, subjective lack of control, an anxiety-mediated increase in somatic symptoms, and dissociation (Golding, 1999). Chronic headaches were significantly more common among sexual assault survivors in one large five-center study (Golding, 1999). Several studies reveal that patients who have a history of sexual or physical abuse have an increased likelihood of irritable bowel–type symptoms (Drossman et al., 1990; Jamieson & Steege, 1997; Talley et al., 1995). Gynecologic disorders, such as dysmennorrhea, dyspareunia, or chronic pelvic pain, are increased among survivors of sexual assault (Golding et al., 1998; Walling et al., 1994). One study that included data from three large population studies found that the probability that previous sexual assault had occurred increased with each additional symptom of dysmenhorrea, menorrhagia, and sexual dysfunction (Golding et al., 1998). Each additional symptom doubled the probability of previous sexual assault. Almost 40% of women with all three symptoms reported prior sexual assault. This association was true for women who were not perimenopausal. Another large study found a statistically significant increase in symptoms of dyspareunia and pelvic pain in women with a history of adult sexual abuse, and an increase in dysmenhorrea, dyspareunia, and pelvic pain in women with a history of childhood sexual abuse

(Jamieson & Steege, 1997). Gynecologic and chronic pain symptoms may also be related to physical and other forms of psychologic abuse, as well as to sexual abuse (Walling et al., 1994).

COMPONENTS OF AN EFFECTIVE RESPONSE

The ideal care of the sexual assault victim includes compassionate treatment by knowledgeable professionals, including rape crisis hotline personnel, police and law enforcement personnel, and prehospital providers to specially trained detectives, skilled medical staff, trained sexual assault examiners, and rape crisis counselors.

Rape crisis centers first began as grass roots efforts, as an outgrowth of the feminist movement in the 1970s. The first rape crisis centers were established in San Francisco (Bay Area Women Against Rape) and Washington, DC (DC Rape Crisis Center). Rape crisis centers are staffed mostly by lay people who are often sexual assault survivors and serve a vital function in the prevention, acute treatment, and ongoing follow-up of rape survivors. The missions of rape crisis centers include educating the public in order to help prevent rape and increase the number of victims seeking assistance, improving the treatment of victims by offering confidential emergency assistance (including hotline and hospital escort) to victims and family members/friends, and offering short-term follow-up crisis counseling.

Prehospital personnel, including police and emergency medical technicians, should be trained to realize that rape or sexual assault is not specific to one gender, race, or socioeconomic status. Prehospital personnel must be trained in evidence preservation and the importance of saving the sheet the patient is transported on, as well as avoiding cutting the patient's clothes and destroying evidence, whenever possible. Prehospital personnel should be trained to listen to the patient with empathy and remind the patient that the assault is never the victim's fault. They should establish a safe environment to transfer the patient (including removing the patient from the scene as soon as possible).

On arrival to the emergency department, rape victims should be given top priority, brought back from triage immediately, and provided a safe, nonthreatening environment. While many medical staff prefer to avoid the patient who has been raped until the examiner arrives, the patient should be immediately screened for serious injuries. An attempt should be made to avoid undressing the patient so that clothing can be collected during the forensic examination, if the patient chooses to have such an examination. The patient should be instructed not to eat or drink anything and not to urinate if possible, if evidence is to be collected. Well-trained emergency department staff should be knowledgeable about, and able to offer appropriate postexposure prophylaxis for pregnancy and STDs, including HIV and hepatitis. Emergency department personnel should realize that there is no single "appropriate" survivor response and be able to recognize and effectively respond to the range of survivor reactions. Acute reactions can range from crying, to anger and yelling, to "numbing" or decreased response, or laughing. A supportive, nonthreatening patient interaction, which allows the patient to retain control, is important to prevent further anxiety in assault survivors. Emergency department personnel should be able to address common concerns that rape victims may not always express, such as whether the injuries will cause permanent damage and the likelihood of becoming pregnant or acquiring an STD (particularly HIV). The health care provider should remember that it is not his or her job to decide if the sexual assault occurred, but rather to examine the victim, collect evidence if the patient consents, offer support, and give medical treatment.

Sexual assault detectives are trained to interview in a nonjudgmental, sensitive, and compassionate manner while obtaining vital information. Specially trained personnel, such as sexual assault nurse examiners (SANE practitioners) and rape crisis counselors are most beneficial in the evaluation and treatment of the victim.

SANEs are specifically trained to counsel the patient, collect a history, examine and obtain forensic evidence in a compassionate manner, and evaluate both the physical and psychologic injuries the patient has suffered. SANEs also receive training in court testimony. Finally, follow-up services, such as mental health care counselors, rape crisis centers, and medical follow-up (including testing for pregnancy, HIV, hepatitis, and STDs), should be arranged.

PREVENTION

Prevention of sexual assault must be made a public health priority. The American Medical Association declared sexual assault "a silent, violent epidemic." Interventions should be aimed at primary, secondary, and tertiary prevention. Primary prevention would include interventions aimed at decreasing the number of sexual assaults. Secondary preventive measures are aimed at early screening and identification of sexual assault survivors, and decreasing future assaults and the sequelae of sexual assault, once it has already happened. Tertiary prevention would include interventions aimed at treating and alleviating advanced disease, or the late effects such as the physical and mental health sequelae of sexual assault.

Although primary prevention is perhaps the most difficult to achieve, it is the most effective means of decreasing the sequelae of sexual victimization. Because the majority of rape victims are young, with half of all rapes occurring before age 18 years, primary prevention interventions must be aimed at the younger population and targeted toward the college-age population (Tjaden & Thoennes, 2000). Previous intervention programs have included women-only, men-only, and mixed audience programs. Intervention strategies for programs include rape-myth based (which focus on dispelling rape myths), victim empathy programs (which focus on the effects on the victim), lecture format courses, discussion groups, interactive improvisational theater presentations, and self-defense strategies. Yeater and O'Donahue (1999) summarize and critique published studies evaluating educational interventions. Most programs have lacked standardized methodology, follow-up, and stringent outcome measures, including endpoints such as measuring decreases in risky behavior and subsequent rapes. Most studies evaluate changes in attitudes after completion. One interesting study aimed at decreasing acquaintance rape in college did evaluate their intervention using an endpoint of subsequent attempted or completed rapes after participation in the program, compared to a control group (Hanson & Gidycz, 1993). The authors found a statistically significant decrease in the number of victimizations in the experimental group (6%) versus control group (14%). In the group of women who had been previously victimized, no statistically significant decrease in the incidence of revictimization was evident following educational intervention (44% for the experimental versus 40% for the control group) (Hanson & Gidycz, 1993). This suggests that interventions aimed at previously victimized individuals may need to be modified.

Primary prevention interventions aimed at women should focus on increasing awareness, addressing rape myths and risk perception, and decreasing risky behaviors. Interventions with men should focus on increasing awareness, increasing respect for women, dispelling "rape myths," and enhancing empathy for victims. Other examples of primary prevention include educating women about the prevention of drug-facilitated rape. Examples include warning young women about accepting drinks from strangers and encouraging women to watch each other's drinks while at parties or in bars. Interventions in acquaintance and intimate partner rape (which unfortunately constitute a large proportion of rapes) are more complex and may differ.

Examples of secondary prevention interventions include efforts to improve the care of rape survivors immediately after the crime, as well as improving follow up services. Institution of SANE or Sexual Assault Forensic Examiner (SAFE) programs, and interventions to decrease the anxiety and acute stress related to rape and the rape examination may decrease future sequelae (Resnick et al., 1999). Prevention of examination-related anxiety and the "second rape" sensation during evidence collection is currently under study. Higher levels of immediate distress are associated with poorer mental health outcomes. In an attempt to decrease forensic examination anxiety, hospital-based video interventions (a videotape is shown to survivors, explaining the evidence collection process) in South Carolina have shown promising results (Resnick et al., 1999). Other studies evaluating the use of beta-blockers to prevent PTSD by blocking imprinting of the event are under investigation. Further innovative, anxiety-reducing interventions are needed to better care for the victim in the immediate post-assault phase. Follow-up is often a weak link in the care of sexual assault survivors. Many regions lack adequate follow-up services, and, when offered, services are often used by less than one third of survivors (Holmes et al., 1998). Both targeted and universal screening policies and protocols to encourage early reporting and help-seeking for rape survivors are crucial. Policies and legal reform to protect the confidentiality of rape victims are vital to encouraging early reporting. Many women surveyed answered that a major barrier to reporting is fear that the press will publish their name and that family and friends will find out about the assault. Most survivors replied that they would be more likely to report early if they could be ensured privacy (Kilpatrick et al., 1992). In addition, rape education for school-age youth should focus on the importance of reporting rape to a supportive role model and emphasize the criminal nature of rape.

Interventions aimed at tertiary prevention include educating medical providers about the importance of asking the questions about previous trauma, and recognizing the signs and symptoms of previous sexual victimization and rape trauma syndrome. This is important in the care of all patients, but is especially important in women who present with multiple somatic complaints, multiple STDs, chronic headaches, abdominal and pelvic pain, substance abuse, depression, and suicide attempts. Despite the fact that many sexual assault survivors do not report the acute incident to law enforcement agencies or medical providers, nearly all sexual assault victims visit their primary care physician within 2 years after assault (Koss et al., 1991). Providers should be trained to recognize signs of sexual and physical abuse, to respond effectively, and to refer to resources available in the area. Widespread screening for trauma and early intervention may have a role in decreasing the silent, violent epidemic of sexual assault.

Numerous recent studies confirm that rape is unfortunately a common experience to many women in the United States. The experience of rape has far-reaching effects on the future health and well-being of the survivor and of his or her family and friends. Future efforts to improve the care of rape survivors should include improving services and encouraging early reporting. Public awareness must be increased in order to dispel the many "rape myths," and protocols must be developed for survivor privacy that encourage early reporting.

REFERENCES

Acierno R, Resnick HS, Kilpatrick DG. Health impact of interpersonal violence, I. Prevalence rates, case identification, and risk factors for sexual assault, physical assault, and domestic violence in men and women. *Behav Med.* 1997;23(2):53-64.

Acierno R, Resnick HS, Kilpatrick DG, Saunders B, Best CL. Risk factors for rape, physical assault and post-traumatic stress disorder in women: examination of differential multivariate relationships. *J Anxiety Disord.* 1999;13(6):541-563.

Bachman R, Saltzman LE. *Violence Against Women: Estimates from the Redesigned Survey.* Washington, DC: US Department of Justice; 1995. Report NCJ-154348.

Burgess AW, Holmstrom LL. Rape trauma syndrome. *Am J Psychiatry.* 1974;131: 981-986.

Drossman DA, Leserman J, Nachman G, et.al. Sexual and physical abuse in women with functional or organic gastrointestinal disorders. *Ann Intern Med.* 1990;113(11):828-833.

Federal Bureau of Investigation (FBI). *Uniform Crime Reports: Crime in the United States 1998.* Washington, DC: US Department of Justice; 1999.

Feldhaus KM, Houry D, Kaminsky R. Lifetime sexual assault prevalence rates and reporting practices in an emergency department population. *Ann Emerg Med.* 2000;36:23-27.

Gidycz CA, Coble CN, Latham L, Layman MJ. Relation of a sexual experience in adulthood to prior victimization experiences: a prospective analysis. *Psychol Women Q.* 1993;17:151-168.

Golding JM. Sexual assault history and headache: five general populations. *J Nerv Ment Dis.* 1999;187:624-629.

Golding JM, Wilsnack SC, Learman LA. Prevalence of sexual assault history among women with common gynecologic symptoms. *Am J Obstet Gynecol.* 1998;179:1013-1019.

Hanson KA, Gidycz CA. Evaluation of a sexual assault prevention program. *J Consult Clin Psychol.* 1993;61:1046-1052.

Holmes MM, Resnick HS, Frampton D. Follow-up of sexual assault victims. *Am J Obstet Genecol.* 1998;179:336-342.

Holmes MM, Resnick HS, Kilpatrick DG, Best CL. Rape-related pregnancy rate: estimates and descriptive characteristics from a national sample of women. *Am J Obstet Gynecol.* 1996;175:320-325.

Jamieson DJ, Steege JF. The association of sexual abuse with pelvic pain complaints in a primary care population. *Am J Obstet Gynecol.* 1997;177:1408-1412.

Kaufman A, Divasto P, Jackson R, Voorhees D, Christy J. Male rape victims: noninstitutionalized assault. *Am J Psychiatry.* 1980;137:221-223.

Kilpatrick DG, Saunders BE. *Prevalence and Consequences of Child Victimization: Results from the National Survey of Adolescents, Final Report.* Washington, DC: US Department of Justice, Office of Justice Programs, National Institute of Justice; 1997.

Kilpatrick DG, Saunders BE, Seymour AK. *Rape in America: A Report to the Nation.* Charleston, SC: Crime Victim Research and Treatment Center; 1992.

Kimerling R, Calhoun KS. Somatic symptoms, social support and treatment seeking among sexual assault victims. *J Consult Clin Psychol.* 1994;62:333-340.

Koss MP, Dinero TE, Seibel CA. Stranger and acquaintance rape: are there differences in the victim's experience? *Psychol Women Q.* 1988;12:1-24.

Koss MP, Gidycz CA, Wisniewski N. The scope of rape: incidence and prevalence of sexual aggression and victimization in a national sample of higher education students. *J Consult Clin Psychol.* 1987;55:162-167.

Koss MP, Koss PG, Woodruff WJ. Deleterious effects of criminal victimization on women's health and medical utilization. *Arch Intern Med.* 1991;151:342-347.

Nadelson CC, Notman MT, Zackson H, Gornick J. A follow-up study of rape victims. *Am J Psychiatry.* 1982;139:1266-1270.

National Institute of Justice. *The Extent and Costs of Crime Victimization: A New Look* (research preview). Washington, DC: US Department of Justice; 1996.

National Violence Against Women Survey. Washington, DC: US Department of Justice; 1995.

Pino NW, Meier RF. Gender differences in rape reporting. *Sex Roles J Res.* 1999;40:979-990.

Ramsay S. Breaking the silence surrounding rape (commentary). *Lancet.* 1999;3564:2018.

Resnick H, Acierno R, Holmes M, Kilpatrick DG, Jager N. Prevention of post-rape psychopathology: preliminary findings of a controlled acute rape treatment study. *J Anxiety Disord.* 1999;13:359-370.

Rothbaum BO, Foa EB, Murdock T, Riggs D, Walsh W. A prospective examination of post-traumatic stress disorder in rape victims. *J Trauma Stress.* 1992;5:455-475.

Sadler AG, Booth BM, Nielson D, Doebbeling BN. Health related consequences of physical and sexual violence: women in the military. *Obstet Gynecol.* 2000;96:473-480.

Sanford J, Cryer L, Christensen BL, Mattox KL. Patterns of reported rape in a tri-ethnic population: Houston, Texas, 1974-1975. *Am J Public Health.* 1979;69:480-484.

Talley NJ, Fett SL, Zinsmeister AR. Self-reported abuse and gastrointestinal disease in outpatients: association with irritable bowel-type symptoms. *Am J Gastroenterol.* 1995;90:366-371.

Tjaden P, Thoennes N. *Prevalence, Incidence and Consequences of Violence Against Women: Findings from the National Violence Against Women Survey.* Washington, DC: National Institutes of Justice; 1998. NCJ-172837

Tjaden P, Thoennes N. *Full Report of the Prevalence, Incidence and Consequences of Violence against Women.* Washington, DC: National Institutes of Justice and Center for Disease Control; 2000. NCJ-183781.

United States Model Penal Code (MPC). The Annual Meeting of the American Law Institute: Philadelphia, Pa; 1962. Quoted by: Epstein J, Langenbahn S. The criminal justice and community response to rape. Washington, DC: US Department of Justice, National Institute of Justice; 1994: 7.

Violence Against Women: Estimates from the Redesigned Survey. Washington, DC: Bureau of Justice Statistics, US Dept of Justice; 1995. Special Report NCJ-154348.

Walker EA, Gelfand AN, Gelfand MD, Koss MP, Katon WJ. Medical and psychiatric symptoms in female gastroenterology clinic patients with histories of sexual victimization. *Gen Hosp Psychiatry.* 1995;17:85-92.

Walker EA, Katon WJ, Roy-Byrne PP, Jemelka RP, Russo J. Histories of sexual victimization in patients with irritable bowel syndrome or inflammatory bowel disease. *Am J Psychiatry.* 1993;150:1502-1506.

Walling MK, Reiter RC, O'Hara MW, Milburn AK, Lilly G, Vincent SD. Abuse history and chronic pain in women, I. Prevalence of sexual abuse and physical abuse. *Obstet Gynecol.* 1994;84:193-199.

Yeater EA, O'Donahue W. Sexual assault prevention programs: current issues, future directions, and the potential efficacy of interventions with women. *Clin Psychol Rev.* 1999;19:739-771.

GENITAL INJURY AND SEXUAL ASSAULT

Donna Gaffney, RN, DNSc, FAAN

Identification and treatment of injury are paramount in the care of sexual assault victims. Recognition of injury requires knowledge of anatomy and physiology; refined skills of observation and examination; and an understanding of the many variables that can contribute to injuries. The clinician must be aware that genital injury can occur in consensual sex, especially among partners who have never been sexually active. In cases of nonconsensual penetration, there may be no indication of any genital injury at all. Therefore, it is imperative for the clinician to remember that each case involves a different set of variables. Because of the complex relationship among contributing factors, it is nearly impossible to predict whether there will be genital injury under a particular set of circumstances. It is also not possible to determine whether sexual contact was consensual given the presence or absence of injury.

TERMINOLOGY RELATED TO SEXUAL CONTACT

In addition to medical terminology and abbreviations used in the patient record it is also important to know the names for sex acts (**Table 13-2**). Victims use these labels for sexual contact and conduct. Clinicians must also be aware of common street names for these activities. In addition to regional differences, common language can change with each generation. A victim often first refers to a sexual act by its street name or uses a euphemism to refer to the sex act. The clinician must clarify the meaning of terms with the victim in order to accurately assess the possibility of injury.

The legal definition of sexual conduct may be more restrictive than the common definitions. Although rape is generally understood to be any unwanted penetration of any orifice, in some states rape is only unwanted penetration, however slight, by a penis into a vagina. Other states refer to "sexual assault" as an umbrella term and do not use the word "rape" at all. In some situations, the law mandates that prosecutors specify which body parts were involved during the encounter.

THE NATURE OF PHYSICAL FINDINGS

Physical findings may be normal, nonspecific, or specific indicators of forceful penetration. Although these terms have been used in discussing child sexual abuse injuries, they are also useful for evaluating the adult victim. Adams (2001) has built on the classification approach developed by Muram et al. (1999) and combined it with information from other elements of the sexual abuse assessment. These investigators proposed a five-category classification system for anogenital findings in children, as follows:

Class 1— Normal

Class 2— Nonspecific findings (may be related to conditions other than sexual abuse)

Class 3— Suspicious for abuse (should prompt examiner to question about sexual abuse)

Class 4— Suggestive of abuse and/or penetration

Class 5— Evidence of penetrating injury

Table 13-1. Male and Female Genital Structures and Characteristics

FEMALE **(Figure 13-1)**

Anus: The terminal opening of the digestive tract, which serves as the opening of the rectum. This area has a concentration of nerve endings. Anal folds, or wrinkles of perianal skin radiating from the anus, are caused by the closure of the external anal sphincter.

Cervix: The lower portion of the uterus that protrudes into the vagina.

Clitoris: A small cylindrical body of erectile tissue situated at the most anterior portion of the vulva. A fold of tissue, called the "hood" or prepuce, covers the clitoris. During arousal, the clitoris enlarges and protrudes from the hood. The clitoris is the most sensitive part of the female anatomy.

Fossa navicularis: The area of the vaginal vestibule located between the posterior attachment of the hymen and the post-erior fourchette. It presents as a shallow depression at the base of the vulva.

Hymen: The circular band of tissue that surrounds (completely or partially) the opening of the vagina. The physical appearance and elasticity of the hymen change over a woman's life span because of hormonal fluctuation (primarily estrogen).

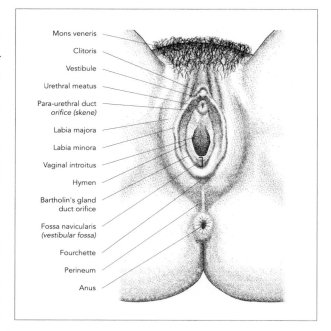

Figure 13-1. *The external genitalia of the adult female.*

Hymen Morphology

   Annular: Circumferential hymen tissue presents 360 degrees around vaginal opening.

   Bump: Solid elevation of hymenal tissue.

   Crescentic: Posterior rim of hymen, with attachments at the 10 to 1 o'clock and 1 to 2 o'clock positions.

   Cribiform: Hymen with multiple small hymenal openings.

   External ridge: Longitudinal ridge (raised area) on the external surface of the hymen from the rim to the fossa navicularis or urethra.

   Fimbriated: A hymen with a ruffled, and/or fringed edge.

   Hymenal cleft: Division or split in the rim of the hymen that does not cross the base of the hymen.

   Longitudinal vaginal ridge: A longitudinal ridge extending from the hymenal rim into the vagina, usually on the posterior or posterolateral walls, and parallel to the vaginal axis.

   Redundant: Hymen of any type that is folded on itself and does not "open" to reveal the orifice, even when multiple positions and methods are used.

   Septate hymen: Two hymenal openings with a band of hymenal tissue in between.

   Imperforate: No hymenal opening.

Labia majora: Latin for "larger lips." These are rounded folds of skin forming the lateral boundaries of the vulva. These outer folds of skin protect the more delicate structures underneath.

Labia minora: Latin for "smaller lips." The longitudinal folds of tissue enclosed within the labia majora that are located on either side of the vaginal orifice. These folds of tissue cover the vaginal orifice and urethral meatus.

Mons pubis: The rounded eminence in front of the pubic symphysis formed by a collection of fatty tissue beneath the integument. It becomes covered with hair at the time of puberty.

Os: The opening located at the center of the cervix, leading to the uterus.

Perineum: The area between the vaginal introitus and anus.

(continued)

Table 13-1. *(continued)*

Rectum: Terminal portion of the lower intestine.

Uterus: A hollow muscular organ, pear shaped, with a small internal cavity. It is where the fetus grows before birth.

Urethral meatus: The opening to the urethra. Its major purpose is the release of urine from the bladder.

Vagina: The structure that opens to the outside of the body at the vaginal introitus and extends 3 to 5 inches inside the body, ending at the cervix.

Vaginal introitus: Located below the urethral meatus and situated behind the labia minora; the entrance to the vagina.

Vaginal vestibule: The space posterior to the clitoris, between the labia minora.

Vulva: The external genitalia of the female, or pudendum. Includes the clitoris, labia majora, labia minora, vaginal vestibule, urethral orifice, vaginal orifice, hymen, fourchette, and posterior commissure.

MALE **(Figure 13-2)**

Coronal ridge: The widest portion around the glans.

Ejaculation: The release of reproductive fluid via the male urethra. The ejaculate may or may not contain spermatozoa.

Foreskin (prepuce): The movable hood of skin covering the glans of the penis. During erection, the foreskin rolls back just below the coronal ridge. In circumcised men, the foreskin has been removed.

Frenulum: On the underside of the penis, with a different texture to its skin, this area is often highly responsive to stimulation.

Glans: The cone-shaped head of the penis. This fleshy "head" of the penis is most sensitive to stimulation. Usually larger in diameter than the shaft, the glans is responsible for the greatest sensation during intercourse.

Penis: The male organ of reproduction and urination.

Perineum: The area between the base of the scrotum and the anus. Beneath the skin are more chambers that fill with blood during arousal, just as the penis does.

Scrotum: The sac encasing the testicles just below the penis.

Semen: A thick fluid released by the male during ejac-ulation. It consists of fluids from various glands plus the spermatozoa.

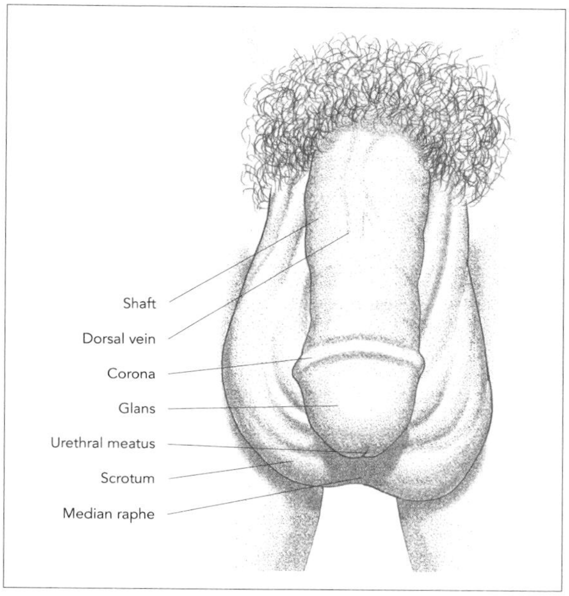

Shaft: The cylindrical part of the penis located between the glans and the body, which is filled with vascular chambers.

Figure 13-2. *Frontal view of the external male genitalia.*

During arousal these chambers fill with blood, causing the shaft to stiffen and producing an erection. Unlike many other animals, the human has no bone or gristle to ensure stiffness.

Testicles: Two spherical glands within the scrotum that produce sperm. The sperm are carried through spermatic cords, joining fluids produced by the prostate gland and seminal vesicles to produce semen, which is then ejaculated. One of the cords is called the epididymis, and the difference in the length of the two epididymides is responsible for one testicle being slightly lower than the other.

Urethral opening: At the end of the penis, this opening serves as the duct through which both urine and ejaculate (semen) flow.

Nonspecific findings can be related to circumstances other than sexual assault in adults as well as children. Many sexual assault victims have normal and nonspecific findings on examination. These findings can include but are not limited to the following: (1) hymenal tags, bumps or mounds, clefts or notches (if the hymen is present at all); (2) labial adhesions; (3) erythema of the genitalia or anus; (4) perianal skin tags; and (5) anal fissures. Findings specific to blunt force trauma in females resulting from forceful penetration include recent or healed lacerations or abrasions of the hymen and vaginal mucosa, posterior fourchette, perineum, labia minora, or labia majora. Examination findings can also be subjective. The victim's experience of pain and tenderness (with or without contact) cannot be documented by visual diagrams or photography. Only examiner observation, documentation, and victim statement can indicate the victim's pain. However, because there are individual differences in how victims perceive and tolerate pain, this subjective finding may not be specific to forceful penetration in itself.

Table 13-2. Definitions of Sexual Conduct

Fellatio: Any mouth to penis contact.

Frottage: Rubbing for the purpose of sexual gratification.

Cunnilingus: Mouth to vulva.

Sexual intercourse: Contact of the penis to the vagina.

Anal intercourse or anal sodomy: Contact of penis to the anus.

Anilingus: Mouth to anus.

Oral sodomy: Mouth to vagina, anus, or penis.

MECHANISMS AND TYPES OF INJURY

Identification of physical findings is not only a critical element in the treatment of the victim but also in the prosecution of most sexual assault trials. Although the law no longer requires proof of resistance, the public, including judges and juries, still perceive physical injury, especially genital injury, as the essential proof the victim did not consent to intercourse. Although this perception is rooted in myth, physical evidence of injury, no matter how small or seemingly insignificant, can corroborate the victim's account of the assault. For example, a pattern of circular bruises on the outer aspect of a victim's upper arm can corroborate the assault history offered by the victim that the offender grabbed her arm in an effort to push her against a wall. With respect to genital injury, new techniques are enabling healthcare providers to identify and document injuries previously not visible to the naked eye. In addition to appreciating the impact that injury can have on the victim's healing and recovery from a sexual assault, it is also important to understand that the victim's entire body, not only the genital area, is a crime scene. When there are no physical findings, nongenital or genital, it is just as important for the clinician to understand why their absence does not indicate consensual sexual contact.

While recognizing that there are adult male as well as female victims of rape, myths and stereotypes primarily center on the woman as victim. They affect how the jury perceives the victim and how they perceive medical and other evidence. These myths are "Rape victims suffer serious physical injury other than the rape itself;" "All rape victims suffer genital injury;" and "A lack of injury findings indicates there was no rape."

The mechanism of injury can explain how an injury occurred, dispel sexual assault myths, and corroborate the victim's account of the assault. Injuries are often

Key Point:
Rape myths include the following:
— Rape victims suffer serious physical injury other than the rape itself.
— All rape victims suffer genital injury.
— A lack of injury findings indicates there was no rape.
These can be dispelled by exploring the mechanism of injury.

classified by appearance and causation (if known). They are never classified by motivation of infliction. The classification categories include abrasions, contusions or bruises, lacerations, and incised wounds such as cuts and slashes. Stab wounds may also be included in the category related to cuts. The different types of injuries are defined by the layer of tissue they affect. The anatomy of the skin includes three layers of tissue: the epidermis, which includes the stratum corneum (keratinized cells) and the basal cell layer; the dermis, which forms the greater part of the skin and contains blood vessels, hair follicles, cutaneous glands, and nerve fibers; and the subcutaneous or fatty layer. Deep fascia or connective tissue and muscle lie beneath the three layers of the skin. The mouth and vaginal vault are lined with mucosal tissue. These areas do not have the same protective layers as the epidermis (keratinized cells) or fatty tissue; therefore, mucosa is more vulnerable to injury.

Victims do not present with a set pattern of typical sexual assault injuries. However, some types of injuries are more indicative of forceful penetration. Injuries primarily fall into the following categories: lacerations, ecchymoses, abrasions, erythema, and swelling. A method for remembering the types of injuries is to use the acronym TEARS (Girardin et al., 1997) as follows:

T: Tear (laceration) or tenderness

E: Ecchymosis (bruising)

A: Abrasion

R: Redness (erythema)

S: Swelling (edema)

ABRASIONS
Abrasions are superficial injuries to the skin limited to the epidermis and superficial dermis. These injuries are normally caused by lateral rubbing, sliding, or compressive forces against the skin in a parallel manner rather than by vertical force. A typical example of abrasion is scraping a knee on cement, as in the case of childhood falls. The outermost layer of skin is scraped away from the deeper layers of the dermis and underlying structures. The shape of the abrasion can vary; a linear abrasion, or a scratch, can result from a thorn or a sharp fingernail, while a graze usually involves a wider area.

CONTUSIONS AND BRUISES
Bruises lie below the intact epidermis and consist of an extravascular collection of blood that has leaked from ruptured capillaries or blood vessels. Contusions may cause far more serious injuries and can occur anywhere in the body. Both of these types of injury result from blood vessel leakage when blunt force is applied to the tissue. With force, a blood vessel is likely to rupture and blood seeps into the surrounding tissue. Bruises do not occur immediately but may take hours or even days to develop. Several factors can influence the size, appearance, and color changes of a bruise: available space for blood to collect, weight of the individual, force of the impact, vascularity of the area, fragility of the blood vessels, and the location of the bruise. More resilient areas that do not have a hard structure (such as bone) beneath the tissue may result in less tissue trauma. For all of these reasons, it is not possible to accurately "age" a bruise using "color" as a guideline. In fact, a number of individual factors determine the appearance and healing of a bruise: impaired blood clotting, immunosuppression, certain malignant diseases, diabetes, alcoholism, malnutrition, and age (Rabkin, 2002). Even the temperature of the environment can influence the appearance of a bruise (Besant-Matthews, 2001). Bruises are also known as ecchymoses (Lee et al., 1993). Petechiae are tiny red or purple spots on skin or other tissue. Petechiae less than 3 millimeters in diameter are pinpoint-sized hemorrhages of small capillaries in the skin or mucous membranes. In all situations, petechiae, ecchymoses, and bruises do not blanch when pressed.

Key Point:
It is not possible to specifically identify the exact "age" a bruise using color as a guideline with absolute accuracy. Factors that can influence the appearance and healing of a bruise include the following:
— Impaired blood clotting
— Immune compromised status
— Certain malignant diseases
— Diabetes
— Alcoholism
— Malnutrition
— Age

ERYTHEMA

Erythema, or redness of the skin, should not be mistaken for bleeding under the skin. Erythema blanches with gentle pressure. Erythema is usually diffuse and does not have a pattern. The cause of redness can be a forceful slap or increased pressure to the skin. With sudden pressure, the blood is momentarily forced out of the capillaries in the area of contact. When the pressure is withdrawn, the blood returns to the capillaries, which may then dilate. The result is redness or flushing of the skin.

LACERATIONS

A laceration occurs when the continuity of the skin is broken and disrupted by blunt force. The force is usually applied in a vertical manner, perpendicular to the plane of the skin. Tearing, ripping, crushing, overly stretching, or pulling apart result in this tear. Often there is a bony surface underneath the tissue, which causes the blunt force to have a particularly damaging impact on the overlying tissue. The edges of the laceration are irregular and can be aligned to fit together. It is important to remember that a laceration is not a cut. A cut is an incision made with a sharp instrument. There may be bruising or crushing of the margins of a laceration and connective tissue strands may "bridge" across the interior of the wound. A laceration frequently contains foreign material including trace evidence such as dirt, fibers, or even grass (Besant-Matthews, 2001).

RESEARCH ON INJURIES AND SEXUAL ASSAULT

As mentioned previously, the presence of rape myths concerning genital injury and nonconsensual penetration requires considerable exploration. The public, juries included, often believes that genital injury occurs in all sexual assault cases. It is incomprehensible to a layperson that an individual who is forcibly penetrated does not sustain some form of injury to the anogenital area. The lay public makes certain assumptions about injury; forcible penetration results in pain, and pain is often related to injury. Nongenital injury, while just as important for a clinician to consider, is often subject to the same misconceptions.

Key Point:
*The majority of sexual assaults **do not** result in genital injury.*

However, research and data collection on injuries resulting from sexual assault seem to suggest that the opposite is true; the majority of sexual assaults do not usually result in genital injury. In the 1992 Rape in America study (CVRTC, 1992), 75% of victims reported no physical injuries and 25% reported minor physical injuries. An even smaller percentage of victims sustain injuries so serious that they require hospitalization. Death as a result of a sexual assault is rare. In 1998 the Research Report from the Violence Against Women Survey found that 31.5% of women (over age 18 years) who were sexually assaulted sustained injuries other than the rape itself. Males reported nongenital injury at a rate of 16.1%.

Since the mid-1980s, a number of studies have examined the incidence of genital injury in female sexual assault victims coming to emergency departments. It is difficult if not impossible to compare or group these studies because of differing methodologies, inconsistent examination techniques, missing data, and poor statistical analyses. Some studies were carried out before the advent of forensic colposcopy. The incidence of genital injuries increases significantly when a colposcope is used for assessment (Lenahan et al., 1998; Slaughter & Brown, 1992; Slaughter et al., 1997). This binocular magnification device is now used to view genital or nongenital injuries in many sexual assault programs.

There are other factors that may prevent comparing data among injury studies. One crucial variable is the time elapsed from assault to examination. Slaughter et al. (1997) found injury in 89% of 171 victims of penile-vaginal penetration when they were examined within the first 24 hours after the assault. After 72 hours, the injury rate dropped to 46%. In other words, the probability of identifying injury decreases as time passes. Healing, especially among younger victims, may be complete in 48 to 72 hours. Adams et al. (2000) conducted a retrospective study on 214 adolescent victims of sexual assault and found that the degree of genital injury was significantly correlated with time elapsed since the assault; injuries were identified in 89% of the cases when the examination was conducted within 72 hours as compared to 46% when the examination was done after 72 hours. All cases used forensic colposcopy as part of the examination process.

In addition to colposcopy, other methods facilitate the identification of injury. Toluidine blue dye is a nuclear stain that adheres to cellular material and enhances the identification of injury. When a 1% solution of toluidine blue dye is swabbed onto human skin and the excess wiped away, the dye then bonds with cellular nuclei. The dye causes the injured area to darken significantly, making visualization of an injury much easier. In one of the first studies using toluidine blue dye, Lauber and Souma (1982) found that their visualization of posterior fourchette tears in sexual assault victims increased to 40% from 34%. McCauley et al. (1987) found tears in only 4% using gross visualization, but after toluidine blue dye was applied, the rate increased to 58%. Neither of these studies used colposcopy for magnification.

Finally, it may be impossible to determine true injury incidence and prevalence rates because most cases go unreported. Therefore, only those victims presenting to law enforcement or healthcare settings are part of the sample studied. As a result, none of these studies is truly representative of the sexual assault victim population.

Bowyer and Dalton (1997) stated that "the relationship between genital injury and rape was questionable" with the incidence of genital injury varying from 10% to 87% in the 13 studies they analyzed. However, it is important to note that of these studies, which were published between 1971 and 1992, only three used enhanced methods of examination (two used toluidine blue dye and one used colposcopy). The studies also focused on different aspects of injury, different classification of injury, unknown elapsed time from assault to examination, and small sample sizes.

Patterns of genital injury in female sexual assault victims have also been the focus of investigation. In 1997, Slaughter et al., using colposcopic examination, found that 68% (213) of a sample of 311 sexual assault victims had some type of anogenital trauma. The percentage of those with genital injury for a specific site were as follows: posterior fourchette (70%), labia minora (53%), hymen (29%), fossa navicularis (25%), anus (15%), cervix (13%), vagina (11%), perineum (11%), periurethral area (9%), labia majora (7%), and rectum (4%). Although this study has been criticized for its methodology (reassigning subjects from the assault group to the consensual intercourse subsample), there are still important findings that need future investigation.

However, there is concern about the validity of some studies. They may be outdated or do not demonstrate appropriate examination procedures or correlate the time interval between the assault and the examination. For example, Penttilia and Karhumen (1990) noted that among the 249 victims in their study only 18% (45) had genital injuries. In this study the method of injury identification was not noted and the elapsed time between the assault and the examination was not factored into the analysis.

By far, the most frequently observed genital injuries are tears and abrasions located at the posterior fourchette. This is called a mounting injury where the penis first touches the perineum. It is usually between the 5 and 7 o'clock positions. The point of contact is often the area of greatest force, causing the tissue to stretch and ultimately tear.

Other sites of injury are the labia minora. Abrasions and bruising or ecchymosis may occur as a result of friction with repeated penetration or attempts to penetrate. Somewhat less frequent are tears and/or ecchymosis to the hymen or the fossa navicularis. The percentage of hymenal injuries may be increased in victims who have never been sexually active. Cervical injury is less common, but it may be seen when the penetrating object is not a penis, such as a finger with a sharp fingernail.

FACTORS INFLUENCING INJURY
CONSENSUAL INTERCOURSE AND EPITHELIAL CHANGES

A concern often addressed in the discussion of injury and sexual assault relates to the possibility of epithelial changes after consensual intercourse. How can a clinician distinguish between physical findings in sexual assault, consensual intercourse, and even intercourse that may be deemed "intense" or "vigorous?" A few studies have addressed physical findings after consensual intercourse. Norvell et al. (1984) examined 18 women within 6 hours of consensual intercourse. Using Lugol's solution and colposcopy, the researchers found microtrauma in 61% of their sample. They defined microtrauma as increased vascularity (telangiectasia), broken blood vessels, and microabrasions. The authors reported these findings were located in the vaginal mucosa, and specifically showed increased vascularity that tended to be widespread and not localized. The study did not identify tears or abrasions of the external genitalia. These findings are in stark contrast in both the location and types of injury found in studies that have investigated sexual assault genital injury.

Fraser et al. (1999) evaluated changes in vaginal and cervical appearance in 107 women (sexually active, age 18 to 35 years) over a 6-month period at 4 research sites (314 total inspections). The study focused on epithelial changes that might correlate with sexual intercourse, tampon use, contraceptive methods, and other environmental factors. Among the study sample there were 103 colposcopic observations made within 24 hours of intercourse. The authors noted that with increased frequency of vaginal intercourse, an increased number of cases had vaginal changes: 14.4% atypical findings in subjects where there was no intercourse in the previous 2 weeks, 17.8% atypical findings when intercourse occurred 1 to 4 times in the previous 2 weeks, and 20% atypical findings when intercourse occurred over four times in the previous 2 weeks. Sexual intercourse in the previous 24 hours was associated with overall epithelial changes. Among 103 observations of vaginal epithelium within 24 hours after intercourse, vaginal changes were noted in 26 inspections (25.2%).

Fraser et al. (1999) used a modification of the World Health Organization (1996) criteria for vaginal epithelial changes. These criteria clearly defined and described atypical findings in the vagina and cervix. Of the 26 atypical findings 24 hours after intercourse, there were five cases of erythema at the introitus or lower third of the vaginal vault, seven observations of petechiae in the fornices or the forniceal surface of the cervix, three cases of abrasions and ecchymosis, and the remainder (11 or 42%) were primarily petechial changes on the vaginal walls. The Fraser findings are consistent with those of Norvell and the preliminary results of the Sommers et al. (2001) study.

Although it is possible that vaginal epithelial changes result from consensual intercourse, the types of changes are remarkable in comparison to the physical findings noted after sexual assault. Studies focusing on sexual assault cases have noted injuries located at the posterior fourchette, labia minora, and fossa navicularis. These structures are part of the external genitalia. The Fraser study (1999) noted changes after intercourse primarily within the vaginal vault; in fact, only five of the 26 observations were located at the introitus or lower third of the vagina. There is also a difference in the type of injuries noted. According to the World Health Organization (1996) criteria, only tears, micro-ulcerations and abrasions result in disrupted epithelium; erthyema, ecchymosis, petechiae, and edema do not result in a break of the epithelial layer. In studies of sexual assault injuries, the physical findings are primarily tears, abrasions, and ecchymoses

(Slaughter & Brown, 1992; Slaughter et al., 1997; Adams et al., 2000)). Fraser et al. (1999) refer to the changes postintercourse as minor surface trauma. The authors describe erythema and petechiae as far more frequent. There were only three observations of abrasions and ecchymosis. Therefore, it is imperative for the clinician to recognize that physical findings for women who have had consensual intercourse can be different from the findings in victims of sexual assault.

Vigorous or intense intercourse is sometimes called "rough sex" in and out of the courtroom. Defense attorneys suggest that a victim's injuries may be the result of more intense and vigorous consensual intercourse, not sexual assault. Fraser et al. (1999) noted that the observations of erythematous introital changes and prominent petechiae were more likely to follow prolonged and intense intercourse, as reported by the subjects. "Rough" sex often involves the tearing of the mucosa of the vaginal vault (Rabkin, 2002). Data concerning physical findings following "vigorous intercourse" is sparse; clinicians tend to rely on anecdotal reports and the patient history. Patients may hesitate to seek medical services when they have sustained injury to the genitalia after episodes of intense sex, unusual positions during sex, or prolonged sexual contact. The clinician will notice during the history that, although the individual may be embarrassed or hesitant to discuss details of the sexual encounter, she is able to recall both her partner's and her own actions that may have led to the injury. Sexual assault victims may not be able to recall the specific actions of the assailant.

THE VICTIM'S HISTORY AND DETERMINANTS OF INJURY

It is necessary to identify any injuries the victim sustains for several reasons:

— To provide appropriate treatment

— To evaluate the need for additional intervention

— To assess the need for referrals

In addition, because the victim's body is a crime scene, the documentation of any injury can offer corroboration of the victim's history of the assault. For example, the victim may report that the assailant grabbed her arm, pulled her into the living room, threw her to the floor, and forced her legs apart. The assessment and examination may reveal that the victim suffered bruising to her upper arm, shoulder, hip, and inner thighs, injuries consistent with being grabbed by the upper arm, hitting her shoulder as she was pulled through the doorway, being thrown to the floor, and having her legs forced apart. A critical point to remember is that while identified injuries may corroborate the victim's account, the absence of such injuries does not mean that a rape did not occur. In addition, two victims with the same assault history may not have the same types of physical findings.

A complex relationship exists among the variables that can influence injury type and location. A comprehensive history is critical to understanding the presence or absence of injury. These variables can be grouped in the following manner: factors related to the victim, the perpetrator, the circumstances, and the environment (**Table 13-3**).

Factors Related to the Victim

Anatomy and Physiology of the Reproductive Organs

The anatomical structure of the vagina is a key factor in understanding how the body may be protected from injury during sexual assault. The vagina is a muscular organ comprising three layers of tissue. There is an internal mucous lining and a muscular coat separated by a layer of erectile tissue. The mucous membrane is continuous with the lining of the uterus. The epithelium covering the mucous membrane is of the stratified squamous variety. The mucous membranes are similar to the lining of the mouth. However, unlike the smooth surface of the mouth lining, the vagina contains folds or wrinkles known as rugae. The submucous tissue is very loose and contains numerous large veins. It contains a number of mucous

Table 13-3. Variables Influencing Injury Type and Location
Factors Related to the Victim:
Anatomy and physiology of the reproductive structures
Health and developmental status
Condition of the genital structures
Previous sexual experience
Lubrication of the vaginal vault (natural or artificial)
Partner Participation
Positioning and pelvic tilt
Psychologic response
Factors Related to the Assailant:
Object of penetration
Lubrication
Male sexual dysfunction
Force of penetration
Factors Related to Circumstances:
Previous history with assailant
Lack of communication
Factors Related to the Environment:
Location of the assault
Materials and surfaces in surrounding area

crypts, but no true glands. The muscular coat (tunica muscularis) consists of two layers: an external longitudinal layer, which is by far the stronger, and an internal circular layer.

The vagina resembles a flattened tube, the sides of which are collapsed on each other. It is not a continually open space, but a potential space. Because of its muscular tissue, the vagina has the ability to expand and contract, much like the cuff of a sweater or glove allowing different sized objects to pass through—a tampon, a penis, or an infant during childbirth.

Key Point:
As the penetrating object moves through the introitus into the lower one third of the vaginal vault, more pain and discomfort result. The vagina is designed to accept an adult penis without injury. Therefore, it is possible that although force was used, no tears, lacerations, or abrasions occurred in the vaginal walls.

The outer one third of the vagina, especially the area near the vaginal introitus, contains nearly 90% of the vaginal nerve endings and therefore is much more sensitive to touch than the inner two thirds of the vaginal vault. This means that the penetration of the vaginal vault is going to result in more pain and discomfort as the penetrating object moves through the introitus into the lower one third of the vaginal vault. The vagina is designed to accept an adult penis without injury. Therefore, it is possible that although force was used, there would be no tears, lacerations, or abrasions to the vaginal walls.

Although the vagina may be protected from lacerations at the time of assault because of its elastic nature, the structures of the external genitalia may not be as immune to blunt force trauma. The labia majora are covered with hair follicles and squamous epithelium. A core of fatty tissue is at the center of each labium. This fatty tissue may serve to protect the labia from blunt force. There are also substantial nerve endings in each labium majora, sensitive to pressure, touch, and pain. The labia minora are much more sensitive than the labia majora; in addition, they are not covered with hair nor do they have a fatty core. The medial sides of the labia minora are covered with mucous membranes, whereas the outer surface is covered with keratinized epithelium (Sanders, 2001). The labia minora may be very susceptible to pressure and friction from the penetrating object. This can result in abrasions on the outer surface and in the crease where the labia minora meet the base of the labia majora.

The posterior fourchette, also known as the frenulum of the labia minora, is a short, flat fold of mucous membrane that forms the posterior border of the vestibule at the junction of the labia minora. This tissue is not elastic and is most prone to irritation and blunt force. In fact, the posterior fourchette is the site for episiotomies during childbirth. The posterior fourchette may also be the site where the penis first touches the female genitalia during attempted penetration.

Health and Developmental Status

Individual health and developmental stage of the victim also play important roles in whether or not the victim suffers any injury. For example, injuries may be observed less frequently in adolescents and younger adult victims, possibly because of the amount of estrogen produced in their bodies. In addition, a younger individual heals faster. There is more resilient tissue, greater elasticity, and more adipose tissue supporting the dermis and epidermis. In older or postmenopausal victims, there is likely to be more injury resulting from decreased estrogen levels and loss of tissue elasticity. In addition, the marked decrease in estrogen directly affects normal cyclical lubrication of the vaginal surface. Injuries suffered by this population usually take longer to heal. A victim of any age who is ill may experience compromised tissue responses and ultimately become more vulnerable to traumatic forces.

Condition of the Genital Structures

There are several considerations a healthcare provider should keep in mind regarding the condition of the victim's genital structures. Healing surgical procedures, such as a new episiotomy, will render the area less stable. Tissue is more vulnerable to pressure and force. Even transsexual surgical procedures or female genital mutilation can contribute to injury in the genital area.

Excessive scarring from a previous operation or lack of perineal elasticity in postmenopausal women can increase the possibility of tears and abrasions. Atrophic vaginitis, or urogenital atrophy, can result in changes to the external genitalia. The epithelium can appear pale, smooth, and shiny. Often, inflammation with patchy erythema, petechiae, and increased friability may be present. External genitalia may have diminished elasticity, loss of skin turgor, sparsity of pubic hair, dryness of labia, vulvar dermatoses, vulvar lesions, and fusion of the labia minora. Introital stenosis may be apparent. These conditions put the individual at considerable risk of injury in a number of circumstances: sexual assault, insertion of the speculum, or intercourse. In addition, there will be considerable pain. Vaginal epithelium that is friable with decreased rugae will be much more prone to traumatic injury. Ecchymoses and minor lacerations at the peri-introital areas as well as the posterior fourchette may also recur after coitus or during a speculum examination (Pandit & Ouslander, 1997).

Any kind of introital lesion puts the victim at risk for significant injury after sexual assault. These lesions can result from a number of inflammatory conditions such as vestibulitis or inflamed labial sweat glands. Abscesses of Bartholin's glands or any infection of the external genitalia can also contribute to tissue damage at the time of assault. Even the use of improperly fitted or inadequately lubricated condoms can

Key Point:
Injuries tend to be observed less often in adolescents and younger adult victims, possibly because of the amount of estrogen produced in their bodies, or the fact that younger individuals heal faster, or the presence of more resilient tissue, greater elasticity, and more adipose tissue supporting the dermis and epidermis. Older or postmenopausal women are more likely to show injuries because of their decreased estrogen levels and loss of tissue elasticity.

cause irritation. Allergic reactions to the contents of contraceptive foams and jellies and to condoms, abnormalities of the female genital tract (e.g., congenital septum, a rigid hymen), and dermatologic disorders (e.g., lichen sclerosis) can further contribute to injury.

Previous Sexual Experience

After the onset of puberty, estrogen causes the hymen to be elastic and easily stretched (estrogenization). As a result, it is possible that a woman will not have any tears or bleeding with intercourse. This may even be true for first-time intercourse or sexual assault. Myths about the hymen may especially impact sexual assault cases. Many jurors believe that the first time a woman has intercourse, there will always be injury to the hymen, and that if the first intercourse is a sexual assault, she will present in the emergency room with visible tears to the hymen. However, this is not necessarily the case.

Prior sexual experience has been associated with different rates of genital injury. Biggs et al. (1998) found that in a sample of 132 women examined within 10 days of their sexual assault, 65% of those without sexual experience exhibited genital injury whereas only 25% of those with prior sexual experience showed similar trauma. Adams et al. (2000) found that acute hymenal tears were more common in subjects who stated they were virgins before the assault (19% versus 3%).

Hymen injury, rupture, or transection as a result of first-time intercourse is very common but not inevitable. The elasticity of the hymenal tissue may allow for penetration of a fully erect penis (Paul, 1984). If the sexual assault victim has not had any previous sexual experience, physical findings may include rupture or hymenal tears. The incidence is higher than the 9% noted by Biggs et al., (1998). However, the Adams study cited above examined 87% of the victims within 72 hours using colposcopy, while the Biggs study examined the victims without magnification within 10 days of the reported sexual assault.

Lubrication

Lubrication can be artificial or natural. The menstrual cycle affects the vaginal environment and the secretions within the vagina. The vagina is lined by nonkeratinizing stratified squamous epithelium, which undergoes hormone-related cyclical changes (Berman et al., 2000). Estrogens stimulate the proliferation and maturation of the epithelium with the accumulation of glycogen in the cells. There is both an increase in vaginal secretions and a change in their consistency at ovulation. The pH balance of the vagina fluctuates during the cycle and is the least acidic on the days just before and during menstruation. Although the vaginal tissue does not contain any secretor glands itself, it is rich with blood vessels.

Vaginal lubrication typically decreases as women age. After menopause, the body produces less estrogen, which, unless compensated for with estrogen replacement therapy, causes the vaginal walls to thin out significantly (Cardozo et al., 1998). The vaginal vault also tends to become slightly shorter and narrower, and the time needed to produce even a reduced amount of lubrication is prolonged. Sometimes a woman who is using a birth control pill that is high in progesterone can experience lessened vaginal lubrication.

Lubrication can also result from vasocongestion, which is an increase in blood volume to the genital area. The blood vessels become engorged with blood and, as a result, pressure inside these blood vessels forces cellular fluid through the vaginal lining into the vaginal vault. The mucosal surface becomes coated with the liquid in a process called transudation. At one time researchers thought that lubrication was the hallmark of the human sexual response, protecting both partners from injury during coitus. This has been a problem for clinicians when working with sexual assault survivors and testifying in court.

The number of studies conducted in the area of human sexual response has significantly increased during the last 10 years. Lubrication, once identified as a crucial element of excitement, or the first stage of the human sexual response (Masters & Johnson, 1966), is not always a harbinger of sexual arousal. Lubrication can be an element of sexual response, but it can also occur as a purely genital response. The reaction of the vaginal mucosa to a penetrating foreign body (pressure and tactile stimulation) is to lubricate. Even in nonconsenting intercourse there will be a certain degree of lubrication (Paul, 1984). It is important to recognize that a sexual response includes both physical and psychologic components. A genital response is only physiologic in nature. Specifically, a genital response is an involuntary, autonomic body response to a sensory stimulus that results in increased blood flow to the pelvic area. The stimulus is most often tactile and can be anywhere on the continuum from the slight brushing of underwear to forceful pushing against the perineum to effect penile penetration.

Key Point:
A sexual response includes both physical and psychologic components. A genital response is only physiologic in nature.

Lubrication does not instantly disappear if the sexual response ends in fear. Take the case of a couple who is engaged in intimate behavior. Their sexual contact and mutual desire serves to initiate the sexual response. The partners agree that they will not have intercourse. However, the boundaries originally agreed upon become violated when forcible penetration is attempted. The victim reacts with fear, yet because she was already sexually stimulated, the lubricating fluid is still present in the vaginal vault. The fact that the woman's vaginal vault did not "dry up" when her partner forced intercourse does not mean that she continued to respond to him sexually. The lubricating fluid was already present.

If a stranger breaks into a woman's home, attacks her, and begins to touch or press her genitals, her body will automatically respond to that tactile stimulus. Blood will begin to move to the pelvic vessels, engorgement is initiated, and she will start to lubricate. This is not a sexual response. The woman is having a purely genital response.

During sexual assault the genital response is affected by the activities of the sympathetic nervous system, which is in the survival mode, sending increased blood to the pelvis and increasing vasocongestion. In times of fear and threat of bodily harm, the sympathetic nervous system becomes activated and mobilizes the "fight, flight, or freeze" responses, putting the individual in survival mode. When this happens, neurochemicals are released, stimulating the body to send blood to the large muscle groups and the pelvis. Nonessential body functions cease, and heart rate, blood pressure, and respirations increase. In fact, the increase in blood flow to the lower part of the body can further increase vasocongestion, resulting in more lubrication (Basson, 2000). This lubrication has nothing to do with sexual response. It is the automatic response of the body to a genital stimulus, which is then exacerbated by fear.

Partner Participation

In consensual situations in which both partners are participating, there is little or no discomfort or injury because of partner cooperation and assistance. The situation is relaxed and the partners assist each other with insertion. However, when there is an absence of cooperation, the muscles may become tense and insertion of the penetrating object is not facilitated. This not only risks pulling the labia minora into the vaginal vault but causes repeated attempts at insertion, prolonging contact, and increasing tissue friction. In addition, there is the possibility of creating a less flexible surface against which the penetrating object forces itself.

Positioning and Pelvic Tilt

Protective positioning facilitates penile insertion. The use of pelvic tilt aligns the penetrating body part with the receiving body orifice. If the pelvic tilt is not maintained, as in the case of a woman who pulls her body away from the penetrating object, the penis will not enter the vaginal introitus on a parallel plane.

Tilting the pelvis allows for alignment of the penetrating object with the vaginal vault, thereby decreasing tension and pressure from misalignment. The perineum posterior to the vaginal introitus and the posterior fourchette will be subject to overstretching. This is often called a mounting injury. In addition, leg positioning can facilitate insertion and lessens muscle tension in the lower body and legs.

Psychologic Response

The victim may not have any identified injuries because she offered no resistance to the assailant. When faced with a life-threatening situation, a victim's brain and body enter a survival mode. The victim reacts with fight, flight, or freezing. Freezing, or tonic immobility, is recognized in the animal kingdom as a "deer in the headlights" or the mouse lying lifeless in the cat's mouth. Levine (1997) describes this response as having an analgesic quality. The victim's terror may also put her into a dissociative mental state. Victims become totally passive as they literally separate their consciousness from the horror of reality (Rothschild, 2000).

Sometimes victims make a deliberate decision not to fight back or resist the assailant. They follow the advice of law enforcement experts and other groups who make recommendations on survival strategies. A victim may follow her own immediate reaction to a dangerous situation. Her instincts may have told her not to fight back because she might suffer far greater injury or even death. It is appropriate for the clinician to explore what the victim felt during the attack. For example, victims frequently say, "I thought I was going to die." Finally, she may have made the conscious decision to avoid infuriating the assailant and risking injury or death of those around her. The victim may explain why she did not scream or try to run away. For example, "My children were in the next room and he said he would kill them if I did not do what he wanted."

Factors Related to the Assailant

Object of Penetration

The penetrating object or perpetrator's finger or penis may be very large, potentially injurious, or not lubricated. This can cause abrasions from increased friction or lacerations from over-stretching, or cuts from sharp or jagged surfaces.

Lubrication

The assailant can supply artificial lubricants. KY jelly, lubricated condoms, or saliva can serve to decrease friction between the penetrating object and the vaginal vault

Sexual Dysfunction

In addition, it is not uncommon for the perpetrator to suffer some type of sexual dysfunction. Groth and Burgess (1980) and other authors suggest that approximately one out of every three offenders shows clear evidence of some type of sexual dysfunction at the time of the offense (Bowker, 1983; Groth, 1979; Rosenbaum & O'Leary, 1981). This leads to prolonged duration of the penetrating object within the vagina or anus. The increased tissue friction can result in abrasions.

Force of Penetration

Increased force and prolonged contact can result in greater probability of injury, especially in a case of anal penetration. This type of contact may be consistent with the victim's account of the incident.

Factors Related to Circumstances

The relationship between the victim and the perpetrator should be factored into evaluating the victim's account of the assault. If the parties were in an intimate relationship, they may have a history of consensual contact with each other. The history of intimacy can influence current, nonconsensual situations. A sexual overture from one partner may cause the other partner's body to respond as it has in the past. If there were objects, props, or tools used during the assault, these may

Key Point:
Victims may make a deliberate decision not to fight back or resist the assailant. This is in line with the advice of law enforcement experts and other groups who make recommendations on survival strategies or may reflect the victim following her own immediate reaction to a dangerous situation. Her instincts may tell her not to fight back because she may suffer far greater injury or even death. It is appropriate for the clinician to explore what the victim felt during the attack.

contribute to nongenital injuries as well as anogenital injuries. Patterned injuries may also corroborate the victim's account of the assault. The shape, size, and pattern of the injury can show the type of instrument used as a weapon.

Factors Related to the Environment

The environment in which the crime took place may increase the likelihood of both genital and nongenital injury to the victim. For example, if the sexual assault occurred in a wooded area, the victim may have pieces of wood or leaves embedded in the creases of her buttocks or labial folds. An assault on a gravel-filled street could result in small pieces of stone embedded in the soft tissue of the victim's back and arms. Debris from these environments can further increase friction between the penetrating object and the victim's body, resulting in abrasions or lacerations. In addition, these materials can be collected as physical evidence and corroborate the victim's history of the assault.

WHEN PHYSICAL FINDINGS ARE NOT OBSERVED

All of the factors mentioned so far can explain lack of injury as well as presence of injury. The clinician must be aware of the complex relationship among the factors. The anatomy of the reproductive structures, delayed reporting, presence of lubrication, and health and age of the victim can all serve to protect her from injury. Many forms of sexual abuse do not cause physical injury. Although the lay public and law enforcement representatives may be fixated on vaginal penetration, sexual abuse may be nonpenetrating contact and may involve fondling; oral-genital, genital, or anal contact; and genital-genital contact without penetration.

Finally, there is also the possibility that a victim may be treated in a hospital where healthcare providers are not specially trained in conducting sexual assault examinations. The examining healthcare provider may not recognize certain injuries. An inexperienced healthcare provider may mistakenly believe that too much time has elapsed from the time of the attack and decide not to do an examination.

Today most sexual assault protocols recommend that evidentiary examinations are completed within 72 hours after a sexual assault. After 72 hours, examinations are sometimes conducted in cases in which there are injuries that can be documented or when the victim has not changed clothes or showered. Naturally, if the victim wants an examination at any time, the clinician should respond accordingly.

DOCUMENTATION

Accurate documentation of injury is essential. Three methods of documenting injury are recommended: a text description, diagrammatic illustration, and, if available, photography (colposcopy). A labeled diagram or traumagram, as well as the photographs taken at the time of the forensic examination, can show relevant genital areas and injury location. Indicating location, size, shape, and color of any injury is imperative. Use of a measuring standard, such as the photomacrograph, will allow for exact measurements of the injury. To effectively communicate injury site to the reader of the medical record, the hours on the face of a clock are used as a locator. (**Figure 13-3**) By using the clock as a locator, descriptive words such as left or right, anterior or posterior, or quadrants do not have to be used, thus ensuring that there will be no confusion or misinterpretation of the injury location. Even if photographs are taken, it is still appropriate to use the clock transparency for courtroom testimony.

REFERENCES

Adams JA. Evolution of a classification scale: medical evaluation of suspected child sexual abuse. *Child Maltreat.* 2001;6:31-36.

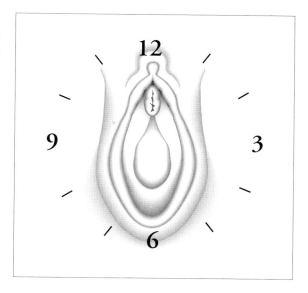

Figure 13-3. *Diagram with clock overlay.*

Key Point:
Although the public and law enforcement personnel may be fixated on vaginal penetration, sexual abuse may be nonpenetrating contact and may include fondling, oral-genital, genital, or anal contact in addition to genital-genital contact without penetration.

Adams JA, Girardin B, Faugno D. Signs of genital trauma in adolescent rape victims examined acutely. *J Pediatr Adolesc Gynecol.* 2000;13(2):88.

Basson R. The female sexual response: a different model. *J Sex Marital Ther.* 2000;26:51-65.

Berman J, Adhikari S, Goldstein I. Anatomy and physiology of sexual function and dysfunction: classification, evaluation and treatment options. *Eur Urol.* 2000; 38:20-29.

Besant-Matthews PE. Blunt Force Trauma. Unpublished paper. Dallas, Tex; 2001.

Biggs M, Stermac LE, Divinsky M. Genital injuries following sexual assault of women with and without prior sexual intercourse experience. *Can Med Assoc J.* 1998;159:33.

Bowker LH. Marital rape: a distinct syndrome? *Soc Casework.* 1983;64(6):347-352.

Bowyer L, Dalton M. Female victims of rape and their genital injuries. *Br J Obstet Gynaecol.* 1997;104:617-620.

Cardozo L, Bachmann G, McClish D, Fonda D, Birgerson L. Meta-analysis of estrogen therapy in the management of urogenital atrophy in postmenopausal women: second report of the Hormones and Urogenital Therapy Committee. *Obstet Gynecol.* 1998;92:722-727.

Crime Victims Research and Treatment Center [CVRTC]. *Rape In America: A Report to the nation.* Charleston, SC: Crime Victims Research and Treatment Center; 1992.

Fraser I, Lahteenmaki P, Elomaa E, et al. Variations in vaginal epithelial surface appearance determined by colposcopic inspection in healthy sexually active women. *Human Reprod.* 1999;14:1974-1978.

Girardin BW, Faugno DK, Seneski PC, Slaughter L, Whelan M. Findings in sexual assault and consensual intercourse. In: *Color Atlas of Sexual Assault.* St. Louis, Mo: Mosby; 1997:19-65.

Groth AN, Burgess AW. Male rape: offenders and victims. *Am J Psychiatry.* 1980;137(7):806-810.

Groth, N. *Men Who Rape.* New York, NY: Plenum; 1979.

Lauber A, Souma M. Use of toluidine blue dye for documentation of traumatic intercourse. *Obstet Gynecol.* 1982;60:644-648.

Lee GR, Foerster J, Lukens J, Wintrobe MM, eds. *Wintrobe's Clinical Hematology.* 9th ed. Philadelphia, Pa: Lea & Febiger; 1993:1302.

Lenahan L, Ernst A, Johnson B. Colposcopy in evaluation of the adult sexual assault victim. *Am J Emerg Med.* 1998;16(2):183-184.

Levine P. *Waking the Tiger.* Berkeley, Calif: North Atlantic; 1997.

Masters W, Johnson V. *Human Sexual Response.* Boston, Mass: Little, Brown; 1966.

McCauley J, Guzinski G, Welch R, et al. Toluidine blue in the corroboration of rape in the adult victim. *Am J Emerg Med.* 1987;5:105-108.

Muram D, Arheart K, Jennings S. Diagnostic accuracy of colposcopic photographs in child sexual abuse evaluations. *J Pediatr Adolesc Gynecol.* 1999;12:58-61.

Norvell MK, Benrubi GI, Thomson RJ. Investigation of microtrauma after sexual intercourse. *J Reprod Med.* 1984;29(4):269-271.

Pandit L, Ouslander JG. Postmenopausal vaginal atrophy and atrophic vaginitis. *Am J Med Sci.* 1997;314:228-231.

Paul D. Medico-legal examination of the living. In: Mant K, ed. *Taylor's Principles and Practice of Medical Jurisprudence.* 13th ed. London: Churchill Livingstone; 1984.

Penttilia A, Karhumen P. Medicolegal findings among rape victims. *Med Law.* 1990;9:725-737.

Rabkin M. HIV in primary care. *General Medicine Clinic.* Available at: http://www.columbia.edu/~am430/HIV.htm. Accessed September 21, 2002.

Rosenbaum A, O'Leary KD. Marital violence: characteristics of abusive couples. *J Consult Clin Psychol.* 1981;49:63-71.

Rothschild B. *The Body Remembers: The Psychophysiology of Trauma and Trauma Treatment.* New York, NY: WW Norton; 2000.

Sanders M. Normal vulva. *PathWeb, the virtual pathology museum* web site. Lindquist RR, Curator. Pathology Department of the University of Connecticut Health Center; 2001. Available at: http://radiology.uchc.edu/eAtlas/GYN/1922.htm. Accessed September, 2002.

Slaughter L, Brown CRV. Colposcopy to establish physical findings in rape victims. *Am J Obstet Gynecol.* 1992;166:1.

Slaughter L, Brown C, Crowley S, Peck R. Patterns of genital injury in female sexual assault victims. *Am J Obstet Gynecol.* 1997;176:609-616.

Sommers MS, Schafer J, Zink T, Hutson L, Hillard P. Injury patterns in women resulting from sexual assault. *Trauma, Violence, & Abuse.* 2001;2(3):240-258.

World Health Organization (WHO) Global Program on AIDS. *Manual for the Standardization of Colposcopy for the Evaluation of Vaginally Administered Products. Update 2000.* Geneva: WHO; 1996.

THE EVALUATION OF THE SEXUAL ASSAULT VICTIM

Iris Reyes, MD, FACEP
Elizabeth M. Datner, MD

Recent studies in the United States reveal that 1 in 6 women and 1 in 33 men will be the victim of a sexual assault during their lifetime (Linden, 1999). Fewer than half of these assault victims report the crime to the police or seek medical care (Feldhaus et al., 2000). Those who do seek medical care most often go to the emergency department or to their private physicians. Some physicians, however, are unprepared to address the issues affecting victims of sexual violence and do not routinely ask their patients about violence in their lives. Both the American Medical Association and American Academy of Pediatrics have called on physicians to become better informed about sexual assault. Guidelines are published by each agency in an attempt to help clinicians better identify, treat, and report sexual assault incidents.

The following review of the evaluation of a sexual assault victim focuses primarily on a female victim. However, men, children, and the elderly are also at risk. (Please see Chapters 7, 3, 21.) Reporting rates of sexual assault for men remain low. Male victims are less likely to report sexual assault than female victims. A review of sexual assault victims in one urban emergency department revealed that 10% were male (Pesola et al., 1999). Male victims were more likely to have physical trauma and were twice as likely as females to have known their assailant less than 24 hours. Sexual abuse in the gay community is also underreported. Societal attitudes contribute to the underreporting of male and gay victimization.

The body of literature addressing the elderly rape victim is meager, but case series do exist. Evaluation can be exceptionally difficult in elderly patients with significant cognitive deficits. Special adjustments in interviewing and examining the elderly victim may by necessary because of underlying medical or psychologic conditions.

Sexual assault can result in serious physical and mental trauma. Identification and intervention soon after its occurrence are imperative. Physicians who are in a position to identify and treat these victims must familiarize themselves with the guidelines and with the local services available to assist them and the victim of sexual assault.

It is clear that only a small percentage of actual cases are reported because this crime is associated with myths, misplaced shame, and social stigmas that incriminate the victim rather than the perpetrator. Unless associated with significant physical trauma, victims of sexual assault rarely seek help within 72 hours. This makes identification, treatment, and conviction of the assailant more difficult.

Performing a sexual assault evaluation can be very difficult for both the patient and the examiner. Ideally, such an evaluation should occur at a rape crisis center. These centers focus on providing a compassionate setting for the victim and skilled medical care and forensic evidence collection. The report of a sexual assault sets a complex process into motion. Preparation is the key to providing comprehensive

Key Point:
Sexual assault victims are often best served at designated rape crisis centers, where personnel are specially trained to provide care and perform detailed forensic evidence.

medical care for the victim and for obtaining appropriate forensic evidence for law enforcement. A standardized rape assessment program such as the sexual assault nurse examiner (SANE) interdisciplinary approach can enhance both care of the victim and improvement in the collection of forensic evidence (Derhammer et al., 2000).

OBTAINING THE HISTORY OF THE SEXUAL ASSAULT

ROLE OF THE HEALTHCARE PROVIDER

The role of the healthcare provider caring for a sexual assault victim is multifaceted. The provider must pay close attention to detail to glean potentially important forensic evidence and also be cognizant of the tremendous psychosocial support the victim needs. A caring, nonjudgmental approach is always important when providing services for a crime victim. The clinician should clearly convey to the victim that (1) no one ever deserves to be raped; (2) the perpetrator, not the victim, is responsible for the assault; (3) the victim made the best choices possible for survival under the circumstances (Linden, 1999). When dealing with adolescent rape victims, it is particularly important to establish trusting relationships and to make the victims aware that regardless of their activity, they are not at fault and that no one had the right to force them to participate in sexual activity against their will (Poirier, 2002). Victims, particularly adolescents, should be made aware of clinician reporting requirements before disclosing information to the provider so that they can choose whether or not to disclose reportable information. All victims, however, should be encouraged to report the assault to police. It is particularly important for reporting and evidence collection to occur within 72 hours of the assault, because physical evidence can rarely be recovered more than 48 to 72 hours after the assault. The victim can decide to not pursue the case at a later time, but evidence cannot be obtained later if it is initially refused. Attempts should be made to collect physical evidence early regardless of whether or not the victim has decided to pursue the case. In addition, most states have crime-victim compensation programs that will cover the financial costs of the evaluation and evidence collection. However, many states require reporting to the police in order to benefit from compensation programs.

Healthcare providers are responsible for treating physical injuries that result from the assault, performing a careful physical examination and collecting legal evidence, documenting all pertinent aspects of the history, and providing care in terms of pregnancy and sexually transmitted disease (STD) prophylaxis and psychologic support. Finally, the clinician is responsible for arranging follow-up care and counseling for the victim (Kobernick et al., 1985). Consent for all procedures should be obtained after thorough explanation. The victim should be informed that refusal of any or all of the procedures or questions is up to the victim and that refusal will not affect the care provided. Victims should also be made aware of reporting requirements before the clinician obtains that information.

Acute medical care is essential for all patients regardless of the severity of their injuries. An evaluation should be performed to rule out any life-threatening conditions, with assessment of the patient's airway, breathing, and circulation (ABCs) as a priority. Treatment of these vital functions supercedes any data collection or gathering of forensic evidence. The forensic examination can be performed after stabilization of the patient or in the operating room in the case that the patient needs immediate operative interventions.

SETTING

A private, quiet environment must be provided for the patient. It is important that the victim feel safe and in control of what is happening to him or her. However, the patient should not be left alone. A nurse or counselor should remain with the patient if he or she comes for medical care unaccompanied. If friends or family members are present, they should be allowed to remain with the victim for emotional support if the victim prefers. It is important to recognize that sexual

Key Point:
Although the clinician should always clearly convey to victims that the rape was not their fault, this is particularly important when the victim is an adolescent.

Key Point:
All victims should be encouraged to allow immediate medical evaluation, forensic evidence collection and reporting to the police regardless of their intention to pursue prosecution because evidence collection is time sensitive and does not obligate the victim to pursue prosecution at a later time.

assault is frequently perpetrated by individuals known to the patient. If the person accompanying the patient is suspected of being the perpetrator, whether a parent, partner, spouse, teacher, etc., the victim should be isolated from that person until the clinician has explored this possibility and the victim has requested the presence of the other person.

The victim's exposure to repetitive questioning by the staff (i.e., triage nurse, examining nurse, intern, resident, and attending physician) is limited. The patient should be informed of what to expect during the evaluation process, give consent for treatment obtained, and be prepared before any procedure is performed.

Key Point:
Individuals accompanying the victim should be present to provide psychologic support only if the victim chooses and if it is determined that they are not potential perpetrators.

The nurse should recognize and inform the victim that this examination will take approximately 30 to 60 minutes. The necessary arrangements should be made to allow for this time. It is important to listen carefully, to speak quietly, and to perform evaluation in an unhurried manner.

Recommendations vary regarding allowing the presence of law enforcement personnel during the history-gathering phase. Whereas some believe that the victim may be intimidated, it is argued that discrepancies in reported details regarding the assault are minimized.

History of the Adult Victim

A history from a patient who has suffered a sexual assault will differ from a routine medical evaluation in several ways. The purpose of the history is to record the events that occurred and to guide the clinician in collecting evidence as well as caring for injuries during the examination. It is important to limit questions to medically relevant history. The patient is informed that it will be necessary to ask some personal questions. A general history is obtained before addressing details about the assault. A general history should include the following information:

— Past history of medical illnesses

— Recent surgery

— Medications

— Allergies

— Tetanus immunization

— History of sexually transmitted diseases

— Contraception use

— Last consensual sexual experience, tampon use, or douching

— Illicit drug use or alcohol ingestion

— Last menstrual period

— Obstetric history

The forensic interview addresses the details of the assault. The nurse should acknowledge that victims sometimes have difficulty talking about the assault. The patient must be informed that he or she may stop the questioning at any time and continue when ready. The following information should be addressed:

— A brief description of the incident

— Number and identity of the attacker(s), if known

— Time of the attack

— Location where the assault took place

— Type of sexual acts that occurred, that is, kissing, fondling, vaginal and/or anal penetration, oral penetration

— Contact with ejaculate, urine, or vaginal secretions

— Use of weapons, restraints, contraceptives, condoms by the perpetrator

— Use of objects to penetrate or coerce the victim

It is important for evidentiary purposes to document whether the patient has changed clothing, bathed, urinated, defecated, or douched since the assault. If the oral cavity was involved, the patient should be asked if he or she has smoked, eaten, had anything to drink, brushed the teeth, or gargled since the assault occurred. All direct quotes made by the patient should be denoted with quotation marks when recorded. It is also important to note any use of alcohol or drugs by the victim. If recollection of the event is poor, the clinician should consider the influence of substances the victim took either intentionally or unintentionally.

Several drugs have been used to facilitate nonconsensual sexual intercourse. Dubbed "date rape drugs," gamma hydroxybutarate (GHB) and flunitrazepam (Rohypnol) are being used increasingly by assailants because of their sedative hypnotic effects (ElSohly & Salamone, 1999). Used initially as an anesthetic agent, GHB has gained popularity as a recreational drug. Although its primary effect is sedation, it can cause memory loss at higher doses (Graeme, 2000). GHB can be detected by crime laboratories in drinking material residue, as well as in the victim's urine up to 4 hours after ingestion. Flunitrazepam can go undetected if added to any drink. It produces sedation, muscle relaxation, and decreased anxiety within 30 minutes of ingestion. It can also produce amnesia during its duration of action, which may be up to 8 to 12 hours after ingestion. In addition, the association of ethanol, cocaine, barbiturates, benzodiazepines, opiates, cannabinoids, and amphetamines with sexual assaults must not be overlooked. Adolescent rape victims, in particular, are more likely than adult victims to have used drugs and/or alcohol. More than 40% of adolescent victims and adolescent assailants have reported drug or alcohol use immediately before an assault (American Academy of Pediatrics [AAP], 2001). Although toxicology tests can screen for most recreational drugs, screening for GHB and flunitrazepam is not routine. If use of these drugs is suspected, a toxicology test specifically screening for them must be requested.

Key Point:
Because screening for GHB and flunitrazepam is not routine, it should be requested, especially if adolescents are involved.

THE PHYSICAL EXAMINATION

The physical examination serves the dual purpose of identifying any injuries requiring medical care and collecting forensic evidence. The physician must be prepared to perform only one physical examination. If a sexual assault is suspected, all materials necessary for the collection of forensic evidence must be readily available. The "rape kit" and its use vary from state to state. Each state has legally mandated procedures for the collection of evidence. The physician should familiarize himself or herself with the guidelines used by the local legal community. The contents of a rape kit are listed in **Table 14-1**.

If a rape crisis center is available, the victim should be transferred in a timely manner once he or she is determined to be medically stable. If no center is available or the victim cannot be transferred for medical reasons, the physician must be prepared to perform a rape examination and gather forensic evidence. To do this, he or she must be familiar with the rape kit contents and the proper use of the materials for the collection of evidence.

A chaperone should be present during the gynecologic examination of any female patient. In the case of child victims, a supportive adult not suspected to be involved in the assault might function in this capacity.

A thorough physical examination should be performed, including assessment for evidence of nongenital physical trauma. Nongenital injuries are common in cases of sexual assault occurring in 25% to 45% of victims. Grossly evident genital injuries

---

Table 14-1. Rape Kit

Recommended contents:

1. Instructions

2. Checklist

3. History and physical documentation forms

4. Equipment for specimen collection:

   — Paper bags (plastic may produce mildew which contaminates evidence)

   — Large paper or cloth sheet

   — Cotton-tipped swabs and tubes for their placement

   — Comb

   — Envelopes

   — Patient discharge information

   — Red- and purple-topped tubes for blood sampling

   — Filter paper

   — Cardboard box

   — Forceps

   — Scissors

   — Labels for clinical samples

---

occur in 15% to 30% of cases (Cartwright, 1987; Solola et al., 1983; Tintinalli & Hoelzer, 1985). Elderly and male victims of sexual assault may sustain more injuries and more severe injuries than premenopausal females (Kaufman et al., 1980; Ramin et al., 1992). Men are also less likely than women to disclose genital trauma to healthcare providers and thus should be carefully examined (Kaufman et al., 1980). The examination should not be a source of further physical trauma.

The patient should first be asked to remove all clothing, particularly underwear, over a clean paper or sheet (contained in the rape kit) to catch any debris that might be used as evidence. The clothing will be kept for forensic evidence. Areas of clothing that have stains or tears should be carefully preserved.

It is best to begin the examination with a nonthreatening approach, such as with the examination of the head, eyes, ears, nose, and throat. The examination may then progress distally with particular attention to signs of injury. It is essential to visualize the entire body. Particular attention should be paid to identify lacerations, bruises, bite marks, etc. Diagrams or photographs of identified injuries are important because clear, objective evidence of trauma increases the chances of successful prosecution (Rambow et al., 1992). Police often are available to take photographs and may have expertise in this area. All photographs should be permanently marked for identification. Forensic evidence may be collected as the examination progresses. All foreign bodies are removed, placed in envelopes, and sealed with a description of the location where they were found on the body and the examiner's initials.

Hair should be combed over a paper towel and debris and loose hair collected and prepared as evidence. Several hair samples are required. Pubic hair is sampled in a similar manner.

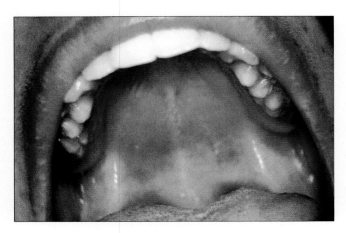

Figure 14-1. *Submucosal hemorrhages at the junction of hard and soft palates, termed fellatio syndrome.*

Key Point:
It is best to collect evidence within 72 hours of the assault, but valid evidence can be collected as late as 5 days after the assault.

The oral cavity should be examined carefully, particularly in the case of oral penetration. Patients may develop small submucosal hemorrhages at the junction of the hard and soft palates, termed fellatio syndrome (**Figure 14-1**). A cotton swab should be used to obtain a sample of fluid between the gum and lips. Several swabs should be made and air dried prior to packaging for evidence. Slides should be used for wet mounts particularly for identification of sperm by a forensic specialist. Any findings from the slides should be noted in the chart, including the presence of sperm, motile or not. After completion of this sampling, a swab is taken for *Neisseria gonorrhoeae*, then the victim rinses his/her mouth with water, waits 5 minutes, and places a filter paper in the mouth to saturate it with saliva to be used for victim blood antigen determination.

Stains on the skin can be scraped with a tongue blade or sampled with a moist cotton tipped applicator. A Wood's light will illuminate semen, which fluoresces, to assist in locating stains. Fingernails must be closely inspected for evidence of foreign material or dirt. Samples of this material should be scraped over a clean paper towel and packaged separately for each hand.

The genital examination follows the general physical examination. Be sure to obtain the victim's consent and prepare him/her for every phase of the examination. Inform him/her of the expected discomfort and of his/her right to stop the examination at any time. It is also important to explain that time plays an important role in the collection of evidence.

Ideally, evidence is best collected within 72 hours of the assault. However, valid evidence can be collected as late as 5 days after the assault. If the victim presents after this interval, a thorough history and physical examination should be performed. The physician should be prepared to gather evidence and document any abnormalities that he or she discovers, particularly those that may be consistent with a sexual assault. Additionally, it is important to proceed with the pelvic examination, even if the victim has no complaints of pelvic trauma or discomfort. Up to one third of victims have evidence of traumatic genital injuries after a sexual assault but do not have symptoms (Rambow et al., 1992).

The time of the examination should be indicated, and all findings clearly documented with proper medical terminology describing location, size, and color of each wound or area of tenderness. When possible, a diagram should be used to indicate sites of injury and, if the patient consents, photographs of the injuries should be included. The external and internal genitalia are carefully examined using adequate lighting and then with a Wood's light to identify semen. The posterior fourchette and fossa, labia, and hymen are particularly susceptible to injury. The majority of genital injuries after sexual assault are minor; however, up to 50% of victims have evidence of vaginal penetration on physical examination (Slaughter & Brown, 1991). Genital trauma is more likely to occur in the postmenopausal female victim, and there is a greater likelihood of requiring surgical repair (Ramin et al., 1992). Either colposcopy or toluidine blue staining can be used to identify microlacerations not evident to the naked eye. A colposcope provides medium-powered binocular enlargement and has been shown to identify microlacerations of the introitus and vagina in 61% of women after sexual intercourse (Norvell et al., 1984). Use of a colposcope has also shown a statistically significant increase in the detection of genital trauma in sexual assault victims (53% vs. 6%, chi2 = 0.64, p = 0.0114) (Lenahan et al., 1998).

Toluidine blue is a nuclear stain that helps to identify breaks in the normally keratinized skin. It is applied to the perineum and then carefully wiped off using lubricating jelly.

The buttocks and anus are carefully examined for evidence of trauma, including fissures, small lacerations, and bruises. Rectal bleeding should be sought in the case of anal penetration. Rectal swabs for gonococcus (GC) and *Chlamydia* should be taken.

The speculum examination should follow the complete external examination of the perineum, vaginal area, and anus. Evidence of trauma to the cervix should be sought. In addition, a suspicion of perforation of the cul-de-sac should alert the clinician to the possibility of bowel injury and an investigation should ensue. Insertion of a foreign body would predispose to this possibility. Samples from the vaginal pool and external cervical os are taken using cotton-tipped swabs. Sperm are known to remain motile in the vaginal pool for up to 12 hours and in the cervical os for up to 7 days (Soules et al., 1978). GC and *Chlamydia* cultures are taken. Vaginal swabs are taken for antigen determination, and seminal factors, including prostatic antigen, p30, acid phosphatase, and DNA testing. Blood group antigens are secreted by 80% of the population and are useful for including or excluding suspects (Cabaniss et al., 1985; Bectel & Podrazik, 1999). Seminal factors are also useful in determining if penile penetration occurred, particularly if sperm are not obtained.

LABORATORY TESTS

Collection of forensic evidence in children is addressed in Chapter 4; forensic issues for the adult victim are addressed in Chapter 15. The examiner should collect laboratory studies necessary for the medical treatment of the victim in addition to what is forwarded to law enforcement under the guidelines of the rape kit. The results of the rape kit will not be returned to the clinician for further treatment of the patient. The nurse must be sure to use only water or saline solution and not standard lubricants during the speculum and rectal examinations. These lubricants can interfere with forensic testing. Wet mount (saline slide) examinations for sperm should be left to forensic experts.

The laboratory studies recommended are as follows:

— Pregnancy testing—either urine or serum testing

— Rapid plasma reagin (RPR) or VDRL—test for syphilis at initial visit and again at 3 months

— Hepatitis serology—testing for hepatitis B is recommended; hepatitis C testing is, as of yet, not generally recommended

— Gonorrhea/*Chlamydia* testing—swab sites potentially exposed during the assault: mouth, throat, vagina, rectum

— HIV testing—at initial visit with locally mandated counseling and again at 3, 6, and 12 months; the site best suited to perform appropriate posttest counseling should perform these studies

— Blood sample for typing to differentiate the victim from the perpetrator

CHAIN OF EVIDENCE

"Chain of evidence" or "chain of custody" refers to the direct line of custody of the evidence from time of collection until it is presented in court. If this direct chain of evidence is not established between the clinician and the court, the evidence could be considered inadmissible. All evidence that is gathered is placed into separate envelopes or containers, sealed, and initialed. All specimens should be labeled with the victim's name, the date, the examiner's name, and the specimen source. All containers and envelopes should be sealed so that it is clear if someone attempts to tamper with the evidence. **Figures 14-2 a and b.** show properly and improperly sealed evidence kits. Once all of the specimens are collected and other evidence is separately packaged, they should be packaged together, sealed, and labeled. The completed package is turned over to the police or placed in a locked cabinet until it is relinquished to the police. A receipt should be obtained for the evidence, and both the person handing over the evidence and the person obtaining it should sign and date the receipt. Laboratory specimens should be refrigerated immediately if a delay in transfer is expected. Most rape kits provide all of the required containers, materials, and instructions needed to provide proper chain of custody.

DOCUMENTATION

Medical records function as legal documents in the event that a case is presented before the judicial system. They may be the key determinants in the outcome of a case. It is crucial to keep clear, organized, and complete records of the evaluation. The records should be legible so that they can be referred to and understood years after the event if necessary. Some states have separate forms for the documentation of child abuse. Records should include the following:

— Date and time of the examination—records should be completed in a timely manner in accordance with routine office procedure

— Standard documentation of a general medical assessment—including history, review of systems, social history, physical examination, and laboratory studies performed

— Historical information relevant to the assault—using the patient's own statements regarding the assault

— Physical examination findings—including detailed descriptions, body charts, and photographs (if applicable) of all injuries

— Laboratory results

— Imaging study results (if applicable)

The role of the clinician is not to determine if a sexual assault occurred; rather it is to determine if the examination findings are consistent with sexual assault. Thus, remarks that imply judgment or belief of the occurrence of the event should not be made in the medical record. Statements that are not supported by facts should be avoided. For example, the victim's affect should be noted in a descriptive manner, "tearful," "nervous," or "giggling," rather than in a conclusive manner, such as, "behavior inconsistent with rape."

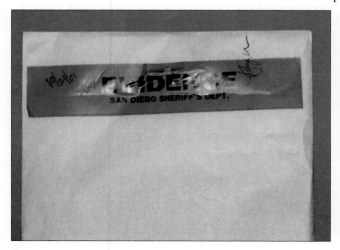

Figure 14-2-a. *Properly sealed evidence envelope seal covers entire opening. Date and examiner's name are indicated. Signature crosses both envelope and seal.*

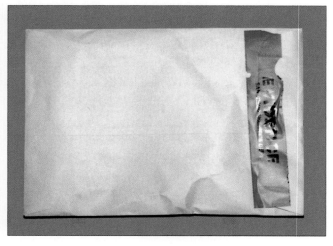

Figure 14-2-b. *Improperly sealed envelope. Seal is ripped, date and name not present, examiner's signature not present.*

FOLLOW-UP CARE

Medical follow-up should be arranged for the victim at 1 to 2 weeks and 2 to 4 months after the initial evaluation. Follow-up evaluation of STDs will occur at this time. Patients should be made aware of all of the physical findings. All injuries, even minor, should be disclosed to patients and assurance of rapid healing should be offered. In addition, reassurance that injuries will not interfere with future reproductive health or sexual function could be offered.

The most significant sequelae after sexual assault are psychologic. All patients should receive counseling and referral for ongoing follow-up either during their initial evaluation or within the next 1 to 2 days. Many local advocacy organizations offer victims counseling services free of charge and work closely with the victim's medical and legal providers. Chapter 24 offers more information on social supports for victims of assault.

PREVENTION EDUCATION

It has been well established that victims of sexual assault are frequently involved in ongoing or recurrent assaults (Walch & Broadhead, 1992). Clinicians should address high-risk behaviors with their patients, particularly adolescents, and provide educational materials to their patients. Many advocacy organizations provide printed materials that may be helpful.

REFERENCES

American Academy of Pediatrics. Committee on Adolescence. Sexual assault and the adolescent. *Pediatrics.* 1994;94:761-765.

American Academy of Pediatrics. Committee on Adolescence. Care of the adolescent sexual assault victim. *Pediatrics.* 2001;107:1476-1479.

American Academy of Pediatrics. Committee on Child Abuse and Neglect. Guidelines for the evaluation of sexual abuse of children: subject review (RE 9819). *Pediatrics.* 1999;103:186-191.

American Medical Association. *Diagnostic and Treatment Guidelines on Child Sexual Abuse.* Chicago, Ill: AMA; 1992.

American Medical Association. *Strategies for the Treatment and Prevention of Sexual Assault.* Chicago, Ill: AMA; 1995.

Bectel K, Podrazik M. Adolescent gynecology, II. The sexually active adolescent: evaluation of the adolescent rape victim. *Pediatr Clin North Am.* 1999;46:809-823.

Burgess AW, Dowdell EB, Brown K. The elderly rape victim: stereotypes, perpetrators, and implications for practice. *J Emerg Nurs.* 2000;26:516-518.

Cabaniss ML, Scott SE, Copeland L. Gathering evidence for rape cases. *Contemp Obstet Gynecol.* 1985;25:160.

Cartwright PS, and the Sexual Assault Study Group. Factors that correlate with injury sustained by survivors of sexual assault. *Obstet Gynecol.* 1987;70:44-46.

Derhammer F, Lucente V, Reed JF III, et al. Using a SANE interdisciplinary approach to care of sexual assault victims. *Jt Comm J Qual Improv.* 2000;26:488-496.

ElSohly MA, Salamone SJ. Prevalence of drugs used in cases of alleged sexual assault. *J Anal Toxicol.* 1999;23:141-146.

Feldhaus KM, Houry D, Kaminsky R. Lifetime sexual assault prevalence rates and reporting practices in an emergency department population. *Ann Emerg Med.* 2000;36:23-27.

Graeme KA. Pharmacologic advances in emergency medicine: new drugs of abuse. *Emerg Med Clin North Am.* 2000;18:625-636.

Kaufman A, Divasto P, Jackson R, et al. Male rape victims: non-institutionalized assault. *Am J Psychiatry.* 1980;137:221-223.

Kobernick ME, Seiferts S, Sanders AB, et al. Emergency department management of the sexual assault victim. *J Emerg Med.* 1985;2:205-214.

Lenahan LC, Ernst A, Johnson B. Colposcopy in evaluation of the adult sexual assault victim. *Am J Emerg Med.* 1998;16:183-184.

Linden JA. Sexual assault. *Emerg Med Clin North Am.* 1999;17:685-697.

Norvell MK, Benrubi GI, Thompson RJ. Investigation of microtrauma after sexual intercourse. *J Reprod Med.* 1984;29:269-271.

O'Neill JF, Shalit P. Health care of the gay male patient. *Primary Care.* 1992;19:191-201.

Pesola GR, Westfal RE, Kuffner CA. Emergency department characteristics of male sexual assault. *Acad Emerg Med.* 1999;6:792-798.

Petter LM, Whitehill DL. Management of the female sexual assault victim. *Am Fam Physician.* 1998;58:920-930.

Poirier, MP. Care of the female adolescent rape victim. *Pediatr Emerg Care.* 2002;18(1):53-59.

Rambow B, Adkinson C, Frost TH, et al. Female sexual assault: medical and legal implications. *Ann Emerg Med.* 1992;21:717-731.

Ramin SM, Saton AJ, Stone IC, et al. Sexual assault in post menopausal women. *Obstet Gynecol.* 1992;80:860-864.

Slaughter L, Brown C. Cervical findings in rape victims. *J Obstet Gynecol.* 1991;164:528.

Solola A, Scott C, Severs H, et al. Rape: management in a noninstitutional setting. *Obstet Gynecol.* 1983;61:373.

Soules MR, Pollard AA, Brown KM, et al. The forensic laboratory evaluation of evidence in alleged rape. *Am J Obstet Gynecol.* 1978;130:142.

Tintinalli JE, Hoelzer M. Clinical findings and legal resolution in sexual assault. *Ann Emer Med.* 1985;14:447-453.

Walch A, Broadhead W. Prevalence of lifetime sexual victimization among female patients. *J Fam Pract* 1992;35:511-516.

Chapter 15

Forensic Issues in Caring for the Adult Sexual Assault Victim

Holly M. Harner, CRNP, PhD, MPH, SANE

Sexual assault is generally defined as any sexual act, including fondling, rape, and attempted rape, performed without the victim's consent (Frampton, 1998). Although a majority of sexual assault victims are female, both males and females of any age may become victims. According to the National Center for Victims of Crime (2001), it is estimated that at least 1 of every 4 women will be sexually assaulted in her lifetime. Thirty-nine percent of victims will be assaulted more than once (Kilpatrick et al., 1992).

Sexual assault is often perpetrated by someone known to the victim, including a current or former intimate partner, acquaintance, or relative (Kilpatrick et al., 1992). Frequently, these rapes are referred to as acquaintance rapes. Linden (1999) described acquaintance rapes as more "emotionally devastating" because the assault not only violates trust but typically is repetitive (p. 686). For many reasons, including the victim's feelings of fear, guilt, and denial about the assault, very few sexual assaults are ever reported to law enforcement (Frampton, 1998).

Over the last decade, there has been increased collaboration between clinicians caring for victims of rape and sexual assault and the criminal justice system prosecuting the perpetrators of such crimes. As a result, nurses specially trained in the forensic evaluation and treatment of victims of rape, commonly referred to as sexual assault nurse examiners and sexual assault forensic examiners, increasingly provide care to victims of rape and sexual assault. The nurses, in collaboration with other clinicians, often practice within emergency room settings (Linden, 1999).

The purpose of this chapter is to outline the medical and forensic healthcare needs after sexual assault. Assessment and treatment of the victim of sexual assault, as well as the basic principles of forensic evidence collection and documentation, are reviewed. The role of the healthcare provider as a collaborative agent with other local victim and criminal justice agencies is also described.

Establishing Victim Safety

The immediate medical needs after sexual assault, including care of the acutely critical physical needs, are similar to those of victims of any trauma. However, when a violent crime such as rape or domestic violence has been committed where the perpetrator may be known to the victim, the clinician must ascertain the victim's level of safety. When the perpetrator is known to the victim, there may be a reasonable fear of retaliation against the victim for seeking medical care. Thus it is important for the clinician to evaluate the victim's level of safety and use available hospital or clinic security measures as indicated (Linden, 1999). When the victim may return to the perpetrator, as in the case of marital rape, a safety plan should be reviewed with the victim before discharge.

MEDICAL AND ASSAULT HISTORY

After non–life-threatening trauma has been ruled out, a basic health history and more detailed assault history should precede physical examination and evidence collection (Hampton, 1995). The healthcare provider should take particular care to present a professional, sensitive, and nonjudgmental manner (Linden, 1999). It is recommended that someone from both the police department and a local victim advocacy organization be present during the assault history, because this coordination will limit the number of interviews the victim must endure. When the treating clinician is a male, some of the female victim's discomfort may be allayed by the presence of a female chaperone during the evaluation.

HEALTH HISTORY

Assessment of the victim's pertinent health history should include an abbreviated history of acute and chronic illnesses, current medications, and allergies to medications (Hampton, 1995). A gynecologic history should document the victim's first day of her last menstrual period, contraceptive method, current pregnancy status, and last consensual coitus within the past 72 hours. The victim should be asked about a history of any chronic psychiatric conditions, including major depression, anxiety disorders, and schizophrenia.

ASSAULT HISTORY

A focused assault history should address several areas, including descriptions of the assault, the perpetrator(s), the crime scene(s), and the victim's post-crime behaviors (Linden,1999). The assault history allows the clinician to facilitate appropriate evidence collection and to later evaluate all injuries. However, according to Hampton (1995), the assault history should not be "excessively detailed" because it may "result in discrepancies with the police report that can adversely affect criminal proceeding" (p. 235). A review of and rationale for these 4 areas is offered here.

The Assault

A description of the sexual assault should be obtained from the victim, including specific violent acts, such as attempted or completed oral, vaginal, and anal penetration by the perpetrator. Although most victims are unable to report if ejaculation occurred, the clinician should inquire about ejaculation as well as the perpetrator's use and disposal of a male condom. In some cases the police may be able to retrieve discarded condoms, thus facilitating evidence collection. In addition to penile and digital penetration, other objects may have been used to sexually assault the victim, including bottles or sticks. Direct questioning about other objects used to assault the victim should be incorporated into the history-taking, because victims may be hesitant to disclose these acts.

Other actual or threatened violent behaviors used in the course of the attack, including kicking, hitting, and punching, should be assessed. Choking and other forms of strangulation, common among sexual assaults, should also be evaluated. Human bite marks, also common among sexual assaults, may offer evidence about the perpetrator. The perpetrator's saliva may also be recovered, providing additional DNA evidence.

Clinicians should inquire about weapons used to subdue, intimidate, threaten, or physically harm the victim during an attack. Weapons can be classified as weapons of opportunity and weapons of choice. Weapons of opportunity are generally found by the perpetrator at the crime scene and may include items such as a rock, kitchen knife, or scissors. Weapons of opportunity indicate a lower level of planning on the perpetrator's part. Weapons of choice, on the other hand, are brought by the perpetrator to the crime scene and may include guns or rope. Weapons of choice indicate the perpetrator's greater level of thought and planning regarding the violent crime.

Key Point:
The healthcare evaluation of a sexual assault victim should include immediate attention to victim safety issues, a basic health assessment, and specific attention to assault history, physical examination, and evidence collection.

Key Point:
The "assault history" specifically includes descriptions of the assault, the perpetrator, the crime scene, and the victim's actions and behaviors since the assault.

The Perpetrator

A description of the perpetrator should be gathered by the clinician during the history. For many victims of sexual assault, the perpetrator may be known, thus facilitating identification. When the perpetrator is known, his name and any other identification, such as Social Security number, or residential or workplace address, should be ascertained. When the perpetrator is unknown, general descriptions should be gathered, including race, if known, height, weight, and body build. Any identifying body marks, such as tattoos, scars, or moles, should be reviewed and reported to the police.

The examiner should also obtain information about the perpetrator's mannerisms and words spoken during the attack. Examples include any comments, threats, or references made during the assault. This information may prove particularly important to law enforcement workers in their attempt to classify the type of rape and profile the perpetrator. Links between the current crime and other crimes may be made based on the type of rape.

The Crime Scene

A detailed description of the crime scene should be obtained from the rape victim. In many cases there may be more than one crime scene, including the initial point of contact with the perpetrator and other locations where the victim was assaulted. Each location may provide evidence helpful in prosecuting the crime. Physical as well as sensory descriptions, including characteristic odors, sounds, and textures (grass, sand, rocks, etc.), may be helpful in documenting unknown locations. The clinician may be able to collect trace evidence, such as grass, sand, and other debris, indicative of the crime scene location.

The Victim's Post-Crime Behaviors

To obtain forensic evidence after a sexual assault, most protocols require the victim to come to the healthcare provider within 72 hours of the incident. Because of the varied time delay between the assault and the victim seeking medical care, clinicians should assess for any post-crime behaviors that may have destroyed evidence of the assault, including showering, bathing, eating, brushing teeth, douching, vomiting, urinating, or defecating. The victim should be asked if she has changed her clothing since the attack. When possible, the police should be notified, thus facilitating the possible retrieval of evidence, including torn or damaged clothing, from the victim's home.

ACUTE CARE OF THE SEXUAL ASSAULT VICTIM

After a complete history of the crime, consent should be obtained to perform a physical examination and to collect evidence. The physical assessment, including pelvic examination, should be performed on adult sexual assault victims in order to identify and document injuries and to collect evidence.

ASSESSING PHYSICAL TRAUMA

The acute care of victims immediately after sexual assault includes the care of nongynecologic and gynecologic injuries as well as injuries inflicted by a weapon. In one study, most victims of sexual assault did not sustain obvious physical injury during an attack (Linden, 1999). Approximately one quarter of the victims sustained minor injuries and 5% sustained major nongenital injuries. However, in another recent study of more than 300 sexually assaulted women (Slaughter et al., 1997), 68% had sustained anogenital trauma and 57% nongenital trauma. In the group with anogenital trauma, tears, ecchymoses, and abrasions were common. When the authors compared these findings with those of women they examined who had had consensual sex, they found that fewer than 11% of women who had had consensual sex had visible or colposcopic evidence of anogenital trauma.

Nongynecologic Injuries

Common ***nongynecologic*** injuries include trauma from kicking, choking, and being tied or otherwise restrained, as well as trauma from human bites. Although these injuries may be classified as nongynecologic, they may be targeted to vulnerable "sexual" body regions, including the breast and genital areas.

Before treating nongynecologic injuries, a thorough description, including the location, size, color, and pattern of injury, should be made. This is best done by using photo-documentation to record each injury. Such documentation can be done with a 35mm camera or other means of photography. In addition, a body map should be used to document the victim's nongynecologic injuries. It is important to note that consent from the victim before photographing her injuries is frequently needed. It is recommended that at least two pictures of each injury be taken. A ruler or other object, such as a coin, should be placed next to the injury when photographed to discern the actual size of the injury. Because injuries, especially contusions, may become more obvious several hours to days after an assault, the clinician should consider having the victim return to the clinic for follow-up photographs.

Gynecologic Injuries
Gynecologic injuries found immediately after sexual assault can include vulvar, vaginal, perianal, and cervical lacerations, contusions, and hematomas. The extent of gynecologic injuries is related to several factors, including the victim's age (Slaughter et al., 1997), the force used to commit sexual acts, and the relationship with the perpetrator (Stermac et al., 1995). Thus, minimal or absent injuries should not be used to rule out sexual assault.

Evaluation of gynecologic injuries should begin with visual inspection of the external genitalia and other surrounding areas, including the inner thighs. This may initially be facilitated by using a handheld magnifying lens (Bechtel & Podrazik, 1999). Trauma to the labia majora and minora, including abrasions, adhesions, swelling, or ecchymoses, should be documented and photographed. Tears to the posterior fourchette and fossa may also be noted (Linden, 1999). Contusions and abrasions to the inner aspect of the thighs may also be evident as a result of violent forcing of the victim's legs open during an attack. Fluid, which may be blood, saliva, or semen, may also be present and should be collected as evidence.

An internal vaginal examination should begin with a thorough inspection of the vaginal introitus, noting introital tears, abrasions, swelling, or ecchymoses. A vaginal examination using a speculum lubricated with warm water should be used to assess for vaginal and cervical bleeding, lacerations, and foreign bodies. Any foreign bodies, such as a tampon, should be removed and appropriately sealed in a plastic, wax-lined bag for later forensic analysis. Additionally, pooled secretions in the posterior vaginal fornix should be aspirated with a syringe without a needle or collected with a cotton swab and included in the evidence kit for forensic evaluation. Inspection of the anus for tears, bleeding, or abrasions should also be performed. Evidence, including rectal swabs, should be collected when evidence of anal assault is present.

Key Point:
The physical examination and evidence collection phase of the healthcare evaluation for the sexual assault victim includes looking for physical trauma in both the anogenital area and non-genital areas of the body.

When available, photographs of external and internal gynecologic injuries should be taken using a 35mm camera. However, smaller, less obvious contusions, abrasions, and tears are better captured through the use of colposcopic imaging (Lenahan et al., 1998). In addition to 35mm camera and forensic colposcopy images, a thorough description of the genital injuries should be documented on the appropriate body map.

PHARMACOLOGIC NEEDS
Prevention of Pregnancy
It is estimated that as many as 25,000 rape-related pregnancies occur each year (Stewart & Trussell, 2000). Included as standard of care practice for the rape victim of childbearing age is making available emergency contraception, also referred to as the "morning-after pill," up to 72 hours after sexual assault. Because the victim may

Table 15-1. Emergency Contraceptive Guidelines	
BRAND	PILLS PER DOSE
Alesse	5 pink pills
Levlen	4 light orange pills
Levlite	5 pink pills
Levora	4 white pills
Lo/Ogestrel	4 white pills
Lo/Ovral	4 white pills
Nordette	4 light orange pills
Ogestrel	2 white pills
Ovral	2 white pills
Preven	2 blue pills
Tri-levlen	4 yellow pills
Triphasil	4 yellow pills
Trivora	4 pink pills
PROGESTERONE-ONLY PREPARATIONS	
Ovrette	20 yellow pills
Plan B	1 white pill

Source: Trussell J, Koenig J, Ellertson C, Stewart F. Preventing unintended pregnancy: the cost-effeciveness of three methods of emergency contraception. Am J Public Health. *1997;87(6):932-937.*

Drug dosage recommendations listed herein are those of the authors and are not endorsed by the US Public Health Service or the US Department of Health and Human Services.

be unable to report if a condom was used during the assault, every woman of childbearing age should be offered emergency contraception when there was any vaginal-penile contact, however slight. Even in cases in which a male condom was used, this added measure of pregnancy prevention may be reassuring to the victim.

Key Point:
The pharmacologic needs of persons being evaluated for sexual assault may include medications for pregnancy prophylaxis and STD treatment and/or prophylaxis.

After determining that the victim is not already pregnant, a combination of oral contraceptive pills, which varies according to specific brand of pills (**Table 15-1**), should be given to the woman twice at a 12-hour interval. In combination, these pills alter the endometrial lining and cervical mucus, making it unlikely for conception to occur. It is important to stress that emergency contraception is not an abortifacient. Because the high levels of estrogen contained in most emergency contraception are likely to cause nausea, anti-nausea medication, such as trimethobenzamide (Tigan), should also be offered. This is especially important for women taking emergency contraception after sexual assault, because autonomic physical reactions after assault can include nausea and vomiting. Instructions to eat before each dose of hormones should be stressed.

Women may be already taking an oral contraceptive regimen as instructed by their prescribing doctor. If a woman misses a dose of her prescribed contraceptive, emergency contraception should be offered in place of one day of her own hormonal pills. She should be instructed to resume her own pills after taking the day of emergency contraception. Virtually all women are able to take emergency contraception on this time-limited basis, including those who would otherwise be considered poor medical candidates for oral contraception. The overall effectiveness of emergency contraception is approximately 75%. Newly available progesterone-only emergency contraception is more effective and associated with fewer side effects than combined estrogen-progesterone preparations.

Prevention of Sexually Transmitted Diseases

In addition to pregnancy, victims of sexual assault are also at risk for contracting sexually transmitted diseases (STDs), including gonorrhea and chlamydia. The Centers for Disease Control and Prevention (CDC) reports that 6% to 12% of adult sexual assault victims acquire gonorrhea after sexual assault. To a similar degree, 4% to 17% of victims acquire chlamydia after assault (Schwarcz & Whittington, 1990).

There remains some controversy regarding the use of screening tests for STDs, including gonorrhea and chlamydia, after sexual assault. Because it can take several days after the exposure to obtain positive culture results, many practitioners omit routine screening and instead treat sexual assault victims prophylactically (**Table 15-2**) (Public Health Service, 1998). Additionally, some clinicians fear that culture results indicating the victim had been infected before the sexual assault may be used to vilify the victim should the criminal justice system become involved. Thus routine screening tests for STDs should be evaluated and used according to hospital guidelines.

In addition to gonorrhea and chlamydia, sexual assault victims may also be at risk for contracting human immunodeficiency virus (HIV) infection. The CDC reports that fewer than 1% of victims acquire HIV as a result of the sexual assault (Schwarcz & Whittington, 1990). Although post-assault screening results do not accurately discern if HIV was contracted after the rape, they do provide baseline data to which 3- and 6-month follow-up testing can be compared. The victim may receive baseline HIV screening within the hospital setting as part of routine care or may be referred to an anonymous, confidential testing site in the area. Hospital protocol should be followed when discussing HIV testing with the victim.

In addition to baseline screening, victims of sexual assault should be informed about the availability of HIV prophylactic medication that should be taken within 72 hours of the attack. Typically, a regimen of zidovudine 200 mg 3 times a day and lamivudine 150 mg twice a day for 28 days is prescribed for the victim after sexual assault (Public Health Service, 1998). Similar preventive pharmacologic measures

Table 15-2. Prophylactic Treatment for Sexually Transmitted Diseases

SEXUALLY TRANSMITTED DISEASE	PROPHYLACTIC TREATMENT
Gonorrhea	Ceftriaxone 125 mg IM
Chlamydia	Azithromycin 1 gram PO
Syphilis	Benzathine Penicillin IM
Bacterial vaginosis	Metronidazole 2 grams PO*
Hepatitis B	1st Dose of Heptavax**

*Nausea from medication may decrease compliance with emergency contraception. Patients are advised to avoid alcohol while taking this medication. Prophylactic treatment should be evaluated on an individual basis. **May be given if not already inoculated.

Adopted from Sexually Transmitted Diseases Treatment Guidlines 2002. MMWR [document online]. 2002. Accessed July 3, 2002.

Drug dosage recommendations listed herein are those of the authors and are not endorsed by the US Public Health Service or the US Department of Health and Human Services.

are frequently recommended for healthcare workers after exposure to blood and other bodily fluids while performing their duties.

FORENSIC EVIDENCE COLLECTION

As noted, the second purpose of the physical examination is collect evidence that may be used to assist the criminal justice system in identifying and prosecuting perpetrators of rape and sexual assault. A general guideline for collecting evidence is provided in **Table 15-3**. It is important to stress that only trained healthcare professionals should undertake evidence collection after sexual assault. Improperly collected and poorly handled evidence may damage the victim's criminal case. When an appropriately trained clinician is unavailable or when hospital protocols differ, referrals to an established sexual assault center, which are designated in most large cities, should be made. When designated sexual assault centers are unknown, most local emergency rooms can guide the clinician to an appropriate site or protocol.

If evidence is collected at the clinic site, a chain of custody must be established (Linden, 1999). In addition to securely collecting, labeling, and sealing all evidence, the clinician responsible for evidence collection must know the location of the evidence kit at all times. When the police do not immediately collect the evidence, the rape kit should be kept in a secure, locked location accessible only to the clinician. Whenever the evidence changes hands, written documentation, including appropriate signatures, badge numbers, license numbers, and time of retrieval/return, should be noted.

DOCUMENTATION AFTER SEXUAL ASSAULT

Medical documentation is an important forensic component in caring for the victim of a violent crime. Because medical documents are considered legal documents, the degree to which the clinician accurately describes the care rendered can greatly affect a legal case. Thus many centers dedicated to caring for sexual assault victims use standardized forms, ensuring that all pertinent medical documentation is addressed.

Key Point:
Careful and accurate documentation of the healthcare evaluation is essential to both the healthcare and legal aspects of the sexual assault evaluation. Many centers use standardized forms to ensure that information gathered during the healthcare interaction is appropriately documented.

Table 15-3. Guidelines for Evidence Collection Following Sexual Assault		
PROCEDURE	MATERIALS NEEDED	INSTRUCTIONS
Clothing Collection	2 Paper sheets 5-10 Paper bags Labels Pieces of paper	Collect all clothing worn at the time of the attack, including shoes. Victim should undress over 2 paper sheets placed on the floor, handing each clothing item to the nurse. Each piece of clothing should be placed in separately labeled paper bags and sealed. Do not shake out clothing or cut through pre-existing rips or tears. If any stains are present on the clothing, place a piece of paper over the stain prior to folding. If clothing is wet/damp, allow to air dry before placing in labeled paper bag. After collecting the clothing, the top paper sheet should be carefully folded and placed in a labeled paper bag and sealed.
Physical Examination and Evidence Collection	Wood's lamp Cotton tipped swabs Normal Sterile Saline (NSS) Labels Sterile water Paper or cardboard containers	Skin: Scan the skin with the Wood's lamp. Areas that react to ultraviolet light may provide biological evidence. Swab these areas with 2 cotton swabs moistened with NSS, air dry, and place in labeled paper or cardboard container. Collect debris from skin and put in labeled container.
	2 Plastic fingernail scrapers Paper towels Labels Envelopes	Nails: Obtain trace evidence from fingernails by scraping nails over a paper towel. Fold evidence in paper towel with fingernail scraper, place in labeled envelope, and seal. Evidence from each hand should be gathered and stored in separate envelopes, labeled "right" or "left" hand.
	2 Red top tubes Gonorrhea/*Chlamydia* culture Cotton tipped swabs Labels Paper or cardboard containers	Oropharynx: Swab buccal mucosa and along the gingiva with cotton swab, air dry, and place in labeled cardboard or paper container. Salivary samples should be collected at least 25 minutes after the victim last ate, drank, or smoked. Collect gonorrhea/*Chlamydia* oropharyngeal cultures per guidelines. Oropharyngeal evidence may be collected if oral-genital contact occured.

(continued)

Table 15-3. *(continued)*

	2 Red top tubes	Genitalia: Swab external genitalia and inner thighs with 4x4 gauze pads moistened with sterile water. Allow to air dry and place in labeled container.
	2 Gonorrhea/ *Chlamydia* culture	
	6 cotton swabs	Swab the vaginal walls and vault with 2 cotton swabs, allow to air dry, and place in labeled container. Repeat with 1 swab each for cervical and anal specimen.
	3 4 x 4 gauze pads	
	2 Envelopes	Place paper towel under victim's buttocks. Comb through pubic hair in downward motion, catching loose hairs in paper towel. Fold paper towel and place in labeled envelope and seal.
	Comb	
	Scissors	Obtain gonorrhea/*Chlamydia* cultures from vagina and rectum when indicated. Label tubes.
	Labels	
	Sterile water	
	Containers	
	Paper towels	
	Paper towels	Head Hair: Pull 15 full-length head hairs, as permitted by patient and by jurisdiction, from back, center, right and left side of the head, catching the loose hairs in a paper towel. Place paper towel in labeled envelope and seal.
	Envelope	
	Labels	
Blood Sample Collection	1 Purple top tube	Collect 3 mL of blood in labeled purple top tube. Blood work for STD testing (HIV, Rapid Plasma Reagin [RPR], and hepatitis B) may be collected in labeled red top tubes if indicated. Some states use buccal swabs, rather than blood, for reference DNA.
	3 Red top tubes	
	Labels	

Adapted from: Sexual Assault Evidence Collection Kit Cat. No. VEC100. Youngsville, NC, Sirchie Finger Print Laboratories, Inc., 2002. Suspected Sexual Abuse Form. Philadelphia, Pa, St. Christopher's Hospital, 2002.

ASSAULT HISTORY

When such standardized forms are not available, the clinician should follow the health history and assault history format described previously. The victim's account of the assault should be described in detail, using the victim's own words, unedited and unsanitized. This includes any pre-crime behaviors of the victim, such as last consensual sex, as well as a description of the crime event, including the date, time, and location of the attack, if known. When the perpetrator's name is known to the victim, this, too, should be included within the medical documentation as a direct quote. Any additional information gathered during the assault history should also be included.

PHYSICAL EXAMINATION

An accurate description of the physical examination follows. This initially begins with information regarding the victim's demeanor at the time of evaluation.

A detailed description of the injuries suffered should be provided by the clinician. Characteristics of the injuries, including the location, size, shape, color, and pattern of injury, should be described in detail. The victim's account of the injury, such as abrasion resulting from being pushed to the ground, should also be included. The description should be supported by 35mm photographs, colposcopic imaging, and body mapping. If appropriate evidence collection and documentation cannot be performed, the patient should be transferred to a facility that can meet the current standard of care for medical and forensic evaluation.

MEDICAL MANAGEMENT

Documentation of the medical management of the victim of sexual assault should include the recording of any laboratory testing done during the course of treatment. This may include culture studies and serologic testing for STDs, as well as urine pregnancy testing. In addition, any pharmacologic measures, such as emergency contraception or prophylactic treatment for STDs should also be recorded in the victim's medical chart.

EVIDENCE COLLECTED

Careful documentation of evidence collected during the examination is of utmost importance. The victim's name and the piece of evidence collected (such as "fingernail scrapings") should be documented on standard labels within the actual rape kit, as noted in **Table 15-3**. Documentation of any evidence collected should also be recorded within the victim's medical chart. The chain of custody of the evidence, that is, a detailed tracking of the location of the evidence, should also be included. When 35mm photographs are taken, the presence of such photographs should be noted within the medical chart. It is often recommended that 2 copies of each view be taken, allowing 1 copy to remain in the victim's medical chart.

SUPPORT SERVICES

A description of supportive services used, including any police involvement, should be included within the victim's medical chart. When the police are involved, the officer's name, badge number, presence/absence during the assault history, and action taken at the time of care should be described. When local victim advocates render services after assault, this should also be included within the victim's medical chart. Any plan for follow-up with either the police or other victim services should be documented.

COLLABORATION WITH OTHER DISCIPLINES

Rape and sexual assault results in a myriad of acute and long-term physical and psychologic sequelae for the victim (Burgess & Holmstrom, 1974). Thus the level of support needed after assault will vary from one victim to the next. Clinicians caring for victims of sexual assault should be aware of and collaborate with local and state agencies available to assist the victim recovering from this violent crime.

With the initiation of medical care, the rape victim will decide the degree to which the criminal justice system will be involved. In some instances the victim may seek medical care after rape or sexual assault while deferring evidence collection as well as additional police involvement. In the case of an adult victim of sexual assault, this request is reasonable and should be respected by the clinician. However, when the victim is a minor, state and federal laws regarding mandatory reporting should be followed.

In addition to collaborating with the local police, clinicians should also refer victims of rape to the local victim advocacy agencies, including domestic violence and rape advocacy resources. When available and appropriate, a victim's advocate should be present, if the patient has given consent, during the initial assault history as well as during the evidence collection procedure. The additional support offered by these specially trained advocates can help comfort the victim during the initial aftermath of the assault as well as offer long-term support and counseling during the recovery period.

Key Point:

Rendering service to patients who have been sexually assaulted is ideally a multi-disciplinary activity. Different service providers and agencies should work together to identify the specific needs of each patient and provide the services that he or she requires.

Sexual assault nurse examiners facilitate the appropriate evidence collection, documentation, establishment of a chain of custody, court testimony, and collaboration with local resources.

CONCLUSION

Since sexual assault is a crime that is rarely witnessed, forensic evaluation and collection of evidence are a crucial part of caring for victims of sexual violence. The examiner/clinician who is collecting the evidence must also do so in a sensitive and compassionate manner and should be mindful of the indications for disease and pregnancy prophylaxis.

REFERENCES

Bechtel K, Podrazik M. Evaluation of the adolescent rape victim. *Pediatr Clin North Am.* 1999;46:809-823, xii.

Burgess AW, Holmstrom L. Rape trauma syndrome. *Am J Psychiatry.* 1974;131:981-986.

Frampton D. Sexual assault: the role of the advanced practice nurse in identifying and treating victims. *Clin Nurse Spec.* 1998;12:177-182.

Hampton HL. Care of the woman who has been raped. *N Engl J Med.* 1995;332(4):234-237.

Kilpatrick D, Edmunds C, Seymour A. *Rape in America. A Report to the Nation.* Charleston, SC: Medical University of South Carolina; 1992.

Lenahan LC, Ernst A, Johnson B. Colposcopy in evaluation of the adult sexual assault victim. *Am J Emerg Med.* 1998;16:183-184.

Linden JA. Sexual assault. *Emerg Med Clin North Am.* 1999;17:685-697, vii.

National Center for Victims of Crime (NCVC) (2001). *Sexual Assault Statistics* [document online]. 2001. Available at: http://www.ncvc.org/stats/sa.htm. Accessed March 11, 2001.

Public Health Service guidelines for the management of health-care worker exposures to HIV and recommendations for post-exposure prophylaxis. *MMWR* [document online]. 1998. Available at: http://www.cdc.gov/mmwr/preview/mmwrhtml/00052722.htm#00003138.htm. Accessed April 13, 2001.

Schwarcz S, Whittington W. Sexual assault and sexually transmitted diseases: detection and management in adults and children. *Rev Infect Dis.* 1990;12:682-690.

Sexual Assault Evidence Collection Kit Cat. No. VEC100. Youngsville, NC, Sirchie Finger Print Laboratories, Inc., 2002.

Sexually Transmitted Diseases Treatment Guidelines 2002. *MMWR* [document online] 2002. Available at: http://www.cdc.gov/mmwr/ PDF/rr/rr5106.pdf. Accessed July 3, 2002.

Slaughter L, Brown CRV, Crowley S, Peck R. Patterns of genital injury in female sexual assault victims. *Am J Obstet Gynecol.* 1997;176:609-616.

Stermac L, DuMont J, Kalemba V. Comparison of sexual assaults by strangers and known assailants in an urban population of women. *CMAJ.* 1995;153:1089-1094.

Stewart F, Trussell J. Prevention of pregnancy resulting from rape: a neglected preventive health measure. *Am J Prev Med.* 2000;19:228-229.

Suspected Sexual Abuse Form. Philadelphia, Pa, St. Christopher's Hospital, 2002.

Trussell J, Koenig J, Ellertson C, Stewart F. Preventing unintended pregnancy: the cost-effectiveness of three methods of emergency contraception. *Am J Public Health.* 1997;87:932-937.

DNA Evidence in Sexual Assault

Patrick O'Donnell, PhD
Joanne Archambault
Kathy Bell, RN
Kathryn M. Turman

Disclaimer: All DNA case histories and information from the San Diego Police Department is courtesy of Joanne Archambault. To protect the privacy of the victims, all names and identifying features have been changed.

IMPORTANCE OF DNA EVIDENCE

Sexual assault has a lasting impact on victims. After an assault, the sense of safety and confidence that is needed to carry out daily activities without overwhelming fear may be shattered. It can be debilitating in many cases. This loss of security is exacerbated and prolonged when the perpetrator is not identified, or when the perpetrator is known but evidence does not exist to successfully prosecute the offender. Although the use of deoxyribonucleic acid (DNA) evidence to identify and convict perpetrators of sexual assault has great value to society, the criminal justice system, and public safety, the greatest potential benefit may be to victims. Effective use of DNA evidence can provide critical resolution to victims, enable them to feel safer in the world, and give them the assurance that other people will not be victimized at the hands of the person who assaulted them. DNA evidence, in conjunction with the development of the Combined DNA Index System (CODIS) and other DNA databases containing convicted offender profiles and DNA profiles obtained from biologic evidence recovered from sexual assault victims and crime scenes, has given new value to the thousands of unanalyzed rape kits sitting in evidence storage facilities around the country. In 1 case, a woman, D.S., was brutally raped near her home in broad daylight while her police officer husband slept in their bedroom. The rapist threatened to come back for her if she told anyone, and for 6¹/₂ years she lived in fear. When processed through Virginia's DNA databank, the DNA left at the crime scene by her assailant produced a match, or "hit," years later with the DNA of an inmate in a Virginia prison. She finally received reassurance that he would not come back for her, and she could begin real healing. Her assailant had gone to jail for another rape 6 months after raping her, but D.S. had to wait 6 years to learn of his identity.

Key Point:
The effective use of DNA evidence can provide critical resolution to victims, enable them to feel safer in the world, and give them the assurance that other people will not be victimized at the hands of the person who assaulted them.

In other cases, the DNA evidence exonerates the alleged perpetrator. Another woman, J.T., was 22 years old when she was raped by a man she described as a tall African American in his early 20s. J.T. identified a 22-year-old man named R.C. from police photos as her rapist, and she later identified him again in a line-up. R.C. was sentenced to life in prison for raping J.T. and another woman. Ten years later, R.C. filed and won a motion for DNA testing. The test showed that R.C. could not have committed the crime, and the state DNA database matched the sample to another inmate who had bragged about committing the crimes for which R.C. was convicted.

Sexual assault victims whose credibility was challenged in court during trial and who believed the conviction was an affirmation of their credibility might resent having their credibility questioned again. Some victims may feel terribly guilty about their part in convicting an innocent person. Victims should be reassured that they did the best they could at the time and that memory can be fallible. Victim services providers and criminal justice officials should emphasize the importance of knowing the truth and identifying the right perpetrator.

There is some anecdotal information that stories in the media, depicting the successful use of DNA evidence to identify perpetrators, are having an impact on how and when victims report an assault. Some victims, aware of the potential presence of DNA evidence, report taking care to preserve evidence by not bathing and by saving items of clothing or bedding for investigators.

Key Point:
Victims need to be provided with a simple, but thorough explanation of how DNA testing may be used in their case, the process and procedures followed, and the potential outcomes of test results. If possible, information should be provided both orally and in writing to give the victim an opportunity to ask questions and to have available for future reference.

Investigators, prosecutors, and victim assistance providers must understand the needs of victims with regard to DNA evidence. This is particularly important if reference samples are to be retrieved from victims or their consensual partners. Victims need to be provided with a simple, but thorough explanation of how DNA testing may be used in their case, the process and procedures followed, and the potential outcomes of test results. If possible, information should be provided both orally and in writing. Providing the information in person will give the victim an opportunity to ask questions. It is equally important for victims to have information on DNA evidence in writing for future reference. It is not unusual for victims to have difficulty absorbing and retaining complex information immediately after an assault, and it would be helpful to have a brochure or fact sheet to read in the future as the case progresses.

UNDERSTANDING THE SEROLOGIC PAST

Before the late 1980s and the introduction of DNA testing, forensic examination of biologic crime scene evidence involved the use of what are commonly referred to as serologic tests. These serologic tests can be classified in 2 broad categories: tests used to identify specific body fluids and those to individualize or type biologic evidence (Gaensslen, 1983; Saferstein, 1982, 1988). The identification of a body fluid is often 2-part, the first involving determining whether a substance is, for example, blood or semen (Gaensslen, 1983; Saferstein, 1982, 1988). Following the probable identification of blood, a second serologic test is often run to demonstrate that the fluid is of human origin. The practice of localizing and identifying body fluids has changed little in the last 30 years.

In stark contrast, the serologic tests used to individualize or type biologic fluid have largely been discarded. The goal of this analysis is to determine the population of individuals who could be a contributor to a particular piece of biologic evidence. In the analysis of sexual assault evidence, few useful serologic markers exist, mainly phosphoglucomutase (PGM), the ABO system, and in some cases peptidase A (Gaensslen, 1983; Saferstein, 1988). These markers are expressed not only in blood but also can be found in other body fluids such as semen and saliva (Gaensslen, 1983; Saferstein, 1982, 1988). Several significant drawbacks exist to employing these serologic markers to type a body fluid. First, these markers are expressed in components of body fluids that cannot be separated, creating complications when analyzing mixtures from 2 or more individuals. For example, during a sexual assault involving vaginal intercourse, seminal secretions will mix with vaginal secretions and there is no method to separate the 2 contributions. Serologic typing results reflect the sum total of the types expressed by the victim and the suspect, thus creating scenarios in which the suspect is completely masked by the victim (Gaensslen, 1983; Saferstein, 1988). A second drawback to using these serologic markers is that there are some individuals termed nonsecretors who do not express their ABO type in their semen or saliva (Gaensslen, 1983; Saferstein, 1988). Finally, the major hurdle to using serologic markers in the identification of the potential source of a body fluid is that it is quite common for 2 individuals to share the same pattern of types for serologic markers. This is easily illustrated by examining the ABO system in which individuals are typically grouped in 4 broad categories consisting of "A," "B," "O," and "AB." Examination of the distribution of type "A" in the Caucasian, African American, and Hispanic populations indicates that it is found in 25% to 40% of individuals (Gaensslen, 1983).

The commonality of these types has important implications for the application of serologic testing to the analysis of sexual assault evidence and the weight these findings should have in a court of law. Due to the high probability that 2 individuals can share the same set of serologic markers, there is a real risk that an individual selected at random will match the serologic suspect profile developed from the analysis of evidence in a particular sexual assault case. In fact, past criminal convictions partly based on the results of serologic testing have created a demand that the judicial system reexamine the evidence using DNA testing (Scheck et al., 2000, 2001; Travis & Asplen, 1999). The results of this DNA testing in some well-publicized cases have revealed that defendants were innocent of the crimes of which they were convicted (Scheck et al., 2000, 2001; Travis & Asplen, 1999). Concerns such as these have led to a moratorium on the death penalty in Illinois, the involvement of defense attorneys and prosecutor's offices in innocence projects, and the implementation of legislation designed to reevaluate criminal convictions when certain objective criteria are met (Travis & Asplen, 1999).

THE FORENSIC DNA REVOLUTION

It is important to appreciate the limitations of serologic testing when analyzing sexual assault evidence because this has been the real driving force behind the forensic DNA revolution. Approximately 60% to 70% of the cases submitted to forensic biology units in crime laboratories throughout the country involve crimes related to sexual assault (P. O'Donnell, personal communication, 2002). Serologic testing offered little hope in solving these cases except in situations in which other evidence strongly implicated a suspect. Because of the low discrimination power of serologic testing, almost no forensic work was conducted on sexual assault cases for which there was no suspect. In fact, it was quite common for crime laboratories not to accept work requests concerning cases without suspects even though these cases make up 20% to 30% of all sexual assaults reported (P. O'Donnell, personal communication, 2002).

In the mid-1980s a dramatic turn of events took place best illustrated by 2 tragic sexual assaults/homicides that occurred in a small village in England and later detailed in the Joseph Wambaugh (1989) novel, *The Blooding*. In late 1983 the raped and strangled body of 15-year-old Lynda Mann was found along a footpath often used as a shortcut in the village of Narborough. A team of 150 law enforcement officers was assigned to the case, but it remained unsolved even though investigators had a strong suspicion that the perpetrator was a local resident. Approximately 3 years later, the raped and strangled body of 16-year-old Dawn Ashforth was found within a short distance of where Lynda Mann had been murdered. In 1984 Dr. Alec Jeffreys, an academic scientist working at nearby Leicester University, was studying a repetitive DNA sequence found in the human myoglobin gene. He discovered that, when this repetitive sequence was used as a probe to analyze human DNA, it revealed an astonishing level of variability and an amazing degree of individuality. Jeffreys termed this repetitive DNA sequence a multi-locus probe and quickly realized the enormous potential of using it to analyze human pedigrees. Significantly, the power of this multi-locus probe to discriminate between humans was far beyond that seen with serologic tests. Jeffrey's work revealed that there was an extremely remote chance that 2 individuals would share the same multi-locus DNA pattern (Jeffreys et al., 1985). The multi-locus probe was incorporated into a technique known as restriction fragment length polymorphism (RFLP), and thus the first generation forensic DNA test was born.

Authorities first applied Jeffery's multi-locus probe to assist in sorting out claims of relatedness in immigration cases, but the forensic science potential was obvious. Jeffreys analyzed sperm evidence from both homicide cases, and the DNA test results revealed that a single individual was responsible for committing both crimes. Police authorities estimated that the perpetrator of the crimes was probably between the ages of early teens to mid-thirties and implemented a program whereby all males within this age-group were asked to give a blood sample for analysis. Four thousand blood samples were collected, screened for serologic types, and a select group analyzed with the multi-locus RFLP DNA test. These RFLP DNA profiles were then compared to the profiles developed from the sperm in both cases. As this enormous effort came to fruition, a coworker came forward and revealed that he had given a blood sample for Colin Pitchfork using altered identification paperwork, which led to Pitchfork's arrest. Analysis of a blood sample from Colin Pitchfork revealed an identical multi-locus RFLP pattern to that seen from the sperm recovered from both homicide victims. Colin Pitchfork was tried and convicted for both murders.

RESTRICTION FRAGMENT LENGTH POLYMORPHISM ANALYSIS

RFLP forensic DNA testing quickly spread from its first application in England and soon was adopted widely by crime laboratories throughout the United States and Europe (National Research Council [NRC], 1992, 1996). Multi-locus probes were replaced by a panel of single locus probes with the distinct advantage of allowing the forensic scientist to calculate how common a particular RFLP pattern would be among the major racial groups such as Caucasians, African Americans, and Hispanics (Inman & Rudin, 1997; NRC, 1992, 1996). Population data was also developed for Asians, American Indians, and other racial groups.

Key Point:
RFLP testing involves the purification of DNA followed by its specific dissection using what are called restriction enzymes. Restriction enzymes recognize a specific sequence in the DNA molecule and cleave the molecule wherever they encounter this sequence.

RFLP testing involves the purification of DNA followed by its specific dissection using what are called restriction enzymes (Inman & Rudin, 1997; NRC, 1992, 1996). These restriction enzymes recognize a specific sequence in the DNA molecule and cleave the molecule wherever they encounter this sequence. The DNA molecules present in a forensic sample are thus cleaved into a collection of fragments of many different sizes. These fragments are separated by size in a process known as electrophoresis and then transferred to a nylon membrane (Inman & Rudin, 1997; NRC, 1992, 1996). The DNA is then fixed to the membrane by heating, and the panel of single locus probes is applied sequentially to the membrane. Each of these single locus probes recognizes a unique site in the human genome. An image is developed on a piece of x-ray film that has a series of bands. These bands differ in position because they represent different DNA fragment sizes. When 4 different single locus probes are used in RFLP testing, it is extremely improbable that DNA samples collected from 2 different individuals would exhibit the same DNA banding pattern. The exception would be identical twins because they inherit the same DNA.

Key Point:
If a suspect's reference blood sample exhibits the same RFLP pattern as the DNA recovered from the sperm on a vaginal swab, it is a virtual certainty that the suspect was the origin of that sample. This is in contrast to previous serologic testing, where the serologic profile present on a vaginal swab might be matched not only by the suspect, but also by 30% of the general male population.

RFLP testing became widely available in crime laboratories in the late 1980s and early 1990s, and rapidly replaced serologic testing for determining the origin of a biologic sample. The test offered, for the first time, scientists and law enforcement the ability to individualize large numbers of people. If a suspect's reference blood sample exhibited the same RFLP pattern as the DNA recovered from the sperm on a vaginal swab, it was a virtual certainty that the suspect was the origin of that sample. This was in contrast to previous serologic testing, where the serologic profile present on a vaginal swab might be matched not only by the suspect, but also by 30% of the general male population. Thus the transition from serologic testing to RFLP DNA testing gave the forensic scientist the ability to provide testimony regarding the identity of a sample with nearly absolute confidence.

Even though RFLP testing represented an enormous breakthrough in the forensic analysis of biologic evidence, 2 significant hurdles still remained (Inman & Rudin,

1997; NRC, 1992, 1996). First, the RFLP test required a relatively large sample in order to obtain a DNA test result. For example, if a knife was recovered that was used in a stabbing and the blade had been wiped clean, so little blood would remain on the knife that it would be impossible to obtain an RFLP test result. Similar challenges were also encountered with many sexual assault cases where there were simply too few sperm present to perform the test. In addition, the RFLP DNA test required that a biologic sample be relatively fresh so that undegraded DNA could be obtained for the test. Many crime scene samples, such as blood exposed to the sun for several months or 10-year-old sexual assault kits, result in very degraded DNA being recovered. These samples proved to be extremely difficult to analyze with the RFLP methodology.

POLYMERASE CHAIN REACTION ANALYSIS

In the 1980s Dr. Kary Mullis et al. (1986), while working for a biotechnology company, invented the polymerase chain reaction (PCR) process. PCR would revolutionize the analysis of small quantities of DNA and profoundly influence molecular biology, medical diagnostics, and forensic science. Before PCR, scientists interested in analyzing a particular sequence of DNA needed to clone that piece of DNA in a labor-intensive process and then replicate the DNA, often using bacterial cultures. The cloning process could take weeks, and there was no guarantee that the sequence of interest would be successfully isolated and replicated. The application of PCR allows a scientist to create millions of copies of a specific DNA sequence within hours, which can then easily be isolated and analyzed.

The PCR process can be thought of as molecular photocopying, with the important distinction being that each copy is of the same quality as the original (Mullis et al., 1986). Scientists interested in the PCR analysis of DNA first design primers that are short, chemically synthesized segments of DNA, typically 15 to 40 nucleotides long. These primers often correspond to unique DNA sequences in the human genome, and a pair of primers is used to flank the designated region of interest. An enzyme involved in the replication of DNA from bacteria found in thermal hot springs is then used in conjunction with a thermocycler to replicate the specific DNA sequence. A thermocycler is an instrument capable of cyclically altering the temperature of a DNA reaction mix, creating denaturation, annealing, and elongation phases for PCR (Inman & Rudin, 1997; NCR, 1996). Theoretically, with each cycle through the denaturation, annealing, and elongation phases of PCR, the number of copies of the targeted DNA sequence is doubled. This exponential growth during the PCR process means that samples containing extremely small quantities of DNA can be analyzed routinely.

Unlike RFLP testing, in which the analysis is carried out on original DNA recovered from a biologic sample, PCR testing only consumes DNA from the sample after it has been duplicated millions of times. Because of this amplification process, PCR typically is 50 to 100 times more sensitive than traditional RFLP testing. In addition, the segments of DNA that are analyzed in the process tend to be relatively short, so the technique works well even with degraded DNA. Forensic scientists routinely employ the PCR process to analyze single hairs, cigarette butts, and as few as 50 to 100 sperm. It also can be used to analyze difficult biologic samples such as those recovered from buried human remains, fire victims, and plane crash victims.

Diversity of PCR Forensic Tests

Crime laboratories have used a large number of PCR-based forensic tests. In 1991 the DQA1 test kit was released, which allowed forensic scientists to characterize a single genetic marker in the human genome (Reynolds et al., 1991). Subsequently, the DQA1/Polymarker test kit was released, which employed the same reverse dot blot hybridization technology as DQA1 but added 5 additional genetic markers.

Key Point:
RFLP tests require a relatively large sample to obtain a DNA test result and require that the samples be relatively fresh so that undegraded DNA can be obtained.

Key Point:
The PCR process can be thought of as molecular photocopying, with the important distinction being that each copy is of the same quality as the original.

The DQA1/Polymarker test kit provided a revolutionary means of analyzing a wide variety of biologic samples. However, these tests drew some criticism because there were few alleles, and these tended to be distributed commonly in the populations. A particular DQA1/Polymarker DNA profile might be found in 1 in every several thousand people. In approximately 1994 the D1S80 test kit was released, and some laboratories used it to complement the DQA1/Polymarker test as a means of providing additional discrimination (Budowle et al., 1991). However, even with the addition of the D1S80 test, PCR forensic testing was not as discriminating as RFLP testing. Crime laboratories were faced with the difficult decision of whether to use the more discriminating RFLP test or the extremely sensitive PCR tests.

It was clear to the forensic community that what was needed was a PCR-based DNA test that achieved the discrimination afforded by RFLP testing. In the late 1990s a forensic test kit based on a new technology known as short tandem repeats (STRs) was released. Using a multiplexing approach, it became possible to analyze a large number of genetic markers using the fluorescence-based detection of flat-based scanners or capillary electrophoresis (Fregeau & Fourney, 1993). When a sufficient number of STR genetic markers are examined, the discrimination power of STR testing is comparable to that offered by RFLP testing. By 2000, STR technology was adopted by most crime laboratories in the United States and Europe, often eliminating the need for RFLP testing. In fact, forensic RFLP testing remains in existence largely because convicted offender databases were constructed using the technology. As states reanalyze their convicted offenders with STRs, RFLP testing will become obsolete.

Key Point:
Forensic RFLP testing remains in existence largely because convicted offender databases were constructed using this technology; as states reanalyze their convicted offenders with STRs, RFLP testing will become obsolete.

CONVICTED OFFENDER DATABASES

In 1983 California became the first state to authorize the collection of blood samples from convicted sex offenders for the purpose of analyzing genetic markers. At that time, analysis was limited to serologic markers, so the database of offenders proved to be of limited value. Local crime laboratories had some success with using the database to track offenders in their areas and to link serial rape cases. With the introduction of RFLP testing in the late 1980s, law enforcement quickly realized the impact offender databases would have if constructed using this powerful new technology. As more state and federal courts accepted DNA testing, the number of states enacting database legislation increased dramatically. As of 1998, all 50 states had authorized legislation requiring certain convicted offenders to provide biologic samples for analysis and entry into the CODIS database (Federal Bureau of Investigation [FBI], 2000b). Legislation in the states varies widely concerning collection, analysis, sample storage, and maintenance of the databases. One of the most controversial aspects of the database legislation involves the offenses that require an offender to provide a biologic sample for the DNA database. In California, only offenders who commit the most serious and violent offenses are required to provide samples (California Department of Justice, 1999). In contrast, in Virginia all individuals convicted of a felony provide samples for the state database. Recently, law enforcement in Virginia indicated that 40% to 50% of the sexual assault cases without suspects that were solved through comparison to the state's DNA database involved offenders required to give samples for previous convictions other than sex crimes (P. O'Donnell, personal communication, 2002). This revelation suggests that the authorization to collect biologic samples will include an ever-expanding list of offenses. In the end, there must be an effort to balance civil rights and privacy concerns with the benefits of using the DNA databases to solve crimes.

COMBINED DNA INDEX SYSTEM

The DNA Identification Act of 1994 formalized the authority of the Federal Bureau of Investigation (FBI) to establish a national DNA index system for law enforcement purposes. This index is known as CODIS and consists of 3 hierarchic levels (FBI, 2000b). All DNA profiles originate at the local level (LDIS), then flow to the state level (SDIS), and finally to the national level (NDIS). NDIS is the highest level in the hierarchy and allows the participating laboratories to exchange and compare DNA profiles between states. SDIS allows laboratories within a state to exchange DNA profiles. The tiered approach allows state and local laboratories to operate their databases in accordance with specific legislative and legal requirements.

There are 2 important parts to the CODIS system (FBI, 2000b). The Forensic Index contains DNA profiles from crime scene evidence, often referred to as forensic unknowns. The Offender Index contains DNA profiles of individuals convicted of crimes that require a biologic sample be provided to law enforcement for DNA profiling. Matches made among DNA profiles in the Forensic Index can link evidence from crime scenes suggesting a serial offender. Using this information, authorities from multiple jurisdictions can coordinate their investigations and share possible leads. Matches made between the Forensic Index and the Offender Index provide investigators with information concerning the identity of the perpetrator. If an offender is identified, an additional reference sample will be obtained and the evidence reexamined to confirm the match.

Key Point:
The DNA Identification Act of 1994 formalized the FBI's authority to establish a national DNA index system for law enforcement purposes, which is known as CODIS. The two important parts of CODIS are the Forensic Index, which contains DNA profiles from crime scene evidence (forensic unknowns), and the Offender Index, which contains DNA profiles of individuals convicted of crimes that require a biologic sample be provided to law enforcement for DNA profiling.

CODIS SUCCESS STORIES

November 1999 (San Diego): In March 1995 a college student returned home to a house she shared with 3 other students after spending the evening studying in a university library only a couple of blocks away. While in the bathroom of the house, she was violently attacked and sexually assaulted. The detective worked the case until all leads were exhausted. Given the type of assault, investigators expected to see the suspect strike again; however, there were no similar cases reported in San Diego County or, to the investigators' knowledge, elsewhere. Evidence was sent to a private laboratory for RFLP analysis. The profile was submitted to CODIS but no match was found. Later in 1995, a few months after the sexual assault, a man was arrested after entering a beach-area tanning salon, masturbating while watching a woman tan, and fleeing with the woman's purse. Semen was found at the tanning salon and had a DNA profile consistent with the suspect in custody. In 1999, after completing a project to enter all DQA1/Polymarker DNA case profiles into CODIS, a criminologist working for the San Diego Police Department noted that the PCR DQA1/Polymarker DNA profile from the suspect in the tanning salon incident was identical to the profile of the perpetrator wanted for the sexual assault of the college student. The sexual assault investigator was provided with the suspect information from the indecent exposure case. The suspect matched the physical description, and he lived within 1 mile of the victim's home at the time of the rape. The suspect was convicted for the incident in the tanning salon and sent to prison 6 months after the rape, which was probably why no similar cases were reported. Although the suspect committed both a petty theft and an indecent exposure, when confronted with the evidence, he had accepted a plea bargain and was sentenced to 6 years in prison for petty theft with a prior. Based on the new information obtained through CODIS, a search warrant was sought to obtain additional blood and saliva samples from the suspect for RFLP analysis to compare with the DNA profile from the rape. The results were a match, and the frequency for the DNA profile in the Hispanic population was 1 in 28 billion.

It should be noted that obtaining DNA analysis on an indecent exposure case is not customary, because there are typically many more heinous sex crimes and child abuse cases waiting for DNA analysis. The suspect was not convicted of a sex offense and thus would not have been required to register as a sex offender in California or to provide a blood or saliva sample. This case would never have been solved without the local PCR database. It illustrates the importance of processing evidence from all types of sex offenses and the need to continue to expand the qualifying offenses for admission into DNA databases across the country. Not surprisingly, when interviewed by the detective, the suspect denied any contact with the victim. However, when faced with the DNA evidence at trial, the suspect said that he met the victim at a liquor store near the university. He said she asked him to buy her alcohol because she was underage and then invited him to her home, where she seduced him. When confronted with the victim's extensive injuries and the fact that she was bound with a telephone cord during the assault, the suspect said she liked rough sex and asked to be tied up. The jury wasn't convinced, and the suspect was sentenced to a term of 85 years to life, requiring him to serve at least 72 calendar years before being eligible for parole.

February 2000 (Florida and Iowa): In 1995 an unidentified woman's body was found on an off-ramp along an interstate in Des Moines, Iowa. After identifying the victim, police began looking at truck drivers as suspects because of the body's location. The Iowa Department of Public Safety sent biologic evidence left at the crime scene to the FBI Laboratory for DNA analysis. The FBI Laboratory analyzed the evidence, and developed a DNA profile of the perpetrator. The profile was uploaded to CODIS, where NDIS matched it to a Florida offender. At the time of the match, the offender was incarcerated in a Florida prison for a sexual assault conviction in early 1999. After identifying the offender, police investigation revealed that he possessed a commercial trucking license (FBI, 2000b).

April 2000 (Virginia): In August 1999 an intruder raped a 20-year-old college student in her house in Charlottesville, Virginia. A man with a gun awakened the woman and a male companion in bed during the early morning hours. The intruder demanded money from the two. He then made the male lie face down on the bed while he raped and sodomized the woman. Afterward, the rapist wiped himself with a towel and made the victim take a long shower. The victim also stated that the rapist drank at least 1 beer from the refrigerator. The Charlottesville Police Department recovered evidence from the scene, including a bed sheet and a beer can found outside the victim's house. The Virginia Division of Forensic Science Laboratory in Richmond conducted DNA analysis of semen recovered from the bed sheet and saliva found on the beer can. In October a CODIS search of the unknown DNA profile matched an offender in the Virginia DNA Database. The offender was subsequently located in the Charlottesville City jail. He had not been convicted of any sex crime previously. The individual was tried in April 2000 and found guilty of rape, sodomy, abduction, and robbery. The jury recommended a 90-year sentence (FBI, 2000a).

THE DNA TESTING RESOURCE CRISIS

Serologic testing of crime scene evidence was mostly limited to blood, semen, and saliva. With the introduction of RFLP DNA testing, forensic analysis grew to encompass all biologic samples containing significant human DNA, including multiple hairs, bone, teeth, tissue, and urine. DNA laboratories soon realized that the demands for their services were outstripping available resources. The introduction of PCR-based analysis only worsened the situation because a whole spectrum of limited samples could now be analyzed routinely. This included single hairs, sweat, dandruff, fingernail scrapings, and miniscule amounts of blood, semen, saliva, and other biologic material. The wide variety of samples the DNA tests could accommodate and the test's incredible discrimination power combined to create an explosion in requests from law enforcement investigators and attorneys.

Because of a shortage of crime laboratory resources, many rape kits have not been examined. On behalf of the National Commission on the Future of DNA, in August and September 1999, the Police Executive Research Forum (PERF) and Eastern Kentucky University (EKU) conducted a survey to estimate the number of rape or sexual assault cases with possible DNA evidence that had not been

Key Point:
Serologic testing of crime scene evidence was mostly limited to blood, semen, and saliva. With the introduction of RFLP DNA testing, forensic analysis grew to encompass all biologic samples containing significant human DNA, including multiple hairs, bone, teeth, tissue, and urine. Then the demands for the services of DNA laboratories outstripped available resources, meaning that many rape kits have not been examined.

submitted for DNA examination and the reasons why that evidence was not submitted for testing. Following the initial faxed survey, 50 agencies were surveyed by telephone. PERF conducted a survey of 122 law enforcement agencies in which each department served a population of 50,000 or more, or employed more than 100 full-time officers and civilian personnel. EKU examined a total of 153 organizations where the population in the jurisdiction did not exceed 50,000 and the department employed 10 or fewer officers. The 275 agencies responding to the survey accounted for approximately 118,000 employees, sworn and civilian, and a service population of nearly 46,000,000 people. Municipal police accounted for 76.4% of the agencies surveyed, while county sheriffs accounted for 18.9%. Within the larger organizations, 85.9% said they would examine evidence for potential DNA analysis, while in the smaller agencies, only 56.9% would assess evidence for potential DNA analysis. Sixty-four percent of the agencies indicated that they submitted evidence to the state laboratory for analysis. A large number (27.3%) either failed to respond to the question or did not know where samples were sent. Six respondents (2.2%) used county laboratories, and private laboratories were used by an equivalent number of agencies (2.5%). In 2.9% of the responses, samples went to combinations of state and private laboratories or state and county laboratories. In the overall analysis, 70.2% of all agencies surveyed revealed that they did assess evidence for potential DNA samples, yet 29.8%, indicated they did not make such assessments. When asked if their respective departments had policies regarding submissions of samples to laboratories, nearly three quarters of the agencies surveyed had no policies.

During 1997, 42 of the 50 agencies surveyed by telephone reported 3133 incidents of forcible rape. The 50 agencies collectively had 8487 untested rape kits in storage over varying periods of time. Reported rapes for 1997, therefore, represent 36.9% of the total number of rape kits in storage. The percentages remain relatively consistent when they considered the entire group (n = 122) of PERF respondents. In 1997 a total of 12,472 forcible rapes were reported in the FBI's Uniform Crime Report (Final Report, National DNA Survey, 2001), and the 122 agencies indicated that they were collectively storing 31,292 untested rape kits. Reported rapes for the entire group represented 39.8% of the total number of stored and untested rape kits. The data show that reported rapes for a given year represent slightly over one third of the total number of rape kits in storage.

Six agencies considered the possibility of DNA evidence when investigating all felonies. Thirty-four agencies considered DNA evidence only when investigating rapes and homicides. The investigating detective determined when evidence would be submitted for DNA analysis 70% of the time. Another 14% said the detective's supervisor would make this determination. Twenty-two agencies said they did not submit a DNA sample unless they had a suspect reference sample with which to compare the evidence. Twenty-five stated they submitted all samples, and 3 respondents did not know if their submissions were limited to those with suspect profiles.

The survey addressed the issue of case backlogs and why DNA evidence may not be processed. In many jurisdictions, some rape kits are not processed because of the case disposition, that is, the prosecutor rejected the case, the report was classified as unfounded, or the victim refused to cooperate with the investigation. In some jurisdictions, DNA analysis rests with the prosecutor's decision to prosecute the identified suspect. Of the 232 agencies that responded to the question, 14 (5.4%) of the total sample retained the largest number of rape kits, a total of 24,943 kits.

DNA laboratories have continued to respond to the resource crisis as the criteria for working cases shifted. Dramatic increases in DNA laboratory personnel have alleviated some of the problem, and DNA testing is now routinely used to evaluate suspects in many jurisdictions. With the emergence of sizable offender databases nationwide, DNA laboratories now face the daunting task of working every criminal case where biologic evidence exists. The challenge is of enormous proportions. Recently in California, a survey of crime laboratories revealed that rape kits from 19,000 sexual assault cases without suspects were collected from 1995 to 2000, yet very few of these have ever been analyzed (P. O'Donnell, personal communication, 2002). The California legislature has recognized the magnitude of the problem, and $50 million was allocated to eliminate the backlog of sexual assault cases without suspects over a 3-year time period. Other communities across the country are exploring their options and coming up with innovative ways to address the problem.

COLLABORATION AMONG LAW ENFORCEMENT, THE JUDICIAL SYSTEM, AND DNA LABORATORIES

Investigators and attorneys need to work with DNA laboratories to make certain that critical DNA testing resources are applied to cases in which the results are most critical. Many DNA laboratories are working under a triage system where limited resources are first directed toward cases with trial dates, and the remainder of resources are expended on sex crime and homicide investigations, where the outcome of the investigation could be dramatically influenced by the test results. The practical reality in many DNA laboratories is if DNA testing resources are wasted on a criminal case where there is questionable merit to the test, another case will undoubtedly suffer as it sits unanalyzed. For example, DNA testing results are generally not going to resolve a sexual assault case where the victim and suspect are not disputing the acts that took place, but whether the victim provided consent. As obvious as this might be, there is a tendency among attorneys and investigators to ask for every possible forensic test simply to bolster the appearance of their case.

The San Diego Police Department's DNA Laboratory has taken 2 important steps to make sure that limited DNA testing resources are expended on the worthiest cases. First, the laboratory supervisor meets weekly with the detectives and supervisors from the sex crimes unit to discuss case priorities, the potential to analyze particular samples, and the projected current resources available to handle incoming cases. Detectives are required to fill out a 4-page work request detailing aspects of the case that must be signed by a sex crimes unit supervisor before being submitted to the DNA Laboratory. (See Appendix II, "Forensic Sciences Lab Services Request," p. 311-312.) Before implementing this protocol, it was common to encounter situations where DNA testing was performed on cases in which the suspect was in the process of pleading guilty or where the district attorney's office had already made a decision against issuing the case even if the DNA test results supported the victim's statement to authorities. Second, the DNA Laboratory supported the creation of a district attorney liaison responsible for discussing the DNA testing needs of attorneys in particular cases as they are scheduled for trial. Implementing this dual-prong protocol has freed up the necessary resources so that in 2001, 30% to 40% of the cases analyzed in the San Diego Police Department's DNA Laboratory were without a suspect. The only hope for solving many of these cases is the development of a DNA profile that can be compared to offender databases currently being constructed. Unfortunately, the traditional view in many jurisdictions has been for laboratories, detectives, and attorneys to operate under the guidelines of minimal communication between parties. This view is often supported on the grounds that it reduces bias in investigations, when instead it results in the misdirected expenditure of limited laboratory resources. If there are concerns about the reliability of DNA testing in a particular case, the clearest means of resolving these concerns is through retesting by a second DNA laboratory (NRC, 1996).

IMPORTANT BIOLOGIC EVIDENCE IN SEXUAL ASSAULTS

Investigators working sexual assault cases must examine the entire range of possible biologic evidence that may prove useful in solving a particular case. Investigators need to make certain that a complete sexual assault kit is collected from the victim. This includes collection of swabbings from possible bite marks; collection of breast swabs and body swabs when a history of kissing, licking, or sucking is involved; fingernail scrapings or swabbings; the collection of clothing worn directly after the assault; and the collection of clothing worn to the hospital. When several days have elapsed since the incident occurred, cervical swabs from the postpubescent victim should be collected. Any loose hairs found on the victim or the victim's clothing should be carefully preserved for future testing.

The importance of collecting biologic evidence from a suspect immediately after his arrest cannot be overstated. If in custody within a day of the sexual assault, penile swabs should be collected from male suspects. The penile swab must include the glans, shaft, and scrotum areas. Fingernail scrapings or swabbings must be routinely collected during suspect examinations because they often prove valuable in alleged situations of digital penetration. Clothing from the suspect must be collected, because it is possible for body fluids from the victim to be transferred to the suspect. If the suspect is not apprehended wearing the clothing believed to be worn at the time of the sexual assault, a warrant or consent should be obtained to search any premise where investigators believe the clothing may be found.

The environment where the sexual assault took place should be also closely examined. Vehicles, apartments, and houses must be examined under appropriate conditions with an alternate light source to detect the presence of possible biologic fluids. Condoms, tissues, and hairs found at the scene should never be overlooked. Finally, reference standards from the victim, suspect, and all consensual partners are essential to the DNA testing process. Failure to collect appropriate reference standards will delay the DNA testing process or make interpretation of test results incomplete.

The shortage of crime laboratory resources in the country has severely limited the ability to evaluate current protocols used by law enforcement and forensic examiner programs to evaluate whether a forensic examination should be obtained; that is, most communities use a 72-hour rule to determine whether a forensic examination should be provided. Little evaluation has been done on the forensic examination itself, and what little evaluation there is has focused on the sexual assault response team (SART) model and the improvement of care for the victim and evidence collection standards. To date, very few studies have looked at what the SART examination and the evidence collected revealed after scientific analysis. It is commonly known that the victim, suspect, and crime scene are the primary sources of physical evidence in sexual assault cases, but little is known about the specific pieces of evidence collected from each of the primary sources (Moreau & Bigbee, 1995). In addition, little is known about the association between the primary sources of physical evidence, forensic DNA analysis, suspect identification, and law enforcement outcomes. Finally, the differences and similarities of the specific pieces of physical evidence collected from the primary sources in adolescent versus adult sexual assault cases have never been examined. It is hoped that by studying each of these elements, an increased understanding of sexual assault evidence can help law enforcement and the medical community evaluate current protocols used to determine if and when a forensic examination should be obtained in the case of a sexual assault. To learn more about what evidence may be obtained from the rape kits, the crime scene, and the suspects themselves, the San Diego Police Department DNA Laboratory and the Sex Crimes Unit worked with Isaac Cain, a forensic science graduate student, to evaluate 77 sexual assault cases where some form of forensic evidence was evaluated. Fifty-one of the cases involved adult victims, age 18 years and older. Twenty-six of the cases were adolescents, age 14 to 17 years. The study was conducted during a period of time when the San Diego Police Department was still using PCR DQA1. (They have since converted to using STR analysis and have since screened and typed DNA on hundreds of sexual assault cases

Key Point:
Investigators working sexual assault cases must examine the entire range of possible biologic evidence offering promise in solving a case. First, a complete sexual assault kit must be collected from the victim. Second, collecting biologic evidence from a suspect immediately after his arrest is imperative. Third, the environment where the sexual assault took place should be closely examined. Fourth, reference standards from the victim, suspect, and all consensual partners are essential to the DNA testing process.

without suspects.) Nevertheless, the analysis is helpful and an example of the work that needs to continue in this area (see **Tables 16-2 a** to **e**, p. 283-287).

DNA Case Histories

Scenario #1

A 32-year-old woman and girlfriend were walking back to their apartment in San Ysidro, California, after spending the evening in Tijuana, Mexico. As they approached a shopping mall parking lot, a man across the street attempted to get their attention and waved for them to come over and meet him. The women ignored the man and continued walking, but the man crossed the street and confronted them. The suspect threw the 32-year-old victim to the ground while the friend looked on. The suspect threatened to hurt both of them if either screamed. The suspect forced the victim to have vaginal intercourse followed by oral copulation. The victim also stated that she was digitally penetrated during the assault. After the assault, the suspect was seen running away from the crime scene. The friend was able wave down a car for a ride to a nearby phone to call the police. Within 1 hour, a subsequent search of the area by police resulted in the arrest of a suspect matching the physical description of the rapist given by the victim. The victim and friend were able to make a positive identification of the suspect during a curbside lineup. The suspect was charged with sexual assault.

The victim was taken to a local hospital for an examination and collection of a sexual assault kit. The victim stated that she and her friend went to party in Tijuana that night and that she had had consensual sex with an individual she only knew by first name. The suspect, after being taken into custody, was also given an examination, and fingernail scrapings and penile swabs were collected. Crime laboratory examination of the vaginal swabs revealed the presence of sperm, but because of the nearly anonymous nature of the prior consensual act and the inability to obtain a reference sample, DNA analysis was focused on other evidence. Examination of the suspect's fingernail scrapings revealed cellular material similar in appearance to vaginal epithelial cells. Examination of the suspect's penile swab revealed the presence of sperm and an abundance of epithelial cells. DNA tests conducted on the suspect's fingernail scrapings indicated that the cellular material originated from the victim and was not from the suspect. DNA tests of the nonsperm fraction of the suspect's penile swab revealed a profile consistent with a mixture of the victim and suspect, assuming a third contributor. Although never proven, this third contributor may have been the result of the victim's previous consensual act.

Outcome: The suspect pleaded guilty to the sexual assault charge and was fined and sentenced to 3 years in prison.

Scenario #2:

A 13-year-old girl was invited over by a friend to help baby-sit for the younger children of a man known as "Rick." Rick returned to the house several hours later and asked the girls if they were thirsty. He served them both orange juice that apparently had been mixed with alcohol. The 13-year-old refused to drink the orange juice because she didn't like the taste. Rick put his children to bed and then gave the baby-sitter some money to go to the local 7-11 store to buy some more orange juice. Rick confronted the 13-year-old while she was on a bed watching television. Rick removed the victim's clothes, licked and fondled her breasts, had vaginal intercourse, and forced the victim to orally copulate with him. After the sexual assault, the victim locked herself in a bathroom and Rick attempted to convince her to take a shower. The baby-sitter returned and Rick began to panic and offered the victim money to keep quiet. The victim and baby-sitter escaped from Rick's house and went to a neighbor's house where the baby-sitter called an aunt and described what happened. The sexual assault was reported to police and Rick was taken into custody hours after the assault.

The victim was taken to a local hospital for an examination and collection of a sexual assault kit and clothing. The victim indicated she was menstruating at the time. The suspect, after his arrest, was also given an examination that included the collection of all clothing that he was wearing at the time of the sexual assault. Crime laboratory examination of the vaginal swabs, rectal swabs, and victim's panties revealed the presence of sperm. Examination of the suspect's boxers indicated the presence of a large bloodstain on the front crotch. DNA tests conducted on the bloodstain indicated the blood originated from the victim and not the suspect. DNA tests of the victim's rectal swab showed that the sperm present were consistent with the suspect.

Outcome: The double link established through DNA testing in which the victim's blood was found on the suspect and the suspect's semen found on the victim proved pivotal. The suspect pleaded guilty to sexual assault and was fined and sentenced to 8 years in prison.

SCENARIO #3:
A 5-year-old developmentally disabled boy described to his mother the details of his molestation. The victim described being fondled and licked in numerous areas. The suspect was the mother's boyfriend and a registered sex offender. Although the mother questioned the validity of her son's story, she called police.

The young victim was taken to Children's Hospital Center for Child Protection where he was interviewed and given a forensic examination. The examination revealed bruising in the area of the upper thigh near the groin and near 1 knee. Wood's lamp testing revealed fluorescence on the victim's penis, left thigh, and right knee. Crime laboratory examination of the victim's penis swabs, left thigh swabs, and right knee swabs suggested the presence of saliva, and nucleated epithelial cells were found. DNA testing of the swabs revealed a profile foreign to the victim was present. Investigators felt they had insufficient probable cause to order a reference sample to be collected from the boyfriend. The Department of Justice DNA Laboratory in Berkeley, California, was contacted because they serve as the depository for convicted offender samples for the state. A portion of the boyfriend's reference sample held in storage was provided to the San Diego Police Department DNA Laboratory for testing. DNA analysis of this reference standard indicated that the suspected boyfriend could be the source of the foreign DNA profile found on the boy.

Outcome: The boyfriend was charged with child molestation and faced third-strike sentencing provisions. A jury found the defendant guilty, and he is now serving a life sentence in prison.

DNA COLLECTION

Evidence is collected during the sexual assault examination that will assist in linking the victim to the suspect, the suspect to the victim, and the victim or suspect to the crime scene. Healthcare professionals most often collect evidence from victims and suspects. Law enforcement collects evidence at the location where the incident occurred which may link the suspect or victim to the crime scene. Medical personnel with little or no training in evidence collection and preservation often have collected the evidence in the past, and this lack of training has led to difficulties in using the evidence because of improper handling and/or collection methods. Many communities are developing programs in which forensic nurses and physicians specially trained in evidence collection perform the forensic medical examinations (Ledray, 1999). The International Association of Forensic Nurses (1996, 1998) has developed a Sexual Assault Nurse Examiner Standards of Practice and Sexual Assault Nurse Examiner Educational Guidelines. These 2 documents outline the minimum standards of nursing practice and level of instruction for the sexual assault nurse examiner (SANE). The SANE Development and Operation

Guide is an excellent resource for communities (Ledray, 1996). It can be accessed via the Office for Victims of Crime, US Department of Justice website, www.ojp.-usdoj.gov/ovc and through the Office for Victims of Crime Resource Center at 1-800-627-6872, reference number NCJ 170609.

GAINING COOPERATION AND CONSENT

The most important step in the collection of DNA evidence from a victim is educating the victim and seeking his or her cooperation during the forensic examination. All patients, whether a small child, an adolescent, an adult, someone with a developmental disability, or an elderly person, will have unique needs. All procedures must be explained so that the patient can better cooperate with the examination. Evidence collected within 72 hours of the assault is more likely to yield DNA material, although there are situations in which it makes sense to collect past this guideline. There is rarely a need for emergency treatment due to severe injury of the victim, and other than this situation, the patient should be examined in a calm, quiet environment.

FORENSIC EVIDENCE COLLECTION

Most communities have access to sexual assault examination kits, also known as "rape kits." These kits contain tools needed to collect evidence. They typically contain numbered sacks and envelopes that will guide an examiner through the collection process. Inside these sacks and envelopes, the examiner may find sheets of white paper that the person being examined stands on during clothing removal. Other envelopes contain cotton swabs that will be used throughout the collection procedure. Still other envelopes contain bindles, which are pieces of clean white paper folded into sections of one third and then into sections of one third again. Bindles are used to contain loose evidence or evidence that cannot be collected using swabs.

Evidence collection involves the collection of known origin and unknown origin samples. Basic evidence collection standards, whether at the crime scene where the assault occurred or from the examination of the victim or suspect, follow the same principles. When collecting from the human body, the examiner should always include the guidelines listed in **Table 16-1**.

Giving control back to the victim of rape is therapeutic and should be used throughout the examination. One way this can be accomplished is by allowing victims to decline any part of the examination. Many times, patients are only hesitant because they do not understand why the examiner is asking to collect a particular sample or perform a certain procedure. With an explanation of the reason and purpose, it is unusual for individuals to continue to decline. Knowledge is control and allows them to make an informed decision about their actions. In cases of children, adolescents, and individuals with developmental disabilities, it is important not to add trauma by forcing or frightening the patient during evidence collection. An unhurried, compassionate, gentle approach is usually all that is needed to gain cooperation. Explaining the process and letting the patient explore the equipment used will alleviate most fears.

Using paper and air-drying all evidence before packaging will prevent the development of a moist environment in which mold and bacteria are likely to grow and subsequently destroy DNA evidence. The use of minimal amounts of water to collect dried specimens facilitates faster drying times. The use of sterile or tap water rather than normal saline solution is recommended for the collection of dried specimens. Because tap water can contain various metals, each community should take that into consideration when deciding on sterile or tap water. The use of normal saline solution is recommended only when there is a wet stain because it prevents lysis of the cells used for serologic tests. Once red blood cells have dried on the skin, they are already lysed (Ledray & Netzel, 1997). Cotton-tipped swabs

Key Point:
The most important step in collecting DNA evidence from a victim is educating the victim and seeking his or her cooperation during the forensic examination. There is rarely a need for emergency treatment because of severe injury to the victim, and unless this is the case, the patient should be examined in a calm, quiet environment.

Key Point:
With children, adolescents, and individuals with developmental disabilities, it is important not to add trauma by forcing or frightening the patient during evidence collection. An unhurried, compassionate, gentle approach is usually all that is needed to gain cooperation. Explaining the process and letting the patient explore the equipment used will alleviate most fears.

Table 16-1. Guidelines for Collecting Samples from the Human Body

— Patients have the right to decline collection of samples.
— Use only paper to package evidence.
— Air dry all evidence 30 to 60 minutes, or until dry, before packaging
   (refer to your state or community protocol).
— Use only one drop of water to moisten swabs.
— Use only cotton-tipped swabs.
— Do not lick sticky seals on evidence envelopes.
— Maintain chain of custody at all times.

---

should be used because cotton has suitable absorption properties for the collection of DNA specimens and does not contain matter destructive to DNA material (Ledray & Netzel, 1997). Licking an envelope seal creates the possibility of contaminating the collected evidence with the DNA of the forensic examiner. It also may expose the examiner to potential infectious agents.

Maintaining chain of custody of the specimens collected is the responsibility of the forensic examiner collecting the samples. If the chain of custody is broken, evidence may not be allowed to be presented in court. Maintaining chain of custody is as simple as documenting who has the evidence, what was done with it, and where and when it went, every time the evidence was handled.

Key Point:
Maintaining chain of custody is as simple as documenting who has the evidence, what was done with it, and where and when it went, every time the evidence was handled.

In crimes of sexual assault, the most common types of body fluids transferred are semen, blood, and saliva. Evidence that might contain these materials includes items such as clothing, and swabs from the skin, external genitalia, or other parts of the body where fluids might be present. The examiner should always be aware that DNA evidence may be present in areas other than the genitalia, such as the hair, abdomen, back, gluteal clefts, face, and neck. Often the patient cannot describe all the sex acts that occurred. Many individuals are vulnerable to sexual assault because they cannot communicate, and the offender counts on this. The victim may have been so fearful for her life that she did not realize all the areas penetrated. Some individuals may be embarrassed and unwilling to talk about oral or anal penetration. The very young, because of lack of development, and the older individual, because of communication difficulties due to disease complications, might not be able to communicate verbally what happened. For these and many other reasons, it is imperative that the forensic examiner conducts a thorough examination.

Key Point:
In crimes of sexual assault, the most common types of body fluids transferred are semen, blood, and saliva.

Altered states of consciousness and inability to remember detail because of drugs and alcohol are commonly a part of sexual assault and another reason why individuals cannot always articulate what happened to them. Unconscious patients present unique situations for evidence collection. When the patient is unconscious, the issue of consent for the examination can be addressed by obtaining consent from a legal guardian or by requesting a warrant from a judge. With life-threatening injuries in the unconscious patient, the hospital protocol regarding medical treatment consent must be adhered to; if the examiner is concerned about liability for the actions taken in collecting evidence, the legal guardian or warrant can be used. Whether or not the unconscious patient has consented will not affect the ability to use the evidence in court. (See Appendix II, "Search Warrant for the Unconscious Victim," p. 309-310).

Key Point:
Altered states of consciousness and inability to remember detail because of drugs and alcohol are commonly a part of sexual assault and another reason why individuals cannot always articulate what happened to them.

There will be little or no history as to what might have happened during the assault. The examiner must use all available critical thinking skills so that valuable evidence is not overlooked and lost. Clothing and swabs from the mouth, external genitalia, anus, and vagina should be collected as well as swabs from the skin where there may have been suspect-victim contact. Swabbing must include areas where a positive Wood's lamp reaction is indicated or where a victim provides a definitive history. Areas to consider are the face, neck, breasts, and any injuries that could be bite or suck marks. Nail swabbings or scrapings should always be performed. A good rule of thumb when collecting evidence from a comatose or deceased victim is when in doubt, collect, because there probably will not be another opportunity for proper collection.

Patient history indicating where the examiner is likely to find evidence is critical. Many times the detection of substances is not possible with the naked eye, and enhancement with other equipment is necessary. Wood's lamps and alternate light sources are the most commonly used pieces of equipment to enhance an examiner's ability to identify areas for collection. A Wood's lamp emits wavelengths of approximately 320 to 400 nm (Santucci et al., 1999). In this long-wave ultraviolet (UV) light, certain substances sometimes fluoresce; semen is one such substance. The room is darkened and the light is shined over the victim's body. Semen stains under UV light may fluoresce. If the semen stains have been subjected to a warm, moist environment, they may appear as a faint light yellow color because of bacterial growth.

Key Point:
Substances other than semen that fluoresce in the presence of UV light include urine, diaper rash medications, and ointments.

There are substances other than semen that fluoresce in the presence of UV light, so it is important that the examiner not assume that semen is present when there is a positive Wood's lamp finding. These include urine, diaper rash medications, and ointments. On the other hand, the examiner should not assume that semen is absent because of a negative Wood's lamp test, especially when victims provide a clear history of events. It is imperative to understand that the Wood's lamp is not a definitive test for the presence of semen but an aid in locating the fluid in some instances.

Questions often arise about whether or not DNA testing of seminal fluid in the absence of sperm can be successfully performed, as in cases where the offender has had a vasectomy. In this situation, male DNA is identified through the analysis of the epithelial cells, white blood cells, or other cell types present in seminal fluid.

Saliva evidence is a common DNA source in sexual assault and is usually placed on the victim through licking, kissing, sucking, and biting. Although saliva will not fluoresce in the presence of a Wood's lamp, an alternate light source that emits a different wavelength can cause saliva to fluoresce. As with semen, it is important for the examiner not to assume anything specific about the type of material that has been enhanced. In the male examination, it is common to collect swabs from the penis to determine the presence of saliva if fellatio was a part of the assault. Swabs collected from the vulva may contain saliva if cunnilingus was part of the assault in the female. Epithelial cells in the saliva are easy to identify in the crime laboratory whenever the possibility of saliva is suspected.

Fingernail scrapings or swabbings are another source of DNA material. If the victim gives a history of scratching the offender, or if there was a struggle between the victim and the suspect and there is a possibility that the suspect's skin or blood may be found under the victim's nails, this evidence should be collected. Some sexual assault examination kits come with labeled envelopes for this collection, or the wooden stick end of a swab can be used to scrape under the nail. One limitation of the scraping method is that it may add many cells from the nails of the person giving the sample, which can complicate the process of identifying the suspect. Another method of collection is to swab under the nails. As with all other evidence, nail scrapings should be properly labeled for location of collection, dried, and packaged to maintain the chain of custody.

One other potential source of DNA material is loose hair. Loose hair may have originated from the head, pubic area, beard, chest, legs, or arms of the suspect. If the hair has the root intact, a DNA profile may be obtained using nuclear DNA testing. In the absence of a root, mitochondrial DNA testing can be performed. Mitochondrial DNA testing provides limited information, but may be very import-ant evidence in some sexual assault cases.

Known reference samples collected to provide the DNA profiles of the victim and suspect may be as simple and noninvasive as collecting a buccal swab from inside the individual's cheek, or may be more invasive, such as drawing a tube of blood. Buccal samples contain epithelial cells and are a quick and painless method to collect a known DNA sample. Caution should be used in collecting buccal swabs from a sexual assault victim where there is a history of oral copulation of the suspect because semen may be present in the victim's mouth.

COLLECTION PROCEDURES

UNKNOWN SPECIMENS

DNA on Clothing

Clothing should be removed 1 item at a time and placed in separate paper sacks. Care should be taken to avoid folding through an observed stain. The stain should be photographed before packaging. The examiner should examine the clothing for any signs of force, such as missing buttons, stretched elastic, or tears. If signs of force are observed, the information must be relayed to the police officers at the scene. Most sexual assault cases result in the defendant claiming that the sexual act was consensual. Therefore any observations or information that corroborates the facts, such as finding the victim's fingernail or missing button at the scene, may be far more critical than obtaining biologic evidence during the forensic examination. It is also critical that the examiner asks whether clothing from the assault may be available at another location, and if so, this information must be relayed to law enforcement so that the clothing or other items of evidence can be recovered. An example of a clothing documentation form is included in Appendix II, "Clothing Documentation Form," p. 315-316. Some sexual assault documentation forms ask for specific information about the clothing. Communication between the examiner and law enforcement is crucial so that the evidence may be collected immediately. If the information is only documented without immediate communication, it may be hours or days before the information is noticed. During this time, valuable evidence may be lost or destroyed.

Oral Swabs in Cases of Oral Copulation

Take two cotton swabs and carefully swab between the cheek and gums, upper and lower lip and gums, where the gum meets the palate, and behind the incisors. Place these two swabs into a labeled holder and air dry before packaging, labeling, and documenting.

Dental Floss in Cases of Oral Copulation

Have the victim floss her teeth and collect the floss in a small envelope or paper bindle.

Biologic Material in Hair

Cut out the suspected area and place it in a paper bindle. The examiner should cut out only what is necessary to obtain an adequate sample and be sensitive to how the collection process will affect the victim's appearance.

Biologic Material on Skin

Semen

Moisten a swab with 1 drop of water and roll the swab over the area of interest to collect the specimen. Then place the swab in a labeled holder and allow to air dry before packaging (American College of Emergency Physicians [ACEP], 1999).

Saliva and Bite Marks

Moisten a cotton swab with 1 drop of sterile water and roll it over the area in question. Set this swab aside in a labeled swab holder. Take another swab that is not moistened and roll it over the same area. Both swabs are then labeled, dried, and packaged. There is no need to identify which was the moistened swab and which was not. This double swab technique has been shown to recover a greater number of cells. It is believed that the moisture present in the first swab rehydrates and loosens the majority of the epithelial cells dried in the saliva and causes them to adhere to the cotton fibers of the swab (Sweet et al., 1997).

DNA on Miscellaneous Items and Surfaces

Condoms

It is not uncommon to find a condom in the vagina when performing the pelvic examination. The examiner should first photograph the condom where it is found, then carefully remove it and place it in multiple paper bags. Because the condom is wet, it should be stored frozen as soon as possible. The crime lab will later collect swabs from both the inside and outside surfaces of the condom.

Shoes

Biologic material may be present on shoes. It may be impossible to tell just by looking at the stain. Photograph the stain with the shoes on, remove the shoes and photograph again from different angles, and then collect the shoes in a paper bag.

DNA from an Unknown Hair

If a loose hair is observed on the person being examined, it should be photographed and collected by picking it up with clean gloved fingers. Post-It® Notes work well, depending on what type of surface on which the hair is located, or a swab may be used and then placed in a paper bindle. Never use forceps or tweezers to collect unknown hair evidence because you may pluck the victim's own hair.

KNOWN REFERENCE SPECIMENS

Known samples typically consist of either a buccal swab or a blood specimen from the person being examined. Oral swabs are collected by rolling cotton swabs on the inside of the cheeks, dried, and then packaged in a labeled holder. One purple top tube of blood is collected for the known blood DNA sample. Different methods of preservation exist. The entire tube should be submitted with the identifying information by placing it into a bubble pack and then sealing it in the kit. This kit should be refrigerated to ensure preservation of the blood sample. Another method used for blood preservation is to place the blood onto a blood preservation card. The cards contain quarter-size circles that are saturated with the sample blood and then air dried. After the blood preservation card has dried, it is labeled, packaged, and sealed in the kit. Once specimens are collected, air dried, properly packaged, labeled, and documented, they must be transported to the police property room or forensic laboratory by law enforcement, maintaining the chain of custody at all times, where they may be analyzed later by crime lab personnel.

Meticulous and thorough evidence collection in the examination of sexual assault victims and suspects is essential. Collected evidence may prove crucial not only to implicate the guilty but also to exonerate the innocent.

LAW ENFORCEMENT INVESTIGATION

DNA AS A PROSECUTORIAL WEAPON

Advances in technology have made DNA testing an essential part of the sexual assault investigation and subsequent prosecution. Traditional serology identity testing methods for blood, saliva, and semen are now obsolete. The role of law enforcement has been limited in the United States, because DNA technology developed primarily as a prosecutorial weapon, not as an investigative tool. DNA evidence has been used to confirm the identity of someone already under suspicion by investigators and to corroborate a victim's history of the sexual assault by identifying evidence of sexual contact. DNA has also exonerated possible suspects and people wrongfully charged, convicted, and sentenced to prison for sexual assault, child molestation, and homicide. The National Institute of Justice published a report that presents case studies of 28 inmates for whom DNA analysis was exculpatory (Asplen, 1999). At the time the report was written in June 1996, at least 57 people had been shown by DNA evidence to have been wrongfully convicted. More recently, the release of Larry Mayes in Indiana on December 21, 2001, marked the 100th person to be freed nationwide because of genetic testing (Tanner, 2002).

Lack of DNA Training for Law Enforcement
and Forensic Examiners

In 1996 there were more than 17,000 cases involving forensic DNA in the United States alone, yet the potential for DNA evidence is far greater than its current use (Weedn & Hicks, 1997). Current limitations in DNA testing resources and the lack of proper training for law enforcement and sexual assault forensic examiners in the identification and collection of possible DNA evidence restrict its use. For example, many police officers and deputies are still evaluating the need for sexual assault forensic examinations based on their outdated understanding of serology. As a result, they often do not obtain forensic examinations unless the victim describes penetration and ejaculation, believing that semen must be present to obtain positive forensic results. Officers must be trained to obtain forensic examinations in a multitude of scenarios even in the absence of penetration and ejaculation, such as oral contact with any part of the victim's body, digital penetration, or oral copulation. In most circumstances, officers should be instructed to collect and impound evidence to be analyzed later by criminologists who have the proper equipment and training to identify and extract biologic evidence. Whenever possible, vehicles, sofa cushions, window screens, bedding, and any other moveable items should be preserved and impounded by police. When the evidence cannot be moved, such as a sidewalk where a suspect is believed to have ejaculated, a criminologist, crime scene specialist, or patrol officer trained in forensic evidence collection procedures should respond to obtain proper swabs of the biologic sample in question and appropriate control swabs. In addition to developing training procedures regarding the identification and collection of biologic evidence, law enforcement agencies must establish protocols for the proper transportation and storage of biologic evidence. It is important to keep biologic samples refrigerated or frozen. Other evidence, such as bedding and clothing, should be kept dry and at room temperature in paper bags or envelopes. Direct sunlight and warm conditions may be harmful to DNA, so evidence should not be placed in locations that may get hot, such as a property room or police car, without air conditioning or refrigeration. For longer storage issues, the general rule is the colder the better. The National Institute of Justice, in cooperation with the National Commission on the Future of DNA, has developed a brochure, "What Every Law Enforcement Officer Should Know About DNA Evidence." The brochure is a valuable resource for first responders and prosecutors and will go a long way toward filling this critical training gap.

DNA testing has been conducted primarily in cases of sexual assault where vaginal sexual assault swabs or semen stain evidence has been obtained. However, saliva, blood, tissue, urine, feces and other biologic specimens may also be sources of DNA found at crime scenes (**Tables 16-2 a** to **e**). For example, a suspect's saliva may be found on a sexual assault victim's bra worn during the assault. It may also be found in chewing gum; cigarette butts; clothing such as underwear, hats, masks, and bandanas; envelopes or stamps; and drinking cups.

Suspect Exams

Many law enforcement agencies recognize the value of a forensic examination for sexual assault victims; however, many still fail to obtain forensic examinations for suspects even if they are arrested within a relatively short period of time after a sexual assault. Law enforcement and forensic examiners must recognize that just as potential evidence was transferred from the suspect to the victim, evidence also may have been transferred from the victim to the suspect. Documentation of genital abnormalities, tattoos, and venereal warts can help to corroborate the identity of the suspect. Any evidence of scratches, bites, and abrasions can be used to overcome a consent defense by corroborating the use of force by the suspect and/or resistance by the victim. Fingernail scrapings or swabbings from a suspect's hands may corroborate digital penetration of the victim's genitals even after the suspect has

Key Point:

Law enforcement and forensic examiners must recognize that just as potential evidence was transferred from the suspect to the victim, evidence may have been transferred from the victim to the suspect.

bathed. Some jurisdictions may require a search warrant or a court order before authorizing a suspect examination to obtain forensic evidence. Prosecutors and law enforcement should create a template to facilitate this important step of the sexual assault investigation. (See Appendix II "Search Warrant," p. 307-308.)

REEXAMINING UNSOLVED SEXUAL ASSAULT CASES

The DNA molecule is long-lived and detectable for many years in bones or body fluid, making it possible for old crimes to be solved and possibly prosecuted using current forensic technology. Investigators and prosecutors, however, must be trained to reevaluate these cases and identify those that lend themselves to DNA testing. On September 28, 2000, California enacted landmark legislation by creating an infrastructure to collect DNA on missing persons and unidentified deceased persons. Currently, in California there are an estimated 3000 persons reported missing to law enforcement that fit the criteria and at least 2100 unidentified deceased persons, of which approximately 150 are children. These numbers were identified from records at the California Department of Justice Missing and Unidentified Persons Unit and span a period of over 20 years (California State Senate Bill 1818, 2000).

Changes in DNA technology have prompted legislative changes across the country regarding the statute of limitations for sexual assault (California Penal Code, 2001). California recently passed a law extending the statute of limitations for sexual assault from 6 to 10 years; in cases in which a DNA profile is obtained but a suspect not yet identified, there is no statute of limitations (California Penal Code, 2001). Wisconsin and other states have managed to successfully work beyond the statute of limitations by using the DNA profile to obtain an arrest warrant for a John Doe. Once an arrest warrant is obtained, the statute of limitations ceases to run until the suspect is apprehended by law enforcement.

CRITICAL SHORTAGE OF CRIME LABORATORY RESOURCES

The potential for DNA evidence is almost unlimited, and although these advances are exciting and extremely valuable for law enforcement and the community, the use of DNA evidence and the technology required for its analysis also exposes the severe budget limitations of our forensic crime labs and the need for additional funds to properly support these labs. Because funding will always be an issue, investigators, criminologists, forensic examiners, and prosecutors must recognize resource limitations and prioritize lab service requests based upon everyone's needs. Representation for victims whose low-profile cases do not receive the attention they deserve, should take priority over individual cases, and those with other overwhelming evidence of a suspect's guilt. In defense of those prosecutors who request DNA work when investigators feel there is more than enough evidence to prove a suspect guilty beyond a reasonable doubt, jurors are generally educated about police procedures, including DNA, by inaccurate portrayals of courtroom proceedings seen on television. Consequently, juries often expect DNA evidence regardless of the defense, and the suspect's attorney will use failure to obtain the expected evidence in court. Because of the severe resource limitations of crime laboratories, prosecutors should consider using experts to explain why laboratory work was not requested rather than leaving the question open.

Currently, DNA evidence often is not collected from the crime scene or not analyzed by crime laboratories because of limited resources. An FBI survey revealed that of all rapes, fewer than 10% had evidence submitted to crime laboratories. As a result of limited resources in crime laboratories, in only 6% of the 250,000 cases investigated was evidence tested for DNA, leaving a backlog of over 200,000 cases waiting to be processed (US Department of Justice, 1999). It is important to note that because of current training issues, potential requests from law enforcement and prosecutors for laboratory work regarding sexual assault cases may be significantly underestimated. In many law enforcement jurisdictions, DNA analysis is never

Table 16-2-a. Crime Scene Evidence: Victim's Clothing

1998 and 1999 SDPD Crime Laboratory Work—25 Female Adolescent Sexual Assault Cases (ages 14-17)

Crime Scene Evidence Associated with the Victim	Individual Pieces of Evidence Examined	Total Number	Semen Found	DNA Work Performed	Suspect Included	Blood Found	DNA Work Performed	Suspect Included	Epithelial Cells Found	DNA Work Performed	Suspect Included
Victim's Clothing:	— Women's underwear	13	8	7	6	1			2	1	
	— Pants/jeans/shorts/skirt	8	3	2	2	1					
	— Shirt/blouse/sweatshirt	7	1	1	1	1					
	— Bra	3	1						1	1	1
	— Night gown	2	1	1							
	— Dress	1	1	1	1	1					
	— Men's underwear	2	1	1		1					
	— Socks	1	1	1	1						
	— Robe	2									
	— Jacket	1									
	Combined Total:	40	17	14	11	5	0	0	3	2	1

1998 and 1999 SDPD Crime Laboratory Work—51 Female Adult Sexual Assault Cases (ages 18+)

Crime Scene Evidence Associated with the Victim	Individual Pieces of Evidence Examined	Total Number	Semen Found	DNA Work Performed	Suspect Included	Blood Found	DNA Work Performed	Suspect Included	Epithelial Cells Found	DNA Work Performed	Suspect Included
Victim's Clothing:	— Women's underwear	25	10	3	1	6	1		1		
	— Pants/jeans/shorts/skirt	14	4	4	1	2					
	— Shirt/blouse/sweatshirt	7	1			1					
	— Bra	4									
	— Men's underwear	1									
	— Dress	1	1	1							
	— Swimsuit	1	1	1							
	— Jacket	1	1	1							
	— Hospital gown	1									
	— Shoes	1									
	Combined Total:	56	18	10	2	9	1	0	1	0	0

Suspect Included = The known suspect is included as a possible contributor of the semen, blood, or epithelial cells found on the individual pieces of evidence that received DNA analysis.

Table 16-2-b. Crime Scene Evidence: Other Evidence Associated with Victim

1998 and 1999 SDPD Crime Laboratory Work—25 Female Adolescent Sexual Assault Cases (ages 14-17)

Crime Scene Evidence Associated with the Victim	Individual Pieces of Evidence Examined	Total Number	Semen Found	DNA Work Performed	Suspect Included	Blood Found	DNA Work Performed	Suspect Included	Epithelial Cells Found	DNA Work Performed	Suspect Included
Other:	— Bedding	6				1	1				
	— Mattress (section)	2									
	— Carpet	2									
	— Car interior	1									
	— Car seat	1									
	— Sleeping bag	1				1					
	— Wall sample	1									
	— Sofa	1									
	— Rug	1									
	Combined Total:	16	0	0	0	2	1	0	0	0	0

1998 and 1999 SDPD Crime Laboratory Work—51 Female Adult Sexual Assault Cases (ages 18+)

Crime Scene Evidence Associated with the Victim	Individual Pieces of Evidence Examined	Total Number	Semen Found	DNA Work Performed	Suspect Included	Blood Found	DNA Work Performed	Suspect Included	Epithelial Cells Found	DNA Work Performed	Suspect Included
Other:	— Bedding	12	1								
	— Car fender	3	1	1	1				1		
	— Car interior	2									
	— Piece of plastic	1	1	1	1	1	1				
	— Tampon/sanitary pad	1									
	— Desenex powder bottle	1									
	— Carpet	1									
	— Car seat	1									
	— Car glove box	1									
	Combined Total:	23	3	2	2	1	1	0	1	0	0

Suspect Included = The known suspect is included as a possible contributor of the semen, blood, or epithelial cells found on the individual pieces of evidence that received DNA analysis.

Table 16-2-c. Crime Scene Evidence: Suspect's Clothing and Other

1998 and 1999 SDPD Crime Laboratory Work—25 Female Adolescent Sexual Assault Cases (ages 14-17)

Crime Scene Evidence Associated with the Victim	Individual Pieces of Evidence Examined	Total Number	Semen Found	DNA Work Performed	Suspect Included	Blood Found	DNA Work Performed	Victim Included	Epithelial Cells Found	DNA Work Performed	Victim Included
Suspect's Clothing and Other:	— Pants/jeans/shorts	1									
	— Shirt/sweatshirt	1				1	1	1			
	— Men's underwear	1				1	1	1			
	— Socks	1									
	— Shoes	1									
	— Belt	1									
	— Condom	1	1	1	1				1	1	1
	— Glass bottle	1				1	1	1			
	Combined Total:	8	1	1	1	3	3	3	1	1	1

1998 and 1999 SDPD Crime Laboratory Work—51 Female Adult Sexual Assault Cases (ages 18+)

Crime Scene Evidence Associated with the Victim	Individual Pieces of Evidence Examined	Total Number	Semen Found	DNA Work Performed	Suspect Included	Blood Found	DNA Work Performed	Victim Included	Epithelial Cells Found	DNA Work Performed	Victim Included
Suspect's Clothing and Other:	— Pants/jeans/shorts	3	1	1		1	1	1			
	— Shirt/sweatshirt	3				1	1				
	— Men's underwear	2									
	— Socks	1									
	— Shoes	1									
	— Belt	1									
	— Jacket	1									
	— Baseball cap	1									
	— Condom	1	1	1	1				1	1	1
	— Tissue	1								1	1
	Combined Total:	15	2	2	1	2	2	1	1	2	2

Suspect Included = The known suspect is included as a possible contributor of the semen, blood, or epithelial cells found on the individual pieces of evidence that received DNA analysis.

Table 16-2-d. SART Exam Evidence: Victim

1998 and 1999 SDPD Crime Laboratory Work—25 Female Adolescent Sexual Assault Cases (ages 14-17)

Crime Scene Evidence Associated with the Victim	Individual Pieces of Evidence Examined	Total Number	Semen Found	DNA Work Performed	Suspect Included	Blood Found	DNA Work Performed	Suspect Included	Epithelial Cells Found	DNA Work Performed	Suspect Included
Swabs/ Specimens of the Victim and Other:	— Vaginal (internal, cervical swab	19	10	8	5	4					
	— External genitalia/vaginal swab	19	10	5	4	2					
	— Rectal/anal (external) swab	16	4			1					
	— External body swab	20	3	1					2	1	
	— Oral/saliva/throat swab	19									
	— Tampon/sanitary pad	2	1			1					
	Combined Total:	95	28	14	9	8	0	0	2	1	0

1998 and 1999 SDPD Crime Laboratory Work—51 Female Adult Sexual Assault Cases (ages 18+)

Crime Scene Evidence Associated with the Victim	Individual Pieces of Evidence Examined	Total Number	Semen Found	DNA Work Performed	Suspect Included	Blood Found	DNA Work Performed	Suspect Included	Epithelial Cells Found	DNA Work Performed	Suspect Included
Swabs/ Specimens of the Victim and Other:	— Vaginal (internal, cervical) swab	49	17	8	4	10					
	— External genitalia/vaginal swab	36	16	4	2	3	1				
	— Rectal/anal (external) swab	22	6	3	1	2					
	— External body swab	46	12	4	2				11	9	7
	— Oral/saliva/throat swab	13	1			1					
	— Tampon/sanitary pad	3	2	1	1	1					
	— Matted public hair cutting	1	1	1	1						
	— Vaginal lavage (2 mm in a tube)	1									
	Combined Total:	171	55	21	11	17	1	0	11	9	7

Suspect Included = The known suspect is included as a possible contributor of the semen, blood, or epithelial cells found on the individual pieces of evidence that received DNA analysis.

Table 16-2-e. Forensic Evidence: Suspect

1998 and 1999 SDPD Crime Laboratory Work—25 Female Adolescent Sexual Assault Cases (ages 14-17)

Crime Scene Evidence Associated with the Victim	Individual Pieces of Evidence Examined	Total Number	Semen Found	DNA Work Performed	Suspect Included	Blood Found	DNA Work Performed	Victim Included	Epithelial Cells Found	DNA Work Performed	Victim Included
Forensic Examination: (Taken at SDPD)	— Penile swab	5	4	3	3				4	4	3
	— External body swab	2								2	1
	— Fingernail scrapings	2									
	Combined Total:	9	4	3	3	0	0	0	4	6	4

1998 and 1999 SDPD Crime Laboratory Work—51 Female Adult Sexual Assault Cases (ages 18+)

Crime Scene Evidence Associated with the Victim	Individual Pieces of Evidence Examined	Total Number	Semen Found	DNA Work Performed	Suspect Included	Blood Found	DNA Work Performed	Victim Included	Epithelial Cells Found	DNA Work Performed	Victim Included
Forensic Examination: (Taken at SDPD)	— Penile swab	10	5	8	7	1	1	1	3	3	3
	— External body swab	6				2	2	2			
	— Fingernail scrapings	7		4	1						
	— Penis ring	1	1	1	1						
	— Pubic swab	1		1							
	Combined Total:	25	6	14	9	3	3	3	3	3	3

Suspect Included = The suspect is included as a possible contributor of the semen found on the suspect's evidence. This is done to show that the semen does match the known suspect.

Victim Included = The victim is included as a possible contributor of the blood or epithelial cells found on the individual pieces of suspect evidence that received DNA analysis.

completed for cases in which no suspect has been identified. Investigators cannot obtain access to the most valuable tool available because of the shortage of resources and the fact that prosecutors have historically driven the allocation of laboratory resources. To illustrate this point, in 1998 and 1999, 355 adult sexual assault victims were examined by sexual assault nurse examiners following sexual assaults within the city of San Diego. Of those 355 cases, only 51, approximately 1%, received some form of laboratory analysis. One case had crime scene evidence available that was examined by the crime laboratory even though a sexual assault examination was not obtained due to the delay in reporting the crime. During that same time period, physicians at Children's Hospital performed 131 sexual assault exams on adolescents (age 14 to 17 years); only 26 of those cases, approximately 20%, had some form of laboratory work completed. Laboratory work may be requested more frequently for cases involving adolescents because consent may not be used as a defense; therefore, sexual contact is usually sufficient evidence to establish the corpus of the crime.

Nationally, 74% of sexual assaults will be perpetrated by non-strangers (US Department of Justice, 1999). The relationship between the victim and the offender and the age of the victim will significantly influence the type of laboratory work requested by the investigating officer. Sixty percent of the cases examined by the San Diego Police Department Forensic Science Unit in 1998 and 1999 involved nonstranger suspects, whereas 40% involved strangers. Of the 51 cases screened for DNA evidence, 32 cases (64%) went on to have DNA work completed, and those cases were equally divided between stranger and nonstranger cases. The District Attorney filed charges in 80% of the cases that had laboratory work. The percentage was even higher when the suspect was a stranger: the District Attorney filed charges in 94.4 % of the cases in which laboratory work was done, but in only half of the cases when no laboratory work was done (LaCoss, 2000). With the increased resources being provided to crime laboratories and the adoption of a PCR technology known as short tandem repeats (STR) as a national DNA standard, drastic changes are occurring in a sex crimes investigator's ability to link cases and identify suspects.

CASE-TO-CASE COLD HITS

Although California has had only a limited number of DNA database hits, several cases in San Diego can provide some insight into the power of STR technology when employed in collective databases. For example, a detective was assigned to investigate the rape of a woman who was walking around a lake with her toddler and her baby in a stroller on a Saturday afternoon in 1997. A suspect matching the description was arrested a short distance from the assault; however, he was excluded by DNA. The case was investigated until all leads were exhausted. In May 2000, a woman was sodomized after the suspect committed a nighttime home invasion. Although detectives would not have linked these two cases based on traditional law enforcement profiling methods, DNA evidence revealed that the same suspect committed both sexual assaults. More recently, an unsolved 1995 case was linked to the same suspect. In that case, the victim was washing her clothes in a public laundromat on a weekend afternoon when the suspect, armed with a gun, raped her. The suspect has yet to be identified, because the DNA profile failed to match an offender in the CODIS database. However, even without a database hit, once cases are linked, investigators can again comb through the investigations to look for clues that might have been missed when looking at each case individually. In addition, geographic maps can be generated, and victims can be profiled to look for any commonalities. A combination of case histories, witness statements, and other associated pieces of evidence may point investigators in a new direction that will result in the identification of a suspect. The DNA profile can be routinely searched in the CODIS database in the hope that the suspect's profile has been entered since the previous search.

RESOURCE MANAGEMENT

Resources and budget constraints will always be an issue for law enforcement agencies. As a result of the demand for DNA analysis, crime laboratories, police investigators, and prosecutors must learn to rethink how and why laboratory service requests are developed. Investigators and prosecutors must learn to assess and interpret all evidence associated with a case, such as the telephone call to police communications; spontaneous statements; the crime scene diagram and photographs; witness statements; the forensic evidence based on the elements of the assault (i.e., child molestation, where consent is not a defense, blitz stranger assault, which is generally a question of identity, or a nonstranger assault, which is generally a question of corroborating a lack of consent; and the suspect's statement(s) and his defense strategy. Investigators and prosecutors often request laboratory work to screen for the presence of semen and DNA analysis even though the suspect admitted to having sex with the victim and the legal issue is one of consent. However, a laboratory service request to evaluate evidence for blood, to analyze fingernail scrapings, or to have hair examined for evidence of being stretched and therefore pulled from the victim's head is more important in establishing the use of force by the suspect or resistance by the victim.

Key Point:
As a result of the demand for DNA analysis, crime laboratories, police investigators, and prosecutors must learn to rethink how and why laboratory service requests are developed.

Most states have child abuse laws making it a felony to engage in any sexual con-duct with a child under age 12 or 14 years, depending on the state. The 1999 National Crime Victimization Survey (US Department of Justice, 2000) reported that in one third of all sexual assaults reported to law enforcement, the victim was younger than 12 years of age. For victims this young, the offender was a family member in 47% of the assaults, an acquaintance in 49%, and a stranger in only 4%. In the case of child molestation or sexual assaults involving children, consent is not a defense. In those cases, if the suspect denies sexual contact, DNA work will be extremely helpful in identifying the perpetrator and establishing sexual contact. Most states have statutory rape laws making it illegal to engage in sexual conduct with a child under age 18 years (or in some states age 16 years), even if the victim "consented." However, penalties are much less severe for statutory rape and, at least in California, it is not an offense requiring sex offender registration upon conviction. If investigators and prosecutors are pursuing allegations of forcible sexual assault or drug-facilitated sexual assault involving an adolescent, the defendant is likely to claim the sexual act was consensual. Because of the high-risk activities of many adolescents and perceived credibility issues, many rapes and other sexual assaults involving adolescents are pleaded out as cases of statutory rape. Therefore, it is imperative that investigators and prosecutors have the skills to identify potential evidence that can be used to overcome the most common defense in a sexual assault case involving a statutory rape defense with an adolescent or a consent defense with an adult.

IMPROVING COMMUNICATION BETWEEN INVESTIGATORS AND CRIMINOLOGISTS

In many jurisdictions, crime scene evidence and forensic evidence kits are submitted directly to crime laboratories, where a criminologist might begin laboratory work without consulting the case detective to obtain a complete history of the assault, suspect statements, or the status of the case. (Many victims decline prosecution or are unable to participate in the criminal justice system as a result of the trauma they continue to suffer caused by the sexual assault.) To improve communication between investigators and criminologists and to guide investigators, the San Diego Police Department created a Preliminary Sexual Assault Information form to help them correctly assess the nature of the sexual assault (i.e., oral copulation, penile vaginal intercourse, or sodomy) and potential evidence sites before submitting a laboratory service request for evidence work. The form includes questions about whether the victim knows if the suspect ejaculated, if he used a condom, or if either the suspect or victim bled during the assault. The investigator is asked specifically about any clothing worn during and after the sexual assault. (See Appendix II, "Preliminary Rape Case Information Form," p. 313-314.) Recent analysis of the 51 cases that received laboratory work during 1998 and 1999 indicated that 60% of the clothing examined was positive for evidence (P. O'Donnell, personal communication, 2002). Therefore, it is imperative that, even in cases beyond the normal 72-hour window of opportunity for an acute forensic examination, first responders determine whether clothing, bedding, or other evidence associated with the assault might still be available. (See Appendix II, "Clothing Documentation Form," p. 315-316.) The form also prompts and reminds an investigator of work that needs to be done prior to submitting a laboratory request. For example, if reference samples are not provided for both the victim and suspect, laboratory work will generally not be initiated. With an adolescent, if the victim engaged in consensual sex with an age-appropriate boyfriend before the sexual assault, laboratory work would also be delayed until the consenting partner's reference sample is obtained. (See Appendix II, "Preliminary Rape Case Information Form," p. 313-314.)

Once the Sexual Assault Case Information Form is completed, the investigating officer is ready to fill out the Lab Service Request. Many veteran officers, detectives, and forensic examiners do not understand the difference between trace evidence (hairs, fibers, paints, glass, shoe prints, gun shot residue, and other physical matches) and biologic evidence (blood, semen, and saliva). In many crime laboratories, these 2 functions are performed in different units. Because of the limitations of serology, trace evidence used to be paramount in a sexual assault investigation. However, because of the advent of DNA analysis and its remarkable sensitivity and power of discrimination, trace evidence evaluation is used only rarely in sexual assault investigations (Scheck et al., 2000). Many investigators and prosecutors are still thinking and prioritizing laboratory requests based on serologic or trace evidence standards. This form helps to differentiate between these 2 types of evidence and then, based on the history of the assault and the evidence impounded, the detective specifically lists in order of priority which item(s) of evidence he or she wants the criminologist to examine. In past years, detectives often would submit only a 1-line request that all the evidence be screened for potential trace and semen evidence without any understanding of the consequence of that request or the impact potential laboratory results might have on the investigation and subsequent prosecution of the case. This practice must cease, and more detailed communication must be encouraged at all levels.

DNA evidence is a double-edged sword that cuts both ways. Victim assistance providers and criminal justice officials must be prepared to help victims understand and cope when DNA evidence points to an individual other than the person the victim identified or investigators suspected.

Post-conviction testing in older cases has the potential to either confirm an identification or indicate that the wrong person was convicted. Many of the cases in which post-conviction testing of DNA evidence showed that the convicted person was not the perpetrator involved convictions based on eyewitness testimony by victims or witnesses. Challenging a conviction with DNA testing in these cases may be the right thing to do, but it may cause great distress to victims and their families, who believe that the crime is behind them. Courts do not accept many requests for post-conviction DNA testing, but criminal justice personnel should ensure that victims are notified of such requests, particularly if it is required by state statute or if it appears likely that the testing will go forward. Notification should be done by the prosecutor's office, preferably by someone who has worked with the victim in the past. Victims should not hear about the request from the media, the defendant, or the defendant's attorney or family. Victims should be provided with an understandable explanation of DNA evidence, the process, and the meaning of potential outcomes. Referrals for counseling and other support should be provided.

Key Point:
It is imperative that, even in cases past the normal 72-hour window of opportunity for an acute forensic examination, first responders determine whether clothing, bedding, or other evidence associated with the assault might still be available.

Key Point:
Victim assistance providers and criminal justice officials must be prepared to help victims understand and cope when DNA evidence points to an individual other than the person the victim identified or who was suspected by investigators.

APPENDIX I: DNA CASE STUDIES

Disclaimer: All DNA case histories and information from the San Diego Police Department is courtesy of Joanne Archambault. To protect the privacy of the victims, all names and identifying features have been changed.

INTRODUCTION

It is important that all sexual assault response team members—physicians, nurses, law enforcement, prosecutors, community based advocates, and state victim witness assistance employees—understand the complexity of a sexual assault investigation. Each of these disciplines may provide an important piece of the puzzle. However, none of these pieces alone provides a clear and credible picture of what happened. Juries must be provided with detailed information that will recreate what the victim experienced during the sexual assault. Only then will sex offenders be held accountable for their violent crimes.

Rape crisis center advocates will be better able to assist their clients if they have a thorough understanding of appropriate investigative procedures and possible criminal justice outcomes. Forensic examiners can do a better examination and collect evidence more effectively if they are provided with crime laboratory results and feedback when the rape kits they collect are screened for evidence and profiled for DNA. Many law enforcement officers and prosecutors believe that a forensic examiner can tell them if the victim was raped. They need to be educated about what information a forensic examination can provide, that is, evidence of sexual contact and documentation of injury that may be consistent or sometimes inconsistent with the history provided by the victim. Most importantly, law enforcement officers and prosecutors must remember that forensic examiners are asked to collect forensic evidence, which then must be examined by a trained criminologist before a conclusion is made as to whether probative evidence exists. However, the detection of forensic evidence and its analysis is only 1 step in an extremely complex investigation. Any evidence identified and subsequently tested then must be assessed and interpreted based on the history provided by the victim, witnesses, and the suspect's own statements. It is essential to evaluate the potential impact of all evidence. For example, the presence of incriminating DNA evidence involving the sexual assault of a child is often all that is needed, because the suspect cannot effectively claim the act was consensual. However, sex offenders frequently use a consent defense in cases involving adolescents and adults. In these cases, the documentation of injuries, witness statements, and investigative tactics are critical to the successful prosecution of the offender.

To date, law enforcement has been provided with limited training opportunities concerning the forensic DNA revolution. Investigators do not understand clearly how DNA technology might assist their investigation, nor do they understand what scientific procedures might be used to screen and profile their cases. Some agencies may only submit the victim's rape kit, whereas others submit the rape kit and other crime scene evidence such as clothing, foreign objects, condoms, or seat cushions. Contributing to the problem is the fact that some law enforcement agencies have their own crime laboratories, others use their state crime laboratories, and still others may use the FBI or private laboratories. As a result, each of these agencies may have access to laboratories using different scientific procedures to screen and profile biologic evidence. It is important to understand what screening methods are available and what methods were used in a particular case (i.e., acid phosphatase, P30, microscopy, visual evaluation, alternate light source examination, Christmas Tree Stain, DNA, etc). In addition to variations in the scientific methods employed by crime laboratories, some hospitals and forensic examiner programs have conducted their own tests (Pap smears or microscopy, for instance) in an effort to identify evidence that might help shed light on the investigation and the possible outcome. When evaluating whether probative evidence exists, it is important to understand the significance of the evidence collected and the methods employed to screen and characterize the evidence.

Many other issues may also surface during the course of a criminal investigation. The crime laboratory may find DNA, but a match in the state and national database cannot be made and law enforcement cannot identify a suspect through traditional investigative means. A DNA match may be made several years after the assault, and the victim cannot be found. If the victim is found and contacted, he or she may be unwilling or unable to participate in a trial, often as a result of the sexual assault. In other cases, the DNA testing results may refute all the other evidence in the case. In many cases, the detective conducts a thorough investigation and the forensic evidence corroborates the victim's allegations. However, the prosecuting agency does not feel that there is enough evidence to prove the case beyond a reasonable doubt and the case is rejected.

Finally, it is important to understand the statistical approach used to express the significance when 2 DNA profiles match. Because of the various DNA typing methods previously available and their continued evolution, cases within the same series and year may contain different DNA profile information. For example, PCR DQA1/Polymarker match frequencies are commonly 1 in several thousand, while STRs are 1 in several billion. In addition, many detectives and prosecutors are surprised and disconcerted when a laboratory report comes back stating only that the suspect could not be excluded or that the suspect can be included when they expect to hear an unequivocal statement of confirmation. It is essential to under-stand the role of criminologists and how they will be required to testify about their findings in court.

The following case summaries are an attempt to offer a complete overview of the critical elements of a sexual assault investigation.

CASE STUDY #1
Victim: M.D. H/F 28
Suspect: H.M. 24
On June 15, 1999, the victim was helping a friend move. The suspect, a coworker, who was also helping, pinned the victim against a wall where he sexually battered her. The suspect was able to get his clothes off while he was on top of the victim. He penetrated her vagina with his finger. He kissed the victim on the mouth and breasts. The victim tried to use her knees to hold him back. The suspect grabbed both of the victim's knees to prevent her from stopping him. He suddenly pene-trated her vagina with his penis. The victim said she was still trying to get away from him while he had sex with her.

Afterward, the victim couldn't leave because she didn't have a ride. She stayed and helped the suspect finish loading the remaining items into his truck. Once they returned, the suspect left and the victim was given a ride to her car by another friend, and then drove home. The next day, the victim told 2 coworkers what had happened. They both encouraged her to call the police. The victim called another friend on June 18. This friend also encouraged her to call the police, which she did. The victim was transported to the SART hospital. The forensic examiner noted redness at the 6 o'clock position of the posterior fourchette with an abrasion and a healing tear that showed toluidine blue dye uptake.

Evidence:

— Victim's rape kit and clothing

— Suspect's buccal swab for DNA reference sample

— Police communications print out

— Polaroid photograph of victim taken by SART nurse

— Polaroid photograph of suspect taken by detective

Suspect's Statement:

The suspect was interviewed in person. He was not in custody, and as such he was not advised of his Miranda rights. The suspect said he met the victim at work. Their relationship was strictly professional other than a couple of occasions when they met socially as part of a softball team. There was never any flirting between them or any indication they were attracted to each other. The suspect is married and lives with his wife.

The suspect said he was helping a coworker move. The suspect and victim were talking. The suspect moved behind the victim and started rubbing her shoulders. She said it felt good and turned around and kissed him on the lips. The suspect kissed her back and moved his hands across the victim's shirtfront, touching her breasts through the shirt material. The victim moved her hand down, groping the suspect's groin through his clothing and then she pulled his shirt free from his pants. The suspect then moved his hands under the victim's shirt, touching her breasts inside her bra, skin to skin. The suspect said the victim pulled his shirt off over his head. The suspect took off the victim's sweatshirt, shirt, and bra. They then helped each other out of their pants and underwear. The victim and suspect both went down to the floor willingly. The suspect used his finger to penetrate the victim's vagina. The suspect then penetrated the victim's vagina with his penis and had sex with her for 2 to 3 minutes. The suspect said he stopped because he realized he is married and got caught up in the moment.

Laboratory Results:

The detective submitted the victim's underwear to the crime lab and asked that they be screened for semen and trace evidence to corroborate sexual activity only. DNA analysis was not requested because there was not a question of identity.

Summary of Analytical Procedures:

— Visual and alternate light examination

— Phenolphthalein presumptive test for blood

— Calcium alpha-naphthyl phosphate presumptive test for semen

— Digestion of the sample by SDS and proteinase K

— Microscopy for the presence of spermatozoa and non-spermatozoa cells

— Crossover electrophoresis for seminal protein P-30

Results:

No semen was found on the pair of white underwear, cervical swabs, or vaginal swabs. A positive presumptive test for blood was obtained on the crotch area of the victim's underwear.

Legal Outcome:

The suspect pleaded guilty to felony sexual battery. The rape and penetration with a foreign object were dropped for the plea. The suspect was sentenced to 3 years probation. He is subject to search and seizure and is required to register as a sex offender for life.

CASE STUDY #2

Victim: J.B. W/F 20

Suspect: D.E. B/M 29

The victim and several of her friends, including the suspect, who was a neighbor, had a small gathering at the victim's condominium. At 2300 hours, the suspect brought alcohol and other ingredients to make alcoholic beverages. The suspect gave the victim 1 of the drinks, which he called a "pink panties," and the victim passed out approximately 20 minutes later. Sometime during the evening, the victim went to her bedroom alone. At 0100 hours, everyone including the suspect left. At approximately 0330 hours, the victim woke up with the suspect orally copulating her vagina. The victim yelled at the suspect to get out and she passed out again. She woke up some time later and the suspect was on top of her having sexual intercourse with her. The victim again yelled at the suspect to stop and get out. She passed out again and didn't wake up until late the next morning. Her legs and vagina were covered with blood. The victim asked her roommate what happened. The roommate told the victim she was really drunk. The victim said she had only 1 drink and it was the drink the suspect gave her.

The night of the party, the roommate confronted the suspect about the victim's level of intoxication and the suspect said the victim had been doing shooters with him in the kitchen. The victim denied having anything else to drink but the 1 drink the suspect provided her. The victim said the suspect had gone into her bedroom during the night because he forgot his shoes and returned to get them. The victim told her roommate that the suspect had oral sex with her against her will. The roommate pointed out some dirt under a window and they decided to call the police.

The victim told the reporting officer that she drinks socially and has always been able to handle the effects of alcohol. The victim said she felt like she had been drugged because she was so incoherent after only 1 drink.

The victim's roommate showed the officer a rear window near the dining area. The witness said the window had been left open the night before but the screen was on. The officer noticed the screen was bent and off its track. There was dirt on the carpet underneath the window. The dirt appeared to be the same dirt as found directly outside the window. The witness/roommate also said she locked the front door when the last person left at 0100 hours but the front door was unlocked in the morning.

Officers contacted the suspect. The suspect said he saw the victim drink 2 to 3 drinks. He noticed that she went to bed sometime between 0100 and 0130 hours. A short time later, everyone left, including the suspect. At approximately 0220 hours, the suspect realized he left his shoes and keys inside the victim's condo. He knocked on the door but no one answered. He walked around to the victim's window and noticed the light was on. He knocked on the window to get her attention. The victim motioned him to go to the front door where she let him in. They talked in the living room for 15 minutes until the victim said she was tired and asked D.E. if he wanted to go to her room. They began talking and one thing led to another. D.E. said the victim told him to "eat her out". D.E. did. She then told him to "put it in," meaning put his penis inside her vagina. D.E. put on a condom and put his penis inside the victim's vagina. Once he was inside her, she asked him to stop and he did. The suspect was not sure if he ejaculated or not. The victim walked him to the front door and said good night. D.E. denied seeing any blood on the victim or hearing her say he hurt her.

The suspect voluntarily gave the officer the clothing he was wearing the night before. Officers photographed the scene, drew a diagram, and collected the evidence.

The victim was examined at the SART hospital. The examiner saw and documented visible trauma to the victim's clitoral hood. Blood was oozing from the victim's cervix, indicating she had started her menstrual cycle.

When Detective O. received this case, she ran a criminal history and discovered that another sex crimes detective had investigated D.E. for a similar sexual assault. That case had been rejected by the District Attorney's office. The urine in that case had been submitted to a private toxicology laboratory, but, due to an error in the report, it was believed that the results were negative at the time.

A search warrant was executed at the suspect's home to look for drugs commonly used to facilitate sexual assault, their packaging, or precursors. Several bottles containing questionable substances were located, seized, and impounded.

— HMB bottle located in kitchen drawer

— Rite Aid eye drop bottle

— Visine eye drop bottle

— Erythromycin stearate bottle

— Universal creatine bottle

— Golden seal bottle

— Androstene bottle

— HMB bottle located in suspect's gym bag

— GNC melatonin bottle located in suspect's gym bag

— Pyruvate pinnacle bottle located in suspect's gym bag

— Insure herbal liquid bottle located in suspect's gym bag

— Daily vitamin pack located in suspect's gym bag

— Hindu Magic Pill bottle located in suspect's gym bag

A laboratory service request was submitted to analyze the vitamins, Visine, and eye drops. A videotape was also recovered. The videotape revealed D.E. engaging in consensual sex with a black adult female. However, toward the end of the tape, there were 2 females completely passed out on a couch. One female was slouched over with her eyes open with a blank look on her face.

Evidence:

Dirt was found on the dining room floor and windowsill. Dirt was taken from outside and from a living room plant for trace analysis and comparison. This was an important point because it proved that the suspect came in through the window and not the front door as he indicated in his voluntary statements to the first reporting officer.

An officer attempted to lift latents from the point of entry, the dining room window, but the window was too dirty.

Three plastic cups were retrieved by the victim's roommate. They were believed to have been used to serve the drinks made by the suspect. They were given to the detective and impounded. The detective submitted a request to the crime laboratory to have the cups analyzed for narcotics residue. The tests were negative for a controlled substance, confirmed by gas chromatography-mass spectrometry (GCMS). She also requested that the plastic cups be checked for fingerprints. Three latent print cards were developed.

A SART examination was obtained. Urine was collected at 1925 hours, approximately 20 hours after ingestion.

Detective O. submitted a laboratory request to have the victim's blood and urine analyzed for controlled substances. A laboratory service request was also submitted for biologic DNA work on the victim's blankets, clothes, and a plastic bag found at the scene.

The victim's urine was screened by immunoassay. The positives were confirmed by GCMS. The test was positive for benzodiazepines, 7-aminoflunitrazepam, indicating further testing was needed. The cut off level was 100/ng/mL.

Once the preliminary toxicology results were obtained, urine and blood samples were submitted to the FBI toxicology laboratory for both victims.

The FBI lab, using pH determination, immunoassays, and liquid chromatography/mass spectrometry, detected flunitrazepam, norflunitrazepam, and 7-aminoflunitrazepam in victim #1's blood and 7-aminoflunitrazepam in her urine.

In the case of the present victim, J.B., victim #2, flunitrazepam, norflunitrazepam, and 7-aminoflunitrazepam were detected in both the victim's blood and urine.

Norflunitrazepam and 7-aminoflunitrazepam are the primary biotransformation products of Rohypnol.

Although the suspect admitted to having sex with the victim, stating that it was consensual, the detective submitted a laboratory service request to have a piece of plastic examined for blood and semen. The victim believed the suspect might have used the plastic bag as a condom. The request was approved because it would help to corroborate lack of consent, in that the victim wouldn't agree to use a plastic bag as a condom.

Summary of Analytical Procedures:

— Visual and Polilight examination

— Calcium alpha-naphthyl phosphate presumptive test for semen

— Phenolphthalein presumptive test for blood

— Digestion of samples with SDS and proteinase K

— Microscopic examination for spermatozoa and nucleated epithelial cells

Results:

Semen was found on the piece of plastic. Positive presumptive tests for blood were obtained on the piece of plastic. Microscopic slides were prepared and stored. A DNA request was then submitted to compare the results to reference samples from the victim and suspect.

Summary of DNA Analytical Procedures:

1. Identification of cellular material using Christmas Tree stain

2. Digestion of non-sperm cells with SDS and proteinase K. Digestion of sperm cell fractions with SDS, proteinase K, and DTT

3. Extraction of the sample digests with phenol/chloroform followed by the additional DNA purification and concentration using Centricon molecular filters

4. Quantitation of DNA using slot blot and/or yield gel

5. Amplification of the DQA1/Polymarker loci using the PCR process

6. Evaluation of amplification with PCR product gel

7. Hybridization probe analysis of the amplified sample DNA with allele specific oligonucleotides (ASOs) for the 7 DQA1 alleles and the alleles associated with the 5 Polymarker genetic markers

Conclusions:

D.E. could be the source of the interpretable DNA types from the sperm-fraction stain taken from the plastic item. The frequency rate in the African American population for this combination of DNA types is 1 in 8200.

The victim was excluded as a possible source of the interpretable DNA types from the stain from the sperm fraction taken from the plastic item.

The DNA results taken from the nonsperm-fraction stain from the plastic indicate a possible mixture from more than one source. The victim could be the source of the predominate DNA types. D.E. is excluded as the source of the predominate DNA types.

No interpretation is provided for trace results.

The calculated frequencies for the DQA1/Polymarker DNA profiles are based on allele frequencies provided with the Perkin Elmer AmpliType PM + DQA1 PCR Amplification and Typing Kit instructions. A theta value of 0.01 was used.

Legal Outcome:

Both cases were submitted to the District Attorney's office. The suspect pleaded guilty to 2 strikes; 2 counts of rape and 1 count of oral copulation. He is required to register as a sex offender for life. The psychologist who conducted the court-ordered evaluation of D.E. said the suspect is not a predator or a danger to the community. The suspect did not do any time in custody. At sentencing, he was given 5 years probation.

Since this incident, he has been convicted of a burglary of an automobile and received 6 months in custody.

CASE STUDY #3
Victim: J.D. W/F 25
Suspect: B.Y. 38

The suspect raped and sodomized the victim while she was unconscious due to intoxication. The victim was visiting her friends in San Diego. They went to a bar in the Gas Lamp Quarter. The victim became extremely intoxicated and passed out. The victim next remembers having 2 drinks with a "foreign" man and another unidentified male. She recalls the "foreign" man being very mean and demeaning. Her next recollection is of walking up and down a street trying to find her way back to her friend's house. The victim felt pain in her elbow and her vagina was very sore.

The victim's friend states that she drove to a grocery store at approximately 0300 hours. The victim stayed in the car because she was very intoxicated. When the friend came out of the store, the victim was gone. The friend contacted a security guard and they searched the area for the victim with negative results. The friend went home and called the police to file a missing persons report. At 0550 hours, the victim's friend received a telephone call from the victim stating that she was all right and she would be home shortly. The friend called the number the victim had called from and a man with an "Arab" accent answered the phone. The man said her friend had been there and had a few drinks with him. The victim arrived home a few hours later and appeared reclusive. The friend was concerned and called the police. Officers transported the victim to the SART hospital for a SART examination. The nurse documented redness and swelling in the labia minora and abrasions with toluidine blue uptake at the 5 and 7 o'clock positions of the posterior fourchette and fossa navicularis. The external rectal examination noted redness and swelling to the surface of the rectum (**Figure 16-1**). The internal rectal examination noted a 0 to 2 inch laceration, bruising, and redness at 5 and 6 o'clock with toluidine blue uptake. Fresh blood was seen around the same area. The Wood's lamp was negative. The nurse also noted a broken fingernail on the right middle finger. No other visible trauma was observed; however, the nurse noted that the victim's underwear had a small tear in the seam and the crotch was stained.

The detective identified the suspect after a search warrant was obtained for phone records from Pacific Bell. A search warrant was then executed at the suspect's residence.

Suspect's Statement:

The suspect said he had been out to several bars drinking with several friends. As he was driving home at 0250 hours, he saw the victim walk across the street in front of his car. He stopped,

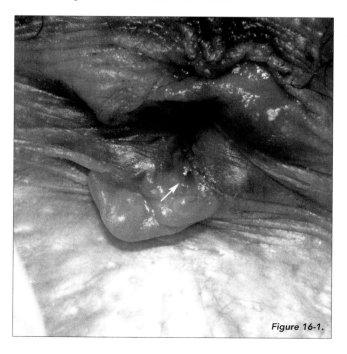

Figure 16-1. *There is perianal swelling, ecchymosis around the anus, and a laceration at 6 o'clock.*

Figure 16-1.

and she said she was cold and lost and could not find her friends. The suspect said she could get in his car to warm up. The woman said she wanted to go to his place. The suspect noticed she had been drinking, but he said he did not have to assist her up the stairs. Once inside his apartment, he offered her something to drink. She asked for wine and they both drank a couple of glasses. A few minutes later, they began kissing and hugging. The woman took her shirt and skirt off and walked upstairs and climbed into his bed. The victim was shivering from the cold and asked the suspect to get into bed with her to keep her warm. The suspect took his clothes off and got into bed with her. He said she was "pretty out of it." He then engaged her in vaginal/penile intercourse and that was all, no other sex acts. The suspect specifically denied engaging in anal intercourse. He said he didn't remember if he used a condom, however, he usually does. The suspect said the woman was very restless and would not lie down and go to sleep. Between 0400 and 0500 hours, the victim asked to use the phone to call a friend. A few minutes later, she grabbed her things and left. The suspect offered to drive her where she needed to go, but she left as though she knew where she was going. The suspect went to sleep. Between approximately 1000 and 1030 hours, a woman called asking where the victim was. The friend was very upset.

The victim's stolen credit card was used at a Vons store on November 21, 1999 at 0300 hours. The store clerk said there were 2 subjects, a Hispanic female and a white male. They purchased groceries totaling $264.90, but the transaction was denied and they began arguing. A person identified as R.O. used a Vons Club discount card at the same time. The case detective attempted to locate this person, but the person had moved from the residence noted on the Vons Club records and computer checks could not identify him further.

Evidence:

— Victim's rape kit and clothing

— Forensic alcohol and narcotic results

— Pacific Bell search warrant

— Property seized from suspect's residence at time of search warrant

— Polaroid photographs of suspect's residence

— Suspect rape kit

— Copy of the stolen credit card transaction at Vons

— Computer forensic laboratory analysis report

— Thirty-nine 35 mm photographs taken at the suspect's residence

DNA laboratory results—Although the suspect admitted to penile vaginal intercourse, he denied anal intercourse. The detective hoped to confirm anal intercourse as a way to show that he was lying about the events that evening. There has not been much success with this however, since vaginal fluid would run into the rectal cavity and therefore is inconclusive.

Victim's matted pubic hair cutting—The clump of hairs was extracted. Sperm and nonsperm cells were identified and differentially extracted for its DNA content.

1. Reference blood samples from victim and suspect

2. Summary of DNA analytical procedures:

3. Identification of cellular material using Christmas Tree stain

4. Digestion of nonsperm cells with SDS and proteinase K. Digestion of sperm cell fractions with SDS, proteinase K, and DTT

5. Extraction of the sample digests with phenol/chloroform followed by the additional DNA purification and concentration of DNA using Centricon molecular filters

6. Quantitation of DNA using slot blot and/or yield gel

7. Amplification of the DQA1/Polymarker loci using the PCR process

8. Evaluation of amplification with PCR product gel

9. Hybridization probe analysis of the amplified sample DNA with ASOs for the 7 DQA1 alleles and the alleles associated with the 5 Polymarker genetic markers

Conclusions:

The suspect could be the source of the interpretable DNA types obtained from the sperm fraction from the matted pubic hair cutting. The approximate frequency rate in the Caucasian population for this combination of DNA types is 1 in 22,000.

The victim is excluded as the source of the interpretable DNA types obtained from the sperm fraction from the matted pubic hair cutting.

The victim could be the source of the interpretable DNA types obtained from the non-sperm fraction from the matted pubic hair cutting. The suspect is excluded as the source.

No interpretation is provided for trace results.

The above calculated frequencies are based on allele frequencies provided with the Perkin Elmer AmpliType PM + DQA1 PCR Amplification and Typing Kit instructions, using equation 4.4a from the 1996 NRC report, and a theta value of 0.01.

Toxicology results—The forensic alcohol analysis report indicated the victim's blood alcohol level was 0.05% at the time the sample was taken at 1655 hours, approximately 12 hours later. The samples were also submitted to a private laboratory for a complete and comprehensive drug panel including Rohypnol and GHB, but were negative.

The regional computer forensic laboratory analyzed the computer seized at the suspect's residence at the time of the search warrant. The search was negative for information regarding any type of sexual assault communication conducted via the computer.

Legal Outcome:

The District Attorney rejected this case because the corpus of the crime could not be established. The suspect presented an affirmative defense that the victim was not unconscious, not unaware, and in fact that she was aware, active, and consented to the acts. A prosecutor cannot file charges when the affirmative defense, if established, would result in a complete exoneration and is not subject to refutation by substantial evidence available to the prosecution at time of issuance. In this case, the suspect's defense meets both these criteria. The single greatest problem with this case is the victim's poor memory as a result of her voluntary intoxication. The victim does not state the facts necessary to establish the elements required for the unconscious victim type rape/sodomy. In fact, her behavior contains numerous instances of her ability to think and engage in conscious choices and actions around the relevant times. There is no other independent, substantial corroboration of the charges sought. The defendant says she was conscious, this cannot be disproved, and in fact is somewhat supported by the victim's own statements. The victim's therapist attempted hypnosis to improve her recall, but it did not help.

CASE STUDY #4
Victims: S. and A.
Suspects: C.L.B. and D.L.
Summary of Prosecution Evidence:
The victim, S., was visiting her boyfriend, A., in Mission Beach. At about 0100, S. went down to her car to get her overnight bag and a video. She saw 2 black males, later identified as the defendants, C.L.B. and D.L., drive by slowly in a Lexus. C.L.B. was wearing a red cap. They were looking at her.

Ten minutes later, the defendants entered the apartment through an unlocked kitchen door. C.L.B. grabbed a butcher knife off the counter. This knife was never located. A butcher-block knife holder with 1 empty slot was photographed in the kitchen **(See Figure 16-2-a)**. It is believed that the suspect took the knife from this location and fled with it. Defendant D.L. simulated a gun under his shirt. The defendants forced the victims into A's bedroom and onto their knees. The defendants continually yelled that they were going to stab or shoot the victims. The defendants demanded money and ransacked the apartment. C.L.B. took some coins and $100 cash from a tin can and $20 from A.'s wallet.

Defendants asked for any drugs and S. offered them a small amount of marijuana from her purse. C.L.B. forced S. into the kitchen. She showed him a small amount of marijuana from her bag. C.L.B. said, "You want to play games. I'll cut you. Strip down!" A. was on the floor and D.L. hit him several times on the head. A. saw S. taking off her clothes. D.L. yelled at him to turn the other way and put his head under the bed. A. complied.

S. removed her clothes and C.L.B. forced her into a second bedroom. C.L.B. took 50-cent pieces, Susan B. Anthony dollars, one-dollar coins and a watch (the victim didn't realize the watch was taken until much later) from a box in the room. C.L.B. told S. to "spread eagle" and attempted to put a bottle of Desenex foot powder in her vagina **(See Figure 16-2-b)**. There was no penetration per the victim. S. began to scream and cry. C.L.B. left the room for a moment and returned. S. was on her stomach. C.L.B. again told her to "spread eagle." He then forced his penis into her vagina and had intercourse with her for about 1 to 2 minutes.

D.L. came to the doorway and said, "What are you doing? Let's go. Let's go. There's no money here." C.L.B. removed his penis and forced it slightly inside S.'s anus for a couple of seconds. He removed his penis and both defendants left. No ejaculation occurred. When the victim got off the bed, she saw blood on her legs and realized she was bleeding from her vagina.

S. and A. called the police. Officers arrived and a description of the suspects and their vehicle was broadcast to all units.

C.L.B. was identified as having been at a party at the Bahia Hotel, a short distance from A.'s apartment in Mission Beach **(See Figure 16-2-c)**. C.L.B. went to the party with a female friend in her Lexus. The friend was dating D.L. at the time but denied D.L. being at the party. Later that night, C.L.B. asked another friend, S.R., for a ride back to C.L.B.'s residence. S.R. was driving a black Mazda.

While driving out of the Mission Beach area, an officer saw C.L.B. and S.R. in the Mazda. The vehicle was stopped because it matched the vehicle description broadcast by officers at the scene: black, tinted windows, and custom wheels. This is ironic because it was actually a different vehicle than the one used in the rape/robbery. The officers initiated a stop. C.L.B. fled from the car. He was caught about an hour later. A fanny pack with $100 cash, coins, and an Italian coin (A. was recently in Italy), 50-cent pieces, Susan B. Anthony dollars, one-dollar coins, the victim's watch (this was not realized until preparing for trial), and a loaded .38 caliber revolver were found in the alley next to the area where C.L.B. was caught **(See Figure 16-2-d)**. C.L.B. was caught by a citizen who got his shotgun and had C.L.B. walk down to the police. C.L.B.'s red baseball hat was found close to the fanny pack. A tentatively identified C.L.B. in a curbside line-up and he was arrested approximately 1.5 hours after the assault.

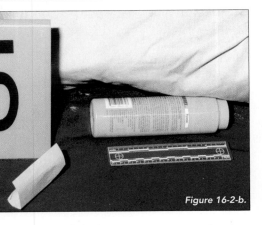

Figure 16-2-a.

Figure 16-2-a. *Knives, one of which was missing, was used to threaten the victim (35 mm).*

Figure 16-2-b. *The foot powder can used in the assault (35 mm).*

A week later, D.L. came to the attention of the police through a crime stopper tip. Both victims tentatively identified D.L. in a photo line-up. S. tentatively identified D.L. in a live line-up. A positively identified D.L. in a live line-up.

Summary of Defense Evidence:

A Forensic scientist testified regarding all the standard eyewitness identification issues. Partygoers testified that C.L.B. was at the party and never left, and that D.L. was not there at all. The defense also focused on the lack of fingerprint and DNA evidence—particularly any blood on C.L.B. at the time of the forensic examination, only a few hours after the assault.

Pertinent Facts of Prior Offenses:

D.L. had a felony conviction in 1996 for assault with the intent to commit forcible penetration by a foreign object. In that case, D.L. assaulted his friend's girlfriend at her apartment in front of her 18-month-old son. He was sentenced to 2 years in prison. He was released from prison on June 11, 1999. D.L. also had priors for narcotics, auto theft, and receiving stolen property. The incident involving the stolen property also included a charge of battery with serious bodily injury and sexual battery. D.L. walked up to a female using a pay phone, told her he wanted to "make love" to her, and grabbed her in the vaginal area.

C.L.B. was on parole for a conviction for sale of cocaine and a parole warrant had been issued for his arrest.

S.R., the driver of the Mazda, was on probation for assault with a deadly weapon; however, the investigation revealed that he was not involved with the sexual assault and robbery.

SDPD Forensic Crime Laboratory Analysis:

A SART examination was obtained for S. at 0320 hours, less than 2 hours after the assault. The nurse noted a scratch to the victim's leg that the victim believes occurred when she bumped into furniture. A Wood's lamp test was positive in the area below the victim's right knee. She also had a small scratch in the small of her back. Upon examination of the genitals, the nurse examiner noted numerous abrasions, lacerations, and tears to the posterior fourchette, labia majora, and hymen **(See Figure 16-2-e)**. Red petechiae were noted at the cervix, and a pool of blood and blood clots were noted in the vaginal canal **(See Figure 16-2-f)**. Due to the amount of blood, the nurse was not able to view vaginal tears in the canal. Redness, swelling, bruising, and a small tear were noted at the anal verge. Due to the amount of bleeding, the victim was referred to the emergency room for treatment by a doctor. (Reports do not indicate the diagnosis, treatment, or source of the bleeding.)

A. had visible injuries from being struck on the head.

Toxicology analysis was requested on S. and defendant C.L.B. S.'s blood and urine were negative for both drugs and alcohol. C.L.B.'s blood was negative for alcohol and positive for cocaine, marijuana, and opiates.

Bedding was collected from the bed where the assault occurred.

Twenty-two latent print cards were collected from the scene. The detective requested that the powder canister be examined for latent prints. Results were negative. Latent prints were also checked for on the male victim's wallet, various items in the

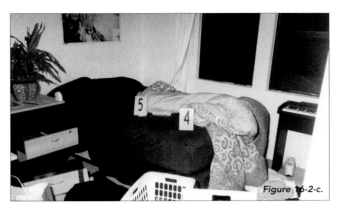

Figure 16-2-c. The victim's bedroom. The assault occurred on the bed (35 mm).

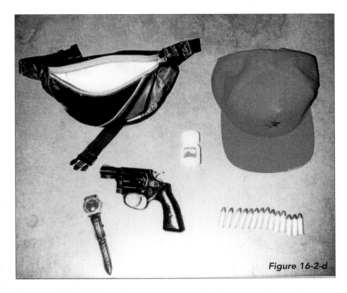

Figure 16-2-d. These items were found in the perpetrators' possession. The watch belonged to the victim, as did some collectable coins that are not present in the photograph (35 mm).

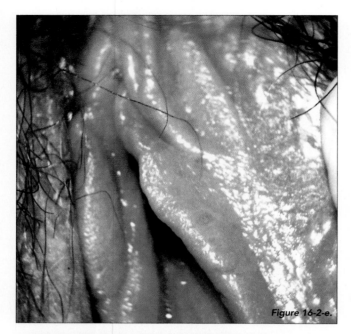

Figure 16-2-e.

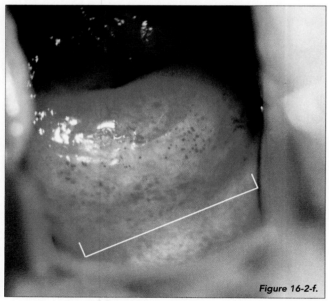

Figure 16-2-f.

Figure 16-2-e. *There is ecchymosis of the labium minus at 9 and 11 o'clock.*

Figure 16-2-f. *Petechiae are visible on the cervix.*

residence handled by the suspects during the robbery, the recovered money, and the window screen. All were negative.

The victim's SART kit was submitted for screening. Specifically, the criminologist looked at the 4 red vaginal swabs, 2 light red external genital swabs, 2 light tan debris swabs, and 1 light red, positive Wood's lamp swab.

With reference to the crime scene evidence, the laboratory looked at the victim's sweatpants, the blue fitted bed sheet, and the Desenex powder bottle (**See Figure 16-2-b**).

A SART examination was obtained for C.L.B.. The laboratory looked at 2 gray penis swabs, 2 white pubic swabs, and fingernail scrapings.

In addition the suspect's boxers, white T-shirt, and plaid shorts were screened for biologic and trace evidence.

The screening procedures included:

Visual and Polilight examination, calcium alpha-naphthyl phosphate presumptive tests for semen, digestion of samples with SDS and proteinase K, microscopic examination for spermatozoa and nucleated epithelial cells. A presumptive test for blood using phenolphthalein was also used.

Results:

Two spermatozoa were found on the vaginal swabs.

Semen was found in the crotch area of the sweatpants and in several areas on the bed sheet.

A positive presumptive test for blood was obtained on the right sleeve of the T-shirt and in the crotch area of the sweatpants. No blood was found on the men's boxers, the shorts, or on the Desenex bottle. Swabs were taken of both ends of the Desenex bottle.

Microscopic slides were prepared and submitted for DNA analysis.

DNA analysis included:

— Microscopic examinations of suspected semen stains and penile swabs for spermatozoa and nucleated epithelial cells

— Differential extraction of suspected semen stains and penile swabs into sperm and nonsperm fractions

— Digestion of sperm fractions with SDS, proteinase K, and DTT

— Digestion of nonsperm fractions, other evidence samples, and reference samples with SDS and proteinase K

— Purification of DNA using phenol/chloroform and Centricon-100 molecular filters

— Quantitation of DNA using slot blot and/or yield gel

— Amplification of the DQA1/Polymarker loci using the PCR process

— Assessment of amplification product using gel electrophoresis

— Reverse dot-blot hybridization of amplified DNA using allele-specific oligonucleotide probe strips

Conclusions:

1. Two portions of a suspected semen stain on the cutting from the sweatpants were differentially extracted. Based on the low number of sperm cells observed, it was determined that the amount of stain on the portions was insufficient for testing.

2. Nucleated epithelial cells were detected in the nonsperm fraction of the penis swab from C.L.B. C.L.B. was included as a possible source of these epithelial cells. The victim was excluded as a possible source of these epithelial cells.

3. No nucleated epithelial cells were detected in the nonsperm fraction of the pubic swab from C.L.B. Although a small amount of DNA was extracted from this sample, the typing results were too weak to interpret.

4. No sperm or epithelial cells were detected in the sperm fraction of the penis and pubic swabs from C.L.B.

5. Although small amounts of DNA were extracted from the fingernail scrapings from C.L.B.'s right and left hands, the typing results were too weak to interpret.

6. The victim and C.L.B. were excluded as possible sources of a bloodstain on the cutting from the T-shirt.

This is a very interesting case forensically. Given the short amount of time between the assault and the forensic examination for both the victim and 1 of the suspects, it seemed likely that this would be an extremely DNA-rich case. The victim's samples might have been affected by the amount of vaginal blood, possibly washing away trace and biologic evidence. It is important to remember that the victim does not believe the suspect ejaculated. There was also a question as to why the victim's blood was not detected on the swabs taken from the suspect's penis during the suspect's forensic examination.

In addition, the length of time the suspects were in the apartment and the amount of ransacking they did would indicate that latent prints would be found, but they were not. It is unknown whether this was pure luck or whether the suspects did something to eliminate this type of evidence.

This case was made because of good police work, demonstrating how everyone must work together and everything must be done to cover all the bases. The fact that the victim's personally engraved watch was found with C.L.B.'s property was one of the strongest pieces of evidence in the case.

Legal Outcome:

The suspects were convicted of conspiracy, forcible rape, rape in concert, forcible sodomy, sodomy in concert, attempted forcible penetration, robbery, and residential burglary. C.L.B. received a sentence of 61 years to life. D.L., because of his prior strikes, received a sentence of 80 years to life. D.L. will be required to serve 85% of his time and C.L.B. 80%.

Case Study #5
Victim: R.J. B/F 24
Suspect: E.B. B/M 32
Forced rape and oral copulation, including charges of rape by threat of authority of a public official.

The suspect was identified in 3 cases involving the rape and forced oral copulation of prostitutes. He is also the suspect in a fourth case; however, the victim could not be located.

On November 1, 1999, Detective R. received a case for investigation. A 25-year-old self-admitted prostitute was raped by an unidentified male impersonating a police officer. The suspect picked up the victim and agreed to pay her $40.00 for sexual intercourse. The suspect drove the victim to a location outside her business area against her will. The suspect said he was "Vice," and the victim would be arrested unless she performed certain sexual acts on him. The victim asked to see his badge, but he said it was in the car. The victim said she guessed she was going to jail then. The suspect walked back to his vehicle and pulled out a pair of handcuffs. He gave the victim one more chance to comply. The victim engaged in oral copulation and sexual intercourse with the suspect out of fear of being arrested. Afterward, the suspect walked away, leaving the victim in the park. The victim flagged down a police sergeant and told him what happened. Officers responded to the crime scene. The victim identified a condom lying in the grass as the one used by the suspect. The officer also recovered 1 unused condom that was left at the scene. The victim recognized the condoms because she had provided them to the suspect. The victim refused to have a forensic examination.

The detective submitted laboratory requests for evidence collection from the used condom and for fingerprints from the condom package. The package was negative for latents.

The detective assigned to this case had not yet been able to locate the victim when she received a second similar case.

In the second case, the victim, also a self-admitted prostitute, age 24 years, was working on El Cajon Boulevard. The suspect offered her $60.00 to get in his Corvette with him. The victim told the suspect where to take her, but the suspect drove to a different area. The victim tried to call the deal off and got out of the car. The suspect grabbed the victim and pulled her to a nearby picnic table. He told her to "suck his dick." The victim said she would, but she wanted to use a condom. The suspect would not allow the victim to use a condom. The suspect forcibly pushed the victim's mouth down on his penis for about 30 seconds. The suspect told the victim he was going to "fuck" her. He agreed to use a condom and the victim provided him with one. The suspect then told the victim to take her clothes off. The victim removed one of her pant legs and lay down on the wood picnic table. The victim was afraid of what the suspect might do if she did not comply. The suspect vaginally raped the victim on the table. The crime was interrupted by a police officer who shined his spotlight on the suspect's parked car. The suspect fled on foot, leaving his vehicle at the crime scene. The victim ran to the officer, crying and screaming that the man who was driving that vehicle had raped her.

The victim identified the crime scene for the officer. The officer recovered a used condom and wrapper, as well as 2 condoms still in their packages. The victim said that the suspect had her pager and cell phone. The pager was identified in the grass near the crime scene. The phone was not located. The suspect's wallet was located in his vehicle. A driver's license identifying the suspect was found in the wallet.

The vehicle was impounded as evidence. The victim was taken to the SART hospital for a forensic examination. She refused the application of toluidine blue dye and an internal vaginal examination.

The suspect was identified by both victims in photo line-ups and subsequently arrested. The suspect invoked his right to have an attorney and was not interviewed.

The detective then received a third case that appeared to be related based on suspect and vehicle description and crime type. On October 7, 1999, the 27-year-old victim was walking toward a bus stop. She accepted a ride from an unidentified black male driving a black Corvette. The suspect agreed to give the victim a ride to her boyfriend's house but said he had to take care of something first. The suspect drove her around, ending up at a school or recreation center. The suspect told the victim he would beat her to death if she didn't do what he said. The victim offered the suspect money if he would leave her alone. The suspect put a condom on his penis and ordered the victim to orally copulate with him. Afterward, he ordered her out of the car. He walked her to a dirt area where he made her get on her hands and knees. The suspect then raped her vaginally. The condom the suspect was wearing broke. The suspect finished the act without a condom and ejaculated onto the dirt next to them. The suspect apologized for raping the victim but said he was fulfilling a fantasy of his. He said he wanted to see the fear in her while he was raping her. The suspect drove the victim back to her hotel and tried to give her $20.00. The victim refused the money. The victim filed a report a month after the rape occurred. She went to Balboa Hospital for a urinary tract infection. She told the doctor she had been raped a month prior. The doctor called the police.

Victim # 1 was eventually located in a rehabilitation program. She was unwilling to discuss the case with the detective. She is required to register as a narcotics offender, and she was on probation. She had failed to report to probation and there was no current address.

Evidence:

— Victim's SART examination and clothing

— Used condom and wrapper, 2 unused condoms, and a Motorola pager

— Blue wallet belonging to suspect

— Ten 35 mm photographs of crime scene

— Two photographs of victim's vehicle, 1989 Chevy Camaro

— Suspect's buccal swab

— Suspect's eyeglasses

— Cell phone

— One Polaroid photograph of cell phone

— Seven photographs of 1982 Chevy Corvette

Used condoms were recovered from both crime scenes. Both were submitted to the crime laboratory for DNA analysis.

Condom recovered from R.J.'s crime scene.

Procedure—Visual examination

Calcium alpha-naphthyl phosphate presumptive test for semen

Microscopy for the presence of spermatozoa and nonspermatozoa cells

Digestion of samples by SDS and proteinase K

Results—Spermatozoa and nucleated epithelial cells were found on the condom. Six airdried swabs were collected from the condom and placed in the laboratory freezer.

The swabs were submitted to a DNA criminologist for further analysis.

DNA procedure:

— Identification of cellular material using Christmas Tree stain

— Digestion of nonsperm cells with SDS and proteinase K

— Digestion of sperm cell fractions with SDS, proteinase K, and DTT

— Extraction of the sample digests with phenol/chloroform followed by the additional purification and concentration of DNA using Centricon molecular filters

— Quantitation of DNA using slot blot and/or yield gel

— Amplification of the DQA1/Polymarker loci using the PCR process

— Evaluation of amplification with PCR product gel

— Hybridization probe analysis of the amplified sample DNA with ASOs for the 7 DQA1 alleles and the alleles associated with the 5 Polymarker genetic markers

Conclusions:

The suspect could be the source of the DNA types from the condom swabs "inside" surface sperm fraction. The frequency rate for the African American population is 1 in 77,000.

The victim was excluded as the source of the DNA types from the condom swabs "inside" surface sperm fraction.

The victim could be the source of the interpretable DNA types from the condom swabs "outside" surface nonsperm fraction. The frequency rate for the African American population is 1 in 780.

The suspect was excluded as the source of the interpretable DNA types from the condom swabs "outside" surface nonsperm fraction.

The DNA results from the condom swabs "inside" surface nonsperm fraction indicate a mixture from more than 1 source. The suspect and victim cannot be excluded as possible contributors to the mixture. However, there is a DNA type present in the mixture that is foreign to both the victim and suspect.

No interpretation is provided for trace results.

The calculated frequencies for the DQA1/Polymarker DNA profiles are based on allele frequencies provided with the Perkin Elmer AmpliType PM + DQA1 PCR Amplification and Typing Kit instructions. A theta value of 0.01 was used.

The suspect was arrested, and a District Attorney interview was scheduled with the victim. The victim failed to show for the interview. The detective made numerous attempts to encourage the victim to cooperate, without success.

In addition to the lack of cooperation from the 3 victims, the District Attorney cited the following reasons for rejecting R.J.'s case.

1. No physical evidence showing a forcible sex act on any incident

2. Other victims are unwilling or not able to be located

3. No SART findings on any incident

4. Each victim has a history of prostitution, which will affect the issue of consent.

APPENDIX II: DOCUMENTATION AND WARRANTS
SEARCH WARRANT

Page 1

1 Numbered Pleading Paper
2 Press [F9] after required entry
3 IN THE SUPERIOR COURT OF CALIFORNIA,
4 COUNTY OF SAN DIEGO CENTRAL DIVISION STATE OF
5 CALIFORNIA
6 AFFIDAVIT FOR SEARCH WARRANT
7
8 (ss. County of San Diego)
9 No._____
10
11 I, Joseph Cristinziani, do on oath make complaint, say and
12 depose the following on this __day of __, 1999: that I have
13 substantial probable cause to believe and I do believe that I
14 have cause to search: the person known as PV, an Hispanic
15 male adult having a date of birth of 01-06-70, being about
16 5'8" in height and 145 lbs. in weight, and is believed to be
17 currently residing and in custody of the State of California
18 under California Department of Corrections number
19 E04294, located at the North Kern State Prison; at 2737
20 West Cecil Avenue, Delano, California; for the following
21 property, to wit: to seize the person and take hair, blood and
22 saliva samples sufficient for comparison purposes using the
23 least amount of force necessary to take said samples.
24
25 I am a peace officer employed by the San Diego Police
26 Department (hereafter SDPD) and have been so employed
27 for about 20 years. I am currently assigned to the Homicide
28 Division and have been so assigned for about 4 years. Prior

Page 2

1 to this assignment, I was assigned to the Sex Crimes Unit.
2 I was so assigned for approximately 14 months. During my
3 career, I have investigated at least 100 Homicide cases as well
4 as approximately 100 sexual assault cases.
5
6 During the course of my duties, I have learned the following
7 information based upon my discussions with the named
8 witnesses or by having read the reports of or talked with
9 other SDPD officers who have spoken directly with the
10 named witness. All references to dates refer to the current
11 calendar year unless otherwise stated.
12
13 I have prepared the attached 17 page report in the course of
14 my duties. I was assigned the case after the victim initially
15 reported the crime to SDPD patrol officers. I hereby request
16 incorporation by reference herein of said report as if fully set
17 forth and identified by SDPD case number 95-091454
18 located in the upper left portion of the front page. This
19 crime was a forcible rape, committed in violation of section
20 261(2) of the California Penal Code. The victim in this case
21 was identified as Ms. JL.
22
23 During the course of the investigation, the victim, JL, was
24 examined by medical personnel following the rape and
25 biological samples were taken from her vaginal vault. The
26 evidence was analyzed by the San Diego Police Department
27 and biological samples sufficient for DNA testing were
28 identified. The San Diego Police Department used a

Page 3

1 polymerase chain reaction (PCR) DNA test to identify the
2 genetic markers of the assailant in JL's assault. The evidence
3 was then sent to Cellmark for RFLP testing with the intent
4 to attempt to identify the suspect using the Combined DNA
5 index system computer database (CODIS) maintained by the
6 FBI. RFLP was obtained, however, there was no match
7 in CODIS.
8
9 In June of 1999, Mr. Brian Burritt was hired by the San
10 Diego Police Department Crime Laboratory as a
11 Criminologist. His specific field of expertise is that of a DNA
12 Analyst. Prior to his employment with the San Diego Police
13 Department, Mr. Burritt was employed as a Criminologist
14 with the California Department of Justice, DNA Laboratory,
15 Berkeley, California. Mr. Burritt has been qualified as an
16 expert witness, in the area of DNA in the Superior Courts of
17 11 different counties within the State of California. The San
18 Diego Superior Court is included in that list.
19
20 Upon his employment with the San Diego Police
21 Department's Crime Laboratory, part of Mr. Burritt's job
22 description was to examine any and all unsolved cases
23 containing DNA evidence and, to create a SDPD database for
24 unsolved cases with PCR evidence.
25
26 On June 20, 1999, Mr. Burritt began an analysis of the PCR
27 profile collected from JL's case. Once the PCR profile from
28 this case was entered into the data base, the data base

Page 4

1 compares the profile against at least 200 other PCR profiles
2 collected from known sex and/or violent crime scenes from
3 within San Diego County. The database compares against
4 other PCR profiles searching for matches. The search
5 revealed a PCR profile match to PV, an identified suspect in
6 an indecent exposure investigation. Mr. Burritt examined
7 PV's PCR profile and found that in the Caucasian popu-
8 lation the frequency is 1 in 2600; in the Hispanic popu-
9 lation the frequency is 1 in 5400 and in the Black population
10 the frequency is 1 in 110,000.
11
12 Utilizing official police computers, I conducted a background
13 investigation on PV. I learned PV was not in custody at the
14 time JL was forcibly raped. I learned PV was living within
15 the City of San Diego at the time the rape occurred. PV's
16 residence was located at 7106 Armadillo Street, in the City
17 and County of San Diego. Armadillo Street is well within a
18 three (3) mile radius of the location where JL was raped.
19 Through my background investigation, I learned PV's
20 physical description matched the suspect description given to
21 me by JL. Additionally, I learned PV has prior convictions for
22 sexually related type crimes.
23
24 A biologic reference sample is now needed from PV for
25 RFLP testing which will provide additional genetic infor-
26 mation to more conclusively include or exclude PV as the
27 person who sexually assaulted JL. By obtaining saliva swabs
28 from PV, forensic laboratory personnel will be able to make

1 further comparisons to the RFLP identified in JL's case. I
2 know that comparisons can be made between fluids found
3 on or in the victim and that of the suspect. By removing
4 blood and saliva, laboratory personnel will be able to make
5 comparisons with those samples taken from the suspect to
6 those taken from the victim using DNA and/or more
7 conventional laboratory comparisons.
8
9 I have been advised that DNA is short for deoxyribonucleic
10 acid. DNA molecules are contained within human cells and
11 hold the genetic "coding" that makes each of us individually
12 distinctive (except identical twins). While forensic DNA
13 technology cannot yet discriminate among human beings to
14 the same extent as fingerprint evidence, it is capable of
15 identification within a very small percentage major popula-
16 tions depending on the type of analysis employed. Forensic
17 DNA evidence has been routinely admitted in courts of
18 California since 1989. Samples taken from the suspect as
19 described more fully above will be compared against that
20 found on the victim. In removing the blood and other samples
21 from the suspect, I will use medically accepted practices, utilize
22 the services of a trained person in drawing the blood, and use
23 the least amount of force necessary to collect the described
24 evidence.
25
26 The suspect was booked into State Prison on an unrelated
27 charge and was booked under the above described California
28 Department of Corrections number.

Page 5

1 I request that this declaration, the affidavit, search warrant
2 and supporting attachments be sealed pending further order
3 of the court. I make the request for the following reason.
4 Without sealing, the affidavit and supporting documentation
5 and warrant become a matter of public record within 10
6 days. Penal Code section 1534(a).
7
8 Also, Penal Code section 293 provides that a victim of a sex
9 offense be advised that his or her name will become a matter
10 of public record unless he or she requests that it not become
11 a matter of public record. The victim in this matter has not
12 yet determined whether or not she wishes her name to
13 become a part of the public record. If the information in
14 these documents is not sealed, the victim's name can be
15 revealed to anyone who wishes to examine the court files,
16 and the victim will be denied her rights under Penal Code
17 section 293. For this reason, I believe all information
18 identifying the victim should remain sealed pending further
19 order of the court.
20
21 Therefore, based on my training, experience, and the above
22 facts, I believe that I have substantial cause to believe the
23 above described property or a portion thereof will be on said
24 person when the warrant is served. Based on the aforemen-
25 tioned information and investigation, I believe that grounds
26 for the issuance of a search warrant exist as set forth in Penal
27 Code section 1524. I, the affiant, hereby pray that a search
28 warrant be issued for the seizure of said property, or any part

Page 6

1 thereof, from said person at any time of the day, good cause
2 being shown therefore, and that the same be brought before
3 this magistrate or retained subject to the order of this Court.
4
5 This affidavit has been reviewed for legal sufficiency.
6 Deputy District Attorney David J. Lattuca.
7 Given under my hand and dated this __day of __, 1999.
8 Joseph Cristinziani ID #2913
9 San Diego Police Department
10 Homicide Section
11
12 Subscribed and sworn to before me
13 this day of _____, 1999
14 at _____ a.m./p.m
15
16 _____
17 Judge of the Superior Court
18 Central Division
19
20
21
22
23
24
25
26
27
28

Page 7

SEARCH WARRANT FOR THE UNCONSCIOUS VICTIM

1 IN THE SUPERIOR COURT OF CALIFORNIA,
2 COUNTY OF SAN DIEGO STATE OF CALIFORNIA
3 AFFIDAVIT FOR SEARCH WARRANT
4 No._____
5 I, ZZ, do on oath make complaint, say and depose the
6 following on this XX that I have substantial probable cause
7 to believe and I do believe that I have cause to search the
8 person known as _____, a _____adult/child approximately
9 __ years old having a date of birth of __, being about __'" in
10 height and __lbs. in weight, and is believed to be currently
11 inside the _____ (Name and Address of Hospital):
12 for the following property, to wit: to seize the person and
13 conduct an examination of said person, including all body
14 cavities with the assistance of hospital staff and "SART"
15 personnel; and, using the least amount of force necessary, to
16 take from the described person the following samples
17 sufficient for comparison purposes: dried and moist
18 secretions; blood, urine; stains; foreign materials from the
19 body including the head, hair, and scalp; to record injuries
20 and findings on diagrams including: erythemia, abrasions,
21 bruises, contusions, induration, lacerations, fractures, bites,
22 burns, and stains and foreign materials on the body; to scan
23 the entire body with a "Wood's Lamp"; and to swab any
24 substance or florescent area with a separate swab; and to
25 preserve the described evidence for later comparison.

26 A short definition of terms follows:
27 "SART"—an abbreviation for Sexual Assault Response Team.
28 Members of this team who perform sexual assault examinations are Registered Nurses and have specialized forensic

Page 1

1 training in the collection of evidence in sexual assault cases.
2 "Wood's Lamp"—An ultraviolet light that enables the user to
3 detect bodily fluids including seminal fluid and vaginal
4 secretions.

5 I am a peace officer employed by the San Diego Police
6 Department (hereafter SDPD) and have been so employed
7 for about __ years. I am currently assigned to the Sex Crimes
8 Unit, and have been so employed for approximately __ years.
9 During my career I have been involved in the investigations
10 of over __ cases involving sexual assault.

11

12 On (date), I was contacted by my supervisor to respond to
13 (Name) Hospital to investigate a possible sexual assault.
14 Upon my arrival I spoke with hospital staff and was advised
15 that the above named person had been brought to the
16 hospital and was unconscious.

17 At the hospital I met with SDPD Officer _____, ID#__,
18 and (Name) who is a certified SART nurse. Officer _____
19 told me the following: (Basis for believing victim was
20 sexually assaulted).

21

22 I advised the hospital that I wished to have the SART nurse
23 perform an examination on the named victim, and to have
24 the SART nurse collect and preserve the above described
25 evidence. I know this type of examination is critical in order
26 to preserve evidence that may serve to identify the
27 perpetrator of the assault on the victim. I know from my
28 training and experience that victims of sexual assault crimes
   are often unable to identify their attackers, and even if they

Page 2

1 are able to do so, evidence which corroborates their
2 testimony is critical to a successful prosecution.
3 Thus, circumstantial evidence of the attacker's identity
4 is critical to a criminal investigation. I know that sexual
5 assaults generally spawn the type of evidence requested, some
6 of which may have come from the suspect, some from
7 the victim.

8 I have been advised that DNA is short for deoxyribonucleic
9 acid. DNA molecules are contained within human cells and
10 hold the genetic "coding" that makes each of us individually
11 distinctive (except identical twins). While DNA technology
12 cannot yet discriminate among human beings to the same
13 extent as fingerprint evidence can, it is capable of identi-
14 fication within a very small percentage population depending
15 on the type of analysis employed. Such evidence has been
16 introduced in evidence within the courts of California and has
17 successfully withstood attack on foundational grounds insofar
18 as the comparison technique is concerned. There is currently a
19 split of opinion as to whether or not accurate statistical
20 predictions can be based upon such testing. However, the
21 California Supreme Court has yet to rule on the admissibility
22 of this new scientific evidence. However, for our purposes
23 herein, I submit that the requested samples are clearly
24 necessary for analysis for probable cause purposes as well as
25 evidentiary purposes. Such samples may also be used for
26 analysis using more traditional scientific techniques. Samples
27 taken from the victim as described more fully above will be
28 compared to any potential suspect. In removing the samples
   from the victim, the SART nurse will use medically accepted
   practices, and use the least amount of force necessary to

Page 3

1 collect the described evidence.

2

3 The hospital staff had no objection to my request to have an
4 examination performed on the victim. However, the SART
5 nurse explained to me that she would not perform the
6 examination without the consent of the victim or a court
7 order. The victim has been unconscious and is unable to
8 communicate whether or not she wishes to submit to this
9 examination. I have been advised by hospital staff, and I know
10 from my own experience, that it is impossible to determine
11 when the victim may regain consciousness. I also know from
12 my experience that the type of evidence to be collected can be
13 lost or will deteriorate with the passage of time. I also know
14 that the medical procedures that the hospital will employ to
15 treat the victim's injuries could result in the loss of this
16 evidence. These procedures often involve cleansing areas of the
17 body which necessarily will result in the destruction of
18 evidence. Therefore, I believe that to delay the examination of
19 this victim until she regains consciousness will result in the loss
20 of evidence that is necessary to identify her perpetrator.

21 I know that Penal Code Section 1530 states that only peace
22 officers may serve a search warrant, but that they may be aided
23 by others when necessary. California case law has upheld the
24 use of experts in the execution of search warrants when non-
25 experts simply could not effectively carry out the execution.
26 (See People v. Superior Court (Moore) (1980) 105.CalApp.3d
27 1001.) I submit that it is critical in this case, since your affiant
28 does not have the training or the license to conduct the
   examination needed to preserve this important evidence.

Page 4

1 Therefore, based on my training, experience, and the above
2 facts, I believe that I have substantial cause to believe the
3 above person will have or be able to produce the requested
4 property or things when this warrant is executed.

5
6 Based on the aforementioned information and investigation,
7 I believe that grounds for the issuance of a search warrant
8 exist as set forth in Penal Code section 1524.

9 I, the affiant, hereby pray that a search warrant be issued for
10 the seizure of said person and property, or portion thereof
11 from said person, at any time of the day, or night, good cause
12 being shown therefore, and that the same be brought before
13 this magistrate or retained subject to the order of this court.

14
15 This affidavit has been reviewed for legal sufficiency by
16 Deputy District Attorney XY.
   Given under my hand and dated this XX.
17 _____
18 Subscribed and sworn to before me
19 this _____,
20 at _____ a.m./p.m.
21
22 _____
23 Judge of the Superior Court
   Central Division
24
25
26
27
28

Page 5

FORENSIC SCIENCES—LAB SERVICES REQUEST

San Diego Police Department
FORENSIC SCIENCES—LAB SERVICES REQUEST

UNIT: _____ M.S.: _____ TODAY'S DATE: _____

1. Victim's Name (Last, First)	2. Suspect's Name (Last, First)	3. Offense Code
4. Detective's Name	5. Telephone Number	6. Case Number
7. Sergeant's Name	8. Telephone Number	

PRIORITY

☐ Preliminary_____ ☐ Trial_____ ☐ Series_____
    (Date)   (Date)   (Date)

☐ Analysis Needed For Case To Be Issued   DDA Assigned/Phone_____

Has a victim reference standard been collected?   ☐ No   ☐ Yes   Property Tag #_____
     B #_____

Has a suspect reference standard been collected?   ☐ No   ☐ Yes   Property Tag #_____
     B #_____

Has a consensual partner reference standard been collected?   ☐ N/A   ☐ No   ☐ Yes   Property Tag #_____
     B #_____

EVIDENCE SUBMITTED

LIST THE ITEM(S) YOU WANT EXAMINED AND POSSIBLE CONSEQUENCES (i.e. "Examine the bottom sheet removed from the suspect's bed and check for trace evidence from the victim.")

TRACE EVIDENCE: Hairs, Fibers, Paint, Glass, Shoeprints, Physical Matches

FORENSIC BIOLOGY: Blood, Semen, Saliva, Fingernail Scrapings, DNA

LIST ITEMS BY ORDER OF PRIORITY DETERMINED BY CASE HISTORY

1. Please Check:_____   _____
     (Item to be Examined)   (Property Tag #)

Screen For Trace Evidence: ☐ Hair   ☐ Fibers   ☐ Other_____

Screen For Biological Evidence: ☐ Blood   ☐ Semen   ☐ Saliva   ☐ Fingernail Scrapings
     ☐ Other_____

☐ **DNA Analysis Requested**

Comments: _____
_____
_____
_____

San Diego Police Department
FORENSIC SCIENCES—LAB SERVICES REQUEST

EVIDENCE SUBMITTED

2. Please Check:_____   _____
　　　　　　　　　　(Item to be Examined)　　　　　　　　　　　　　　　　　　　　　(Property Tag #)

Screen For Trace Evidence:　　　☐ Hair　　☐ Fibers　　☐ Other_____

Screen For Biological Evidence:　☐ Blood　☐ Semen　☐ Saliva　☐ Fingernail Scrapings

　　　　　　　　　　　　　　　　　☐ Other_____

☐ **DNA Analysis Requested**

　　Comments: _____
　　_____
　　_____
　　_____
　　_____

3. Please Check:_____   _____
　　　　　　　　　　(Item to be Examined)　　　　　　　　　　　　　　　　　　　　　(Property Tag #)

Screen For Trace Evidence:　　　☐ Hair　　☐ Fibers　　☐ Other_____

Screen For Biological Evidence:　☐ Blood　☐ Semen　☐ Saliva　☐ Fingernail Scrapings

　　　　　　　　　　　　　　　　　☐ Other_____

☐ **DNA Analysis Requested**

　　Comments: _____
　　_____
　　_____
　　_____
　　_____

4. Please Check:_____   _____
　　　　　　　　　　(Item to be Examined)　　　　　　　　　　　　　　　　　　　　　(Property Tag #)

Screen For Trace Evidence:　　　☐ Hair　　☐ Fibers　　☐ Other_____

Screen For Biological Evidence:　☐ Blood　☐ Semen　☐ Saliva　☐ Fingernail Scrapings

　　　　　　　　　　　　　　　　　☐ Other_____

☐ **DNA Analysis Requested**

　　Comments: _____
　　_____
　　_____
　　_____

_____　　_____
Requesting Unit's Supervisor Approval　　　　　　　　Date

FORENSIC SCIENCES—PRELIMINARY RAPE CASE INFORMATION

San Diego Police Department
FORENSIC SCIENCES—PRELIMINARY RAPE CASE INFORMATION

CASE#: _____   TODAY'S DATE: _____   DETECTIVE: _____

1. Victim's Name (Last, First)	2. Suspect's Name (Last, First)	3. Suspect in Custody? ☐ No ☐ Yes

1. Did the victim have consensual sex within 96 hours (4 days) prior to the time the hospital samples and/or clothing were collected?   ☐ No   ☐ Yes

   Specify: ☐ 1 day before   ☐ 2 days before   ☐ 3 days before   ☐ 4 days before

   If yes, can a reference sample be obtained from the consensual partner(s)?   ☐ No   ☐ Yes

   (Reference standards from all consensual partners should be collected before submitting a request to the laboratory for testing.)

2. Was oral activity involved in the sexual assault?   ☐ No   ☐ Yes   ☐ Unknown

   If yes: ☐ Fellatio   ☐ Victim on suspect   ☐ Suspect on victim
   ☐ Cunnilingus   ☐ Victim on suspect   ☐ Suspect on victim
   ☐ Other?   Specify:_____

3. Was anal activity involved in the sexual assault?   ☐ No   ☐ Yes   Type:_____   ☐ Unknown

4. Did the suspect ejaculate?   ☐ No   ☐ Yes   ☐ Victim Unsure   ☐ N/A

   If yes, where did ejaculation occur?
   Internal?   ☐ Vagina   External?   ☐ Victim's body (location)_____
   ☐ Mouth   ☐ Clothing item (describe)_____
   ☐ Rectum   ☐ Other (specify)_____

5. Was a condom worn during the assault?   ☐ No   ☐ Yes   ☐ Victim Unsure   ☐ N/A

6. Was victim or suspect bleeding during the assault?
   Victim: ☐ No   ☐ Yes   ☐ From what area(s) of the body?_____
   Suspect: ☐ No   ☐ Yes   ☐ From what area(s) of the body?_____
   Was the victim menstruating?   ☐ No   ☐ Yes

7. Was clothing collected other than items worn to the hospital (e.g. from the scene)?   ☐ No   ☐ Yes
   If yes, describe_____
   Describe clothing worn during and any clothing put on immediately after the assault.   ☐ Same
   During:_____   After:_____
   Based on information from the victim, which item(s) of clothing is/are most likely to have seminal fluid stains from the suspect? _____
   _____
   _____

San Diego Police Department
FORENSIC SCIENCES—PRELIMINARY RAPE CASE INFORMATION

8. Was bedding collected? ☐ No ☐ Yes   If "No" go to Question #11.

9. Based on information from the victim, which item of bedding is most likely to have seminal fluid stains from the suspect?

   ☐ Bottom bed sheet ☐ Top bed sheet ☐ Bedspread ☐ Blanket ☐ Pillowcase
   Other_____

10. Did any type of consensual sex act take place on the bedding since the last time it was washed?

Bottom bed sheet:	☐ No	☐ Yes	Top bed sheet:	☐ No	☐ Yes
Bedspread:	☐ No	☐ Yes	Blanket:	☐ No	☐ Yes
Pillowcase:	☐ No	☐ Yes	Other:	☐ No	☐ Yes

   (If yes, unless the seminal fluid stain(s) related to the assault can be identified for the Criminologist, it will be necessary to obtain blood and saliva standards from all individuals involved before any comparative analysis is performed.)

   Note: If the above information concerning the history of the bedding is not obtained, the bedding will not be examined.

11. Were any other items collected from the scene? ☐ No ☐ Yes
    If yes, list items collected:_____
    _____
    _____
    _____

12. Has a suspect been identified? ☐ No ☐ Yes
    Are suspect reference samples available? ☐ No ☐ Yes   Property Tag#:_____

13. Do the suspect and victim know each other? ☐ No ☐ Yes
    If yes, at the time of the assault, were they involved in a consensual sexual relationship? ☐ No ☐ Yes

    Note: Bedding that has not been washed since the consensual sex act(s) between the victim and the suspect will not be examined for semen.

14. Other relevant information: _____
    _____
    _____
    _____
    _____
    _____
    _____
    _____
    _____
    _____
    _____

SART Clothing Documentation

San Diego County SART
ADDENDUM TO 923
CLOTHING DOCUMENTATION

Obtain a complete history prior to evidence collection and documentation. Complete all blanks. If not applicable, write N/A. When specific evidence is not required, write "deferred." Document accurately. **Write clearly and neatly.**

Patient Presented at Hospital Wearing Clothing Worn During Assault:

Describe clothing, (With minimal handling) carefully noting condition (clean, dirty, rips, tears, stretched out elastic, missing buttons) and visible signs of foreign material (grass, fiber, hair, twigs, soil, splinters, glass, blood, dry or moist secretions).

Procedure for wet clothing: Items must be dry to preserve evidence. If clothing is wet, lay on a sheet of clean, unused, white paper and cover with another sheet of white paper. Gently fold each article of clothing and place in a labeled, sealed paper bag. Give to the officer. Advise that the clothing is wet.

Bra:_____

Shirt:_____

Undershirt:_____

Sweater:_____

Jacket:_____

Pants:_____

Underwear:_____

Socks (state one or two socks present):_____

Shoes (state one or two socks present):_____

Other:_____

Patient Presented at Hospital Wearing Clothing Put On Immediately After the Assault:

Describe clothing put on after the assault, (with minimal handling) carefully noting any visible signs of foreign material (grass, fiber, hair, twigs, soil, splinters, glass, blood, dry or moist secretions). Focus on clothes worn closest to the genitals or areas where the suspect's mouth made contact, i.e., breasts/bra.

Bra:_____

Shirt:_____

Undershirt:_____

Sweater:_____

Jacket:_____

Pants:_____

Underwear:_____

Socks (state one or two socks present):_____

Shoes (state one or two socks present):_____

Other:_____

San Diego County SART
ADDENDUM TO 923
CLOTHING DOCUMENTATION

Patient's Description of Clothing Worn During the Assault:

_____ Patient brought clothing worn during assualt. Collected by forensic examiner.
(Initial)

_____ Clothing worn at the time of the assault collected by law enforcement prior to arrival of the forensic examiner.
(Initial)

_____ Patient provides location of clothing worn at the time of the assault and/or additional evidence and law enforcement
(Initial)
is notified at _____ hours.

_____ Clothing collected by law enforcement.
(Initial)

In cases involving non-acute exams where clothing, bedding, or other evidence has been identified and collected, a DNA reference sample must be collected from the patient.

Buccal Swab _____   Blood _____

Based on the patient's history, note any areas that need to be evaluated by the Crime Lab and/or investigating officer for foreign material, i.e., blood, dry or moist secretions, and/or tears, stretched out material, and missing buttons.

Bra:_____

Shirt:_____

Undershirt:_____

Sweater:_____

Jacket:_____

Pants:_____

Underwear:_____

Socks (state one or two socks present):_____

Shoes (state one or two socks present):_____

Other:_____

REFERENCES

American College of Emergency Physicians. *Evaluation of Patients with Complaint of Sexual Assault and Sexual Abuse.* Washington, DC: Health and Human Services, Maternal and Child Health Bureau, Department of Health and Human Services; 1999.

Asplen CH. Forensic DNA evidence: national commission explores its future. *Natl Inst Justice J.* January 1999;238:17-24.

Budowle B, et al. Analysis of the VNTR locus (D1S80) by the PCR followed by high-resolution PAGE. *Am J Hum Genet.* 1991;48:137-144.

Cain I. National University Forensic Science Graduate, San Diego Police Department Sex Crimes Unit Student Intern. 2002.

California Penal Code, 2001.

California State Senate Bill 1818. *DNA data base.* September 28, 2000.

California Department of Justice. Information Bulletin: *Legislative Changes to Sex and Violent Offender Requirements to Provide Blood and Saliva Samples for DNA and Other Forensic Identification.* Sacramento, Calif: Bureau of Forensic Services; 1999. 99-02-BFS.

Federal Bureau of Investigation (FBI). *Combined DNA Index System Bulletin Board for CODIS Laboratories.* Washington, DC: US Department of Justice; 2000a.

Federal Bureau of Investigation (FBI). *The FBI's Combined DNA Index System (CODIS) Program Brochure.* Washington, DC: US Department of Justice; 2000b.

Federal Bureau of Investigation (FBI). Uniform Crime Report 1997. Washington, DC: US Department of Justice; 1997.

Final Report, National DNA Survey, submitted by the Police Executive Research Forum, 1120 Connecticut Avenue, Suite 930, Washington, DC. 20036, (202)466-7820. Commissioned work by the National Commission on the Future of DNA Evidence, Office of Science and Technology, National Institute of Justice, US Department of Justice.

Fregeau CJ, Fourney RM. DNA typing with fluorescently tagged short tandem repeats: a sensitive and accurate approach to human identification. *Biotechniques.* 1993;15:100-119.

Gaensslen RE. *Sourcebook in Forensic Serology, Immunology, and Biochemistry.* Washington, DC: National Institute of Justice; 1983.

Inman K, Rudin N. *An Introduction to Forensic DNA Analysis.* New York, NY: CRC Press; 1997.

International Association of Forensic Nurses (IAFN). *Sexual Assault Nurse Examiner Standards of Practice.* Pitman, NJ: IAFN; 1996.

International Association of Forensic Nurses (IAFN). *Sexual Assault Nurse Examiner Educational Guidelines.* Pitman, NJ: IAFN; 1998.

Jeffreys AJ, Wilson V, Thein SL. Individual specific fingerprints of human DNA. *Nature.* 1985;316:76-79.

LaCoss J. *A Study of the Association Between DNA Analysis and Law Enforcement Outcomes in Cases of Sexual Assault Reported to the San Diego Police Department* [master's thesis]. San Diego, Calif: National University; 2000.

Ledray LE. *SANE Operation and Development Guide.* Washington, DC: Office for Victims of Crime, US Department of Justice; 1996.

Ledray LE. *Sexual Assault Nurse Examiner Development and Operation Guide*. Washington DC: Office for Victims of Crime, US Department of Justice; 1999.

Ledray LE, Netzel LN. DNA evidence collection. *J Emerg Nurs*. 1997;23:156-158.

Moreau DM, Bigbee PD. Major physical evidence in sexual assault investigations. In: Hazelwood RR, Burgess AW, eds. *Practical Aspects of Rape Investigation: A Multidisciplinary Approach*. Boca Raton, Fla: CRC Press, Inc; 1995:75-113.

Mullis KB, et al. Specific enzymatic amplification of DNA in vitro: the polymerase chain reaction. *Cold Spring Harbor Symp Quant Biol*. 1986;51:263-273.

National Institute of Justice (NIJ), National Commission on the Future of DNA. *What Every Law Enforcement Officer Should Know About DNA Evidence*. Washington, DC: National Institute of Justice; Sept. 1999.

National Research Council (NRC). *DNA Technology in Forensic Science*. Washington, DC: National Academy Press; 1992.

National Research Council (NRC). *The Evaluation of Forensic DNA Evidence*. Washington, DC: National Academy Press; 1996.

Reynolds R, et al. Analysis of genetic markers in forensic DNA samples using the polymerase chain reaction. *Analytical Chem*. 1991;63:2-15.

Saferstein R, ed. *Forensic Science Handbook*. Englewood Cliffs, NJ: Prentice-Hall Inc; 1982.

Saferstein R, ed. *Forensic Science Handbook*. Vol 2. Englewood Cliffs, NJ: Prentice-Hall Inc; 1988.

Santucci KA, Nelson DG, McQuillen KK, Duffy, SJ, Linakis JG. Wood's lamp utility in the identification of semen. *Pediatrics*. 1999;104:1342-1344.

Scheck B, Neufeld P, Dwyer J. *Actual Innocence: Five Days to Execution, and Other Dispatches from the Wrongly Convicted*. New York, NY: Doubleday; 2000.

Scheck B, Neufeld P, Dwyer J. *Actual Innocence: When Justice Goes Wrong and How to Make it Right*. New York, NY: Signet; 2001.

Sweet D, Lorente M, Lorente JA, Valenzuela A, Villanueva E. An improved method to recover saliva from human skin: the double swab technique. *J Forensic Sci*. 1997;42:320-322.

Tanner R. DNA frees 100th inmate as advocates call for movement to reform. *Associated Press*. January 17, 2002.

Travis J, Asplen C. *Post-Conviction DNA Testing: Recommendations for Handling Requests*. Washington, DC: National Institute of Justice; 1999.

US Department of Justice, Bureau of Justice Statistics. *Criminal Victimization 1998: Changes 1997-98 with Trends 1993-98*. Washington, DC. 1999: 7.

US Department of Justice, Bureau of Justice Statistics. *1999 National Crime Victimization Survey*. Washington, DC. 2000

Wambaugh J. *The Blooding*. New York, NY: Bantam Doubleday Dell Publishing Group; 1989.

Weedn VW, Hicks JW. The unrealized potential of DNA testing. *Natl Inst Justice J*. December 1997;234:17-23.

Chapter 17

Sexually Transmitted Diseases and Pregnancy Prophylaxis in Adolescents and Adults

Margot Schwartz, MD
Jeanne Marrazzo, MD, MPH

Male and female victims of sexual assault frequently fear the acquisition of sexually transmitted diseases (STDs), including human immunodeficiency virus (HIV) infection. In addition, women who are victims of sexual assault may fear becoming pregnant as a result of the attack. STDs in child victims of assault are discussed in Chapter 5 and are not addressed in this chapter. This chapter will (1) review STDs and related syndromes in adolescents and adults and their evaluation in the victim of sexual assault; (2) cover treatment and prevention strategies for STDs and HIV in victims of sexual assault; and (3) discuss options for emergency contraception.

A limited number of studies have addressed the incidence of STD after sexual assault. In victims who were sexually active before the assault, the question may arise as to whether an STD found at the time of the initial physical examination after the assault was present previously. If the victim comes for medical care within 72 hours of the assault, many STDs will not have had sufficient time to incubate and thus will not be detected. However, if *Chlamydia trachomatis* is present in the semen of the assailant, it may be detected in a female assault victim immediately after the assault (Glaser et al., 1991). Evaluation of the assault victim may also be complicated if sexual intercourse occurred between the initial evaluation and a follow-up medical visit a few weeks later; STDs may have been acquired after the assault. Although it is rarely possible to determine whether an STD was present before the assault, proving that an STD was acquired as the result of an assault may have important emotional or legal ramifications.

Several factors may predict the risk of acquiring an STD from an assailant. These include whether or not penile penetration and ejaculation occurred, what type of sexual assault occurred (vaginal, anal, or oral penetration), the number of assailants, the susceptibility of the victim to infection, the inoculum size for a given pathogen, and the infectivity of the organism (Glaser et al., 1986, 1989; Jenny et al., 1990). For example, the rate of transmission of *C. trachomatis* from male to female partner has been estimated at 0.35; that is, one third to one half of women engaging in coital acts with men infected with *C. trachomatis* will also become infected (Katz, 1992; Quinn et al., 1996).

Because victims of assault may have preexisting STDs, the prevalence of STD at the initial post-assault evaluation, usually performed within the first few days after an assault, tends to reflect the baseline rates of STDs in the community or population under study. Studies that have evaluated rates of STD prevalence among victims of sexual assault have generally involved women. Gonorrhea has been found in 0% to

Key Point:
Some factors that can predict the risk of acquiring an STD from an assailant include the following:
— *Whether or not penile penetration and ejaculation occurred*
— *The type of sexual assault that occurred (vaginal, anal, or oral)*
— *The number of assailants*
— *The victim's susceptibility to infection*
— *The size of the inoculum for a given pathogen*
— *The organism's infectivity*

20% of victims (median 3.3%), chlamydia in 0% to 8% (median 3.3%), trichomoniasis in 2% to 20% (median 9.4%), bacterial vaginosis in 2% to 38% (median 18.3%), genital warts in 2% to 20% (median 5.6%), and syphilis in 0% to 3% (Beck-Sague & Solomon, 1999; Schwarcz & Whittington, 1990). One study reported that 18% of male victims of sexual assault had an STD (Hillman et al., 1991).

A decision to provide treatment for STD at the initial evaluation depends on whether an STD-related syndrome is present, the pathogen involved, and the underlying prevalence of STD in the community. Some STDs, such as genital herpes and genital warts, are chronic and recur with or without treatment, so many sexually active adults will have preexisting infection. Thus, preventive therapy after sexual assault for these viral STDs is not routinely offered. If recognized at the post-assault examination, gonorrhea, *Chlamydia*, and trichomoniasis can be treated. Postexposure prophylaxis for HIV, one exception in which preventive therapy for a chronic sexually transmitted infection is sometimes offered after sexual assault, will be discussed later in this chapter. In addition, vaccination for preventable STDs, such as hepatitis B, should be considered.

RECOGNITION AND TREATMENT OF COMMON SEXUALLY TRANSMITTED DISEASES AND ASSOCIATED SYNDROMES

STDs can be caused by bacteria, such as *Neisseria gonorrhoeae* or *C. trachomatis*; viruses, such as herpes simplex virus, hepatitis viruses or human papilloma virus (HPV), protozoa, such as *Trichomonas vaginalis*; and treponemes such as *Treponema pallidum*, which causes syphilis. In addition, ectoparasites such as lice (*Phthiriasis pubis* or "crabs") or scabies (*Sarcoptes scabiei*) are parasites that live on skin or hair. Some STDs cause well-described clinical syndromes, including mucopurulent cervicitis, pelvic inflammatory disease (PID), and nongonococcal urethritis (NGU). Individual STDs will be discussed in detail. **Table 17-1** summarizes treatment options for STDs commonly diagnosed after sexual assault.

GONORRHEA

Gonorrhea refers to the clinical syndromes caused by the gram-negative intracellular diplococcus, *N. gonorrhoeae*. Although rates of gonorrhea declined in the United States between 1985 and 1997, rates began to rise again in 1998 (Centers for Disease Control and Prevention [CDC], June 23, 2000). In men, gonorrhea causes urethritis, characterized by urethral discharge or dysuria (painful urination), epididymitis (fever and epididymal or testicular pain), proctitis (rectal pain and discharge), and pharyngeal infection (usually asymptomatic). In women, gonorrhea causes infection of the cervix that is frequently asymptomatic, but may present with mucopurulent vaginal discharge consequent to mucopurulent cervicitis. Gonorrhea may also cause PID, characterized by lower abdominal pain and sometimes fever, nausea and vomiting, or abnormal vaginal bleeding. Untreated gonococcal or chlamydial infection of the upper genital tract in women frequently leads to tubal infertility, ectopic pregnancy, and chronic pelvic pain; thus recognition and early treatment of these pathogens is extremely important. Gonococcal conjunctivitis, pharyngitis, and disseminated gonococcal infection (mainly affecting the joints and skin) can occur in both men and women. The incubation period for gonorrhea is typically 2 to 7 days; therefore, acute infection may be present at the initial post-assault evaluation. The diagnosis can often be made within minutes using a Gram stain of secretions obtained from the affected area (endocervical, urethral, or conjunctival swab). The Gram stain is >95% sensitive and 95% specific for the diagnosis of gonococcal urethritis in men; although less sensitive (about 50%) for the diagnosis of cervicitis or proctitis, it is highly specific (Hook & Handsfield, 1999). Specific diagnostic testing, such as culture or nucleic acid amplification (NAA) tests, including polymerase chain reaction (PCR) and ligase chain reaction (LCR) assays, are required to make a definitive diagnosis of cervical, rectal, or

Key Point:
Untreated gonococcal or chlamydial infection of a woman's upper genital tract can produce tubal infertility, ectopic pregnancy, or chronic pelvic pain. Recognition and early treatment of these pathogens is extremely important.

pharyngeal infection. However, NAA tests are not yet approved for use with pharyngeal or rectal specimens.

For treatment of uncomplicated gonorrhea of the urethra, cervix, or rectum, a single oral dose of cefixime 400 mg, ciprofloxacin 500 mg, or levofloxacin 500 mg can be used, or ceftriaxone 125 mg can be given intramuscularly (IM) (**Table 17-1**). Fluoroquinolones are not recommended for pregnant women or for persons who may have acquired gonorrhea from Hawaii or Southeast Asia, where resistance rates to these drugs are high (CDC Guidelines, 2002). Spectinomycin (2 g IM) is an alternative if there are contraindications against using cephalosporins (such as allergy) or fluoroquinolones (such as allergy or pregnancy), but it is not reliable treatment for gonococcal pharyngeal infection. The supply of spectinomycin is now limited.

Table 17-1. Antibiotic Regimens Used to Treat Common STDs Found After Sexual Assault

STD	Antibiotic	Dose and Route	Duration
Gonorrhea* (uncomplicated urethritis, cervictitis, or proctitis)	Ceftriaxone	125 mg IM†	Single dose
	Cefixime	400 mg PO	Single dose
	Ciprofloxacin	500 mg PO	Single dose
	Levofloxacin	250 mg PO	Single dose
Chlamydia (uncomplicated cervictitis, or proctitis)	Azithromycin	1 g PO	Single dose
	Doxycycline	100 mg PO bid**	7 days
	Alternatives:		
	Levofloxacin	500 mg qd	7 days
	Ofloxacin	300 mg bid	7 days
	Erythromycin base	500 mg qid	7 days
Trichomoniasis	Metronidazole	2 g PO	Single dose
	Metronidazole	500 mg bid	7 days
Bacterial vaginosis	Metronidazole	500 mg PO bid	7 days
	Metronidazole gel (0.75%)	5 g intravaginally qd	5 days
	Clindamycin cream (2%)	5 g intravaginally qhs	7 days
	Clindamycin	300 mg PO bid	7 days
Primary herpes simplex virus (HSV) infection (first clinical episode)	Acyclovir	400 mg PO tid	7-10 days
	Acyclovir	200 mg PO 5 times daily	7-10 days
	Famciclovir	250 mg PO tid	7-10 days
	Valacyclovir	1 g PO bid	7-10 days

*When treating for gonorrhea, also treat empirically for chlamydia.

†IM = intramuscularly, PO = orally, mg = milligrams, g = gram.

**qd = once daily, bid = twice daily, tid = three times daily, qid = four times daily, qhs = at night.

Drug dosage recommendations listed herein are those of the authors and are not endorsed by the US Public Health Service or the US Department of Health and Human Services.

For gonococcal conjunctivitis, a single dose of 1 gram of ceftriaxone is given IM, and for disseminated gonococcal infection, higher and more prolonged doses of ceftriaxone are used. All individuals with a diagnosis of gonorrhea should be presumptively treated for coexistent chlamydial infection, because these two infections frequently occur simultaneously.

CHLAMYDIA INFECTION

C. trachomatis is an obligate intracellular bacteria. Asymptomatic infection is common with *C. trachomatis*, occurring in approximately 90% of infected women and about 60% of infected men (Marrazzo & Stamm, 1998). Important syndromes associated with *C. trachomatis* include urethritis, cervicitis, PID, epididymitis, proctitis, and conjunctivitis. Infection of the urethra with *C. trachomatis* can mimic a urinary tract infection in men and women by causing dysuria and pyuria. *Chlamydia* is most common in adolescents and young adults in the United States, infecting 12% to 25% of female adolescents (Burstein et al., 1998; Marrazzo et al., 1997). *C. trachomatis* has been associated with a reactive arthritis (previously termed Reiter's syndrome, a constellation of urethritis, arthritis, conjunctivitis, and skin lesions [keratoderma blennorrhagica and circinate balanitis]). The incubation period for *C. trachomatis* is longer than for *N. gonorrhoeae*, on the order of 1 to 2 weeks (Stamm, 1999).

The diagnosis of *C. trachomatis* can be made in several ways, these including, in decreasing order of sensitivity, NAA tests (such as LCR and PCR), culture, antigen detection tests (direct fluorescent antibody and enzyme linked immunoassay), and nonamplified DNA probe. *C. trachomatis* cannot be seen by Gram stain, but the presence of polymorphonuclear leukocytes (PMN) on a Gram stain of urethral exudate (≥5 per high power field), mucopurulent cervical discharge, or easily induced endocervical bleeding suggests a compatible clinical syndrome.

For uncomplicated chlamydial infection of the urethra, cervix, or rectum, a single dose of azithromycin (1 g orally [PO]) is as effective as a 1-week regimen of doxycycline (100 mg bid) (Martin et al., 1992; Stamm et al., 1995). Although a single dose of azithromycin is more expensive than doxycycline, compliance is markedly enhanced with single-dose therapy (Katz et al., 1992; Brookhoff, 1994). Alternative regimens for *C. trachomatis* include levofloxacin or ofloxacin; less effective is erythromycin. Ciprofloxacin is not adequately effective against *C. trachomatis*. Levofloxacin, ofloxacin, and doxycycline are contraindicated in the pregnant patient; erythromycin or amoxicillin should be used to treat *Chlamydia* in pregnancy. Extensive data on the use of azithromycin, although widely used in pregnancy, are not available. Regardless of which antibiotic is used to treat *Chlamydia* in pregnancy, a test of cure should be performed 3 weeks after completion of therapy.

SYPHILIS

Syphilis is caused by the spirochete *Treponema pallidum*. Although rates of syphilis declined in the United States through the 1990s, with reported rates as low as 2.5 per 100,000 in 1999 (Division of STD Prevention, 2000), rising rates in some urban areas have been reported among men who have sex with men (CDC, Feb 23, 2001). The incubation period varies from 10 days to 3 months. Thus, early syphilis is not frequently diagnosed at the initial patient evaluation after a sexual assault. Many patients are asymptomatic during the early phase of infection and do not notice a primary lesion (chancre) or secondary rash. The primary syphilitic chancre is typically a painless ulcer, but cannot be reliably distinguished from genital ulcers caused by other pathogens, such as herpes or chancroid. Secondary syphilis, which occasionally overlaps primary infection, may cause a generalized macular and papular rash involving the palms and soles. Mucocutaneous lesions, including condyloma lata, a moist, flat, wartlike lesion, and lymphadenopathy may accompany this rash.

Key Point:
Usually, early syphilis is not diagnosed at the initial patient evaluation after a sexual assault. Most patients are asymptomatic during this early phase and do not notice a primary lesion or a secondary rash.

The diagnosis of syphilis can be made with a darkfield examination or performance of fluorescent antibody test of fluid from a primary syphilitic chancre, or by serologic testing. Non-treponemal tests such as the rapid plasma reagin (RPR) and Venereal Disease Research Laboratory (VDRL) tests have high false positive rates and must be confirmed by treponemal tests. Treponemal tests include the fluorescent treponemal antibody absorption (FTA-ABS), the treponemal pallidum particle agglutination, and the microhemagglutination assay for antibody to *T. pallidum* (MHA-TP). Quantification of non-treponemal tests is used to follow response to treatment.

Penicillin is the drug of choice for treating syphilis. Primary, secondary, and early latent syphilis are treated with a single intramuscular shot of 2.4 million units of benzathine penicillin G. For the nonpregnant patient with a history of allergy to penicillin, doxycycline or tetracycline can be substituted except for patients with neurosyphilis. Penicillin is the gold standard, especially for neurosyphilis, and penicillin skin testing and desensitization should be considered for patients with allergy to penicillin. Patients treated with regimens other than penicillin should be monitored closely for treatment failure. A single 1-gram dose of azithromycin, which is part of the recommended prophylactic antibiotic regimen for the victim of sexual assault, is efficacious in combating syphilis during the incubation period following exposure (Hook et al., 1999).

CHANCROID

Chancroid, caused by the bacteria *Haemophilus ducreyi*, is an uncommon cause of genital ulcer in most areas of the United States. Unlike syphilis, the ulcers of chancroid are often painful, and tender regional lymphadenopathy is common. Culture (which is not readily available) is required for diagnosis. If chancroid is suspected, an expert should be consulted. Effective antibiotics for chancroid include azithromycin, ceftriaxone, ciprofloxacin, and erythromycin.

TRICHOMONIASIS

Trichomoniasis, caused by the protozoan *Trichomonas vaginalis*, is a common cause of vaginitis in women and a less frequent cause of urethritis in men. In women, it is one of the most prevalent STDs found during the sexual assault evaluation. Its incubation period is 4 to 20 days. Vaginal discharge caused by *T. vaginalis* may be purulent and malodorous, and women may also complain of external dysuria, itching, genital irritation, or dyspareunia. As with bacterial vaginosis, the pH of the vaginal exudate is high ($\geq$5.0). Cervical petechiae ("strawberry cervix") may be noted on examination.

Key Point:
Trichomoniasis is one of the most prevalent STDs found during the sexual assault evaluation.

The diagnosis of trichomoniasis may be made by finding motile trichomonads on a saline preparation of vaginal exudate or by culture. Although the wet mount is the most common tool for diagnosing trichomoniasis, its sensitivity when used with vaginal fluid is only 60% compared to culture (Krieger et al., 1988). *T. vaginalis* infection should be suspected if PMNs are prominent in the absence of trichomonads on the saline wet prep. Men with trichomoniasis may be asymptomatic or have symptoms of NGU (urethral discharge and/or dysuria). *T. vaginalis* is not transmitted between men.

The drug of choice for trichomoniasis is oral metronidazole, either as a single 2-g dose or as a twice-daily dose of 500 mg for 1 week. Metronidazole gel, which is used for the treatment of bacterial vaginosis, is ineffective for trichomoniasis and is not recommended. Although a single 2-g dose of metronidazole is included in the recommended antibiotic prophylaxis regimen for female victims of sexual assault, some experts recommend deferring empiric therapy until the follow-up visit 2 weeks later because metronidazole-induced nausea may interfere with pregnancy prophylaxis (Linden, 1999). In support of this approach, *T. vaginalis* does not cause ascending pelvic infection and infertility, and therefore, delaying empiric therapy may not have long-term consequences. However, *T. vaginalis* has been associated with premature rupture of membranes in the pregnant patient (Minkoff et al., 1984). Because many victims of assault will not return for follow-up visits, the opportunity for preventing this complication as well as the infection itself may be missed if prophylactic drug therapy is not offered at the initial visit.

HERPES SIMPLEX

Approximately one in five adults in the United States is infected with herpes simplex virus (HSV) type 2, which is responsible for most genital herpes (Fleming et al., 1997). HSV type 1 usually causes oral cold sores, but may account for up to 30% of genital herpes in the United States (Corey & Wald, 1999). Clinically, genital infections caused by HSV-1 and HSV-2 may be initially indistinguishable, but genital HSV-1 infection follows a more benign course with less frequent and less severe recurrences (Corey & Wald, 1999). The incubation period after exposure to HSV ranges from 2 to 12 days. Most infected individuals are asymptomatic on most days and have localized recurrences with symptoms. Even in the absence of genital blisters or ulcers characteristic of herpes, infected individuals may shed the virus and transmit it to another person (Wald et al., 1995). The primary or initial outbreak of HSV-1 or HSV-2 in an individual is usually worse than subsequent episodes and should be sought specifically in the victim of sexual assault. Symptoms of primary HSV infection may be systemic, especially in women, and include fever, headache, malaise, and myalgia (Corey et al., 1983). Aseptic meningitis, symptomatic urethritis, and cervicitis may also occur. For persons with anal exposure, herpes proctitis can occur as part of a primary or recurrent infection. Recurrences are characterized by localized blisters on an erythematous base, which usually occur in clusters. When the vesicular or pustular lesions break open, an ulcer is seen, which on a dry surface, forms a crust or a scab after a few days. Herpes lesions may be atypical, especially in people co-infected with HIV. Thus, any genital lesion, especially with the appropriate history, should be evaluated appropriately. However, unless a lesion is typically "herpetic," one should always consider ruling out syphilis in the evaluation, particularly in the post-assault evaluation.

Viral culture, direct fluorescent antibody testing, or PCR are commonly used for the diagnosis of genital herpes infections. The base of the lesion should be swabbed with a Dacron-tipped swab, which is then inoculated into the appropriate media. Antigen detection is less sensitive than culture; the Tzanck prep is insensitive and should not be used. PCR is highly sensitive and specific, but expensive. Type-specific serologic tests are now available for the diagnosis of HSV. Newer serologic tests based upon glycoprotein G reliably distinguish HSV-1 from HSV-2, whereas older tests did not accurately make this distinction. It may take up to 3 months for an individual to show evidence of HSV antibodies on serologic testing; thus, testing should be deferred in recently exposed persons.

Although most recurrent episodes of genital herpes are self-limited, all patients with primary or initial episodes of genital herpes should receive antiviral therapy. In patients with recurrent episodes, antiviral therapy may decrease the symptoms and duration of outbreaks (Wald, 1999). Systemic therapies commonly used for the treatment of genital herpes include acyclovir, famciclovir, and valacyclovir. Acyclovir is less expensive than the famciclovir and valacyclovir, but is less well absorbed and must be taken more frequently. Topical acyclovir has not been proven effective for genital herpes.

HUMAN PAPILLOMAVIRUS

HPVs commonly cause anogenital warts and infrequently cause cervical and anal neoplasia. More than 70 subtypes of HPV can infect the genital tract; types 16 and 18 confer the highest risk for neoplasia, and types 6 and 11 are commonly found in genital warts. Most HPV infections are asymptomatic and chronic. External genital

Key Point:
Even without the detection of genital blisters or ulcers characteristic of herpes, infected persons can shed the virus and transmit it to another person.

warts are usually diagnosed based on appearance alone. They are commonly papular rather than flat (unlike condyloma lata) and are hyperkeratotic or cauliflower-like in appearance. HPVs are the most common cause of cervical neoplasia. Women with genital warts should have a Papanicolaou smear in accord with routine guidelines. Women or men with visible perianal warts should undergo anoscopy. Available treatments for genital warts include cryotherapy with liquid nitrogen, topical podophyllin, trichloroacetic acid, or patient-applied podofilox or imiquimod. Alternative treatments for extensive warts or for those not responding to therapy include surgical excision or CO_2 laser surgery.

BACTERIAL VAGINOSIS

Bacterial vaginosis is the most common cause of vaginitis in women and is frequently found in women after sexual assault. It is associated with a history of a new sex partner and of douching (Hawes et al., 1996), but has not been associated with a sexually transmitted pathogen. The overgrowth of common vaginal anaerobes, including *Prevotella* sp., *Mobiluncus* sp., *Bacteroides* sp., and *Gardnerella vaginalis*, cause bacterial vaginosis and its attendant malodorous discharge. On examination, a homogeneous, uniformly adherent, milky-white discharge may be seen. The diagnosis of bacterial vaginosis is made if 3 of the following 4 criteria are met (Amsel et al., 1983):

— PH of vaginal discharge >4.5

— Fishy or amine odor after addition of 10% potassium hydrochloride (KOH) (whiff test)

— Presence of >20% clue cells on examination of saline preparation of discharge

— Presence of homogeneous discharge

Treatment regimens can be oral (metronidazole 500 mg or clindamycin 300 mg twice daily for 1 week) or intravaginal (metronidazole 0.75% gel for 5 days, or clindamycin cream for 7 days, both used at night). A single 2-g dose of metronidazole, as used for *Trichomonas*, is associated with higher relapse rates than the other regimens, but may be useful in the patient who is unlikely to adhere to longer regimens.

MUCOPURULENT CERVICITIS

Mucopurulent cervicitis is characterized by the presence of mucopurulent endocervical exudate. Easily induced cervical bleeding and edematous cervical ectopy may also occur. Although *C. trachomatis* and *N. gonorrhoeae* are well-known causes of mucopurulent cervicitis, more than half of cases have no known etiology; however, many relevant studies were performed before the advent of highly sensitive diagnostic tests for *Chlamydia* and gonorrhea. The criteria for establishing the diagnosis of mucopurulent cervicitis are somewhat controversial. In women younger than 25 years old, the presence of ≥30 PMNs per 1000¥ field on examination of endocervical exudate is suggestive of but not definitive for the diagnosis, and many experts recommend against performing this test (Sellors et al., 1998). All women should be tested for gonorrhea and *Chlamydia* if mucopurulent cervicitis is noted. Treatment for mucopurulent cervicitis is directed against *C. trachomatis* and, depending on the individual's risk and the baseline gonorrhea prevalence in the population, *N. gonorrhoeae*. In the sexual assault victim, preventive regimens as described in **Table 17-2** are adequate for treating this syndrome.

PELVIC INFLAMMATORY DISEASE

PID describes any combination of endometritis, salpingitis, tubo-ovarian abscess, and pelvic peritonitis. It is associated with sexually transmitted pathogens, such as *C. trachomatis* and *N. gonorrhoeae*, as well as bacteria that normally colonize the vagina, including anaerobes associated with bacterial vaginosis. PID is important to

Key Point:
HPVs are the most common cause of cervical neoplasia.

Key Point:
Bacterial vaginosis is the most common cause of vaginitis in women and is often found in women after sexual assault.

recognize and treat early, as its sequelae include infertility, chronic pelvic pain, and ectopic pregnancy. Vaginal douching has been associated with an increased risk of PID and ectopic pregnancy (a sequela of PID) (Daling et al., 1991; Scholes et al., 1993). Symptoms include lower abdominal pain, nausea and/or vomiting, fever, vaginal discharge, and sometimes a change in the menstrual pattern. On examination, abdominal tenderness, adnexal tenderness, and cervical motion tenderness may be present. Fever and abnormal cervical or vaginal discharge are sometimes found. If the patient is pregnant; is unable to take oral therapy, has a suspected tubo-ovarian abscess; has severe illness with nausea, vomiting, or high fever; or if another surgical diagnosis (such as appendicitis) is in question, then hospitalization may be required. Recommended treatments include antibiotics to cover *C. trachomatis*, *N. gonorrhoeae*, and anaerobes (**Table 17-2**). Women with PID should have follow-up examinations 2 to 3 days after starting treatment to assess for improvement.

Key Point:
Women with PID should have follow-up examinations 2 to 3 days after they begin treatment to evaluate the effectiveness of the regimen.

PROCTITIS AND PROCTOCOLITIS
Sexual assault victims who have had anal penetration by the assailant's penis are at risk for proctitis and proctocolitis. Proctitis refers to inflammation of the rectum and may cause anorectal pain or itching, tenesmus (a sensation that one must defecate when stool is not passed), or rectal discharge. STD pathogens that commonly cause proctitis include *N. gonorrhoeae*, *C. trachomatis*, *T. pallidum*, and herpes simplex virus. Proctocolitis refers to inflammation of the colon and rectum.

Table 17-2. Recommended Treatment for Pelvic Inflammatory Disease

OUTPATIENT

— Levofloxacin 500 mg once daily or ofloxacin 400 mg twice daily
  PLUS
  Metronidazole 500 mg twice daily for 14 days

  OR

— Cefriaxone 250 mg or Probenecid 1 g with cefoxitin 2 g IM (once)
  PLUS
  Doxycycline 100 mg orally twice daily for 14 days, with or without
    metronidazole 500 mg twice daily for 14 days

— Intravenous cefoxitin or cefotetan
  PLUS
  Doxycycline 100 mg IV or orally twice daily for 14 days

  OR

— Intravenous cefoxitin or cefotetan
  PLUS
  Doxycycline 100 mg IV or orally twice daily for 14 days

  OR

— Intravenous clindamycin plus gentamicin initially, followed by clindamycin
    450 mg orally 4 times daily or doxycycline 100 mg orally twice daily to
    complete 14 days of therapy

Drug dosage recommendations listed herein are those of the authors and are not endorsed by the US Public Health Service or the US Department of Health and Human Services.

Symptoms include those listed for proctitis, plus diarrhea and/or abdominal cramping. Pathogens that cause proctocolitis are more commonly enteric pathogens from fecal-oral contact, such as *Campylobacter* sp., *Shigella* sp., *Entamoeba histolytica*, and, less commonly, some serovars of *C. trachomatis*. The evaluation for proctitis/proctocolitis in the symptomatic patient includes anoscopy to look for mucosal erythema or edema, rectal ulcers, or bleeding. An abdominal examination should be done to look for left lower quadrant tenderness, sometimes present in proctocolitis. A Gram stain should be prepared from any exudate or mucus obtained on an anoscopically obtained swab to look for gram-negative intracellular diplococci consistent with *N. gonorrhoeae* or for abundant PMNs. In addition, rectal cultures for *N. gonorrhoeae* and *C. trachomatis* should be performed. Cultures for HSV should be done if suspected, especially if any suspicious lesions are seen. In addition, any perianal ulcers should be suspect for syphilis, and a darkfield examination and RPR should be performed. If severe cramps or diarrhea is present, or if the patient is HIV positive, stool samples should be obtained for evaluation of enteric pathogens, including ova and parasite examination.

Key Point:
Patients who have symptoms of proctitis or proctocolitis should undergo anoscopy to detect mucosal erythema or edema, rectal ulcers, or bleeding, and an abdominal examination to detect left lower quadrant tenderness.

Treatment for proctitis/proctocolitis should be directed at any pathogens identified, using the guidelines described earlier. If no clear pathogen is identified, and if anorectal pus or PMNs are present, then a single dose of cefixime (400 mg PO) or ceftriaxone (250 mg IM) plus 7 days of doxycycline (100 mg bid) is the recommended treatment for the nonpregnant patient.

PUBIC LICE

Pubic lice (pediculosis pubis, *Phthirus pubis*) cause itching and/or visible lice or nits in the pubic hair. They may also affect other areas of the body with hair, including the thighs, eyelashes, eyebrows, or trunk. Treatments include permethrin 1% cream rinse (Nix) or pyrethrin lotion (Rid, and others). Lindane 1% shampoo (Kwell, Scabene) is also effective but should not be used in pregnant or lactating women, young children, individuals with severe dermatitis or open skin lesions, or those with seizure disorders. It should also not be used after a bath. These regimens should not be used around the eyes.

SCABIES

Scabies (*Sarcoptes scabiei*) causes itching and a papular erythematous rash, often with excoriation. It is transmitted by close physical contact. Common areas include the finger webs and arms, trunk, inguinal area, labia majora, penis, scrotum, or buttocks. The diagnosis can be confirmed by microscopic examination obtained by scraping a fresh papule. Examination under oil or KOH may reveal the mite, eggs, or feces of *S. scabiei*. Permethrin 5% cream (Elimite) is the recommended treatment. Lindane 1% lotion or cream is an alternative, but the same precautions must be used as when treating pubic lice. For individuals with scabies or pubic lice, clothing and bedding should be washed and dried at high temperatures for prevention of reinfection.

VIRAL HEPATITIS

Both hepatitis A and hepatitis B viruses may be transmitted by sexual contact. Hepatitis A is shed in the feces, and transmission is fecal-oral. Men who have sex with men are at higher risk of sexually acquired hepatitis A (CDC, 2002). Infection with hepatitis A is self-limited, and treatment is supportive. Sexual transmission accounts for 30% to 60% of new cases of hepatitis B in the United States (CDC, 2002). Unlike hepatitis A, hepatitis B may become chronic in 1% to 6% of cases (CDC, 2002). Preventive vaccination after sexual assault is recommended for hepatitis B, and can be considered for hepatitis A if a high-risk exposure has occurred. In addition, for the highest risk exposures from an assailant believed to be a carrier of hepatitis B, hepatitis B immunoglobulin can be administered to the nonimmune victim.

Key Point:
Preventive vaccination after sexual assault is recommended for hepatitis B.

HISTORY AND PHYSICAL EXAMINATION

Medical providers should obtain a detailed, objective, nonjudgmental history of the assault with attention to the sensitive nature of the history and emotional state of the victim. This offers an opportunity for the examiner to gain the trust of the victim before obtaining any physical evidence. Pertinent historical information should include details regarding the assault and the assailant(s), any physical injury that may have occurred, menstrual history, history of recent consensual intercourse prior to the assault, and contraceptive history. **Table 17-3** lists important information to obtain from the assault victim regarding the sexual history. Further details of taking a comprehensive history from the adult victim of sexual assault are discussed in Chapter 14.

A careful physical examination of the assault victim should be performed. In addition to examining for signs of trauma, as described elsewhere in this textbook, a targeted examination for STDs should be performed, along with collection of specimens for STD testing and forensics. Some experts argue against routine testing for common STDs at the initial examination in the victim who has been sexually active previous to the assault if the patient is to be treated with prophylactic medications that treat these STDs (Linden, 1999). Most centers, however, routinely test for STDs at the initial and follow-up visits (see Specimen Collection).

Informed consent should be obtained before the medical examination and collection of specimens. Examination of the genitals, mouth, throat, and anus should be performed. The lower abdomen, inguinal areas, thighs, hands, palms, and soles should also be inspected for rashes or lesions. The inguinal and femoral areas should be examined for lymphadenopathy. In women a speculum examination of the vagina and cervix and bimanual pelvic examination should be performed. Colposcopy can aid in the evaluation of internal genital trauma in women. In men and women the anus should be evaluated for seminal fluid and signs of trauma, such as a relaxed external sphincter, fissures, and hemorrhoids. If anorectal injury is suspected, proctoscopy or anoscopy may be necessary. The penis should be inspected, including retraction of the foreskin and visualization of the urethral meatus. In addition, the prostate gland should be examined during a digital rectal examination.

DIAGNOSTIC EVALUATION

The diagnostic evaluation for STDs in women at the initial examination should include a microscopic analysis of a cervical Gram stain for evidence of gram-negative intracellular diplococci (indicating gonorrhea), and a saline preparation and trichomonas culture (if available) of vaginal fluid (**Table 17-4**). Culture for *T. vaginalis* helps to identify this organism relative to saline microscopy (Krieger et al., 1988). Saline microscopy should also be used to look for clue cells (evidence of bacterial vaginosis) or yeast. Other indicators of bacterial vaginosis are a homogeneous white discharge with a high pH (>4.5). A "whiff test" may detect a fishy odor to the vaginal discharge before or after adding 10% KOH. If rectal or urethral discharge is present, a Gram stain should be done to look for PMNs and gram-negative intracellular diplococci. Cultures of a cervical, urethral, pharyngeal, or rectal specimen obtained by a cotton-tipped swab for *N. gonorrhoeae* should be performed when penetration or attempted penetration have occurred. To detect *C. trachomatis*, a Dacron-tipped swab of the above areas, except the throat, should be performed.

NAA tests are sensitive in detecting *C. trachomatis* and *N. gonorrhoeae*. False positive results rarely occur; however, in a sexual assault evaluation, it may be necessary to confirm nonculture tests by a second FDA-approved nucleic amplification test that targets a different molecule from the initial test (CDC, 2002). LCR and PCR tests for gonorrhea and *Chlamydia* are approved using specimens only from the cervix, urethra, and urine; results from other sites should be interpreted with caution.

Other nonculture tests for *C. trachomatis* include the DNA probe (GenProbe), fluorescent antibody, and enzyme immunoassay (EIA) tests. These tests are more rapid and less expensive than culture, but less sensitive and specific. For this reason, the CDC does not recommend nonamplified DNA-based tests, fluorescent antibody, and EIA to evaluate victims of sexual assault (CDC, 2002). A DNA probe is also

---

Table 17-3. Important Information to Assess STD Risk for Sexual Assault Victims

1. Date and time of the assault

2. Interval between the assault and the initial medical evaluation

3. Number of assailants

4. Description and identification, if possible, of the assailant(s)

5. If the assailant is known, is his/her HIV status known?

6. Are the assailant's history of STD and risk behaviors such as intravenous drug use known?

7. Description of the assault, including type of sexual contact (vaginal, anal, and oral), penetration by a body part or other object, ejaculation, condom use, extragenital contact (vaginal, anal, and oral), trauma or threats that occurred, use of weapons by the assailant. Include a description of any contact with the assailant's blood or body fluid (especially on mucosal surfaces or breaks in the skin).

8. History of consensual sexual intercourse (ever, most recent, including any voluntary sexual intercourse that occurred between the assault and the initial evaluation, or between the initial evaluation and follow-up examination)

9. Last menstrual period and pregnancy status (for female victims)

10. Use of contraception (for female victims)

11. History of bathing, urinating, defecating, douching, changing clothes, or brushing teeth between the assault and the initial examination

12. History of sexually transmitted disease in the victim

13. History of previous sexual assault

14. Any symptoms including vaginal or rectal discharge; pelvic or rectal pain; genital, perianal, or oral lesions

15. History of prior or chronic medical conditions, including thrombosis, liver disease, or hypertension, which are theoretical contraindications to pregnancy prophylaxis

16. Medication allergy

> ### Table 17-4. Recommended Evaluation for STDs in Adult and Adolescent Victims of Sexual Assault
>
> #### WOMEN
>
> — Saline preparation of vaginal fluid to examine for motile trichomonads, clue cells, and yeast
>
> — Culture of vaginal fluid for *T. vaginalis*
>
> — Culture or NAA tests for *N. gonorrhoeae* and *C. trachomatis*
>
> — Serum testing for HIV, hepatitis B (surface antigen and antibody), and syphilis
>
> — Culture of suspicious lessions for herpes simplex virus if diagnosis was not established
>
> — Optional: pH of vaginal fluid and "whiff test" for evidence of bacterial vaginosis: cervical Gram stain for evidence of gram-negative intracellular diplococci and PMNs
>
> #### MEN
>
> — Culture or NAA tests for *N. gonorrhoeae* and *C. trachomatis* from any site of penetration or attempted penetration
>
> — Gram stain of any rectal or urethral discharge for evidence of gram-negative intracellular diplococci and PMNs
>
> — Serum testing for HIV, hepatitis B, and syphilis
>
> #### FOLLOW-UP EXAMINATIONS
>
> — 2 weeks after the assault or sooner (1 week) if no prophylactic therapy was provided
>
> — Repeat tests as above, unless prophylactic treatment was provided or if symptoms are reported
>
> — Follow-up serologic testing for HIV, hepatitis B, and syphilis 6, 12, and 24 weeks after the assault if initial results were negative

Key Point:
Because specificity of DNA-based tests is not 100%, these tests may not be admissible as legal evidence. In addition, prophylactic treatment after nonculture techniques were used during the initial evaluation makes retesting for legal evidence problematic. Every effort to perform diagnostic testing adequate for legal evidence should be made, but this should not override appropriate and timely therapy.

available to detect *N. gonorrhoeae*, but again it is less sensitive and specific than both culture and DNA amplification tests (LCR and PCR). Culture for gonorrhea and *Chlamydia* remains the gold standard for legal evidence because false positive tests are very unlikely. In addition, in the rare instance when both the victim and the assailant have had positive cultures for an STD, the strain can be compared between the victim and the assailant for similarity. Because specificity of DNA-based tests approaches but is not equal to 100%, these tests may not be admissible as legal evidence. Prophylactic treatment after nonculture techniques were used during the initial evaluation makes retesting for legal evidence problematic. Every effort to perform diagnostic testing adequate for legal evidence should be made, but this should not override appropriate and timely therapy.

Male victims of sexual assault may be at greater risk for syphilis, HIV, and entero-pathogens such as *Shigella* sp., amebiasis, *Giardia* sp., and hepatitis A. They should be tested and treated for these illnesses if symptomatic.

Baseline serologic tests should be performed for hepatitis B (if the victim has not previously been vaccinated) and syphilis. Victims should also be offered serologic testing for HIV. Women should have a serum or urine pregnancy test.

A follow-up examination should be performed about 2 weeks after the assault to detect newly acquired infections and to continue efforts to counsel and treat victims of sexual assault. Tests should include repeat testing for gonorrhea and *Chlamydia*, as well as saline microscopy of vaginal fluid in women if they did not receive prophylactic therapy against specific STDs or if they have any new symptoms of STDs. Follow-up serologic testing for syphilis (RPR or VDRL) and HIV should be done 6, 12, and 24 weeks after the assault, if test results were negative at the initial examination. Follow-up pregnancy tests should be offered to women.

TREATMENT AND PROPHYLAXIS OF STDs

Sexual assault victims should be treated for any STDs diagnosed at the initial or follow-up examination. Both experience and formal studies have shown that follow-up rates for victims of sexual assault are poor (Glaser et al., 1991; Putz et al., 1996). Efforts should be made at the initial examination to offer routine prophylaxis of STDs (**Table 17-5**). If the female victim is pregnant, doxycycline (or tetracycline) and quinolones (ciprofloxacin, levofloxacin, gatifloxacin, and others) should be avoided. Some experts recommend considering waiting until the 2-week follow-up visit for administering metronidazole because the nausea from metroni-dazole can interfere with pregnancy prophylaxis (Linden, 1999). Use of antiemetics or alternative dosing schedules may also be considered. Victims should be instructed to abstain from sexual intercourse until prophylactic therapy is completed.

Key Point:
Sexual assault victims should receive treatment for any STDs diagnosed at the initial or follow-up examination, recognizing that follow-up rates for victims of sexual assault are poor. Victims should be told to avoid sexual intercourse until prophylactic therapy is completed.

HIV POSTEXPOSURE PROPHYLAXIS

Women commonly report fear of acquiring HIV after a sexual assault (Baker et al., 1990). Although there are guidelines for postexposure prophylaxis for sexual exposure to HIV, these are extrapolated from postexposure prophylaxis guidelines in occupationally exposed individuals. In occupationally exposed individuals, antiretroviral therapy is thought to decrease the risk of HIV acquisition by 79% (CDC, 1995). The risk for HIV acquisition through sexual assault is considered low, but there have been documented cases of HIV seroconversion after sexual

---

Table 17-5. STD Prophylaxis in the Adult Victim of Sexual Assault

— Ceftriaxone 125 mg IM once
    PLUS
    Azithromycin 1 PO once, or doxycycline 100 mg bid for 7 days
    PLUS
    Metronidazole 2 g once (for women, or men who were assaulted by women)

— Hepatitis B vaccine if no prior history of vaccination or natural immunity; first dose at intial examination, second dose at 1 to 2 months, and third dose at 4 to 6 moths after the initial dose

— HIV prophylaxis (optional): see **Table 17-6**

Drug dosage recommendations listed herein are those of the authors and are not endorsed by the US Public Health Service or the US Department of Health and Human Services.

assault. Decisions regarding postexposure prophylaxis in victims of sexual assault depend on several factors, including the likelihood that the assailant is infected with HIV and, if so, what stage of HIV illness the assailant may have (Bamberger et al., 1999). Individuals with high viral loads of HIV in the blood are more likely to transmit HIV through sexual intercourse than are those with low viral loads (Quinn et al., 2000). Serum levels of HIV are generally highest immediately after seroconversion during the acute or primary HIV illness, or in the late stages of AIDS (Fauci et al., 1996). If the HIV status of the assailant is not known, one should determine if the assailant has any known risk factors for HIV, such as intravenous drug use or being a male with other male sex partners. Other factors to consider include what type of contact occurred during the assault and to which body fluids (including blood) the victim may have been exposed. Also, the number of assailants may be a factor or may add to the uncertainty of the risk of acquiring HIV. The type and severity of physical trauma may play a role in the sexual transmission of HIV because of potential blood exposure or disruption of protective mucosal surfaces. In addition, STDs are cofactors for HIV transmission and thus the presence of an STD, especially a genital ulcer, may increase the likelihood that HIV transmission will occur (Fleming & Wasserheit, 1999; Greenblatt et al., 1988; Gray et al., 2001; Kreiss et al., 1989; Telzac et al., 1993).

Estimates for the rate of HIV acquisition are highest with receptive anal intercourse, estimated at 10 to 30 new infections per 10,000 exposures among men who have sex with men, and receptive vaginal intercourse, estimated at 8 to 20 new infections per 10,000 exposures (Bamberger et al., 1999; Gray et al., 2001; Peterman et al., 1988). Although the risk of HIV acquisition from receptive oral intercourse is much lower, transmission has been reported via this route and is thought to be higher if ejaculation has occurred (Schacker et al., 1996).

Healthcare workers counseling victims of assault should thus try to assess the level of risk exposure to the victim. If the victim did not know the assailant, this may be impossible to determine. Other important factors in making decisions regarding postexposure prophylaxis include the length of time since the exposure, the health and reproductive status of the victim, the local epidemiology of HIV, and, most importantly, the victim's attitude toward postexposure prophylaxis. A clear discussion of risks versus benefits of postexposure prophylaxis should occur before prescribing postexposure prophylaxis. Initiating postexposure prophylaxis within 72 hours of exposure is recommended for occupational exposures to HIV, such as needle stick exposures with infected blood (CDC, June 29, 2001). Although this 72-hour cutoff is somewhat arbitrary, data in animals suggest that beginning postexposure prophylaxis within 4 hours of a blood exposure is most effective (Katz & Gerberding, 1997; Tsai et al., 1998).

The choice of antiretrovirals used in postexposure prophylaxis is based on both the guidelines for occupationally exposed individuals and established guidelines for treating patients with known HIV infection. Once the antiretrovirals are initiated, they should be continued for 4 weeks unless (1) the assailant was confirmed to be HIV negative and is not likely to be in the process of seroconversion or (2) a prohibitive side effect has occurred. Side effects are common, and victims receiving HIV postexposure prophylaxis should be counseled as to which side effects to expect. Similarly, a follow-up appointment within 2 weeks should be made, and patients should be told whom to call if side effects develop.

Suggested regimens for HIV postexposure prophylaxis are listed in **Table 17-6** (Bamberger et al., 1999; CDC, June 29, 2001; Katz & Gerberding, 1997). The standard regimen includes two nucleoside analogues; a third medication, usually the protease inhibitor indinavir or nelfinavir, is offered for the highest risk exposures. The recent CDC guidelines for occupational exposures also include efavirenz, a

Key Point:

The risks versus benefits of postexposure prophylaxis should be openly and clearly discussed before prescribing postexposure prophylaxis. All victims should be informed of the symptoms of primary HIV infection to be alert for (prolonged febrile or flu-like illness, fatigue, lymphadenopathy, rash, pharyngitis), and they should understand that postexposure prophylaxis is not 100% effective. Condoms must be used with regular sex partners until the testing for HIV is completed 6 months after the victim's potential exposure.

Table 17-6. Recommended Regimens for Postexposure Initiated Within 72 Hours of Sexual Exposure to HIV

Treatment regimen (4 weeks)
— Zidovudine (AZT) 300 mg orally twice daily or 200 mg orally 3 times daily
 PLUS
 Lamivudine (3TC) 150 mg orally twice daily
  (Zidovudine 300 mg/Lamivudine 150 mg are available in a
  combination pill)
 OR
 Stavudine (D4T) 40 mg orally twice daily
 PLUS
 Didanosine (ddI) 200 mg orally twice daily

Consider adding to either regimen for highest risk exposures (assailant with a viral >50,000 copies/mL or suspected advanced HIV disease or has suspected resistance to the one or both nucleoside analogue medications in the regimen):

— Nelfinavir 1250 mg orally every 12 hours or 750 mg every 8 hours
 OR
 Indinavir 800 mg orally every 8 hours
 OR
 Alternatives; efavirenz, abacavir, lopinavir/ritonavir

Drug dosage recommendations listed herein are those of the authors and are not endorsed by the US Public Health Service or the US Department of Health and Human Services.

nonnucleoside reverse transcriptase inhibitor; abacavir, a nucleoside analogue; and lopinavir/ritonavir as alternative third drugs. Adding a protease inhibitor will increase the potential for side effects. Although the nonnucleoside reverse transcriptase inhibitor nevirapine has been used in a single dose to prevent mother to child transmission of HIV, it should not be used for postexposure prophylaxis because significant hepatotoxicity has been reported in this situation (CDC, January 5, 2001; Guay et al., 1999). Prescribing and managing antiretroviral protocols is complicated, and expert consultation should be considered, especially in the highest risk exposures when three drug regimens are used. Some states have laws permitting disclosure of information regarding a known assailant's HIV status (Gostin et al., 1994).

If HIV postexposure prophylaxis is initiated, a complete blood count and liver function tests should be performed approximately 2 weeks into the therapy to monitor for side effects. If a protease inhibitor is used, serum glucose levels should be assessed, and amylase evaluation and urinalysis should be done if indinavir is prescribed. Amylase should also be tested if didanosine (ddI) is used. A baseline HIV test should be performed as well as a follow-up test in 6 weeks, 3 months, and 6 months.

Antiretroviral medications are expensive, and in many victims of assault, it is not clear who will pay for HIV postexposure prophylaxis. Optimally, for high-risk exposures, postexposure prophylaxis should be offered regardless of cost. For a 2-drug antiretroviral regimen, the cost is approximately $500 for a 4-week supply. If a protease inhibitor is added, the cost is roughly doubled.

All victims should be educated regarding symptoms of primary HIV infection, including a prolonged febrile or flu-like illness, fatigue, lymphadenopathy, rash, and pharyngitis (Schacker et al., 1996). In addition, victims should be counseled that postexposure prophylaxis is not 100% effective, and until they have completed testing for HIV 6 months after their potential exposure, they should use condoms with regular sex partners.

EMERGENCY ORAL CONTRACEPTION

In the United States, it has been estimated that 5% of women of reproductive age who are raped will become pregnant (Holmes et al., 1996); over 32,000 rape-related pregnancies occur annually in the United States. Immediate access to emergency oral contraception should be made available to all female victims of sexual assault who seek medical care. Commonly recommended regimens include two doses of oral contraceptives taken 12 hours apart. A regimen originally described by Yuzpe et al. (1982) containing ethinyl estradiol and norgestrel (Ovral) is one of the most commonly prescribed regimens; however, a progestin-only regimen consisting of levonorgestrel is reported to have similar efficacy with fewer side effects (**Table 17-7**) (Ho & Kwan, 1993). Other regimens, including the antigonadotropin danazol, the antiprogestin mifepristone, and nonhormonal methods including insertion of an intrauterine contraceptive device are less commonly used. The first dose of emergency oral contraception should be administered within 72 hours of unprotected intercourse (ACOG, 2001). The sooner emergency oral contraception is initiated after unprotected intercourse, the more effective it will be (WHO, 1998). In a study sponsored by the World Health Organization (WHO), the levonorgestrel regimen was slightly more effective in

---

Table 17-7. Recommended Regimens for Emergency Oral Contraception

Levonorgestrel regimen:
— Levonorgestel 0.75 mg within 72 hours of assault, and repeated 12 hours later

Yuzpe regimen:
— 100 μg of ethinyl estradiol and 1 mg of norgestrel (2 Ovral) within 72 hours of assault, and repeated 12 hours later

---

Drug dosage recommendations listed herein are those of the authors and are not endorsed by the US Public Health Service or the US Department of Health and Human Services.

---

preventing pregnancy than the Yuzpe regimen (85% of pregnancies prevented versus 57%) (WHO, 1998). This result differs from most other studies in which the two regimens were roughly equivalent; in one review the reported average effectiveness of the Yuzpe regimen was 74% (ACOG, 2001; Ho & Kwan, 1993; Trussell et al., 1996).

Hormonal emergency oral contraception interferes with conception before implantation occurs. Thus, it is considered contraception rather than an abortifacient. Possible mechanisms by which these hormonal methods interfere with conception include interference with fertilization or inhibition of endometrial implantation (Glasier, 1997).

The most common side effects of emergency oral contraception are nausea and vomiting. In the study conducted by WHO, only 6% of women who took a levonorgestrel only regimen vomited, compared to 19% who took the Yuzpe regimen (WHO, 1998). In addition, only 23% who took levonorgestrel reported nausea, compared to 50% who took the Yuzpe regimen. Because nausea and vomiting are the most common side effects of emergency oral contraception some providers routinely prescribe antiemetics 1 hour before the contraceptive pills. Other less common side effects include delayed return of menses, fatigue, headaches, breast tenderness, and abdominal pain (WHO, 1998). Although there is a theoretical risk of thromboembolism, which is a known side effect of long-term use of oral contraceptives, no increased risk of thromboembolism with the short courses of emergency oral contraception has been described. Women who receive emergency oral contraception should be counseled regarding the predicted efficacy and potential side effects. They should be reminded that emergency oral contraception or hormonal contraceptives do not prevent STDs. If menses does not resume within a week of the expected date, women should seek pregnancy testing.

CONCLUSION

STDs are common sequelae of sexual assault. Providing evaluation and preventive treatment for STDs and counseling patients concerning the signs and symptoms of STDs are essential roles for the medical provider conducting the post-assault evaluation. Emergency oral contraception and postexposure prophylaxis against HIV should be offered to victims of assault on an individual basis.

REFERENCES

American College of Obstetricians and Gynecologists. *Emergency Oral Contraception*. ACOG Practice Bulletin. Number 25. Washington DC: The American College of Obstetrics and Gynecologists; March, 2001.

Amsel R, Totten PA, Spiegel CA, et al. Non-specific vaginitis: diagnostic and microbial and epidemiological associations. *Am J Med*. 1983;74:14-722.

Baker TC, Burgess AW, Brickman E, et al. Rape victims' concern about possible exposure to HIV infection. *J Interpers Violence*. 1990;5:49-60.

Bamberger JD, Waldo CR, Gerberding JL, et al. Postexposure prophylaxis for human immunodeficiency virus (HIV) infection following sexual assault. *Am J Med*. 1999;106:323-326.

Beck-Sague CM, Solomon F. Sexualy transmitted diseases in abused children and adolescent and adult victims of rape: review of selected literature. *Clin Infect Dis*. 1999;28(suppl 1):S74-S83.

Brookhoff D. Compliance with doxycycline therapy for outpatient treatment of pelvic inflammatory disease. *South Med J*. 1994;87:1088-1091.

Burstein GR, Gaydos CA, Diener-West M, et al. Incident Chlamydia trachomatis infections among inner-city adolescent females. *JAMA*. 1998;280:521-526.

Centers for Disease Control and Prevention (CDC). Case-control study of HIV seroconversion in health-care workers after percutaneous exposure to HIV-infected blood: France, United Kingdom, and United States, January 1988-August 1994. *MMWR*. December 22, 1995;44:929-933.

Centers for Disease Control and Prevention (CDC). Chlamydia trachomatis genital infections: United States, 1995. *MMWR*. March 7, 1997;46:193-198.

Centers for Disease Control and Prevention (CDC). Gonorrhea: United States, 1998. *MMWR*. June 23, 2000;49:538-542.

Centers for Disease Control and Prevention (CDC). Serious adverse events attributed to nevirapine regimens for postexposure prophylaxis after HIV exposures: worldwide, 1997-2000. *MMWR*. January 05, 2001;49:1153-1156.

Centers for Disease Control and Prevention (CDC). Outbreak of syphilis among men who have sex with men: Southern California, 2000. *MMWR*. February 23, 2001;50:117-120.

Centers for Disease Control and Prevention (CDC). Updated US Public Health Service guidelines for the management of occupational exposures to HBV, HCV, and HIV and recommendations for postexposure prophylaxis. *MMWR*. June 29, 2001;50(RR11):1-42.

Centers for Disease Control and Prevention (CDC). 2002 guidelines for the treatment of sexually transmitted diseases. *MMWR.* 2002;51(RR-6):1-78.

Corey L, Adams HG, Brown ZA, et al. Genital herpes simplex virus infections: clinical manifestations, course, and complications. *Ann Intern Med.* 1983;98:958-972.

Corey L, Wald A. Genital herpes. In: Holmes KK, Sparling PF, Mårdh P-A, et al., eds. *Sexually Transmitted Diseases.* 3rd ed. New York, NY: McGraw-Hill; 1999:285-312.

Daling JR, Weiss NS, Schwartz SM, et al. Vaginal douching and the risk of tubal pregnancy. *Epidemiology.* 1991;2:40-48.

Department of Health and Human Services. Division of STD Prevention. *Sexually Transmitted Disease Surveillance, 1999.* Atlanta, Ga: Centers for Disease Control and Prevention (CDC), September 2000.

Fauci AS, Pantaleo G, Stanley S, et al. Immunopathogenic mechanisms of HIV infection. *Ann Intern Med.* 1996;124:654-663.

Fleming DT, McQuillan GM, Johnson RE, et al. Herpes simplex virus type 2 in the United States, 1976 to 1994. *N Engl J Med.* 1997;337:1105-1111.

Fleming DT, Wasserheit JN. From epidemiological synergy to public health policy and practice: the contribution of other sexually transmitted diseases to sexual transmission of HIV infection. *Sex Transm Infect.* 1999;75:3-17.

Glaser JB, Hammerschlag MR, McCormack WM. Sexually transmitted diseases in victims of sexual assault. *N Engl J Med.* 1986;315:625-627.

Glaser JB, Hammerschlag MR, McCormack WM. Epidemiology of sexually transmitted diseases in rape victims. *Rev Infect Dis.* 1989;11:246-254.

Glaser JB, Schachter J, Solomon B, et al. Sexually transmitted diseases in postpubertal female rape victims. *J Infect Dis.* 1991;164:726-730.

Glasier A. Drug therapy: emergency postcoital contraception. *N Engl J Med.* 1997;337:1058-1064.

Gostin LO, Lazzarini Z, Alexander D, et al. HIV testing, counseling, and prophylaxis after sexual assaualt. *JAMA.* 1994;271:1436-1444.

Gray RH, Wawer MJ, Brookmeyer R, et al. Probability of HIV-1 transmission per coital act in monogamous, heterosexual, HIV-1-discordant couples in Rakai, Uganda. *Lancet.* 2001;357:1149-1153.

Greenblatt RM, Lukehart SA, Plummer FA, et al. Genital ulceration as a risk factor for human immunodeficiency virus infection. *AIDS.* 1988;2:47-50.

Guay LA, Musoke P, Fleming T, et al. Intrapartum and neonatal single-dose nevirapine compared with zidovudine for prevention of mother-to-child transmission of HIV-1 in Kampala, Uganda: HIVNET 012 randomised trial. *Lancet.* 1999;354:795-802.

Hawes SE, Hillier SL, Benedetti J, et al. Hydrogen peroxide-producing lactobacilli and acquisition of vaginal infections. *J Infect Dis.* 1996;174:1058-1063.

Hillman R, O'Mara N, Tomlinson D, et al. Adult male victims of sexual assault: an underdiagnosed condition. *Int J STD AIDS.* 1991;2:22-24.

Ho PC, Kwan MS. A prospective randomized comparison of levonorgestrel with the Yuzpe regimen in postcoital contraception. *Hum Reprod.* 1993;8:389-392.

Holmes MM, Resnick HS, Kilpatrick DG, et al. Rape-related pregnancy: estimates and descriptive characteristics from a national sample of women. *Am J Obstet Gynecol.* 1996;175:320-325.

Hook EW III, Handsfield HH. Gonococcal infections in the adult. In: Holmes KK, Sparling PF, Mårdh P-A, et al., eds. *Sexually Transmitted Diseases*. 3rd ed. New York, NY: McGraw-Hill; 1999:451-466.

Hook EW III, Stephens J, Ennis DM. Azithromycin compared with penicillin G benzathine for treatment of incubating syphilis. *Ann Intern Med*. 1999;131:434-437.

Jenny C, Hooton TM, Bowers A, et al. Sexually transmitted diseases in victims of rape. *N Engl J Med*. 1990;322:713-716.

Katz BP. Estimating transmission probabilities for chlamydial infection. *Stat Med*. 1992;11:565-577.

Katz BP, Swickl BW, Caine VA, et al. Compliance with antibiotic therapy for Chlamydia trachomatis and Neisseria gonorrhoeae. *Sex Transm Dis*. 1992;19:351-354.

Katz MH, Gerberding JL. Postexposure treatment of people exposed to the human immunodeficiency virus through sexual contact or injection-drug use. *N Engl J Med*. 1997;336:1097-1100.

Kreiss JK, Coombs R, Plummer R, et al. Isolation of human immunodeficiency virus from genital ulcers in Nairobi prostitutes. *J Infect Dis*. 1989;160:380-384.

Krieger JN, Tam MR, Stevens CE, et al. Diagnosis of trichomoniasis. *JAMA*. 1988;259:1223-1227.

Linden JA. Domestic violence. *Emerg Med Clin North Am*. 1999;17:685-697.

Marrazzo JM, Stamm WE. New approaches to the diagnosis, treatment, and prevention of chlamydial infection. In: Remington JS, Swartz MN, eds. *Current Clinical Topics in Infectious Diseases*. 18th ed. Boston, Mass: Blackwell Science; 1998:37-59.

Marrazzo JM, White CL, Krekeler B, et al. Community-based urine screening for Chlamydia trachomatis with a ligase chain reaction assay. *Ann Intern Med*. 1997;127:796-803.

Martin DH, Mroczkowski TF, Dalu ZA, et al. A controlled trial of a single dose of azithromycin for the treatment of chlamydial urethritis and cervicitis. *N Engl J Med*. 1992;327:921-925.

Minkoff H, Grunebaum AN, Schwarz RH, et al. Risk factors for prematurity and premature rupture of membranes: a prospective study of the vaginal flora in pregnancy. *Am J Obstet Gynecol*. 1984;150:965-972.

Peterman TA, Stoneburner RL, Allen JR, et al. Risk of human immunodeficiency virus transmission from heterosexual adults with transfusion-associated infections. *JAMA*. 1988;259:55-58.

Putz M, Thomas BK, Cowles KV. Sexual assault victims' compliance with follow-up care at one sexual assault treatment center. *J Emerg Nurs*. 1996;22:560-565.

Quinn TC, Gaydos C, Shepherd M, et al. Epidemiologic and microbiologic correlates of Chlamydia trachomatis infection in sexual partnerships. *JAMA*. 1996;276:1737-1742.

Quinn TC, Wawer MJ, Sewankambo N, et al. Viral load and heterosexual transmission of human immunodeficiency virus type 1. *N Engl J Med*. 2000;342:921-929.

Schacker T, Collier AC, Hughes J, et al. Clinical and epidemiologic features of primary HIV infection. *Ann Intern Med*. 1996;125:257-264.

Scholes D, Daling JR, Stergachis A, et al. Vaginal douching as a risk factor for acute pelvic inflammatory disease. *Obstet Gynecol*. 1993;81:601-066.

Schwarcz SK, Whittington WL. Sexual assault and sexually transmitted diseases: detection and management in adults and children. *Rev Infect Dis*. 1990;12(suppl 1):S682-S690.

Sellors J, Howard M, Pickard L, et al. Chlamydial cervicitis: testing the practice guidelines for presumptive diagnosis. *CMAJ*. 1998;158:41-46.

Stamm WE. Chlamydia trachomatis infections of the adult. In: Holmes KK, Sparling PF, Mårdh P-A, et al., eds. *Sexually Transmitted Diseases*. 3rd ed. New York, NY: McGraw-Hill; 1999:407-422.

Stamm WE, Hicks CB, Martin DH, et al. Azithromycin for empirical treatment of the nongonococcal urethritis syndrome in men. *JAMA*. 1995;274:545-549.

Telzac EE, Chiasson MA, Bevier PJ, et al. HIV-1 seroconversion in patients with and without genital ulcer disease. *Ann Intern Med*. 1993;119:1181-1186.

Trussell J, Ellertson C, Steward F. The effectiveness of the Yuzpe regimen of emergency contraception. *Fam Plann Perspect*. 1996;28:58-64.

Tsai C-C, Emau P, Follis KE, et al. Effectiveness of postinoculation (R)-9-(2-phosphonylmethoxypropyl) adenine treatment for prevention of persistent simian immunodeficiency virus (SIV) infection depends critically on timing of initiation and duration of treatment. *J Virol*. 1998;72:4265-4273.

Wald A. New therapies and prevention strategies for genital herpes. *Clin Infect Dis*. 1999;28(suppl 1):S4-S13.

Wald A, She J, Selke S, et al. Virologic characteristics of subclinical and symptomatic genital herpes infections. *N Engl J Med*. 1995;333:770-775.

World Health Organization, Task Force on Postovulatory Methods of Fertility Regulation, Special Programme of Research Development and Research Training in Human Reproduction. Randomised controlled trial of levonorgestrel versus the Yuzpe regimen of combined oral contraceptives for emergency contraception. *Lancet*. 1998;352:428-433.

Yuzpe AA, Smith RP, Rademaker AW. A multicenter clinical investigation employing ethinyl estradiol combined with dl-norgestrel as a postcoital contraceptive agent. *Fertil Steril*. 1982;37:508-513.

Chapter 18

Dating Violence and Acquaintance Rape

Janice B. Asher, MD
Christine M. Peterson, MD

Acquaintance rape is unusual among crimes in that it is often not considered to be a crime by the perpetrator, by the criminal justice system, by society, and sometimes even by the victim. As one investigator put it, "Acquaintance rape has a status somewhere between accepted practice and unacceptable crime" (Ellis, 1994).

Nonetheless, acquaintance rape is a crime that is common and that may have devastating consequences for the victim. In this chapter we will discuss acquaintance rape and how the clinician's response to the victim can effectively address the medical and psychosocial implications of this crime.

Epidemiology

Rape statistics are difficult to obtain because of overall underreporting of sexual assault. It is not surprising, therefore, that data about the incidence of acquaintance rape are limited. The National Institute of Justice estimates that there are approximately 1 million sexual assaults per year in the United States, two thirds of which are not reported to the police, and two thirds of which are committed by a perpetrator known to the victim (Tjaden & Thoennes, 1998).

In a review article on this subject, Peipert and Domagalski (1994) reported that adolescents and young adults are four times more likely to be victims of sexual assault than are women in all other age-groups. It is more likely that adolescents rather than adults will be raped in the context of a voluntary social encounter such as a date. It has been estimated that 60% of adolescent rapes and 44% of adult female rapes occur in the context of social encounters.

Another study estimates that the lifetime prevalence of date rape ranges from 13% to 27% among college women and 20% to 68% among the general adolescent population (Rickert & Wiemann, 1998). Other studies indicate 25% of college women and 6% of college men have been victims of sexual assaults that meet the legal definition of rape (Fisher et al., 2000; Tanzman, 1992). The highest incidence of rape in this study occurred during the senior year of high school and the freshman year of college. Forty one percent of the women who had been raped stated that they were virgins at the time of the assault.

Key Point:
25% of college women and 6% of college men have been victims of sexual assaults that meet the legal definition of rape.

Risk Factors

Several factors appear to increase the risk for acquaintance rape. For example, dating violence is associated with early sexual activity and prior sexual victimization. Dating violence and acquaintance rape are also associated with increased alcohol and substance abuse, increased suicidality, and increased high-risk sexual behavior (Wilson & Joffe, 1995). In one study of college women, the highest incidence of sexual assault was seen in those women who had been previously assaulted in early adolescence. These women were 4.6 times more likely to be sexually assaulted than women with no prior history of assault (Humphrey & White, 2000).

Women are at greater risk for assault under conditions where rape myths are more widely accepted, violence toward women is tolerated, and sex role stereotypes are followed. For example, a girl may be taught that if she voluntarily engages in any sexual activity, then she is a "tease" if she tries to stop further activity. She may be taught that girls who dress in a sexually provocative manner "deserve what they get." She may be taught that a man who is sexually aroused "can't control himself."

Finally, factors associated with the date itself may also increase the risk of acquaintance rape. Dating violence is more likely if a male pays for the date, if the date occurs in an isolated location, and if alcohol and/or drugs are used (Rickert & Wiemann, 1998).

THE ROLE OF DRUGS AND ALCOHOL IN ACQUAINTANCE RAPE

Acquaintance rape is associated with drug and alcohol use by both the perpetrator and the victim. As many as 73% of assailants and 55% of victims have used alcohol and/or drugs immediately before the episode of sexual assault (Warshaw, 1988).

Interestingly, several studies have demonstrated that society as a whole—the police, perpetrators, and even victims—hold male perpetrators of date rape less accountable if they committed the rape when they were intoxicated (Hammock & Richardson, 1997; Lopez, 1992; Richardson & Campbell, 1982; Schuller & Stewart, 2000). Female victims, on the other hand, are more likely to be held more accountable if they were intoxicated at the time. While the assailant was seen as unable to control his actions due to intoxication, the victim's willingness to become intoxicated is interpreted as a signal of sexual interest.

One reason for this discrepancy may be the common misconception that alcohol causes people to become violent. In fact, alcohol is a disinhibitor and is associated with increased violence, but alcohol use is not a cause of violence. One explanation for this association is that, in addition to alcohol having a physiologic effect, people use alcohol with the expectation of and as an excuse for the disinhibition (Caetano et al., 2001).

Whereas alcohol is certainly the most common substance implicated in acquaintance rape, other drugs are quickly gaining prominence in sexual assaults. They include flunitrazepam (Rohypnol), a fast-acting benzodiazepine, ketamine, and gamma-hydroxybutrate (GHB) and its cogeners (Schwartz et al., 2000; Smith, 1999). These drugs are added to the intended victim's drink without her knowledge or consent. In addition to causing disinhibition, one of the effects of such drugs is anterograde amnesia, which makes it difficult to obtain a history of the event. Clinicians need to suspect the use of these drugs, which may cause symptoms similar to those of alcohol. Many emergency departments have established protocols for urine or blood sample collection to test for the presence of such drugs. In the absence of protocols, the drug manufacturers can be contacted (Anglin et al., 1997).

A VICTIM'S RESPONSE TO DATING VIOLENCE AND ACQUAINTANCE RAPE

JENNIFER'S STORY

I met Michael at a fraternity party. Actually, I'd seen him a few times before in some classes and with other friends, but I didn't know him well before. We really hit it off at the party. After a while, after I'd had pretty much to drink, we were dancing together, and he asked me to go up to his room with him. I wanted to. I wanted to be alone with him and be close to him. But I didn't want to have sex. He started pulling off my clothes, and I told him I didn't want to do that, that I wasn't ready. But he said that I was and that it would feel good. I felt so drunk and dizzy and out of it—I don't know—I just couldn't think straight. And I was afraid to make a scene. As soon as it was over, I pulled on my clothes and ran back to my dorm. You know, I can't believe it happened. I can't believe that I got that drunk and that I was stupid enough to go to his room with him. What did I think was going to happen? I don't want to tell any of my friends—they'll think I'm so unbelievably stupid. I just want to forget the whole thing.

Key Point:
The relationship of alcohol and dating violence:
— *Dating violence is associated with drug and alcohol use by both the perpetrator and victim.*
— *Intoxication is often used to excuse the perpetrator and to blame the victim of date rape.*
— *Alcohol is a disinhibitor, but not a cause of violence.*

All too frequently, the victim of acquaintance rape blames herself for the incident. She feels embarrassed and ashamed for having been drinking alcohol, for dressing in a "sexy" manner, or for being "a tease" when she did not desire intercourse, even though she was interested in other sexual activity. Because of her shame, she may not want to tell anyone about the assault.

Another reason that the victim of an acquaintance rape may not want to report the incident, particularly to police, is that she may not want the perpetrator to be charged with a serious crime and be sentenced to prison. She herself may not want to go through the difficult, and sometimes humiliating, ordeal of a trial. In fact, many victims of acquaintance rape state that they are not looking for a criminal investigation by the police, but for an acknowledgment and apology by the perpetrator.

Psychologic Consequences

In the end, the victim may decide to just "forget that it ever happened." However, psychologic sequelae of date rape, including depression and social isolation, may be evident as long as 15 years after the assault (Kilpatrick et al., 1988). Self-blame is associated with greater psychologic distress and an even longer recovery period (Katz & Burt, 1988).

One of the most severe consequences that occurs commonly among victims of sexual assault is posttraumatic stress disorder, which is chiefly characterized by 4 symptoms:

1. Involuntary re-experiencing of the traumatic event through thoughts, nightmares, and/or flashbacks

2. Avoidance of activities, including those that were previously pleasurable

3. Avoidance of circumstances in which the rape occurred

4. A state of increased psychomotor arousal, which may be associated with sleep disturbances and panic attacks

Depression, difficulty forming emotional attachments, and decreased appetite are also commonly associated with posttraumatic stress disorder. Women who have a past history of depression or alcohol abuse, as well as women who are injured during the rape, are more likely to suffer subsequent posttraumatic stress disorder (Acierno et al., 1999). Victims of date rape are 11 times more likely to be clinically depressed and 6 times more likely to experience social phobia than are nonvictims.

WHEN THE VICTIM IS MALE

According to 1 estimate, 5% of rape victims are male (Grevalamus et al., 1987). The actual number is probably much higher, because underreporting by male victims is likely to be even more common than by female victims.

Male victims are more likely to have had multiple assailants and to have had weapons used against them (Lacey & Roberts, 1991). Nevertheless, they are even more likely than are females to blame themselves for not being able to fend off their attackers. In contrast to women, men may also feel more anxious that any emotional response they may have could be a sign of weakness or decreased masculinity (Laurent, 1993). The result is the same pattern of shame that keeps female victims from reporting sexual assault.

Male victims of rape are also less likely to report the event because there are fewer options for support. The vast majority of rape crisis intervention programs are in place to support and assist female victims.

A PERPETRATOR'S RESPONSE TO DATING VIOLENCE AND ACQUAINTANCE RAPE

MICHAEL'S STORY

I was really happy to run into Jennifer at our fraternity party, since she was someone I wanted to get to know better. We played some chug-a-lug games with a bunch of other

people and then danced for a while. She was really leaning up against me, and I knew she was as interested in hooking up as I was. I invited her to my room, and she said yes. One thing led to another and then we had sex. She said no at first, but that's just what girls think they're supposed to say, right? She pretended to push me away, but I guess she just didn't want me to think she was "easy." Afterward, she just sort of got up and left. I guess maybe she felt a little sick from all that beer. She's a really nice girl, though, and I'll probably call her and ask her out for this weekend.

The perpetrator (and for that matter the victim) may have grown up in a family, peer group, or culture where manhood is defined as being sexually aggressive. He may think that women are "supposed" to refuse sex and that men are "supposed" to pressure, coerce, or even force them.

Key Point:
Many cultural stereotypes and values support the notion that acquaintance rape does not occur or that it can be justified.

In order to truly understand the full impact of acquaintance rape on a victim, it is important to understand how the perpetrator and society at large perceive it. Many cultural stereotypes and values support the notion that it simply does not exist, or that if it does, it is justifiable under a variety of circumstances.

For example, in a study of high school students, 60% of boys interviewed thought that forcing sex on a girl was appropriate in certain circumstances, such as if she has gotten him sexually excited or if she is wearing sexy clothing. (Davis et al., 1993). A survey of children ages 11 through 14 years revealed the following (Humphrey & White, 2000):

—Fifty-one percent of boys and 41% of girls said that forced sex was justified if the boy "spent a lot of money on the girl."

—Thirty percent of boys and girls said that forced sex is justified if the girl is not a virgin.

—Eighty-seven percent of boys and 79% of girls said that forced sex is justified between married couples.

—Sixty-five percent of boys and 47% of girls said forced sex was justified if a couple had been dating for 6 months or longer.

AN EFFECTIVE CLINICAL RESPONSE
THE NEED FOR ACTIVE SCREENING

Because of shame and self-blame, the victim of acquaintance rape may never even seek medical or forensic evaluation. For this reason, clinicians need to routinely raise the subject of relationship violence and acquaintance rape with patients.

The possibility of dating violence, particularly in the context of drug and alcohol use, should be included in routine visits with adolescent patients. Clinicians should also remember that male rape is not uncommon and that male victims may be even less forthcoming than are female victims in reporting the incident or discussing it in the context of medical symptoms.

Very specific screening questions are necessary:
—Have you ever felt hurt or threatened by a sexual partner?
—Has anyone ever forced you to have sex?
—Are you concerned that someone you're dating may try to make you have sex when you don't want to?
—Do you feel that someone has ever tried (or might try) to get you to use drugs or alcohol so that you will be more likely to have sex with him/her?

This discussion should also include information about sexually transmitted diseases and emergency contraception. According to the Council on Child and Adolescent Health, such preventive counseling is particularly important at the pre-college visit (Committee on Adolescence, 1994). Any patient who comes for emergency contraception should be asked if the sexual activity was consensual.

AFTER AN ASSAULT HAS OCCURRED

As with other types of rape, the clinician's approach to acquaintance rape should include identification and treatment of injuries, prevention of sexually transmitted diseases (STDs) and pregnancy, psychologic assessment with appropriate referral for counseling, and collection of forensic evidence if the assault has occurred within 72 hours (See also Chapter 15, Forensic Issues in Caring for the Adult Sexual Assault Victim).

Preventing Sexually Transmitted Diseases

The incidence of STDs resulting from rape has been estimated to be between 3.6% and 30% (Resnick et al., 1997). Specimens from appropriate sites should be obtained for *Neisseria gonorrhoeae* (gonorrhea) and *Chlamydia trachomatis* (chlamydia). Visible vesicles or ulcers may be cultured for herpes. A wet mount of vaginal secretions can be examined for *Trichomonas*, as well as for sperm. The patient must be advised that seroconversion for syphilis and hepatitis B takes 6 weeks and to return for testing at that time. All patients who have not received the hepatitis B vaccine should be offered vaccination. Human immunodeficiency virus (HIV) testing may be done at 6 weeks as well, but must be repeated at 3 and 6 months.

Adolescents in almost all states may consent to the confidential diagnosis and treatment of STDs (Centers for Disease Control and Prevention [CDC], 1998). The American Academy of Pediatrics recommends offering adolescent rape victims antibiotic prophylaxis for syphilis, gonorrhea, and chlamydia.

Preventing Pregnancy

All female rape victims should undergo baseline pregnancy testing and be offered emergency contraception. Emergency contraception reduces the risk of pregnancy when used within 72 hours after intercourse.

Providing Psychologic Support

The importance of psychologic support on the part of the clinician cannot be overemphasized. The victim, whether male or female, is likely to feel traumatized and ashamed. A compassionate, nonjudgmental response by the clinician is crucial in helping the victim of rape begin the process of psychologic healing.

It is usually appropriate and helpful to the patient to state directly that acquaintance rape is indeed a crime and that the rape was not her fault. (*Editor's note*: While the female pronoun is used here, our recommendations apply to all victims of rape, regardless of gender.) In this context, it is crucial to help the patient understand the difference between taking responsibility for ensuring as much personal safety as possible and taking the blame for the assault, which rests solely with the perpetrator.

For example, it is important to stress to a patient that she can minimize the risk of being the victim of acquaintance rape by not drinking excessive alcohol or by not going to a secluded place with a date. This is by no means the same as saying that if she does not practice these risk-reduction behaviors, a rape is her fault. *The responsibility for a crime always rests with the perpetrator of the crime.*

Letting the victim know that she will heal both physically and emotionally can also be encouraging to her. A simple statement from the clinician that he or she is available to the patient to help her with her current and future medical needs decreases her sense of isolation.

PREVENTING DATING VIOLENCE AND ACQUAINTANCE RAPE

There is increasing interest in involving adolescent and young adult males in sexual assault prevention efforts. School and college-based programs are endeavoring to educate males about their ethical and legal responsibility to be certain they have their sex partner's consent before engaging in intimate activity (Avert-Leaf et al.,

Key Point:
People can take safety precautions to minimize their risk of being raped, but the responsibility for rape rests solely with the perpetrator.

1997; Foshee et al., 1998; Hong, 2000). Some programs also train young men to relate in specific empathic and supportive ways to their girlfriends, friends, and acquaintances who have been the victims of assault. Visionary leaders of such programs communicate the message that men must help other men learn to respect a woman's right to determine when, where, and with whom she will engage in sexual activity. A fascinating emphasis in some of these programs concerns the redefinition of "masculine" behavior (Hong, 2000).

Similarly, young women are learning that they have a right to refuse sex under any circumstances and that there are ways to increase their safety (see Appendix).

CONCLUSION

Dating violence is common and yet inadequately recognized by victims, perpetrators, clinicians, and society. Issues ranging from sex role stereotypes, alcohol as an excuse for violence, and appropriate expectations in dating relationships all come into play. Clinicians may be the only professionals with whom victims will discuss dating violence and are therefore in a position to offer pregnancy and sexually transmitted disease protection, support, and safety strategy information.

APPENDIX: SAFETY TIPS FOR ACQUAINTANCE RAPE PREVENTION

— If someone is trying to force you into behavior you prefer to avoid, don't worry about being polite or nice—tell him NO forcefully.
— Always carry enough money for cab fare and change for a pay phone.
— If possible, carry a cell phone with you.
— Don't go off alone to a secluded place with someone you don't know well.
— Don't drink so much alcohol that you are at risk for passing out or not using your good judgment.
— Don't leave a drink unattended so that someone can slip something into it.
— If you're dating someone who seems overly jealous or controlling, consider that to be a warning sign that he may become violent.
— Above all, trust your instincts—if you don't feel comfortable in a situation, get out of it as best you can.

REFERENCES

Acierno R, Resnick H, Kilpatrick DG, Saunders B, Best CL. Risk factors for rape, physical assault, and posttraumatic stress disorder in women: examination of differential multivariate relationships. *J Anxiety Disord*. 1999;13:541-563.

Anglin D, Spears KL, Hutson HR. Flunitrazepam and its involvement in date or acquaintance rape. *Acad Emerg Med*. 1997;4:323-326.

Avery-Leaf S, Cascardi M, O'Leary KD, Cano A. Efficacy of a dating violence prevention program on attitudes justifying aggression. *J Adolesc Health*. 1997;21:11-17.

Caetano R, Schafer J, Cunradi CB. Alcohol-related intimate partner violence among white, black, and Hispanic couples in the United States. *Alcohol Res Health*. 2001;25:58-65.

Centers for Disease Control and Prevention (CDC). 1998 guidelines for treatment of sexually transmitted diseases. *MMWR*. 1998;47(No. RR-1):1-116.

Committee on Adolescence. Sexual assault and the adolescent. *Pediatrics*. 1994;94:761-765.

Davis TC, Peck GQ, Storment JM. Acquaintance rape and the high school student. *J Adolesc Health*. 1993;14:220-224.

Ellis GM. Acquaintance rape. *Perspect Psychiatr Care*. 1994;30:11-16.

Fisher BS, Cullen FT, Turner MG. The sexual victimization of college women. *NCJ 182369*. Washington, DC: National Institute of Justice, Bureau of Justice Statistics; 2000.

Foshee VA, Bauman KE, Arriga XB, Helms RW, Koch GG, Linder GF. An evaluation of Safe Dates, an adolescent dating violence prevention program. *Am J Public Health*. 1998;88:45-50.

Grevalamus DE, Shaw RD, Kennedy EL. Examination of sexually abused adolescents. *Semin Adolesc Med*. 1987;3:59-66.

Hammock GS, Richardson DR. Perceptions of rape: the influence of closeness of relationship, intoxication and sex of participant. *Violence Vict*. 1997;12:237-246.

Hong L. Toward a transformed approach to prevention: breaking the link between masculinity and violence. *J Am College Health*. 2000;48:269-279.

Humphrey JA, White JW. Women's vulnerability to sexual assault from adolescence to young adulthood. *J Adolesc Health*. 2000;27:419-424.

Katz B, Burt M. Self-blame in recovery from rape. In: Burgess AW, ed. *Rape and Sexual Assault II. Garland Reference Library of Social Science*, Vol 361. New York, NY: Garland; 1988:151-190.

Kilpatrick DG, Best CL, Saunders BE, Veronen LJ. Rape in marriage and in dating relationships: how bad is it for mental health? *Annals NY Acad Sci*. 1988;528:335-344.

Kilpatrick DG, Edmunds CN, Seymour AK. *Rape in America: A Report to the Nation*. Washington, DC: National Victim Center; 1992.

Lacey HB, Roberts R. Sexual assault on men. *Int J STD AIDS*. 1991;2:258-260.

Laurent C. Male rape. *Nurs Times*. 1993;89(6):10-16.

Lopez P. He said . . . she said . . . an overview of date rape from commission through prosecution through verdict. *Criminal Justice*. 1992;13:275-302.

Peipert JF, Domagalski LR. Epidemiology of adolescent sexual assault. *Obstet Gynecol*. 1994;84:867-871.

Resnick, HS, Acierno R, Kilpatrick DG. Health impact of interpersonal violence. 2: medical and mental health outcomes. *Behav Med*. 1997;23:65-78.

Richardson D, Campbell JL. Alcohol and rape: the effect of alcohol on attributions of blame for rape. *Pers Soc Psychol Bull*. 1982;8:468-476.

Rickert VI, Wiemann CM. Date rape among adolescents and young adults. *J Pediatr Adolesc Gynecol*. 1998;11:167-175.

Schuller RA, Stewart A. Police responses to sexual assault complaints: the role of perpetrator/complainant intoxication. *Law Hum Behav*. 2000;24:535-551.

Schwartz RH, Milteer R, LeBeau MA. Drug-facilitated sexual assault ('date rape'). *South Med J*. 2000;93:558-561.

Smith KM. Drugs used in acquaintance rape. *J Am Pharm Assoc*. 1999;39:442-443.

Tanzman ES. Unwanted sexual activity: the prevalence in college women. *J Am College Health*. 1992:40:167-171.

Tjaden P, Thoennes N. *Prevalence, Incidence and Consequences of Violence Against Women: Findings from the National Violence Against Women Survey*. Washington, DC: Research in Brief, US Department of Justice, National Institute of Justice; 1998.

Warshaw R. *I Never Called It Rape: The Ms. Report on Recognizing, Fighting, and Surviving Date and Acquaintance Rape*. New York, NY: Harper and Row; 1988.

Wilson MD, Joffe A. Adolescent medicine. *JAMA*. 1995;273:1657-1659.

Chapter 19

DOMESTIC VIOLENCE AND PARTNER RAPE

Elizabeth M. Datner, MD
Janice B. Asher, MD
Bruce D. Rubin, MD

The common denominator in all forms of domestic violence, including rape, is the intent to exert power and control over an intimate partner. Domestic violence and rape are common in a society that fosters the dominance of males over females (Marsh, 1993). In this chapter we will discuss partner rape as one manifestation of domestic violence within an intimate relationship where maintaining power and control within that relationship is paramount. We will provide a means by which clinicians can identify and assess victims of domestic violence who have experienced marital rape and how to help women begin to make self-protective changes in their lives.

DOMESTIC VIOLENCE OVERVIEW

Domestic violence is a means for one intimate partner, usually male, to maintain power and control over another intimate partner, usually female. At the outset, episodes of domestic violence may occur infrequently but may subsequently occur with great regularity. The severity of domestic violence varies and may begin as simple verbal or emotional assaults intended to intimidate and isolate the victim. These assaults can escalate to the intentional infliction of brutal physical injuries. Incredibly, intentional injury is the leading cause of trauma of young women, and trauma is the leading cause of death (Council on Scientific Affairs, 1992; Farley, 1986; Grisso et al., 1991; McAfee, 1995). Although death is the most serious sequelae of domestic violence, there are many forms of domestic abuse, including partner rape, that result in significant short- and long-term physical and mental health problems for women.

Key Point:
Domestic violence, including marital rape, is not about "losing control," but about maintaining power and control.

Although the occurrence of domestic violence crosses all lines of socio-economic status, race, ethnicity, and gender preference, certain risk factors have been identified. Domestic violence tends to be associated with poverty, substance abuse, depression, unintended pregnancy, short inter-pregnancy intervals, history of child abuse of the victim and/or perpetrator, and the concurrent presence of child abuse in the family. Likewise, marital rape does not appear to be limited to any specific socio-economic or racial group.

Domestic violence is a major public health concern, and healthcare providers are frequently the only professionals with whom victims of domestic violence come in contact. Thus, it is within the realm of clinicians to address and prevent ongoing violence to women.

RAPE AND DOMESTIC VIOLENCE

Marital or partner rape is less well understood than is "stranger rape" and is not well studied from epidemiologic perspectives. Only in the last few decades has research on marital rape been published. Before that time, sexual relations within the context of marriage were commonly considered the "right" of the husband and the "obligation" of the wife.

Before 1980, not a single state in the United States recognized marital rape as a crime. Based on 18th century English Common Law, husbands were provided with "spousal immunity" from sexual assault laws. Such immunity reflected ignorance of the dynamics of sexual assault, threats, and coercion as tactics of terror and control in an abusive relationship.

The acts described by victims of marital sexual assault are varied. They include vaginal intercourse against one's will, being forced to imitate acts from pornographic movies or magazines, performing or enduring oral and anal sex, being beaten and insulted during intercourse, being forced to have sexual activity with a third person, and having foreign objects penetrated into the vagina or anus. In a study of women who had endured marital rape, approximately half of them reported being threatened with a weapon if they attempted to refuse sex. The same number described being forced to have sex immediately after having been beaten. Forty-four percent reported being hit, kicked, or burned during sex. Almost 29% reported having objects forcibly inserted in the vagina and anus. Others reported being forced to have homosexual sex, to have sex with animals, to engage in prostitution, and to be involved in sex acts with their children (Campbell & Alford, 1989).

Whereas a few studies have documented rape in the absence of other forms of domestic violence, marital rape occurs most commonly within the context of other types of ongoing battering. In a study done in 1988, 37.5% (6 of 16) of women studied who indicated a history of physical abuse within the prior 12 months had also been raped by a male intimate during the same period. Further, 41% (28 of 69) of women studied who sought help from abusive relationships had experienced at least one type of sexual abuse in the past 6 months (Eby et al., 1995). Furthermore, a study of sexually abused battered women described sexual abuse occurring along with other forms of domestic violence, including physical, emotional, financial, and property abuse (Grams et al., 1997).

As with other forms of domestic violence, marital rape is a recurrent event. In one study, 63.6% of women who disclosed marital sexual assault noted that the episodes occurred more than five times in the prior 12 months. In only one case was the rape an isolated event (Grams et al., 1997).

Prevalence

Although marital rape is clearly a more common occurrence than previously thought, reported prevalence rates vary significantly. The prevalence of marital rape is not well delineated. One reason for such varied prevalence rates is the lack of commonly accepted definitions applicable to sexual assaults within marriage. For example, the definition of "forced sex" can vary from unwanted rough and painful sexual acts to threatened violence if sexual demands are not met, to actual beatings before, during, or after sex, and/or sex with objects. (Campbell & Alford, 1989). Without a common definition of what constitutes marital or partner rape, it is difficult to determine the full extent of the problem. Because clinicians lack a clear understanding of the problem's extent, both researchers and practitioners are limited in their recognition of marital rape cases.

Prevalence rates also vary widely depending on the population studied and the method of survey utilized. A national survey of women in the general US population describes a 7.7% (7.75 million) lifetime prevalence rate of rape by an intimate partner (defined as current and former spouses, opposite and same-sex cohabiting partners, or dates/boyfriends). The 1-year prevalence rate was 0.2% of all women surveyed (Tjaden & Thoennes, 1998). Russell (1982) studied a random sample of women and found that 12% of the 644 married women surveyed reported having been raped by their husbands. Doran (1980) found a prevalence of 23% in a similar sample. A later study of women coming to a social service agency reported a 1-year prevalence rate of marital rape of 10%. Marital rape in this

Table 19-1. Types of Acquiescence	
Unwanted turns to wanted	In these cases, the women did not desire sex initially, but were able to enjoy it after a few minutes. This were reported by 10% of women and occurred almost exclusively in relationships that were current, happy, and healthy according to the women.
It's my duty	This concept of a "wifely obligation inherent in the marital contract" is a common belief. The unwanted sex was considered an "inconvenience of married life" in an effort to "keep peace" and the wife's inherent "responsibility" or "duty." Seventy-six percent of the respondents participated in sex for this reason, and 34% reported this as the main reason they had unwanted sex.
Easier not to argue	The respondents described this circumstance as occurring when verbal or nonverbal behavior from a partner became overwhelming and giving in to sex was the easiest way out of the situation. This was frequently associated with other forms of "emotional manipulation, pressure, and in some instances, control." Twenty-seven percent of the respondents reported this experience.
Don't know what might happen if I don't	In these cases, women acquiesced to unwanted sex due to fear of negative reactions, including threats of violence, from their partners. Verbal threats and elements of emotional control were also present in these relationships. Seven percent of women reported this reason for submitting to unwanted sexual acts.
Know what will happen if I don't	These women had experienced physical abuse in their relationships and submitted to unwanted sex in an effort to avoid more physical abuse from their partner. Twenty percent of respondents fit into this category. A statement from one respondent is illuminating: "When you're intimidated by someone and they want to have sex no matter what the reason or what the situation, you do it, otherwise, you get the hell beat out of you, to be quite honest . . . you just let him do it. It's not him actually holding you down and forcing you, but it is being forced because you can't say no."

population was highly correlated with concomitant emotional and physical abuse within the relationships (Yegidis, 1988). A recent study published by Feldhaus et al. (2000) reported a lifetime prevalence rate of sexual assault of 39% in an emergency department population; 18% of these cases were perpetrated by an intimate partner. In a population of battered women, prevalence rates of sexual assault have been reported as high as 55% (Campbell & Soeken, 1999; Frieze, 1983; Shields & Hanneke, 1983; Wingood et al., 2000).

Another reason for such varied prevalence rates is that marital rape is a dramatically underreported event. Despite the best efforts of researchers and law enforcement agencies to quantify the frequency of rape, most cases are never reported. A report by Kilpatrick et al. (1992) estimates that only 10% to 15% of rapes are ever reported to law enforcement agencies or medical professionals. The study performed in an emergency department setting by Feldhaus et al. (2000) found that only 46% of rape victims reported the crime to law enforcement officials and only 43% sought medical care.

There are many reasons why rape victims do not report the incidents to authorities. These include embarrassment, feelings of guilt, fear of retaliation, lack of faith in the legal system, fear of police involvement, lack of knowledge of rights, and concerns about confidentiality, particularly if the victim is an adolescent who has limited access to healthcare (Kilpatrick et al., 1992; Beebe, 1991).

The Role of Coercion

Sexual coercion, in the absence of actual physical force or violence, is another method of maintaining power and control over an intimate partner. A woman may subsequently submit or "give in" to unwanted sex with a husband or stable relationship partner. Basile (1999) studied cases in which women admitted to engaging in unwanted sex. The reasons for acquiescence were explored. Each case involved elements of coercion, yet did not involve any physical force and may not have involved threats or even discussion between the partners. These cases of "rape by acquiescence" were characterized as unwanted sexual contact in which a woman submits, against her wishes, to a husband or partner. The study was done through return telephone calls of 41 women previously randomly selected in a national telephone poll of 1108 women in 1997. The study population was small but sufficient to provide insight into types of acquiescence. Corroboration of the basic results were found in an earlier national poll, which found that 76% of the general public believes some husbands use force to make their wives have sex, and 80% believe use of force occurs often or somewhat often. The current study classifies acquiescence into 5 types (**Table 19-1**).

Key Point:
Sexual coercion, in the absence of actual physical force, is another method of maintaining power and control over an intimate partner.

In each of the circumstances outlined in **Table 19-1**, physical force was not used during the sexual act; rather, some form of coercion occurred to cause the women to acquiesce. However, more than half of the women in this survey did not characterize their experiences as rape. Most women consider their experience as rape only when there is the clear use of physical force at a time when they did not give consent.

Both "not interested at first" and "wifely duty" are generally viewed as innocuous in our culture. Inherent in both is the societal notion that women should be sexually available to their partners. This was termed "social coercion" by Finkelhor and Yllo (1985) and is the result of a society that dictates "proper" behavior for women and roles for wives. The last 3 types of acquiescence are coping strategies used to avoid confrontation or a physically threatening situation. "Don't know what will happen" and "know what will happen" were seen as ways to avoid potential and real physical danger while surviving the situation.

CLINICAL PRESENTATION AND SEQUELAE

The clinical presentation of victims of domestic violence can be quite varied. Scenarios range from injuries directly resulting from violence to chronic complaints that neither the patient nor clinician recognizes as a manifestation of domestic violence. In addition to the physical injuries, over 50% of abused women have somatic complaints such as headache, abdominal pain, pelvic pain, fatigue, shortness of breath, gastrointestinal disturbances, sleep disorders, and other chronic complaints (Sutherland et al., 1998). Many women who are victims of domestic violence seek help through both primary medical care and emergency care visits. In fact, more women come for medical care as the result of battering than stranger rapes, car accidents, and muggings combined (Council on Scientific Affairs, 1992; McGrath et al., 1997). Unfortunately, these women usually are not identified by health care providers as abused, so their abuse-related symptoms also go unrecognized. This is true even for acute trauma. For example, in one study, only 13% of women coming to the emergency room for abuse-related injuries were asked about domestic violence (Abbott et al., 1995).

Women who experience marital rape suffer more severe physical injuries than do either acquaintance rape victims or victims of domestic violence without concomitant sexual assault (Bowker, 1983; Easteal & Easteal, 1992). In addition to the physical injuries, marital rape victims also report increased physical health symptomatology and increased mental health problems (Eby et al., 1995).

Physical Injuries and Symptoms

Victims of domestic violence suffer a broad range of physical injuries. Women who are victims of marital rape in the context of other forms of domestic violence may suffer the same types of injuries and symptoms. They also describe various gynecologic complaints, including vaginal and anal tearing or pain, bladder infections, dysmenorrhea, dyspareunia and other forms of sexual dysfunction, pelvic pain, urinary tract infections, and increased frequency of sexually transmitted diseases (Campbell & Alford, 1989). Two of the most frequently recounted health concerns of these women were painful intercourse (72%), and vaginal pain (63%) (Campbell & Alford, 1989). In a recent study sexually abused women reported significantly more gynecologic problems than abused women who were not sexually assaulted, including abdominal cramping and pain, urinary problems, decreased sexual desire, and genital irritation and pain (Campbell & Soeken, 1999).

Sexually abused domestic violence victims are also at greater risk for death. There is a higher risk of homicide among women who are battered and sexually abused as compared to non–sexually abused battered women as measured by the Danger Assessment Scale (Campbell, 1986). Using this assessment tool, women who were sexually assaulted by their partners had significantly higher scores for homicide risk factors than abused women who were not sexually assaulted. These data remained unchanged even when controlling for the seriousness of physical abuse and demographic variables. The detection of marital rape in a woman's experience should heighten a practitioner's concern for the safety of that individual.

Psychologic Effects

The psychologic effects of marital rape can be significant, although not as outwardly evident as the physical trauma suffered by the victim. The prevalence rate of depression in abused women ranges from 10.2% to 21.3% (Kessler et al., 1994; Weissman & Klerman, 1992). In comparison, the prevalence rate of depression in women, in general, is estimated at 9.3%. Intensity of depression appears to be correlated with the level of abuse. The number of forced sex experiences was found to correlate significantly with depression; women who experienced more sexual assaults reported increased levels of depression (Campbell & Soeken, 1999). In the absence of a diagnosis of clinical depression, lower self-esteem, especially poor body image, is also frequently reported (Campbell, 1989). Even women who experienced other forms of battering without sexual assault expressed a more positive physical self-image than women who experienced sexual assault.

Key Point:
More than 50% of abused women do not spontaneously disclose the abuse. Rather, they come with varied somatic complaints that they and their examining clinicians may not recognize as being related to abuse.

Key Point:
Women who are sexually assaulted by their partners are at increased risk for being murdered by their partners.

Most investigators have found depression to be frequently associated with relationship violence. It is worth noting here there is no simple cause-and-effect relationship between abuse and depression. Some women, particularly those with a history of child abuse, enter abusive relationships in a depressed, vulnerable state. Others become depressed only as a result of the abuse; these women do not suffer persistent depression if they ultimately leave the abuser and go on to have successful nonabusive relationships. Depression, "learned helplessness," and erosion of self-esteem are particularly common sequelae of relationship violence (See also Chapter 23, Revised Trauma Theory: Understanding the Traumatic Nature of Sexual Assault).

A particularly cruel irony of depression associated with domestic violence is that if the woman receives psychiatric care and/or is treated with antidepressant medications, she may be labeled as a "mental patient" or "crazy." If she ultimately does decide to leave her abuser, this label may then be used against her in a custody battle, where she may be portrayed as an "unfit mother." Such court battles are another arena where the power and control mechanisms of abuse are played out. Abusers often seek custody of children as another tactic to use against their partners.

Health Status and Disease Prevention

In addition to sustaining physical injuries and psychologic stresses associated with violent assaults, women who are victims of domestic abuse also experience significant negative effects on their health and well-being, including perceived evaluation of their own health. The Commonwealth Fund national random survey found that women abused by spouses were significantly more likely to rate their health as fair or poor compared to women who were not battered (Plichta, 1996). This perception, along with a desire to obtain help in dealing with the violent behavior, may account for abused women's increased frequency of medical visits as compared with non abused women. Additionally, the ability to enhance one's own health and prevent disease is compromised in abusive relationships. Women in abusive relationships are less likely to use condoms, more afraid to ask their partner to use condoms, and more likely to be emotionally abused or threatened with physical abuse when discussing safe sex than women in nonviolent relationships (Wingood & DiClemente, 1997). Campbell and Soeken (1999) also suggest that women experiencing partner rape have a significantly higher mean number of somatic symptoms. This study differentiated sexually abused from non–sexually abused battered women. The authors describe detrimental physical and mental health effects on women who had been sexually abused that differ from those incurred by women who had been physically and emotionally, but not sexually, abused.

Key Point:
Women in abusive relationships cannot negotiate safer sex practices.

Associated Behaviors

Drug and alcohol abuse are more common in both victims and perpetrators of abuse. Victims of violence, whether current adult victims or adult survivors of child abuse, often use drugs and alcohol as a form of self-medication in response to abuse. A drug-using abusive partner may also coerce or force his partner to use drugs or alcohol in order to "keep him company." The abusive partner may use drugs or alcohol during times of assault and then blame the violent behavior on the use of drugs. Weingourt (1990) found that 75% of women who were raped and battered by their husbands reported that spousal alcohol use was a factor in their rapes.

IDENTIFICATION OF ABUSE

It is frequently difficult for a clinician to discover that a patient has suffered from marital rape unless physical abuse has also taken place. Victims are sometimes reluctant to discuss the situation, even in a safe medical setting. Many women still consider that they have an obligation to accept sex within marriage. Others do not want to talk about what may have occurred because they are embarrassed to raise the issues themselves. The professionals involved may feel that initiating a conversation about sexual matters when a patient does not show related signs of trauma is an invasion of privacy. However, women are more likely to discuss abuse with their health care providers than with anyone else, including family members, friends, and clergy, but only when asked.

Most victims of sexual assault, whether partner, acquaintance, or stranger rape, do not file a police report or seek emergency medical treatment. However, victims of partner rape are even less likely to report events or to seek additional services. In the Feldhaus et al. (2000) study of women evaluated in an emergency department setting, victims of partner rape were significantly less likely to report the event to police (79% vs. 18%), obtain medical care (70% vs. 29%), or contact a social service agency (30% vs. 24%) compared to victims of stranger rape.

The vast majority of women in abusive relationships do not spontaneously disclose that they are being abused. Because of this lack of reporting, clinicians should practice routine screening of their female patients for partner violence, including rape. Unfortunately, few clinicians routinely screen patients for domestic violence, despite its common occurrence and its association with medical sequelae.

Abuse crosses all racial, ethnic, religious, and socioeconomic lines; therefore many abused women will not be identified if screening is aimed only at those who fit a certain "profile." Numerous studies have shown the value of universal screening for relationship violence with regard to increasing the detection rate (Feldhaus et al., 2000; Norton et al., 1995). The rate is much greater when the screening is performed by the clinical provider, as opposed to using a self-assessment tool (McFarlane & Gondolf, 1998).

Recommended screening questions include the following:

1. Are you in a relationship in which you have been hit, pushed, or kicked?
2. Are you in a relationship in which you have been forced to have sex?

Providers should also make information available to all female patients about domestic violence, partner rape, and the availability of sexually transmitted disease (STD) prophylaxis, emergency contraception, and long-term contraception.

It is imperative that the patient be interviewed alone. This may be particularly difficult in the context of domestic violence, because controlling behavior is a hallmark of abusive relationships.

Strategies used by clinicians to separate patient and partner may include the following:

1. Posting a sign stating a policy of having partners leave during physical examinations
2. Ordering tests and accompanying the patient to the test site while the partner is asked to wait
3. Having a staff member ask the partner to come outside the examining room in order to provide additional insurance information

An abusive partner may still refuse to leave the examining room. This refusal is another form of exerting control and also ensures that the victim will not disclose information about the violence. For this reason, abuse-related materials, particularly safety planning information, should be kept in all patient bathrooms. Insisting that the partner leave the room is not advisable; he may become hostile or threatening to the clinician, or he may refuse to allow his partner to return to the office, thereby increasing her isolation and sense of helplessness.

The patient may deny being abused, but the clinician still strongly suspects abuse has occurred. If, for example, a woman has a black eye and states that she walked into a wall, *it may be helpful to return to questions about abuse with introductory statements such as the following:*

1. "An injury like yours often occurs because of being punched. Is that what happened?"

Key Point:
Because victims of partner rape rarely report the incident or seek emergency treatment, clinicians must routinely screen for partner violence and sexual assault.

2. "Because abuse is so common, we are asking all our patients about it. Has someone hurt you?"

When there is physical abuse, it is not uncommon to find out that sexual abuse has also occurred. In fact, in such situations interviewing the patient about whether sexual abuse has also occurred is vital. The clinician must be able to recognize symptoms that may be indicative of spousal rape. Without this first-line assessment, there may not be other opportunities to introduce interventions to aid the victim. If the clinician is not conscious of the possibility of unwanted sexual acts, effective treatment is not possible.

THE CLINICIAN'S RESPONSE TO DOMESTIC VIOLENCE

After obtaining the victim's history regarding the nature and severity of the abuse, the clinician must communicate to the patient a concern for her safety and an appreciation of the complex dynamics of an abusive relationship. Physicians and other clinicians often overlook how powerful their words are to their patients. In no other situation is the power of words more noteworthy than in the context of domestic violence. A hallmark of abuse is that the victim, rather than the perpetrator, feels embarrassed, ashamed, and blameworthy for the abuse. The abuser has told the victim that the abuse is her fault, that his violent behavior is because of something that she did or said, or that she "makes him lose his temper." He has warned her that there will be dire consequences if she tells anyone and that no one will believe her anyway. She has been isolated from her family and friends and has lost confidence in her intelligence, her competence, and her very self-worth. She may blame herself for not feeling able to leave the relationship. For all these reasons, the role of the clinician in supporting and validating the patient who discloses abuse cannot be overstated.

Particularly effective may be such comments as the following:

1. I'm glad you told me about this.
2. I believe what you've told me.
3. The abuse is not your fault.
4. No one deserves to be assaulted.
5. The situation is likely to get worse, not better.
6. If you are not safe, your child cannot be safe.
7. Help is available.

By taking a non-judgmental, compassionate approach, the clinician does more than just offer support. He or she also validates the patient's sense of worth and offers a measure of optimism that her situation can change.

DOCUMENTATION

Part of ensuring patient safety is to document the patient's statements regarding abuse and to document the physical findings associated with battering. Documentation is critical because it may eventually be useful in a court of law, particularly if custody issues arise. The clinician should document the abuse in the patient's own words. For example, "Patient states, 'My husband, John Smith, hit me with his fists,'" is preferable to "Patient reports being punched." Documentation should include the name of the perpetrator and nature of the weapon used. For description of injuries, dated photographs are ideal, but body maps or written descriptions are also acceptable. The clinician should also document, when possible, whether injuries appear recent or old (See also Chapter 15, Forensic Issues in Caring for the Adult Sexual Assault Victim).

INTERVENTION

Clinicians do not need to be experts in domestic violence in order to provide appropriate interventions. Once a victim of domestic violence is identified, it is important that the clinician be able to refer the patient to a domestic violence expert.

Key Point:
A clinician's supportive, non-judgmental attitude toward an abused patient is, in itself, a powerful intervention.

Key Point:
The clinician's documentation is vital, because there are rarely witnesses to episodes of assault.

That individual may be a hospital-based or community-based social worker, a colleague who is knowledgeable about domestic violence, a local domestic violence advocacy organization, or the national domestic violence hotline at 1-800-799-SAFE.

Sexually assaulted women must be offered emergency contraception as pregnancy prophylaxis within the first 72 hours of sexual assault, even when the assault occurs within the context of marriage. The only absolute contraindication to emergency contraception is a current pregnancy. Even women not ordinarily considered to be good candidates for oral contraception because of concurrent medical problems may be safely offered emergency contraception. Injectable contraception that can be used surreptitiously may protect women in abusive relationships by eliminating the need for the partner's consent or cooperation (Heise, 1993). In addition, victims of sexual assault should be offered STD screening and sexual assault forensic examinations.

Key Point:
It is important to discuss contraception, including emergency contraception, with women in abusive relationships.

Caution should be used in prescribing any sedatives to a domestic abuse victim. These medications can impair the patient's ability to adequately defend herself, escape, or seek immediate help if necessary.

Safety Is the Paramount Goal in Abuse Intervention

Insisting that an abused woman leave her partner is neither the responsibility nor the right of the clinician. Rather, the victim must decide whether or not she leaves the abusive relationship. An understandable, but dangerous, response by the clinician may be to urge the patient to leave the violent relationship at once. Abundant data show that the most dangerous time for a woman to be seriously injured or killed by her violent partner is when she attempts to leave the relationship. An abuse victim's attempt to leave the relationship before having a well-thought-out safety and exit plan is fraught with danger. In addition, the clinician must ensure that he or she does not attempt to be yet another controlling person in the patient's life, trying to coerce or force her into taking action for which she must bear responsibility.

Key Point:
The clinician should not urge an abused woman to "just get out" because she is more likely to be seriously injured or killed at the time she leaves her abuser than at any other time.

Safety Assessment Is Essential

Questions about violence are logical in the context of questions about personal and home safety.

Such questions may include:

1. Do you wear a seat belt?
2. Do you have working smoke detectors in your home?
3. Is there a gun in your home? If so, is it kept in a place safe from children? Is there a safety mechanism on it?
4. Do you have concerns that someone might hurt you or your children?

Key Point:
Questions about violence are logical in the context of questions about personal and home safety.

Instead of encouraging the patient to leave the abuser at once, the clinician should assist the victim in taking the necessary steps to ensure her safety and that of her children. The clinician is in an ideal position to offer validation and support to the patient. A statement such as, "I understand that you can't just leave, but no one deserves to be beaten, and it's important that we begin to think about your safety" may be the first step in constructive safety planning for an abused woman who feels isolated, terrified, and even blameworthy.

Safety assessment falls into 2 categories: immediate and long-term.

Immediate Safety

It is incumbent upon the clinician to assess whether there is an immediate threat to the abused patient's safety. There are some indicators that it may not be safe to return to her home that day.

Among these are the following:

1. He has recently obtained a gun.
2. He has increased the frequency and/or severity of attacks.

3. He has made suicidal and/or homicidal threats.
4. He has threatened the children.
5. He has displayed violence toward a pet.
6. He has escalated drug and/or alcohol abuse.

All these behaviors are indicative of a dangerously escalating risk of severe violence and danger toward the patient. In such a situation, the clinician may suggest to the patient that it may be unsafe for her to go home that day.

Long-Term Safety Issues
If the patient maintains that it is safe to go home, the clinician must respect her autonomy as a survivor and must make available safety-related information. Assessment can take the form of asking, "What will you do if this happens again?" Such a question can assist the patient in planning safety and/or exit strategies. The clinician may wish to review safety measures or give out printed material, such as the example found in Appendix II.

The clinician does not need to be a "domestic violence expert," but he or she does need to know who the experts are in his or her institution and in the community at large. In-house social workers and women's advocacy groups in the community can assist the clinician in obtaining referral information. Most communities have pocket cards available to give out to patients with safety information and phone numbers for shelters, other hot lines, and community advocacy resources.

Issues of confidentiality have probably been overstated in the context of relationship violence, but they may be of concern nonetheless. For patients who wish to maintain confidentiality regarding abuse, clinicians should take the same precautions as they do for other similarly sensitive health care issues, such as human immunodeficiency virus (HIV) status.

Key Point:
Routine referral for couples counseling is not recommended.

Routine referral for couples counseling is not recommended. If the patient discloses feelings of anger, for example, in a counseling session, her partner's abusive behavior may escalate. After the violence and threat of violence has ceased, joint counseling may then be an option in some cases.

A useful clinical tool for domestic violence assessment is the RADAR model. *RADAR is an acronym named by the Massachusetts Medical Society, as follows:*

R = Routine screening
A = Ask direct questions
D = Document findings
A = Assess safety
R = Review options and refer

An algorithm for using RADAR can be found in Appendix I.

SOCIETAL REACTION TO MARITAL RAPE
Laws have only recently reflected an understanding of marital rape as a crime. Many states had previously defined rape as when a man has "sexual intercourse with a female, not his wife, by force and against her will" (Finkelhor & Yllo, 1985). Under such an interpretation of law, it was not possible to charge a man with the rape of his wife. Nevertheless, our society has made progress in recognizing that rape within a relationship can have the same components of forcible sex that occur in acquaintance rape—coercion, physical force, and physical and mental trauma to the victim. Since 1993, rape within the marriage is a violation of the criminal code under some circumstances in every state. As of 1996, 32 states still had some exemptions from prosecuting husbands or cohabitants for rape in one or more of the sex offense laws (Bergen, 1996).

Social awareness of the prevalence of marital rape has been accompanied by corresponding legal aid to its victims in recent years. Many states now provide financial compensation to victims of sexual assault in addition to the social services in order to alleviate the financial burden of the medical care required.

SPECIAL POPULATIONS

Immigrants

A woman who is an immigrant may be particularly vulnerable to abusive relationships for many reasons. She may come from a culture in which the subordination of women is the norm, she may be completely dependent economically on her partner, and she may be particularly isolated because of an inability to speak English comfortably.

In the context of immigrant populations, there may be particularly onerous tactics associated with abuse. For example, an abusive partner may hide her immigration papers and other vital documents. He may threaten to have his abused partner deported (even if he has no ability to do so) if she discloses the violence to anyone. He may prevent her from learning English in order to maintain her isolation and dependence.

Furthermore, there are particular disincentives for an abused woman who is unfamiliar with the language, culture, and laws to disclose abuse. As already noted, she may be entirely dependent on her partner economically and have little means of supporting herself and children, particularly if she speaks little or no English. Her partner may serve as her translator, thereby offering her no opportunity to disclose the violence in a private setting. In a survey of Latina women who were outpatient clinic attendees, of those who identified themselves as abused, 34% identified language barriers, and 21% reported concerns about the immigration authorities as reasons for not wishing to disclose the abuse (Rodriguez et al., 2000).

Key Point:
Abused immigrant women most often cite language difficulties and fear of immigration authorities as reasons for not disclosing violence.

In addition, an abused woman from another country and/or culture may have fewer options for escape. She may not have the financial resources to return to her family, or she may feel ashamed or even fearful of punishment if she returns to her family with a "failed" marriage. If her partner is American or is a legal US citizen, she may fear losing her children if she attempts to leave the relationship.

Clinicians caring for women from other cultures must be aware of the importance of cultural sensitivity and knowledge of those cultures. Clinicians also need to be familiar with local resources for women of other countries and cultures. Peer counselors from the same cultural community may be particularly helpful. Clearly, it is important to try, whenever possible, to avoid using family members as interpreters.

Women with Disabilities

While there have been few studies concerning abuse and assault against disabled women, it seems that the prevalence of physical, sexual, and emotional abuse is the same among women with and without disabilities (Young et al., 1998).

Disabled women are particularly vulnerable to physical and sexual abuse and assault.

The reasons for their increased risk include:

1. Physical vulnerability
2. Dependence on caretakers, including family members, healthcare workers, and attendants
3. Difficulty making and carrying out a safety/escape plan (Nosek et al., 1998)
4. Lack of accessibility to services (Nosek et al., 1998)

Sexual abuse has been documented in 25% of mentally retarded adolescent girls and 31% of adolescent girls with congenital physical disabilities (Brown, 1998; Chamberlain et al., 1984).

Gay and Lesbian Relationships

Same-sex physically and/or sexually abusive relationships are fraught with the same problems as heterosexual relationships (Merrill & Wolfe, 2000). However, additional issues may make terminating a same-sex violent relationship even more difficult or dangerous than terminating a heterosexual violent relationship.

Additional barriers to terminating the relationship include:

1. The abusive partner may threaten to "out" the victim, that is, disclose his or her status as being homosexual. This threat may have tremendous real or perceived implications for employment and family relationships.
2. Gays and lesbians may live within small social frameworks. Leaving an abusive partner may entail leaving an entire social network and can increase the sense of isolation.
3. In male same-sex relationships, the abusive partner may threaten the victim with exposure to HIV (although this potential threat is clearly not limited to same sex relationships).
4. The abusive partner may claim to be the victim. Particularly in relationships in which one member of the couple is larger or appears physically stronger or more "masculine," outsiders may draw erroneous conclusions as to who is the batterer.
5. There is perceived and real lack of resources for abused partners in same-sex relationships. This is particularly true for males (Merrill & Wolfe, 2000).

In a study of homosexual and bisexual men attending an STD clinic, a history of sexual abuse was associated with mental health hospitalization, depression, suicidality, and HIV risk behavior (Bartholow et al., 1994).

Overall, physical and sexual violence are more common in heterosexual and homosexual male relationships than in lesbian relationships (Tjaden & Thoennes, 1998). Men are more likely to perpetrate physical and sexual violence than are women, regardless of the gender of the partner.

Key Point:
Violence exists in both heterosexual and same-sex relationships. In general, regardless of the gender of the partner, males are more likely to perpetrate violence than females.

FUTURE STUDY AND INTERVENTIONS FOR INTIMATE PARTNER RAPE

Clearly, there is a tremendous need for both research and effective interventions to address intimate partner rape.

The interventions of greatest priority include the following:

1. Training for clinicians in the identification and counseling of victims.
2. Intervention programs for abusers.
3. Social agency resources that are made known to providers. A recent survey of 621 rape crisis centers and battered women's shelters, for example, found that only 4% included wife rape as an issue of concern in their mission statements (Bergen, 1996).
4. Cross-disciplinary services for victims when there is both child abuse and domestic violence in the home.
5. Shelters and advocacy resources for abused women that can address not only the physical symptoms of abuse, but also the psychologic ones.
6. Assistance and counseling for the ancillary victims, such as small children in the household or aged parents living with the couple.

The incidence of partner rape and its consequences for the victim and for society are much greater than previously believed. The rape of a spouse, which once was considered under the law to be an oxymoron, has become recognized as a problem that the physician or other clinician is likely to encounter in his or her practice. It behooves us to be able to recognize it where it exists and to treat it effectively, with compassion, and in coordination with advocacy, legal, social, and other resources, as we would any other social problem with medical ramifications.

APPENDIX I: RADAR ALGORITHM

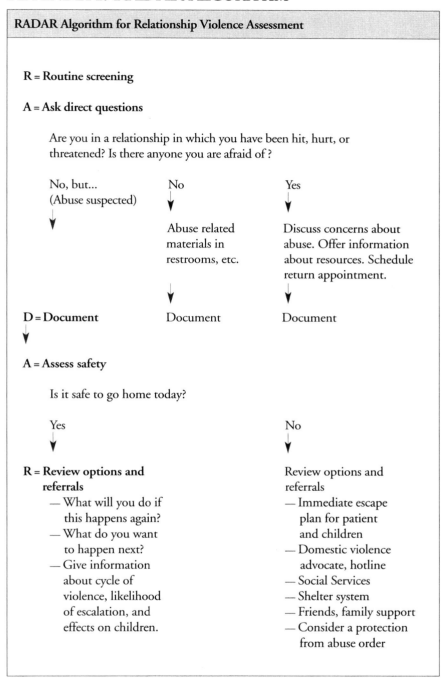

RADAR Algorithm for Relationship Violence Assessment

R = Routine screening

A = Ask direct questions

Are you in a relationship in which you have been hit, hurt, or threatened? Is there anyone you are afraid of ?

No, but...
(Abuse suspected)

No

Yes

Abuse related materials in restrooms, etc.

Discuss concerns about abuse. Offer information about resources. Schedule return appointment.

D = Document   Document   Document

A = Assess safety

Is it safe to go home today?

Yes

No

R = Review options and referrals
— What will you do if this happens again?
— What do you want to happen next?
— Give information about cycle of violence, likelihood of escalation, and effects on children.

Review options and referrals
— Immediate escape plan for patient and children
— Domestic violence advocate, hotline
— Social Services
— Shelter system
— Friends, family support
— Consider a protection from abuse order

APPENDIX II: SAFETY TIPS WHEN THERE IS VIOLENCE IN THE HOME

1. Let people know what's happening to you—your friends, family, doctor, minister, the police. An abuser is NOT entitled to privacy.
2. Remove weapons from your home. If there is a gun that must remain in the home, make sure there is a "safety" on it.
3. Teach your children to dial 911 during an emergency.
4. Hide money (e.g., in your purse in a tampon container). If possible, open your own bank account.

5. Keep a copy of important papers, rent receipts, birth certificates, insurance policies, important phone numbers, with a friend.
6. Keep extra personal items such as clothes for you and your children, house and car keys, etc., with a friend.
7. Notify your children's school that there is a problem. This may be important to protect your children's safety.
8. If you and your partner get in a fight, try to get out of the kitchen or garage. There are too many objects that can be used as weapons in these places.
9. If you need to leave at once, do whatever you can to take your children with you.
10. Avoid alcohol and drugs, which may slow your reflexes and impair your judgment.
11. If you have visible injuries, show them to a doctor or a nurse. A photograph may be very helpful if you go to court at some time.
12. Even if you don't have injuries that show, tell your doctor or nurse what happened. A statement in the medical chart will be helpful to you if there is ever a custody battle.
13. If you have a protection from abuse order, keep it with you at all times.

Keep available the number of the child abuse hotline (1-800-932-0313) and that of a local emergency shelter.

REFERENCES

Abbott J, Johnson R, Koziol-McLain J, Lowenstein SR. Domestic violence against women: incidence and prevalence in an emergency department population. *JAMA.* 1995;273:1763-1767.

Bartholow BN, Doll LS, Joy D, et al. Emotional, behavioral and HIV risks associated with sexual abuse among adult homosexual and bisexual men. *Child Abuse Negl.* 1994;18:747-761.

Basile KC. Rape by acquiescence: the ways in which women "give in" to unwanted sex with their husbands. *Violence Against Women.* 1999;5:1036-1058.

Beebe DK. Initial assessment of the rape victim. *J Miss State Med Assoc.* 1991;32:403-406.

Bergen RK. *Wife Rape: Understanding the Response of Survivors and Service Providers.* Thousand Oaks, Calif: Sage; 1996.

Bowker L. Marital rape: a distinct syndrome? *Soc Casework.* 1983;64: 347-352.

Brown DE. Factors affecting psychosexual development of adults with congenital physical disabilities. *Phys Occup Ther Pediatr.* 1998;8:43-58.

Campbell JC. Nursing assessment for risk of homicide with battered women. *Am J Nurs.* 1986;8:36-51.

Campbell JC, Alford P. The dark consequences of marital rape. *Am J Nurs.* 1989;89:946-949.

Campbell JC, Soeken KL. Forced sex and intimate partner violence: effects on women's risk and women's health. *Violence Against Women.* 1999;5:1017-1035.

Chamberlain A, Rauh J, Passer A, McGrath M, Burket R. Issues in fertility control for mentally retarded female adolescents, I: sexual activity, sexual abuse, and contraception. *Pediatrics.* 1984;73:445-450.

Council on Scientific Affairs, American Medical Association. Violence against women: relevance for medical practitioners. *JAMA.* 1992;267;3184-189.

Doran J. Conflict and violence in intimate relationships: a focus on marital rape. Paper presented at: Annual Meeting of the American Psychological Association; August 1980; Montreal, Canada.

Easteal PW, Easteal S. Attitudes and practices of doctors toward spouse assault victims: an Australian study. *Violence Vict.* 1992 Fall;7:217-28.

Eby KK, Campbell JC, Sullivan CM, et al. Health effects of experiences of sexual violence for women with abusive partners. *Health Care Women Int.* 1995;16:563-576.

Farley R. Homicide trends in the United States. In: Hawkins DF, ed. *Homicide Among Black Americans.* New York, NY: University Press of America; 1986:13-27.

Feldhaus KM, Houry D, Kaminsky R. Lifetime sexual assault prevalence rates and reporting practices in an emergency department population. *Ann Emerg Med.* 2000;36:23-27.

Finkelhor D, Yllo K. *License to Rape: Sexual Abuse of Wives.* New York, NY: Free Press; 1985.

Frieze IH. Investigating the causes and consequences of marital rape. *J Women Cul Soc.* 1983;8:532-553.

Grams AC, Carneiro de Sousa MJ, Roesh R, et al. Sexual abuse within the marital relationship. *Med Law.* 1997;16:743-751.

Grisso JA, Wishner AR, Schwartz DF, et al. A population-based study of injuries in inner city women. *Am J Epidemiol.* 1991;134:59-86.

Heise LL. Reproductive freedom and violence against women: where are the intersections? *J Law Med Ethics.* 1993;21:206-216.

Kessler R, McGonagle K, Nelson C, Hughes M, Swartz M, Blazer D. Sex and depression in the National Comorbidity Survey, II. cohort effects. *J Infect Dis.* 1994;30:15-26.

Killpatrick DG, Edmunds CN, Seymour AK. *Rape in America: A Report to the Nation.* Charleston, SC: Crime Victim Research and Treatment Center; 1992.

Marsh CE. Sexual assault and domestic violence in the African American community. *West J Black Studies.* 1993;17(3):149-155.

McAfee RE. Physicians and domestic violence: can we make a difference? *JAMA.* 1995;273:1790-1791.

McFarlane J, Gondolf E. Preventing abuse during pregnancy: a clinical protocol. *MCN Am J Matern Child Nurs.* 1998 Jan-Feb;23(1):22-6.

McGrath ME, Bettachi A, Duffy SJ, Peipert JF, Becker BM, St Angelo L. Violence against women: provider barriers to intervention in emergency departments. *Acad Emerg Med.* 1997;4:297-300.

Merrill GS, Wolfe VA. Battered gay men: an exploration of abuse, help seeking, and why they stay. *J Homosex.* 2000;39:1-30.

Norton LB, Peipert JF, Pierler S, Lima B, Hume L. Battering in pregnancy: an assessment of two screening methods. *Obstet Gynecol.* 1995;85:321-325.

Nosek MA, Howland CA, Young ME. Abuse of women with disabilities: policy implications. *J Disab Policy Studies.* 1998;8:158-175.

Plichta, SB. Violence and abuse: implications for women's health. In: Falik MM, Collins KS, eds. *Women's Health: The Commonwealth Survey.* Baltimore, Md: Johns Hopkins University Press; 1996:237-272.

Rodriguez MA, Sheldon WR, Bauer HM, Peréz-Stable EJ. The factors associated with disclosure of intimate partner abuse to clinicians. *J Fam Pract.* 2000;50:338-344.

Russell D. *Rape in Marriage.* New York, NY: Macmillan Publishing Co; 1982.

Shields NM, Hanneke CR. Battered wives reactions to marital rape. In: Finkelhor D, Gelles RJ, eds. *The Dark Side of Families*. Newbury Park, Calif: Sage Publications Inc; 1983:131-148.

Sutherland C, Bybee D, Sullivan C. The long-term effects of battering on women's health. *Women's Health: Research on Gender, Behavior, and Policy*. 1998:4;42-70.

Tjaden P, Thoennes N. *Prevalence, Incidence and Consequences of Violence Against Women: Findings of the National Violence Against Women Survey*. Washington, DC: US Department of Justice, National Institute of Justice; 1998. NCJ Publication No. 172837.

Weingourt R. Wife rape in a sample of psychiatric patients. *Image: J Nurs Sch*. 1990;22:144-147.

Weissman M, Klerman G. Depression: current understanding and changing trends. *Annu Rev Public Health*. 1992;13:319-339.

Wingood GM, DiClemente RJ. The effects of abusive primary partner on the condom use and sexual negotiation practices of African-American women. *Amer J Pub Health*. 1997;87:1016-1018.

Wingood GM, DiClemente RJ, Raj A. Identifying the prevalence and correlates of STDs among women in rural domestic violence shelters. *Womens Health*. 2000;30:15-26.

Yegidis B. Wife abuse and marital rape among women who seek help. *Affilia*. 1988;3:62-68.

Young, ME, Nosek MA, Howland CA, Chanpong G, Rintala DH. Prevalence of abuse of women with physical disabilities. *Arch Phys Med Rehabil*. 1998;78(special issue):S34-S38.

Chapter 20

SEXUAL ASSAULT AND PREGNANCY

Janice B. Asher, MD
Elizabeth M. Datner, MD

Violence in pregnancy represents a unique challenge in that there are two victims: mother and fetus. However, pregnancy is also a time of tremendous opportunity in terms of availability of medical, social, and community supports. Three potential situations exist with regard to sexual assault and pregnancy: sexual assault in the context of domestic violence, sexual assault of pregnant women, and sexual assault resulting in pregnancy. In this chapter, we will address medical and obstetric sequelae, the role of the clinician, and public health issues associated with sexual assault in pregnancy. Adolescent pregnancy, which has special concerns for both obstetric and pediatric providers, will be addressed as well.

SEXUAL ASSAULT IN THE CONTEXT OF DOMESTIC VIOLENCE DURING PREGNANCY

EPIDEMIOLOGY

An abuser employs many tactics to maintain power over his partner, including physical violence, emotional abuse, intimidation, and isolation. In this context, sexual assault and/or coercion is yet another tactic for exerting control over a partner.

The leading cause of maternal mortality is homicide, and the most likely perpetrator is the pregnant woman's partner (Horon & Cheng, 2001; Martin et al., 2001). More pregnant women die as a result of domestic violence than of any medical complication of pregnancy, yet its detection rate is woefully low (Fildes et al., 1992). Results of a recent study indicate that more than 60% of obstetrician-gynecologists do not routinely screen pregnant patients for violence, even though domestic violence during pregnancy is more common than pre-eclampsia, gestational diabetes, and placenta previa (Gazmararian et al., 1996). This lack of assessment for violence is particularly striking when we consider the amount of time, money, and resources used to screen for these other common obstetric complications. In one study, fewer than 3% of physically abused pregnant women were identified as abused by their medical practitioners, even though the injuries were often visible (Wilson et al., 1996).

The single greatest risk factor for partner violence in pregnancy and postpartum is a history of violence by that partner within the year before pregnancy (Campbell & Alford, 1989; Martin et al., 2001; Stewart, 1994). The incidence of domestic violence in pregnancy has been estimated at between 4% and 20%, depending on the methods used and the population studied (Gazmararian et al., 1995). Domestic violence tends to escalate in frequency and intensity during pregnancy. Of women who were abused in the year before pregnancy, 40% to 60% of them are abused during pregnancy as well (McFarlane, 1993).

Several studies have concluded that violence in the postpartum period is more common than it is during pregnancy. In one study, 90% of women who were battered during pregnancy were abused by their partner within 3 months of the

Key Point:
The single greatest risk factor for partner violence in pregnancy and postpartum is a history of violence by that partner within the year before pregnancy.

baby's birth (Stewart, 1994). With regard to sexual violence, another study of abused pregnant women found that 46% of married women were coerced or forced to have intercourse immediately following hospitalization, most often after childbirth (Campbell & Alford, 1989).

INCREASED ABUSE DURING PREGNANCY

Many reasons have been put forth to explain the increased incidence and severity of domestic violence during pregnancy. One is that pregnancy represents a new opportunity for the maintenance of power and control that characterizes an abusive relationship. Violence is a particularly chilling and effective tactic for maintaining control over a woman who is pregnant and feeling physically, emotionally, and financially vulnerable for herself and for her baby.

Another plausible explanation for abuse during pregnancy is the phenomenon of jealousy toward the baby (Campbell et al., 1993). Intense and pathologic jealousy is a hallmark of many abusive relationships; it is easy to understand how an abusive partner might feel threatened and incensed at the prospect of his displacement as the most important person in his partner's life. The abuser might also feel anger toward the baby in the context of an unintended or unwanted pregnancy.

Finally, there are often other stresses resulting from pregnancy, including obstetric complications and financial concerns. It is important to appreciate that stress does not cause violence; rather, increased stress may be a precipitating factor in the escalation of violence.

In the postpartum period, increased stress is accompanied by increased fatigue and increased attention to the baby on the part of the woman. This accumulation of stresses makes clear why the incidence of abuse is higher in the postpartum period than at any other time. The increased incidence of abuse coupled with the overlap of domestic violence and child abuse make it imperative that pediatricians, as well as obstetricians, screen mothers of infants for domestic violence (Duffy et al., 1999; McKibben et al., 1989; Thompson & Krugman, 2001; Wright, 2000). According to the American Academy of Pediatrics (1998):

> Pediatricians are in a position to recognize abused women in pediatric settings. Intervening on behalf of battered women is an active form of child abuse prevention. Knowledge of local resources and state laws for reporting abuse are emphasized (p. 1091-1092).

PREGNANCY AS A WINDOW OF OPPORTUNITY FOR INTERVENTION

The rationale for violence prevention and intervention efforts in pregnancy is based on the unique window of opportunity that pregnancy represents for both mother and child. Factors that increase the opportunity to address violence include:

— Under no other circumstances do healthy young women have repeated, ongoing contact with the medical system (McFarlane, 1993). Health care professionals are often the first, and sometimes the only, caregivers with whom abused women come into contact. The numerous visits with clinicians that pregnancy affords and the common goal of delivering a healthy baby provide the opportunity for a trusting relationship between patient and provider.

— During pregnancy, women are concerned about their own well-being and that of their unborn babies. Ordinarily, an abused woman may feel that she cannot leave an abusive relationship, that the abuse is her fault, that her partner needs help, or that she hopes the situation will get better. During pregnancy, an abused woman may do on behalf of her baby what she would not otherwise do for herself. The prenatal period represents an ideal opportunity to begin the comprehensive linkage of services that are likely to be needed for successful outcome for an abused woman and her baby.

Key Point:
Violence increases postpartum depression. Pediatricians who screen for domestic violence may be able to help prevent child abuse.

Key Point:
Because of frequent visits with healthcare professionals and a mother's concern for the well-being of the baby, pregnancy offers a unique opportunity for the assessment of relationship violence on behalf of both mother and child.

— Social, economic, and community support systems are already in place for pregnant women and can be used to greater advantage with a well-designed collaborative model. "Pregnancy is a time when societal values coincide with a woman's desire to bring a healthy baby into the world" (Mayer & Liebschutz, 1998).

INTERSECTION OF DOMESTIC VIOLENCE AND CHILD ABUSE

Child abuse and maternal abuse are inextricably linked. Nearly 60% of abused children have mothers who are also abused (McKibben et al., 1989). Women who were abused as children have a much greater incidence of severe depression, drug and alcohol abuse, and earlier first pregnancies than women without such a history (McCauley et al., 1997). With specific regard to sexual assault and abuse, women who were sexually abused as children are almost five times as likely to be sexually abused as adults (Duffy et al., 1999).

Key Point:
There is a significant correlation between domestic violence and child abuse: 60% of abused children have mothers who are also abused.

Children who witness abuse in the home are at as much risk for poor emotional, social, behavioral, and academic achievement as are those who are abused themselves (Wright et al., 1997). A particularly chilling observation is that witnessing abuse of a parent is one of the principal risk factors for becoming an abusive or abused adult oneself (Dodge et al., 1990; Wilson et al., 1996).

Unintended pregnancy is a common outcome in abusive relationships (Dietz et al., 1999) because abused women may not be able to negotiate sexual activity or contraceptive use. Numerous studies have demonstrated that unintended pregnancies are also more common in women who were sexually abused as children (Boyer & Fine, 1992; Dietz et al., 1999; Fiscella et al., 1998; McCauley et al., 1997). Children who live in families of several unplanned pregnancies are up to 4.6 times more likely to be abused than are children in families where there are no unplanned pregnancies (Zurawin, 1991).

Because it is well documented that abused women are much more likely to have children who are abused as well, a lack of systems continuity represents a missed opportunity to intervene in the intergenerational cycle of violence. Most importantly, when clinicians provide effective interventions, including offering support and encouragement, making referrals to appropriate sources, and providing assistance with developing safety strategies, abused pregnant women adopt more safety behaviors to protect themselves and their babies both during and after pregnancy (McFarlane et al., 1998).

A painful irony is that particular barriers may exist to addressing domestic violence in pregnancy. A pregnant woman may feel more vulnerable emotionally and financially, including being dependent on her partner's health insurance. She also may be particularly anxious at this time to try to keep the family together (Mayer & Liebschutz, 1998). She may hope that the situation will improve after the baby is born and that her most intense fears are groundless. The obstetric clinician must be aware of such barriers and offer support and safety planning within these parameters.

SEXUAL ASSAULT AND ABUSE OF PREGNANT WOMEN

The most serious sequela of assault and abuse is death. More pregnant women die as a result of partner violence than from any complication of pregnancy (Fildes et al., 1992). Several studies have indicated that pregnant women who are abused may be at increased risk for various obstetric, medical, and psychosocial complications. All of these problems have direct and indirect consequences for both mother and fetus. Although abusers usually claim that their acts of violence occur because of a loss of control, in fact, the converse is usually true: abuse is a tactic of control.

CLINICAL MANIFESTATIONS

Inadequate Prenatal Care

In several studies, abused women had significantly later entry into prenatal care (Dietz et al., 1997; McFarlane, 1993). One reason is that because a pregnancy is more likely to be unintended in the context of abuse, a woman may delay beginning prenatal care until she has decided whether or not to continue the pregnancy. As a correlate of this, she may be in a psychologic state of denial about an unintended and unwished-for pregnancy. She may be terrified of disclosing the fact of the pregnancy to her partner, even if the pregnancy resulted from his refusal to allow contraception or because of nonconsensual intercourse.

Abused women are also more likely to miss prenatal visits than nonabused women are. This is partly because of late entry into prenatal care but may also result from the abusive partner's refusing to allow the woman needed access to medical care as another tactic of control and isolation. A patient who is a frequent "no-show" may be missing appointments because she is not being allowed to attend them, not because she is noncompliant.

Abdominal and Genital Trauma

Along with causing injury to the mother, abdominal trauma may also result in serious harm to the fetus, including fetal fractures, dermal scars, and even death (Peterson et al., 1997; Ribe et al., 1993). In addition, blunt abdominal trauma may result in a placental abruption and other manifestations of fetomaternal hemorrhage. It is incumbent on the clinician to assess for the necessity of administering RhoGam to the Rh-negative pregnant woman who has sustained abdominal trauma (Mayer & Liebschutz, 1998). Forced sex with a woman who has a placenta previa puts both her and the fetus at risk for life-threatening hemorrhage.

Because of increased vascularity that exists during pregnancy in general, as well as vulvar varicosities that are more common in pregnancy in particular, genital trauma may result in vulvar hematomas and other bleeding in the genital area that may be difficult to control. The clinician must obtain a detailed history when there is genital trauma. If objects have been used to cause the trauma, irrigation, antibiotics, and/or tetanus prophylaxis may be indicated.

Adverse Outcome of Pregnancy

Some studies show an increased incidence of premature delivery, low birth weight, abdominal trauma, cesarean sections, and pyelonephritis in women who are battered during pregnancy (Cokkinides et al., 1999; Fraser et al., 1995; Jolly et al., 2000; Parker et al., 1994). Medical consequences may result from an abusive partner limiting the pregnant patient's access to medical care, medications, or even food.

Unintended Pregnancy and Sexually Transmitted Diseases

Pregnancy may be, in itself, a manifestation of abuse and assault. The correlation between abuse and unintended pregnancy is high. Both pregnancy and sexually transmitted diseases (STDs) result from the inability of abused and assaulted women to negotiate condom use and other methods of contraception (Gazmararian et al., 1996; Wingood & DiClemente, 1997). The sexually assaulted woman should be offered emergency contraception as pregnancy prophylaxis within the first 72 hours of sexual assault. Progesterone-only emergency contraception, which has recently become available, is more efficacious and has fewer side effects (Gainer et al., 2001).

STDs and unintended or mistimed pregnancies are also much more common in women in abusive relationships. These findings are not surprising when we consider the basis for all STD and unintended pregnancy prevention: the ability to negotiate with one's partner. Abused women do not have this option, and numerous studies have borne out the increased incidence of unintended pregnancies and STDs in abused pregnant women compared with pregnant women who are not abused (Wingood & DiClemente, 1997).

Depression

In one study, 20% of abused pregnant women reported attempting suicide (Hilliard, 1985). The inextricable link between depression and interpersonal violence has been noted. (See also Chapter 19, Domestic Violence and Partner Rape.)

Drug and Alcohol Abuse

Abuse of drugs and alcohol, which is more common in both perpetrators and victims of domestic violence, is especially problematic in pregnancy because of the effects on the fetus (Berenson et al., 1992). In particular, fetal alcohol syndrome is associated with congenital malformations, mental retardation, and behavior problems. Maternal ingestion of cocaine is associated with placental abruption and fetal cerebrovascular accidents.

Pregnancy should be viewed as a uniquely opportune time to address substance abuse because of the pregnant woman's concern for her baby. For example, women are more likely to stop smoking when they become pregnant than when they are not pregnant (Dolan-Mullen et al., 1994; Kendrick & Merritt, 1996).

Pregnancy Termination

As many as 39.5% of women seeking elective pregnancy termination report being in a violent relationship. Abused women are less likely to inform their partners about the pregnancy or to involve them in the decision to terminate the pregnancy (Glander et al., 1998).

STEPS IN IDENTIFYING ABUSE AND ASSAULT IN PREGNANCY

Despite how common violence is during and after pregnancy, abused women are reluctant to spontaneously bring up the topic, and obstetricians do not routinely screen for domestic violence (Durant et al., 2000; Horan et al., 1998; Plichta et al., 1996; Stewart & Cecutti, 1993). This lack of assessment seems particularly ironic when we consider the enormous attention and resources devoted to screening for such disorders of pregnancy as pre-eclampsia, placenta previa, and gestational diabetes that are much less common than battering in pregnancy. Numerous studies have shown the value of universal screening for relationship violence with regard to increasing the detection rate.

Ideally, screening should be performed at each trimester of pregnancy. Screening questions can be the same as those for non-pregnant patients:

— Are you in a relationship in which you have been hit, pushed, or kicked?
— Are you in a relationship in which you have been forced to have sex?

Screening should be done with the woman alone because she may not feel safe to disclose abuse with her partner present. Sometimes it may be impossible to separate the partner and patient. For this reason, abuse-related materials, particularly safety planning information, should be kept in all patient bathrooms.

Studies have demonstrated that the rate of disclosure increases with frequency of screening (Covington et al., 1997; McFarlane, 1993). There are many reasons for this. For example, a woman may not wish to disclose violence until she has established a trusting relationship with her provider. She may not feel emotionally prepared to discuss violence the first time the issue is raised. Also, because the incidence of violence increases as pregnancy progresses, a negative response at the initial prenatal screening visit may not be predictive of a negative response later in the pregnancy.

The 36-week screen, when signs and symptoms of labor are reviewed, is an ideal time to review safety, and abuse-related questions easily lend themselves to this context.

CLINICIAN RESPONSE TO ABUSE DURING PREGNANCY

The most important feature of responding to abuse in pregnancy is to first identify it. Assessment is, in itself, a powerful form of intervention (McFarlane & Parker, 1994). The clinician must obtain a history about the nature and severity of the abuse to be able to adequately assess danger and potential lethality. It is crucial to maintain a nonjudgmental and compassionate demeanor when discussing relationship violence. The importance of the clinician's role in supporting and validating the patient who discloses abuse cannot be overstated.

Key Point:
Red flags for risk of abuse and assault in pregnancy:
— *History of abuse in the year prior to pregnancy*
— *Unintended pregnancy*
— *Late entry into prenatal care*
— *Poor compliance with appointments, medical recommendations*
— *Maternal trauma, particularly breast, abdomen, genitals*
— *Fetal trauma, particularly fractures*
— *Poor weight gain*
— *Sexually transmitted disease*
— *Depression*
— *Substance abuse*
— *Partner refuses to leave or answers questions for patients*
— *Adolescent pregnancy*

Pregnancy is an especially opportune time to facilitate linkages necessary to support, assist, and advocate on behalf of abused women. Federal, state, and local programs are in place for pregnant women to a greater extent than for non pregnant adults.

The pelvic examination and the experience of labor may be particularly traumatic for women who have been sexually abused or assaulted as children or adults (Grant, 1992; Mayer, 1995; Rhodes & Hutchinson, 1994). Clinicians must consider this response in two contexts:

Key Point:
Thirty-six-week home safety screening questions:
— Do you have a car seat for the baby?
— Do you have working smoke detectors in your home?
— Is there a gun in your home? Is it in a place safe from children?
— Do you have concerns that someone might hurt you or the baby?

— The patient who has reported sexual abuse and who needs extra psychosocial support.
— The patient who has not disclosed abuse or who has no memory of abuse, but who seems more terrified than expected when she undergoes pelvic examination or labor.

When a woman seems particularly frightened while being examined, the clinician should make the examination as patient-driven as possible. For example, the provider should ask permission to begin the examination and should tell the patient that she may ask to stop the examination at any time. Judicious use of analgesia and anesthesia during labor is recommended (Committee on Health Care, 2000).

SAFETY IS THE CRITICAL ISSUE

As with all victims of abuse, the clinician's role is to assist the pregnant patient to take necessary steps to ensure her safety and that of her baby. The frequency of prenatal appointments provides ample opportunity to offer assistance. Safety assessment and planning can and should be part of every prenatal visit for the pregnant woman who is being abused during pregnancy or who has a history of being abused by her partner in the year before pregnancy. (See also Chapter 19, Domestic Violence and Partner Rape.) Safety information and lists of local resources, hotlines, and shelters should be offered. Some patients do not feel safe taking such information or deny needing it. For this reason, abuse and assault-related information should be kept in all lavatory areas, where it can be read in private by patients.

Part of ensuring patient safety is to document the patient's statements regarding abuse, including the name of the perpetrator and the weapons used. It is also important to document the physical findings associated with battering and sexual assault, ideally using photographs. (See also Chapter 19, Domestic Violence and Partner Rape.)

THE ROLE OF PEDIATRICIANS IN PREVENTING BOTH CHILD ABUSE AND DOMESTIC VIOLENCE

Domestic violence screening by pediatricians has the potential of an enormous effect on child health as it may protect children from child abuse and neglect as well as psychological and behavioral dysfunction throughout the life cycle. Identifying and responding appropriately and sensitively to battered mothers may be the most effective means of intervening on behalf of the children (Wright, 2000, p. 432).

Domestic violence assessment is particularly vital for pediatricians to embrace as part of their role. Traditionally, pediatricians and other pediatric care providers, while very aware of the importance of child abuse recognition, have not concerned themselves with partner abuse. Fortunately, domestic violence is becoming recognized as a pediatric issue (American Academy of Pediatrics, 1998). The link between domestic violence and child abuse has been abundantly documented (Duffy et al., 1999; McKibben et al., 1989). In one study performed at a pediatric sexual abuse evaluation clinic, there was a 54% incidence of domestic violence in the homes of children being evaluated. Forty-two percent of the mothers reported a history of childhood sexual abuse to themselves (Bowen, 2000). Pediatric practitioners who do not assess for domestic violence are missing a crucial opportunity to assess for indicators of child abuse and to initiate preventive measures.

Questions about domestic violence can be asked in the child's presence as long as the child is sufficiently young enough that he or she will not report the content of the discussion back to the abusive partner. The topics of child and domestic abuse may be logically raised in the context of discussions about discipline. Questions may also be incorporated into more general home safety questions.

When both maternal and child abuse are suspected, the pediatric practitioner, in addition to reporting the child abuse, is obliged to take steps to help ensure the safety of both the mother and child (Schecter & Gary, 1992). In this context, an interdisciplinary, collaborative approach is of highest importance (Wright et al., 1997).

ABUSE AND ASSAULT IN ADOLESCENT PREGNANCY

I met him when I was 14 and he was 19. I liked him because he showed so much interest in me and had a car and enough money to take me to get food. We talked about having a baby for a while, and he was happy when I got pregnant. He said he would stop using drugs as soon as the baby was born. But he didn't. When the baby was 2 weeks old, he said he had waited long enough to have sex, and he made me do it. It hurt my stitches. I got pregnant again when the baby was 2 months old. When I was 4 months pregnant, we were riding in the car. My boyfriend was high. He hit a post. Now the baby is paralyzed from the neck down. She's only 6 months old. It's all my fault.

Adolescents are over-represented among abused pregnant women, with as many as 29% of pregnant adolescents experiencing abuse, including sexual abuse and assault (Berenson et al., 1992; Martin et al., 2001). Abuse is particularly increased in pregnant adolescents whose partners are 4 or more years older than they are (Harner et al., 2001; Males, 1995). A particularly chilling observation is that pregnant teens, compared with those who are not pregnant, have a much greater history of having been sexually abused as children (Boyer & Fine, 1992; Fiscella et al., 1998; Raj et al., 2000). This intergenerational cycle of abuse should serve as a compelling reason for all clinicians to take a role in preventing and intervening in family violence and sexual assault (**Figure 20-1**).

Teen parenthood is associated with particularly painful outcomes for both mother and baby. Studies have shown that teen mothers display more aggressive, inappropriate, and abusive behavior toward their babies (Elster et al., 1990; Flanagan et al., 1995; Stier et al., 1993). The two major risk factors for infanticide are associated with maternal age under 15 years and short interpregnancy interval with maternal age under 17 years (Overpeck et al., 1998). School-aged children of adolescent mothers have been shown to have more cognitive and behavioral problems than do children of adult mothers (Stevens-Simon & McAnarney, 1994).

Abused teens are also more likely to smoke cigarettes and abuse drugs and alcohol during pregnancy (Boyer & Fine, 1992; Martin et al., 1999). In addition, they have twice the school drop-out rate as do those who are not abused. They have a much higher rate of sexually transmitted diseases during pregnancy than do non-abused pregnant teens (Asher et al., 2000). Some studies have reported later entry into prenatal care among abused teens.

The positive side of this picture, however, is that pregnant teens also benefit the most from intensive intervention (Parker, 1993). Teens are less likely than adult women to have long-term emotional, financial, and familial attachments to their partners. As a result, they may feel less compelled or threatened to remain in abusive relationships. If they are in school, systems and social supports are in place to assist them and their children.

Clinicians caring for female adolescents, pregnant and non pregnant alike, must screen for past and current sexual abuse. Specifically, they should ask the patient if she is involved in a relationship in which she is being coerced or forced to engage in sexual activity. If she is sexually active and is not using contraception, the reasons

Key Point:
The paramount role of the clinician is increasing the safety of the patient, not getting her to leave her partner.

Key Point:
Pregnant adolescents are more likely to be physically and sexually abused than are pregnant adult women.

Key Point:
Teen parents are more likely to abuse their children, use tobacco, drugs and alcohol, drop out of school, and have children with cognitive and behavior problems.

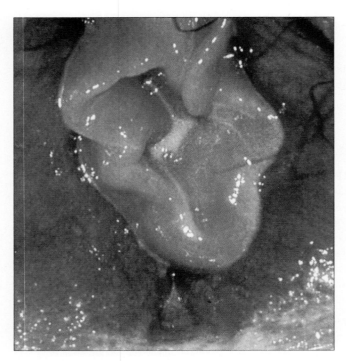

Figure 20-1. *Normal hymen of adolescent 8 months pregnant with her stepfather's baby. (Courtesy of Linda Ledray, RN, PhD, SANE).*

Key Point:
The use of emergency contraception could prevent 22,000 rape-related pregnancies each year in the United States.

for this behavior need to be explored with her. The patient must have a sense of assurance of confidentiality (unless child abuse laws are being violated) and of a compassionate attitude on the part of the clinician. Detection of exposure to violence among pregnant adolescents has been shown to increase significantly when multiple, direct violence assessments are carried out as a routine part of prenatal care (Covington et al., 1997).

SEXUAL ASSAULT RESULTING IN PREGNANCY

Pregnancy resulting from rape is not rare. Holmes et al. (1996) estimate that approximately 32,000 pregnancies per year in the United States result from sexual assault. This number may be considerably lower than the actual number, because rape is a seriously underreported crime (Bureau of Statistics, 1998). Unfortunately, most women who have been raped do not seek medical care and therefore do not have access to emergency contraception or STD prophylaxis. It is estimated that 22,000 pregnancies in the United States that result from rape could be prevented if all women who had been raped had emergency contraception available to them within 72 hours of the assault (Stewart & Trussel, 2000).

Because most rapes are not reported, and because the baseline prevalence of STDs varies among different groups, it is difficult to accurately determine the incidence of newly acquired STDs resulting from sexual assault. According to the Centers for Disease Control and Prevention (CDC) (1998), the most frequently diagnosed infections in women who have been sexually assaulted are chlamydia, gonorrhea, and trichomoniasis. What is more difficult to determine is whether these infections were present before the assault. Thus, identification of these infections is more important for medical than for forensic and legal purposes.

In a recent study, the prevalence of STDs resulting from rape was as follows (Reynolds et al., 2000):

C. trachomatis (chlamydia)	3.9% to 17%
N. gonorrhoeae (gonorrhea)	0.0% to 26.3%
T. pallidum (syphilis)	0.0% to 5.6%
T. vaginalis (trichomonas)	0.0% to 19%
Human papillomavirus (HPV, or genital warts)	0.6% to 2.3%

Every one of these infections, along with genital herpes, has important clinical implications in pregnancy.

Sexual assault of the pregnant woman who has a placenta previa places both her and the fetus at risk for potentially fatal hemorrhage. In addition, genital trauma in the pregnant woman may be much more severe than in the nonpregnant woman because of the area's increased vascularity during pregnancy.

PROPHYLAXIS AND TREATMENT OF STDS IN PREGNANCY
Because of the effects of certain antibiotics and other medications on the fetus, the treatment of pregnant women with STDs may differ from that of nonpregnant women. These STDs are listed in order of most to least common in most pregnant populations.

GENITAL HERPES (HERPES SIMPLEX VIRUS [HSV] TYPE II)
Acyclovir has not been approved for routine use for recurrent herpes or herpes prophylaxis in pregnancy, but it may be used to treat a primary outbreak and for any outbreak at term.

HPV (Condyloma Accuminata, or Genital Warts)

Podophyllin is contraindicated in pregnancy. Cryotherapy and acid preparations may be safely used.

Trichomonas

Pregnant women may be treated with a 2g single-dose regimen of metronidazole during pregnancy.

Chlamydia

Due to limited experience with azithromycin in pregnancy, the CDC (1998) still lists erythromycin and amoxicillin as the drugs of choice for treating chlamydia during pregnancy. Nonetheless, azithromycin appears to be safe in pregnancy and is associated with markedly improved compliance because it is a one-dose treatment. Consequently, azithromycin is used in many centers to treat chlamydia. Doxycycline, like all tetracyclines, is contraindicated in pregnancy because of damage to fetal bones and teeth. Erythromycin estolate is also contraindicated because of its association with drug-induced hepatotoxicity.

Gonorrhea

Pregnant women with gonorrhea should be treated with an appropriate cephalosporin, such as cefixime or ceftriaxone. For pregnant women who cannot receive cephalosporins, spectinomycin may be safely administered. Like tetracyclines, quinolones are contraindicated in pregnancy.

Syphilis

Penicillin is the drug of choice for pregnant women with syphilis, as it is for non-pregnant women. However, pregnant women who are allergic to penicillin cannot take tetracycline, which is the alternative drug of choice for treating syphilis in non-allergic, nonpregnant patients.

Until the last few years, pregnant women with syphilis who were allergic to penicillin were treated with erythromycin. Unfortunately, however, erythromycin does not adequately cross the placenta to treat fetal syphilis. Fetal syphilis is an infection associated with fetal and neonatal death, as well as other potentially devastating complications. For this reason, the current CDC recommendation for penicillin-allergic pregnant women with syphilis is that they undergo penicillin desensitization in a hospital setting and then receive a therapeutic course of penicillin.

While the Jarisch-Herxheimer reaction is rare, it may be associated with uterine contractions if it occurs in pregnant women. For this reason, some clinicians recommend that patients remain for a few hours for monitoring in the clinic or wherever they are being treated with their first dose of penicillin.

Hepatitis B

Use of the hepatitis B and hepatitis B immunoglobulin vaccines is not contraindicated in pregnant women.

Human Immunodeficiency Virus (HIV)

It is of particular importance to offer HIV-positive pregnant women treatment with zidovudine (ZDV) because the drug reduces the risk for HIV transmission from mother to infant from approximately 25% to 8% (CDC, 1998). HIV-positive women should also be advised against breastfeeding, because the HIV virus does cross into breast milk. There is no increased maternal morbidity or mortality associated with pregnancy among HIV-positive women (CDC, 1998).

Conclusion

Sexual abuse and assault of the pregnant woman, whether in the context of an established intimate relationship or as a stranger attack, can have serious medical implications for both mother and fetus. Psychologic consequences may be equally devastating, and the likelihood of perpetuating an intergenerational cycle of physical and sexual violence is great when abused women have children.

REFERENCES

American Academy of Pediatrics Committee on Child Abuse and Neglect. The role of the pediatrician in recognizing and intervening on behalf of abused women. *Pediatrics.* 1998;101:1091-1092.

Asher J, Berlin M, Petty V. Abuse of pregnant adolescents: what have we learned? *Obstet Gynecol.* 2000;95:41S.

Berenson A, SanMiguel VV, Wilkinson GS. Prevalence of physical and sexual assault in pregnant adolescents. *J Adolesc Health.* 1992;13:466-469.

Berenson AB, Stiglisch NJ, Wilkinson GS, et al. Drug abuse and other risk factors for physical abuse in pregnancy among white non-Hispanic, black, and Hispanic women. *Am J Obstet Gynecol.* 1991;164;1491-1499.

Bowen K. Child abuse and domestic violence in families of children seen for suspected sexual abuse. *Clin Peds.* 2000;39:33-40.

Boyer D, Fine D. Sexual abuse as a factor in adolescent pregnancy and child maltreatment. *Fam Plann Perspect.* 1992;24(4):4-19.

Bureau of Statistics. Criminal victimization in the United States, 1998 statistical tables. Available at http://www.ojp.usdoj.gov/bjs/pub/pdf/cvus98.pdf. Accessed March 27, 2002.

Campbell JC, Alford P. The dark consequences of marital rape. *Am J Nurs.* 1989;89:946-949.

Campbell JC, Oliver C, Bullock L. Why battering during pregnancy? *AWHONNS Clin Issues Perinat Womens Health Nurs.* 1993;4:343-349.

Centers for Disease Control. *MMWR.* 1998;47(RR-1):1-128.

Cokkinides VE, Coker AL, Sanderson M, Addy C, Bethea L. Physical violence during pregnancy: maternal complications and birth outcomes. *Obstet Gynecol.* 1999;93:661-666.

Committee on Health Care for Underserved Women. Adult manifestations of childhood sexual abuse. *ACOG Educational Bulletin.* 2000;259:1-9.

Covington DL, Dalton VK, Diehl SJ, Wright BD, Piner MH. Improving detection of violence among pregnant adolescents. *J Adolesc Health.* 1997;21:18-24.

Dietz PM, Gazmararian JA, Goodwin MM, Bruce FC, Johnson CH, Rochat RW. Delayed entry into prenatal care: effect of physical violence. *Obstet Gynecol.* 1997;90:221-224.

Dietz PM, Spitz AM, Anda RF, et al. Unintended pregnancy among adult women exposed to abuse or household dysfunction during their childhood. *JAMA.* 1999;282:1359-1366.

Dodge KA, Bates JE, Pettit GS. Mechanisms in the cycle of violence. *Science.* 1990;250:1680-1683.

Dolan-Mullen P, Ramirez G, Groff JY. A meta-analysis of randomized trials of prenatal smoking cessation. *Am J Obstet Gynecol.* 1994;171:1328-1333.

Duffy SJ, McGrath ME, Becker BM, Linakis JG. Mothers with histories of domestic violence in a pediatric emergency department. *Pediatrics.* 1999;103:1007-1013.

Durant T, Gilbert BC, Saltzman LE, Johnson CH. Opportunities of intervention: discussing physical abuse during prenatal care visits. *Am J Prev Med.* 2000;19:238-244.

Elster AB, Ketterlinus R, Lamb ME. Association between parenthood and problem behavior in a national sample of adolescents. *Pediatrics.* 1990;85:1044-1050.

Feldhaus KM, Liziol-McLain J, Amsbury HL, et al. Accuracy of 3 brief screening questions for detecting partner violence in the emergency department. *JAMA.* 1997;277:1357-1361.

Fildes J, Reed L, Jones N, et al. Trauma: the leading cause of maternal death. *J Trauma.* 1992;32:643-645.

Fiscella K, Kitzman JH, Cole RE, Sidora KJ, Olds D. Does child abuse predict adolescent pregnancy? *Pediatrics.* 1998;101:620-624.

Flanagan P, Coll CG, Adreozzi L, Riggs S. Predicting maltreatment of children of teenage mothers. *Arch Ped Adolesc Med.* 1995;149:451-145.

Fraser AM, Brockert JE, Ward RH. Association of young maternal age with adverse reproductive outcomes. *N Engl J Med.* 1995;332:1113-1117.

Freund KM, Bak SM, Blackhall L. Identifying domestic violence in primary care practice. *J Gen Intern Med.* 1996;11:44-46.

Gainer E, Mery C, Ulmann A. Levonorgestrel-only contraception: real-world tolerance and efficacy. *Contraception.* 2001;64:17-21.

Gazmararian JA, Adams MM, Saltzman LE, et al. The relationship between pregnancy intendedness and physical violence in mothers of newborns. *Obstet Gynecol.* 1995;85:1031-1038.

Gazmararian JA, Lazorick S, Spitz AM, Ballard TJ, Saltzman LE, Marks JS. Prevalence of violence against pregnant women. *JAMA.* 1996;275;1915-1920.

Glander SS. Moore ML, Michielutte R, Parsons LH. The prevalence of domestic violence among women seeking abortion. *Obstet Gynecol.* 1998;91:1002-1006.

Grant LJ. Effects of childhood sexual abuse: issues for obstetric caregivers. *Birth.* 1992;19:220-221.

Harner HM, Burgess AW, Asher JB. Caring for pregnant teenagers: medicolegal issues for nurses. *Obstet Gynecol Neonatal Nurs.* 2001;30:139-147.

Hilliard PJA. Physical abuse in pregnancy. *Obstet Gynecol.* 1985;66:185.

Holmes MM, Resnick HS, Kilpatrick DG, Best CL. Rape-related pregnancy: estimates and descriptive characteristics from a national sample of women. *Am J Obstet Gynecol.* 1996;175:320-325.

Horan DL, Chapin J, Klein L, Schmidt LA, Schulkin J. Domestic violence screening practices of obstetrician-gynecologists. *Obstet Gynecol.* 1998;92:785-789.

Horon IL, Cheng D. Enhanced surveillance for pregnancy-associated mortality—Maryland, 1993-1998. *JAMA.* 2001;285:1455-1459.

Jolly MC, Sebire N, Harris J, Robinson S, Regan L. Obstetric risks of pregnancy in women less than 18 years old. *Obstet Gynecol.* 2000:96:962-966.

Kendrick JS, Merritt RK. Women and smoking: an update for the 1990s. *Am J Obstet Gynecol.* 1996;175:528-535.

Males MA. Adult involvement in teenage childbearing and STD. *Lancet.* 1995;346:64-65.

Martin SL, Clark KA, Lynch SR, Kupper LL, Cilenti D. Violence in the lives of pregnant teenage women: associations with multiple substance use. *Am J Drug Alcohol Abuse.* 1999;25:425-440.

Martin SL, Mackie L, Kupper LL, Buescher PA, Moracco KE. Physical abuse of women before, during, and after pregnancy. *JAMA.* 2001;285:1581-1584.

Mayer L. The severely abused woman in obstetric and gynecologic care: guidelines for recognition and management. *J Reprod Med.* 1995;40:13-18.

Mayer L, Liebschutz J. Domestic violence in the pregnant patient: obstetric and behavioral interventions. *Obstet Gynecol Survey.* 1998;53:627-635.

McCauley J, Kern DE, Kolodner K, et al. Clinical characteristics of women with a history of childhood abuse: unhealed wounds. *JAMA.* 1997;277:1362-1368.

McFarlane J. Abuse during pregnancy: the horror and the hope. *AWHONN's Clin Issues.* 1993;4:350-362.

McFarlane J, Parker B. Preventing abuse during pregnancy: an assessment and intervention protocol. *MCN Am J Matern Child Nurs.* 1994;19:321-324.

McFarlane J, Parker B, Soeken K, Silva C, Reel S. Safety behaviors of abused women after an intervention during pregnancy. *J Obstet Gynecol Neonatal Nurs.* 1998;27:64-69.

McKibben L, De Vos E, Newberger E. Victimization of mothers of abused children: a controlled study. *Pediatrics.* 1989;84:531-535.

Norton LB, Peipert JF, Zierler S, et al. Battering in pregnancy: an assessment of two screening methods. *Obstet Gynecol.* 1995;85:321-325.

Overpeck MD, Brenner RA, Trumble AC, Trifletti LB, Berendes HW. Risk factors for infant homicide in the United States. *N Engl J Med.* 1998;339:1211-1216.

Parker B. Abuse of adolescents: what can we learn from pregnant teenagers? *AWHONN's Clin Issues.* 1993;4:363-370.

Parker B, McFarlane J, Soeken K, Torres S, Campbell D. Physical and emotional abuse in pregnancy: a comparison of adult and teenage women. *Nurs Res.* 1994;4:29-37.

Petersen R, Gazmararian JA, Spitz AM, Rowley DL, Goodwin MM, Saltzman LE, et al. Violence and adverse pregnancy outcomes: a review of the literature and directions for future research. *Am J Prev Med.* 1997;13:366-373.

Plichta S, Duncan M, Plichta L. Spouse abuse, patient-physician communication, and patient satisfaction. *Am J Prev Med.* 1996;12:297-303.

Raj A, Silverman JG, Amaro H. The relationship between sexual abuse and sexual risk among high school students: findings from the 1997 Massachusetts youth risk behavior survey. *Matern Child Health J.* 2000;4:125-134.

Reynolds MW, Peipert JF, Collins B. Epidemiologic issues of sexually transmitted diseases in sexual assault victims. *Obstet Gynecol Surv.* 2000;55:51-57.

Rhodes N, Hutchinson S. Labor experiences of childhood sexual abuse survivors. *Birth.* 1994;21:213-220.

Ribe JK, Teggatz JR, Harvey CM. Blows to the maternal abdomen causing fetal demise: report of three cases and a review of the literature. *J Forensic Sci.* 1993;8:1092-1096.

Schechter S, Gary LT. *Health Care Services for Battered Women and Their Abused Children: A Manual About Advocacy for Women and Kids in Emergencies (AWAKE).* Boston, Mass: Children's Hospital; 1992.

Stevens-Simon C, McAnarney ER. Childhood victimization: relationship to adolescent pregnancy outcome. *Child Abuse Negl.* 1994;18:569-575.

Stewart DE. Incidence of postpartum abuse in women with a history of abuse during pregnancy. *Can Med Assoc J.* 1994;151:1601-1604.

Stewart DE, Cecutti A. Physical abuse in pregnancy. *Can Med Assoc J.* 1993;149:1257-1263.

Stewart FH, Trussell J. Prevention of pregnancy resulting from rape: a neglected preventive health measure. *Am J Prev Med.* 2000;19:228-229.

Stier DM, Leventhal JM, Berg AT, Johnson L, Mezger J. Are children born to young mothers at increased risk of maltreatment? *Pediatrics.* 1993;91:642-648.

Thompson RS, Krugman R. Screening mothers for intimate partner abuse at well-baby care visits; the right thing to do. *JAMA.* 2001;285:1628-1630.

Wilson LM, Reid AJ, Midmer DK, Biringer A, Carroll JC, Stewart DE. Antenatal psychosocial risk factors associated with adverse postpartum family outcomes. *Can Med Assoc J.* 1996;154:785-796

Wingood GM, DiClemente RJ. The effects of abusive primary partner on the condom use and sexual negotiation practices of African-American women. *Am J Pub Health.* 1997;87:1016-1018.

Wright RJ. Identification of domestic violence in the community pediatric setting: need to protect mothers and children. *Arch Pediatr Adolesc Med.* 2000;154(5):431-433.

Wright RJ, Wright RO, Isaac NE. Response to battered mothers in the pediatric emergency department: a call for an interdisciplinary approach to family violence. *Pediatrics.* 1997;99:186-192.

Zurawin SJ. Unplanned childbearing and family size: their relationship to child neglect and abuse. *Fam Plan Perspect.* 1991;23:155-161.

Chapter 21

RAPE AND SEXUAL ABUSE IN OLDER ADULTS

Michael Clark, MSN, CRNP
Hannah Ufberg Rabinowitz, MSN, CRNP

Rape and sexual assault of older adults is a poorly understood phenomenon. It has been the subject of only scattered and limited scientific study. Because of the limits of existing methods of data collection, the true prevalence of rape committed against older adults can only be inferred from the existing literature.

As the size and proportion of the United States population over age 65 years increase, how we understand and respond to the rape and sexual assault of older adults becomes increasingly important. Existing social services for sexual assault victims are generally not designed to meet the needs of older adults and do not address the vulnerabilities, exposure patterns, and physical and emotional responses that are unique to older victims. Moreover, although there is a paucity of research on the quality of care of older victims, there is clearly significant room for improvement regarding the detection and clinical care of such victims. A proper clinical care response to elder sexual abuse should address the cognitive, physical, and emotional issues unique to elder sexual assault victims.

Key Point:
Existing social services for sexual assault victims are generally not designed to address the needs presented by older adults, especially their vulnerabilities, exposure patterns, and physical and emotional responses.

This chapter reviews the existing knowledge on the occurrence of elder sexual assault, explores the current literature, discusses the limitations of the current data collection methods, and describes shortcomings of these data. In addition, the chapter reviews the clinically relevant aspects of elder sexual assault, including vulnerability of this special population, evaluation of potential victims, sequelae of sexual assault of the older victim, and resources available for victims and their families.

INCIDENCE OF SEXUAL ABUSE AMONG OLDER ADULTS

America is aging. During the next 30 years, the proportion of the population over age 65 years will grow from about 13% to about 20% of the total US population. The population age 85 years and older is currently the fastest growing segment of the older population. By the year 2050, the percentage in this age-group is projected to increase to almost 5% of the US population.

The US Department of Justice obtains national statistics on rape and sexual assault. The Department of Justice employs two approaches in collecting national data on sexual assault. First, through the Federal Bureau of Investigation (FBI), the Department of Justice publishes the Uniform Crime Reports. The Uniform Crime Reports is a compilation of data from 90% to 96% of our nation's law enforcement agencies regarding the incidence of rape and six other categories of violent crime. It is designed primarily to follow trends in the incidence of major crimes. The Uniform Crime Reports does not include incidents of rape involving male victims.

Second, the Department of Justice seeks to gather information regarding the sexual victimization of adults in a more comprehensive manner through its National Crime Victimization Survey (NCVS). In this survey a random sample of approximately 100,000 individuals residing in 50,000 households is interviewed. A series of seven interviews are conducted over a 3-year period. The survey does not include children under age 12 years or those who are incapacitated and unable to answer for themselves. In these cases, another member of the household may answer as a proxy.

The NCVS includes questions about sexual assault as well as rape. It seeks to identify perpetrators and victims of both genders. It also tries to capture both attempted and completed incidents of sexual victimization as well as those not reported to authorities.

Key Points:
Older adults may experience violent crime less often than younger individuals, but those age 50 years and older are victims of 7% of the serious violent crimes.

Based on the data gathered by the Department of Justice, older adults are less likely to experience violent crime than younger individuals. It is estimated that those age 50 years and older represent about 30% of the population (US Department of Justice, 2000). Yet, this same group represents about 7% of the serious violent crime victims.

The overall incidence of elder abuse is thought to be significant. The NCVS (1997) estimates the incidence of rape committed against older adults at 10 per 100,000 per year. The NCVS estimates that those over age 50 years represent about 3% of sexual assault victims.

The National Elder Abuse Incident Study (1998) estimated that about 450,000 community-residing older adults are victims of abuse. This study also suggests that many incidents of abuse remain undetected by sentinels (those intimately involved in the care of older adults who are generally responsible for identifying and responding to suspected abuse) or state investigative agencies.

Data on the incidence of rape among older men is extremely limited. For all age-groups the incidence of rape of males is thought to be significantly less than that of females. The FBI estimates that one in three women and one in seven men will experience rape over the course of their lifetime. The NCVS estimates the incidence of female rape as one in 270, while that for males is one in 5000. Riggs et al. (2000), in an analysis of 1076 rape cases in a level-one trauma center, found that about 4% of the rape victims were male. The limited data on the incidence of sexual victimization of males is most often not broken down by age-group. Chapter 7 offers a further discussion of sexual victimization of males.

The limited research studies that collected data from select emergency departments and rape crisis centers produced figures that are fairly consistent with results of the NCVS. Cartwright and Moore (1989) performed a 2-year retrospective review of the records of one Nashville, Tennessee emergency department to determine the number of visits of women who reported sexual assault. They found that in 1 year, 21 of 493 victims were over age 60 years. This represents about 4% of those treated. However, they found no older women among the 247 victims recorded in the following year. To explain this yearly variance, they hypothesize that rapes in this community were of a serial nature and involved relatively few rapists.

Ramin et al. (1992) performed a 5-year retrospective chart review of female victims of sexual assault who were treated at a Dallas, Texas emergency department between 1986 and 1991. They found that postmenopausal women represented 2.2% of women reporting sexual assault. Simmelink (1996) reports that 3% of clients treated in a sexual assault nurse clinician program in Minneapolis, Minnesota were older than age 55 years.

DEFINING RAPE AND SEXUAL ASSAULT OF OLDER ADULTS

One reason that rape and sexual assault of older adults is a poorly understood phenomenon is that we currently lack a common definition of the terms rape, sexual assault, and sexual abuse. A historical review of the terms rape, sexual assault, and sexual abuse demonstrates an evolving societal perspective on these issues. In the past the definition of rape focused more exclusively on forced vaginal intercourse by a male with a female who was not his wife. Currently, the definitions of the terms rape, sexual assault, and sexual abuse include victims and perpetrators of both genders, and the definition of the nature of the sexual contact includes both oral and anal penetration.

With respect to older adults, Ramsey-Klawsnik (1998) defined sexual abuse of older adults as sexual activity that occurs when a person over age 60 years is forced, tricked, coerced, or manipulated into unwanted sexual contact. It also includes situations in which the older adult is incapable of giving consent because of cognitive and other impairments, including impairments associated with aging. However, the terms rape, sexual assault, and sexual abuse are sometimes used in variable and overlapping ways. A particular incidence of sexual violation of the older adult can sometimes be described using different and/or more than one term. Sexual assault can include rape but also includes other forms of unwanted sexual contact (i.e., fondling and other forms of physical contact that do not involve penetration). Sexual abuse often involves situations in which the victim is somehow dependent on a perpetrator who is entrusted either professionally or personally with the care of the victim.

How we define the terms rape, sexual assault, and sexual abuse is important because such definitions may shape efforts to identify and prevent violations as well as develop effective responses for older individuals and those caring for them. In fact, several authors point out that both society as a whole and older individuals may be slow to recognize and respond to the problem of sexual assault because of certain common misperceptions and beliefs (Burgess et al., 2000a). Younger adults may not recognize the sexuality of older adults. Seeing older adults as asexual may inhibit their ability to recognize and respond to patterns of sexual victimization. Several reports indicate that older adult victims state confusion about the motive of the attacker (i.e., "why are you interested in an old lady?"). Older adults may be less comfortable talking about sexuality in general. As a cohort group they were raised during an era when sexuality was not openly discussed. Values, attitudes, and beliefs about sexuality may predispose the victim of sexual assault to increased guilt and shame.

The incidence of sexual abuse is also difficult to determine in part because of conceptual differences among those who report and study the phenomenon. Some consider sexual abuse as part of a larger phenomenon of elder abuse, while others consider it separately as a form of sexual assault.

LIMITS OF EXISTING DATA COLLECTION METHODS

A second reason that rape and sexual assault of older adults are poorly understood phenomena is the limitations of existing methods of data collection regarding rape and sexual assault of older adults. The survey method employed by the NCVS is inherently weak for several reasons. First, the survey does not accurately identify victimization that occurs when the perpetrator and victim live in the same household. Because the survey includes interviews of all mentally competent members of a household over age 12 years, attempts to capture the incidence of sexual assault by household members may either be unsuccessful or, worse, present further safety risk for the victim. In the case of domestic violence, for instance, the survey is terminated once domestic violence is suspected. Second, the NCVS method is poorly designed to capture the experiences of those with cognitive impairments and does not capture the experiences of older adults residing in institutional settings.

Moreover, as with younger age-groups, the number of reported sexual assault incidents is thought to be a fraction of the actual numbers. Tyra (1993) asserted that the reporting rates among elderly victims of sexual assault were estimated to range from 10% to 100%.

Key Point:
The definitions of rape, sexual assault, and sexual abuse include victims and perpetrators of both genders. The nature of sexual contact includes both oral and anal penetration. These definitions are important because they may shape efforts to identify and prevent violations as well as develop effective responses for older individuals and those who care for them.

Estimates of reporting rates among all age-groups range from 16% to 30% according to the US Department of Justice, Bureau of Justice Statistics (2000). The NCVS estimates that 32% of rapes and sexual assaults are reported to law enforcement agencies. The most common reason for reporting is that the victims wanted to prevent further assaults against themselves. The most common reason for not reporting was that the victims considered the assault a "personal matter." Although differences in reporting by age-group are not known, it is clear that the incidence rate of sexual victimization of older adults is underreported.

Another general problem with existing survey methods is that researchers often use different inclusion criteria for age in reporting the incidence of sexual assault among older adults. In some cases age criteria are selected to study particular effects of rape. For instance, some studies intend to contrast the physical effects of rape on premenopausal versus postmenopausal women. One such study by Tyra (1993) defines "older adults" as women over age 50 years. Other studies and data sources may define "older adults" differently and/or do not clearly explain their rationale regarding their selection of age criteria. The variability in defining older adult populations among studies limits attempts at estimating the incidence and prevalence of sexual victimization for the older adult population.

Yet another limitation of existing survey methods is the problem of estimating the overall rate of sexual assaults of males. This problem is just beginning to be addressed. The literature and information on sexual assault of older men are extremely limited and consist mostly of anecdotal reports. Data and research on the problem of sexual assault of older men must be included to improve survey methods.

With more accurate information regarding the true incidence rate of sexual assaults against older adults, we shall be better able to address services for such victims.

EXPOSURE TO SEXUAL ABUSE

Older adults differ significantly from younger victims in characteristics that leave them vulnerable and exposed to the threat of sexual assault. Sexual abuse in the older adult often implies a violation of a relationship between caregiver and dependent. Often older adults must rely on the perpetrator because of physical or cognitive limitations or impairments. They may also differ from younger victims in terms of ability to report and respond to assaults based on their relative degree of isolation and physical or cognitive impairments. These factors affect the incidence and patterns of assault as well as the coping responses of the victims.

Data on perpetrators include only those who are both caught and convicted. Conviction occurs in about half of rape cases that are prosecuted. Of those cases that go to trial, about 80% of those convicted plead guilty. Based on limited data, the typical profile of a rapist is a young single male. About 7% of rapists and 12% of sexual assailants are older than age 50 years (US Department of Justice, Feb 1997).

Unlike younger victims, many older adult victims do not know their assailants (Cartwright & Moore, 1989; Deming et al., 1983; Groth, 1978). It is not clear whether this profile is accurate, or whether it represents underreporting of rape and sexual assault incidents in which the victim knows the assailant.

A few small qualitative studies look at perpetrators who assault community-residing, functionally independent older women. In a small sample of 170 convicted assailants referred for treatment, Groth (1978) found that 18% had selected female victims who were significantly older than the assailants. The majority of the crimes took place in the victim's home or automobile.

These attacks by strangers more frequently involved higher levels of violence. In a small study done by Pollock (1988), five male sexual offenders who assaulted women age 60 years and older were compared with seven offenders who assaulted younger women. Generally, the assaults on the older women were more violent, brutal, and sadistic.

Key Point:
Often, sexual abuse of an older adult implies a violation of the relationship between the caregiver and the dependent elderly individual.

SEXUAL ABUSE OF OLDER ADULTS RESIDING IN INSTITUTIONAL SETTINGS

At any given time in the United States, about 5% of the adult population over age 65 years reside in a nursing home or other long-term care facility. The proportion of elderly adults residing in nursing homes increases with age and reaches 20% for those over age 85 years. Longitudinal studies indicate that a person age 65 years has a 40% chance of living in a nursing home at some point in life. Those who reside in nursing homes, however, actually represent two very distinct sub-populations. Some residents are admitted for short stays from hospitals in order to undergo rehabilitation associated with acute illness, while other residents stay for much longer periods due to disabilities that cannot be managed in the community (Kane et al., 1999). This latter population may be more vulnerable to sexual assault. In addition, women represent 58% of those age 65 years and older and 70% of those over age 85 years. Older female nursing home residents have physical and/or cognitive limitations that impair their ability to fend off an attacker.

Burgess et al. (2000a) conclude that while sexual assault has received increased attention over the past 25 years, the literature on sexual assault and abuse of older adults has been minimal. In addition, sexual assault of older adults residing in institutions has been addressed the least. Information that does exist is mostly retrospective and descriptive, and is based on individual cases. Much of what is known can be found in investigations of complaints made to ombudsman groups and through the analysis of information generated in criminal and civil legal proceedings.

Burgess et al. (2000b) studied 20 nursing home residents who were sexually assaulted. Most victims were cognitively impaired and many suffered from other debilitating physical conditions that left them vulnerable to assault. Despite the fact that the majority of victims had severe cognitive impairment, in 18 of the 20 incidents the perpetrator was eventually identified. None of the victims reported the assaults directly to nursing home administrators. Instead, incidents were reported to staff and family members in a direct, indirect, or fragmented fashion. Often the resident would allude to the incident indirectly or complain of symptoms related to the assault, such as genital, anal, or other bodily pain suggestive of sexual assault.

Incidents also came to the attention of staff and family through changes in the victim's behavior. Ramsey-Klawsnik (1991, 1993) notes that there may be subtle changes in the victims' behavior. Therefore, it is essential for healthcare providers to assess and fully understand their elderly patients. Indicators of sexual abuse include psychologic manifestations such as sleep disorder, irritability, mood swings, and depression. Such symptoms are nonspecific and may be associated with menopausal changes in addition to other psychosocial problems. Other psychologic warning signs that may alert healthcare providers that their patient may be a victim of sexual assault are as follows:

— Aggressive/regressive behavior

— Mistrust in others

— Disturbed peer interactions

— Nightmares

For example, nursing home residents might refuse to be washed or react with fear when a particular staff member approaches them. They might exhibit new behaviors such as crying, nightmares, and a need to be near the nursing station. Some may withdraw and stop engaging in previous activities or refuse further general care and treatment. In some cases, incidents are discovered by physical findings such as signs of trauma to genital or surrounding tissue. Occasionally, abuse has been detected through signs and diagnostic findings that confirmed the presence of sexually transmitted infections.

Key Point:
Among the indicators of sexual abuse of the older adult are psychosocial manifestations (sleep disorder, irritability, mood swings, depression) that may also accompany menopausal changes or other psychosocial problems.

Staff attitudes and knowledge of sexual assault may be a significant barrier in terms of both recognizing and responding to the problem of sexual assault in nursing homes. Burgess et al. (2000b) found that nursing home staff might be reluctant to take effective action even when clues to assault and abuse are present. In their review, some incidents evoked an effective response only after family members became directly aware of symptoms or reports from victimized residents.

Effective response begins with the ability of nursing home staff to recognize and respond to verbal, behavioral, or physical evidence suggestive of possible sexual assault. Family members must also be alert for this potential problem in the event that nursing home staff fails to recognize or to respond effectively to the problem. In some cases in the Burgess study, (1991) nursing home staff seemed to "blame the victim." This was exhibited through changes in portrayal of the resident in reports and documentation. Residents alleging sexual assault were described more negatively after incidents of sexual assault were reported.

Perpetrators are frequently present in nursing home facilities. Burgess et al. (2000b) found in their review that the majority (15 of 18) of perpetrators worked for the facility in which the victim resided. Four of these perpetrators had previous records of sexual assault despite a requirement that nursing homes perform criminal background checks on their employees.

Hazelwood and Burgess (1995) have described three styles of approach used by perpetrators in assaulting frail older adults:

1. The "confidence" approach is used with mobile, more highly functional victims and involves gaining the victim's confidence through verbal manipulation or coercion.

2. A "blitz" approach involves overtaking the victim through injurious force.

3. A "surprise" approach employs the use of threats but no force when the victim is either unsuspecting or incapacitated.

Nursing homes are obligated to investigate suspected abuse within 5 days of a report to the nursing home administration. If sexual abuse is suspected, it is important for the nursing home staff and administration to take care to avoid subjecting the victim to unnecessary further trauma during the investigation process (Capezuti & Swedlow, 2000). The potential for a "second assault" on the victim exists in such situations.

The guidelines for interviewing should be carefully considered and are described later. The location of the interview may be a particularly sensitive issue. If the interview must take place in the nursing home, extra effort should be taken to establish that the interview process is as safe as possible for the resident. If the interview cannot be conducted in an office, extra effort should be taken to ensure privacy as well as the absence of interruptions.

The sexual assault examination may be problematic because of reluctance on the part of the victim to have a thorough physical assessment. This may be compounded by the difficulty in gaining the cooperation and consent as a result of issues associated with cognitive impairment. In addition, speculum examination of debilitated females may be problematic because of joint contractures. When the resident will permit a speculum examination, a posterior approach is sometimes more successful. Forensic evidence may be difficult to obtain if the incident is discovered in a delayed manner.

Legal perspectives on the issue of sexual abuse within nursing homes have evolved significantly over the last 25 years. A number of states have made the commission of assault or battery on an older adult nursing home resident an aggravated offense with enhanced penalties (Capezuti & Swedlow, 2000). Increasingly, nursing homes have been held responsible for providing a safe environment that minimizes the likelihood of sexual abuse. The current standard seems to indicate that the nursing home can be held liable when foreseeable risks may have contributed to a sexual assault (Loggins, 1985).

SEXUAL ABUSE OF OLDER ADULTS RESIDING IN NONINSTITUTIONAL SETTINGS

Family members perpetrate the majority of abuse and violence inflicted upon older adults outside of an institutional setting. Ramsey-Klawsnik (1998) describes five types of offenders who commit violence against family members, with sexual abuse rarely occurring among the first two types:

1. The otherwise competent but overwhelmed caregiver.

2. The willing but physically or cognitively impaired caregiver.

3. The caregiver with a "user mentality" who expects to gain something from the caregiving relationship.

4. The unstable, angry, and volatile caregiver who "lashes out" toward those less powerful than themselves.

5. The sadistic caregiver who gains pleasure by harming or intimidating others.

Ramsey-Klawsnik (1991) outlines two distinct phases of sexual abuse: covert sexual abuse and overt sexual abuse. In covert sexual abuse there may be expressed sexual interest or discussion of sexual activity. The perpetrator treats the victim as a sex object or potential sexual partner.

Overt abuse may progress from activities such as voyeurism and inflicting pornography on the victim to various degrees of sexual contact, from kissing and fondling to oral-genital contact to various forms of oral, vaginal, or anal penetration. The most extreme forms of sexual abuse involve overt exploitation (i.e., offering the victim in a sexual way to others for the gratification or financial gain of the perpetrator), sadistic activity, or ritual abuse. Groth (1978) has described a sexual abuse continuum. Those who commit sexual abuse often progress from milder to more severe forms over time. The abuse often goes undetected for long periods of time and, once detected, more pronounced patterns of abuse may be evident.

Ramsey-Klawsnik (1991) suggests that sexual assault on elders by friends and family has not received the same public and professional attention afforded to younger individuals. Riggs et al. (2000) report that there has been an overall increase in the reporting of rapes of younger victims committed by known assailants. They posit that increased awareness and willingness to report may be driving this trend. Older adults, however, may be less knowledgeable and less willing to report rape by known assailants. The ability of the victim to report the assault depends on a number of factors, including assault history, physical status, and cognitive ability of the victim. Social values of older adults may lead the victim to view the assault as shameful and thus reduce the likelihood of reporting (Groth, 1978).

Limited qualitative reports note sexual assault of higher-functioning older adult females by assailants known to the victim. In the cases reported, the victim knew her assailant but was not involved in a sexual relationship (Simmelink, 1996; Tyra, 1993).

IMMEDIATE AND LONG-TERM RESPONSES OF OLDER SEXUAL ASSAULT VICTIMS

Burgess and Holmstrom (1974) introduced the concept of rape trauma syndrome to describe a model for a victim's emotional and behavioral response to rape. Rape trauma syndrome predicts that a victim's response typically has two phases: an acute phase followed by a long-term reorganization process. The rape trauma syndrome is described in detail in Chapter 12.

Key Point:
The two distinct phases of sexual abuse are covert and overt. In covert sexual abuse, sexual interest may be expressed or sexual activity discussed. The perpetrator treats the victim as a sex object or potential sexual partner. In overt abuse, activities such as voyeurism and inflicting pornography on the victim may escalate to various degrees of sexual contact ranging from kissing and fondling to oral-genital contact to various forms of oral, vaginal, or anal penetration.

Key Point:
The first, or acute, phase of the rape trauma syndrome is characterized by disorganization and fear. The second, or reorganization, phase involves the process of stabilization after the initial acute disequilibrium.

The acute phase is one of disorganization and fear. Common emotions are shock and disbelief. Survivors who experience rape trauma syndrome may exhibit two different emotional response styles. Some survivors exhibit an expressive style. Their behavioral-emotive style is typically demonstrative and may include crying, sobbing, and overt displays of anger. Other victims may exhibit a more controlled manner. They may be calm and subdued. Emotions are often masked and may go unrecognized.

Somatic symptoms may be seen in all survivors of sexual abuse. Common symptoms seen within the first weeks are tension headaches, fatigue, sleep disturbances, and gastrointestinal irritability.

The second, or reorganization, phase of the rape trauma syndrome involves the process of stabilization after the initial acute disequilibrium. This phase may begin 4 to 8 weeks after the assault (Tyra, 1996). Symptoms of the reorganization phase are often consistent with those of posttraumatic stress disorder (PTSD) as described in the DSM-IV. Burgess and Holmstrom (1974) show that a good deal of overlap exists in the symptoms of rape trauma syndrome and those of PTSD.

Common criteria for PTSD and rape trauma syndrome include the following:

1. A stressor of significant magnitude such that it would likely evoke distinguishable symptoms in most individuals.

2. The victim reexperiencing the trauma through recurrent and sometimes intrusive recollection of the event.

3. The victim developing a constricted view of and reduced involvement with the environment.

Other symptoms are also often present in patients experiencing the rape trauma syndrome. There is often an exaggerated startle response or hyperarousal state, particularly when people or situations remind victims of the assault. The victim may feel guilt about either survival or the perception that he or she did not sufficiently resist the attacker. Even among otherwise cognitively intact individuals, victims may have an impairment of memory surrounding the event. They may experience problems with concentration and attention. Rothbaum et al. (1992) report that PTSD is underdiagnosed because of symptoms that are ascribed to aging instead of response to trauma. Davis and Brody (1979) indicate that the normal losses of self-efficacy and power experienced by older women are compounded by the experience of sexual assault.

FRAMEWORK FOR WORKING WITH OLDER SEXUAL ASSAULT VICTIMS

Key Point:
The concepts, theories, and practices characteristic of victimology and those related to gerontology must be integrated to address the needs of older victims of sexual assault.

Existing services for those experiencing sexual victimization are by and large not designed to meet the needs of older adults. Those trained in rape counseling and emergency care often have little or no training in gerontology. On the other hand, workers who deal with older adults often have little training in dealing with sexual victimization. Concepts, theories, and practice associated with both victimology and gerontology must be integrated to meet the needs of older sexual assault victims.

Victimology addresses selected aspects of the phenomenon of sexual victimization. These aspects include the vulnerability patterns of the victim, the exposure patterns associated with the victimization incident, and factors that influence the degree of adaptation on the part of the victim after the traumatic event.

Gerontology addresses selected aspects associated with the aging process. Instead of defining old age strictly in terms of chronology, gerontologists often find greater utility in defining age in terms of the ability of an individual to respond to stressors. This approach looks at the older adult in a more holistic way. It focuses on the quality of life of the individual as exhibited by how well day-to-day functioning is in accord with the values and expectations of the older adult. It also takes into account the coping strategies and supports that help the older adult maintain optimal functioning.

Older adults differ in their ability to adapt successfully to stress. Although there is an overall decline in adaptive capacity with age, there is great variability in the rate of decline among individual older adults. This variability can be seen in the ability to fend off stressors as well as in the ability to successfully cope with stressors and results from differing rates of decline in the functional reserve of various organ systems. Some experts refer to this phenomenon as "homeostenosis."

Gerontologists attempt to view aspects of successful aging. Baltes (1991) describes this process of successful aging as selective optimization with compensation. The individual optimizes the adaptation process by employing successful chosen and practiced behaviors to respond to stressors. He or she also accommodates by modifying conditions to meet ability level. The older individual employs compensation strategies to deal with age-related and other losses. This includes the use of physical and social supports to compensate for loss of functioning.

Health care providers often frame their interactions with older adult patients using a problem-oriented perspective. The common endpoint in considering the adaptive capabilities of an older adult revolves around an assessment of the overall frailty of the individual. Ory et al. (1993) describe frailty as a "state of reduced physiological reserves associated with increased susceptibility to disability" (p. 283). Assessment of frailty encompasses consideration of physiologic impairments and their impact on the functional disabilities and handicaps in role performance of the older individual. It also considers the individual within the context of the physical and social environments. Environmental factors that challenge and support the individual are assessed. Simmelink (1996) defines several factors that result in increased vulnerability to the threat of sexual assault, including declining health and strength, financial limitations, housing conditions, limited sensory capacity, change in mental faculties, dependence on caregivers, and increased burdens on family members.

Appreciation of the altered responses to stress as well as the need to look at contextual factors involved in supporting the quality of life for older adults are central to providing effective care for the older adult victim of sexual assault. Unfortunately, no known resources exist for victims that link the perspectives of victimology, gerontology, and healthcare.

EFFECTIVE CLINICAL RESPONSE TO ELDER SEXUAL ABUSE

There is significant room for improvement in clinical care for the older sexual assault victim. An effective clinical care response involves prompt detection of sexual abuse and an understanding of the cognitive, physical, and emotional issues unique to elder sexual assault victims that allows a nonjudgmental and caring approach to interviewing, examining, and providing care to the victim. An effective response also supports adaptation and optimal return of functioning. Throughout the evaluation and assessment, clinicians should avoid the possibility of causing a "second assault" on the older adult victim in the form of insensitive care that further traumatizes the individual.

SCREENING

Sexual abuse may be detected directly, indirectly within a larger pattern of abuse, or through screening when it is not suspected. Ramsey-Klawsnik (1993) points out that detection begins with suspicious behaviors and physical findings. Caregivers should become involved based on any suspicion of sexual assault or abuse. Triggers may be physical findings or direct or indirect verbal indications on the part of the older individual.

Key Point
The components of an effective clinical care response include the following:
— Prompt detection of sexual abuse
— An understanding of the cognitive, physical, and emotional issues unique to elder victims of sexual abuse
— A nonjudgmental and caring approach to interviews, examinations, and other caregiving activities
— Support for the adaptation and optimal return of functioning

Fulmer et al. (2000) recommend that an initial evaluation of geriatric patients should include a social history and assessment. The social assessment should include screening for indicators of all types of abuse, even in the absence of suspicion of abuse. Screening for sexual abuse should also be part of this process. Fulmer and Wetle (1986) outline a detailed elder abuse assessment that includes an evaluation for sexual abuse. Their method explores indicators of abuse, neglect, exploitation, and abandonment. It categorizes indicators according to a level of evidence scale ranging from no evidence to possible evidence to probable evidence to definite evidence. Regardless of the method of detection, it is important that health care providers who work with older adults maintain a high level of suspicion for abuse. Using a comprehensive screening method such as that described by Fulmer and Wetle allows clinicians to perform comprehensive evaluations of all of their patients.

Many older adults will come to the emergency department for evaluation through an emergency medical system. Because these individuals will typically arrive via ambulance, EMTs, paramedics, and other transport personnel should receive training regarding the needs of the older adult victim of sexual assault or abuse. In particular, such personnel should be alert to and make note of residential conditions, physical signs, and verbal or other behaviors that may indicate sexual assault or abuse. They should also be aware of the need to preserve evidence that may be important to a forensic investigation. Generally, the patient should not be washed, and clothing should not be changed. If clothing is removed, it should be kept in a paper bag to prevent bacterial overgrowth that might interfere with subsequent forensic analysis. Chapter 15 outlines the details of forensic evidence collection; Chapter 28 gives information on the role of prehospital care providers.

INTERVIEW

Before conducting an interview of the sexual assault patient, the clinician should evaluate several details based on the circumstances of the individual case, as follows:

— Who should interview the individual?

— Where should the interview take place?

— How should the interview be conducted?

— What actions need to be taken as a result of information gathered during the interview?

— What information should the interviewer share and with whom?

To avoid secondary trauma, it is generally suggested that the interviewer be of the same gender as the victim, particularly when the assailant is thought to be of the opposite sex. Although holding the interview away from the site of the suspected assault is preferable, this is not always possible because of physical impairments that make travel impractical. However, interviews can be conducted in the victim's residence as long as the interviewer provides a sense of safety and privacy. When the assailant has free access to the victim, it is especially important that the victim be assured that the assailant will not overhear the interview, nor will he or she be privy to what is said by the victim.

It is important to build rapport with the victim. The clinician should address the older adult by her or his last name unless otherwise directed by the patient. "Caretaker speech" in which the patient is addressed in familiar terms such as "honey," "dear," or other terms of endearment should be avoided. It is sometimes helpful to have a family member or other trusted individual present during the interview. Allowing the older adult as much control as possible over the interview process can help the victim regain a sense of control. The interviewee should know that he or she has the right to terminate the interview at any time or decline to answer any question. The interviewer should explain his or her role carefully before beginning the interview.

Questions should be initiated in an open-ended manner. The older adult may require more time to answer questions or provide details than a younger patient might and should be accommodated. He or she may also have subtle sensory impairments not immediately apparent to the interviewer; therefore, older adults should be asked directly if they have any difficulty seeing or hearing. A brief mini-mental status examination should be performed if there is any question regarding cognitive impairment that could hinder the interview. Hogstel and Curry (1999) outline several strategies that promote the psychosocial support of older adult patients in the emergency department setting, particularly key communication and teaching strategies that may enhance patient care. Speaking in a well-modulated, slower-paced, and lower-pitched voice, for instance, may counter the effects of age-related hearing loss. Some clinicians place the earpieces of a stethoscope in the ears of the older patient and speak through the diaphragm. Also, small portable amplifying devices are available at low cost. It is important to ask one question at a time and give the patient ample time to respond to each question.

Older adults, particularly those who are cognitively impaired, may make indirect references to sexual assault. Indirect verbal cues that indicate fear, guilt, shame, or inappropriate sexual references should be explored further.

Based on the results of the interview, the clinician must decide if there is reason to suspect sexual assault or abuse. If action must be taken, emotional support of the victim should be a top priority. Crisis intervention, rape counseling, or other acute mental health interventions may be indicated. If the interview takes place in the residence of the older individual, he or she will often need to be transported to an emergency department for further care. The interviewer may choose to accompany the patient to the emergency department or provide for a safe, comfortable transport, possibly with a trusted escort or family member.

EXAMINATION

Older adult female sexual assault victims have an increased incidence and degree of genital trauma. Most of this results from normal postmenopausal changes. A good understanding of these normal changes allows clinicians to appropriately assess physical consequences of sexual assault in older female victims. In addition, some victims may not allow the healthcare provider to touch them during a physical examination. This is associated with phobic behavior after an assault in which a person may have the intense fear of individuals or a person. It is imperative to note that only persons with training and expertise along with compassion and exceptional communication skills should examine the sexual assault victim (Capezuti & Swedlow, 2000).

Menopause generally occurs between age 45 and 55 years. Many structural changes in the female sexual organs result from a decrease in the hormone levels after the cessation of ovulation (Yurick et al., 1989). As estrogen levels begin to fall, the labia and clitoris become smaller, and the uterus and ovaries diminish in size (Bickley, 1999). There is a loss in the elasticity of breast tissue. There is also a loss of fatty tissue deposits and elastic tissue of the labia majora. Pubic hair becomes thinner. Bartholin's glands, which produce vaginal secretions, have reduced activity, causing a decrease in lubrication during intercourse and resulting dyspareunia (painful intercourse).

The vaginal walls of women with functioning ovaries appear reddish, thickened, and well-corrugated, while the postmenopausal woman's vaginal walls may be light pink or pale and appear tissue paper thin and dry (Bickley, 1999; Yurick et al., 1989). In addition, the vaginal walls become thinner and lose some capacity for expansion. Some older females also develop urinary frequency or urgency, or stress incontinence.

Two studies have evaluated sexually assaulted postmenopausal women and have reported similar findings. Cartwright and Moore (1989) found that a significant number of older female sexual assault victims sustained genital trauma. They reviewed the medical records of 21 female patients age 60 to 90 years who were treated in an emergency room for sexual assault. Eleven of the victims had genital injuries and lacerations, one of which required surgical repair. Cartwright and Moore asserted, however, that genital trauma should not be taken as an unequivocal sign of rape. Older women may experience genital trauma with consensual sexual activity or may have no evidence of genital trauma in the case of a sexual assault.

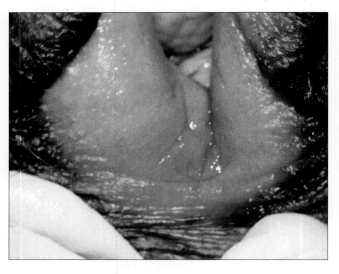

Figure 21-1. *46-year-old nonpost-menopausal woman 2 hours after assault.*

Ramin et al. (1992) compared the medical and forensic records of 129 postmenopausal victims of sexual assault over age 50 years with 129 non-postmenopausal victims age 14 to 49 years. The groups were compared for the presence of genital and extragenital trauma, patterns and type of injuries, forensic evidence, and interval to emergency department examination. They found no difference in the frequency of trauma in general in both groups (**Figures 21-1** and **22-2**). However, significant differences were seen in the patterns of injury. Genital trauma was more frequent and more severe in the postmenopausal group. Surgical repair was required in 6 of 24 women with lacerations (Ramin et al., 1992). Younger rape victims were more likely to experience trauma to the head and neck. Despite these differences, younger and older groups both experienced a significant incidence of injuries to the trunk and extremities. Surgical repair of non-genital lacerations was required in about 3% of both younger and older patients.

It is also important to recognize that less serious injuries have more serious consequences in terms of both morbidity and mortality among older adult patients. Schwab and Kauder (1992) report that outcome differences between older and younger trauma patients are most disparate at the lower end of the injury scale. Thus, it is seemingly minor injuries that may need increased attention.

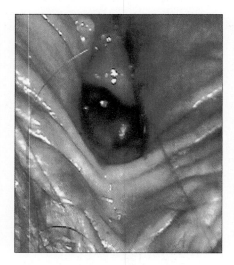

Figure 21-2. *80-year-old postmenopausal woman 5 hours after assault (Courtesy of Linda Ledray, RN, PhD, SANE).*

Key Point:
It must be recognized that less serious injuries can produce more serious consequences in terms of morbidity and mortality among older adult patients. Thus, seemingly minor injuries may require increased attention.

According to Clarke and Pierson (1999), when sexual assault is being considered, evidence of bruising to the perineum, pain with micturation, vaginal bleeding, and discharge are all ominous signs. When proceeding with the pelvic and rectal examination, it is important to proceed slowly and cautiously. The practitioner must continue to reassure the patient and realize it may take longer than expected. While continuing to assess and examine the suspected victim, the clinician should be alert especially for difficulty walking or sitting, and torn, stained, or bloody clothing. Pain or itching of the genital area; recurrent vaginal infections; bruising or bleeding of the external genitalia, vaginal, or anal area; and unexpected or unreported reluctance to cooperate with toileting or the physical examination of the genitalia are red flags for the healthcare provider to further suspect sexual assault (Clarke & Pierson, 1999). For examples of vaginal and anal trauma see **Figures 21-3** to **21-5**.

PROVISION OF CARE AND RESOURCES

Older adults are twice as likely as younger patients to experience functional status decrements as a result of problems associated with their emergency visit. Yet the emergency department staff addresses functional status issues in less than one quarter of visits (Sanders, 1992). This is problematic because the effects of illness and trauma in older adults may present in a delayed and sometimes atypical manner, with the final common pathway being an overall change in functional status. Sanders points out that specialized training in geriatrics is a minimal requirement among emergency department staff.

Explanations and instructions should be given to the patient as indicated. In some instances the patient will need to have the procedures surrounding the interview and examination, as well as ongoing legal and follow-up care issues, adequately reinforced. Specific educational interventions include providing written instructions using large bold lettering. Time must be provided and questions encouraged. New information and tasks should be related to previous experiences. The clinician should use language familiar to the patient. A follow-up phone call is made within 24 hours. Plans for follow-up referrals must be clear. The patient's family is included whenever possible in any educative effort.

REPORTING REQUIREMENTS

Clinicians should familiarize themselves with their state elder abuse reporting laws. Most states require that clinicians report suspected elder abuse to state adult protective services systems. With few exceptions, the mistreatment need only be suspected. Most mandatory and voluntary reporting laws grant immunity from civil and criminal liability to those who report in good faith (Capezuti et al., 1996).

The Joint Commission for the Accreditation of Health Care Organizations requires that hospital emergency departments provide training to staff regarding the detection and management of elder abuse. Resources, including access information for the local adult protective services agency and other services such as those provided by the local agency on aging, should be readily available.

CONCLUSION

Although rape and sexual assault of older adults is a poorly understood phenomenon, how we explore and respond to it will become increasingly important as the size and proportion of the US population over age 65 years increases. Clear definitions of elder sexual assault and more precise data collection methods would provide a greater understanding of the scope of the problem. In addition, the development of social services for sexual assault victims that address the vulnerabilities, exposure patterns, and physical and emotional responses unique to older victims would not only allow a richer understanding of the complex issues surrounding elder sexual assault but would also provide experience from which better and more comprehensive clinical care can be developed. Most importantly, however, clinicians who may be faced with the older sexual assault victim would benefit from new knowledge and training in caring for these victims, particularly focusing on prompt detection as well as the cognitive, physical, and emotional issues unique to elder sexual assault victims.

REFERENCES

Baltes PB. The many faces of aging: toward a psychological culture of old age. *Psychol Med.* 1991;21(4):837-854.

Bickley LS. *Bates' Guide to Physical Exam and History Taking.* 7th ed. Philadelphia, Pa: JB Lippincott; 1999.

Burgess AW. *Rape Sexual Assault III: A Research Handbook.* New York & London: Garland Publishing, Inc; 1991.

Burgess AW, Dowdell EB, Brown K. Sexual assault: Clinical issues. The elderly rape victim: stereotypes, perpetrators and implications for practice. *Emerg Nurs.* 2000a;26(5):516-518, 526-530.

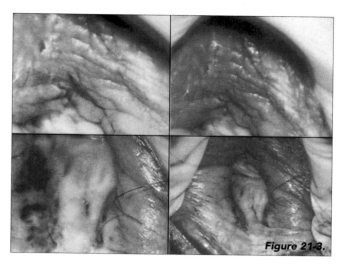

Figure 21-3.

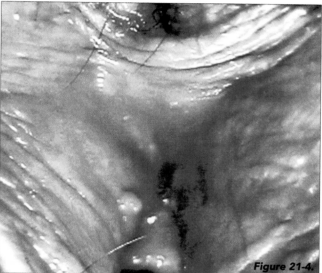

Figure 21-4.

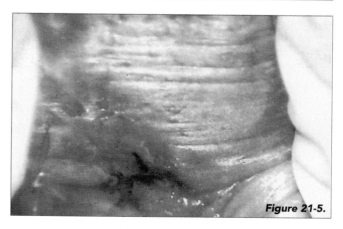

Figure 21-5.

Figure 21-3. *60-year-old woman 5 hours after assault (Courtesy of Linda Ledray, RN, PhD, SANE).*

Figure 21-4. *80-year-old woman 10 hours after assault (Courtesy of Linda Ledray, RN, PhD, SANE).*

Figure 21-5. *57-year-old woman 5 hours after assault (Courtesy of Linda Ledray, RN, PhD, SANE).*

Burgess AW, Dowdell EB, Prentky RA. Sexual abuse of nursing home residents. *J Psychosoc Nurs Ment Health Surv.* 2000b;38(6):11-17.

Burgess AW, Holmstrom LL. Rape trauma syndrome. *Am J Psychiatry.* 1974;131(9):981-986.

Capezuti EA, Swedlow DJ. Sexual abuse in nursing homes. *Elder Advisor J Elder Law.* 2000;2(2):51-61.

Capezuti E, Yurkow J, Goldberg E. Meeting the challenge of elder mistreatment. *Home Care Provid.* 1996;1(4):190-193.

Cartwright PS, Moore RA. The elderly victim of rape. *South Med J.* 1989;82:988-989.

Clarke ME, Pierson W. Management of elder abuse in the emergency department. *Emerg Med Clin North Am.* 1999;17(3):631-644.

Comijs H. Elder abuse in the community: prevalence and consequences. *Am Geriatr Soc.* 1998;46:885-888.

Davis L, Brody E. *Rape and Older Women: A Guide to Prevention and Protection.* (DHEW Publication No. 78-734). Bethesda, Md: National Institute of Mental Health; 1979.

Deming JE, Mittleman RE, Wetli CV. Forensic science aspects of fatal sexual assaults on women. *J Forensic Sci.* 1983;28(3):572-576.

Fulmer T, Paveza G, Abraham I, Fairchild S. Elder neglect assessment in the emergency department. *J Emerg Nurs.* 2000;26(5):436-443.

Fulmer T, Wetle T. Elder abuse screening and intervention. *Nurse Pract.* 1986;11(5):33-38.

Groth AN. The older rape victim and her assailant. *J Geriatr Psychiatry.* 1978;11:203-215.

Hazelwood RR, Burgess AW. *Practical Rape Investigation.* Boca Raton, Fla: CRC Press; 1995.

Hogstel MO, Curry LC. Elder abuse revisited. *J Gerontol Nurs.* 1999;25(7):10-18.

Kane RL, Ouslander JG, Abrass IB. *Essentials of Clinical Geriatrics.* 4th ed. New York, NY: Mc-Graw-Hill; 1999.

Loggins SA. *Rape as an intentional tort.* Trial, 1985 Oct, 45-55.

National Center on Elder Abuse. The National Elder Abuse Incidence Study. Washington, DC:1998.

Ory MG, Schechtman KB, Miller JP, et al. Frailty and injuries in later life: the FICSIT trials. *J Am Geriatr Soc.* 1993;41(3):283-296.

Pollock NL. Sexual assault of older women. *Ann Sex Res.* 1988;1:523-532.

Ramin SM, Satin AJ, Stone IC, Wendel GD. Sexual assault in postmenopausal women. *Obstet Gynecol.* 1992;80:860-864.

Ramsey-Klawsnik H. Elder sexual abuse: preliminary findings. *J Elder Abuse Negl.* 1991;3(3):73-89.

Ramsey-Klawsnik H. Interviewing elders for suspected sexual abuse: guidelines and techniques. *J Elder Abuse Negl.* 1993;5(1):5-18.

Ramsey-Klawsnik H. Speaking the unspeakable: an interview about elder sexual abuse. *Nexus.* 1998;4(1):4-6.

Riggs N, Houry D, Long G, Markovchick V, Feldhause KM. Analysis of 1,076 cases of sexual assault. *Ann Emerg Med.* 2000;35(4):358-362.

Rothbaum BO, Foa EP, Riggs WA. A prospective examination of posttraumatic stress disorder in rape victims. *J Trauma Stress*. 1992;5:455-475.

Sanders AB. Care of the elderly in the emergency department: conclusions and recommendations. *Ann Emerg Med*. 1992;21(2):830-834.

Schwab CW, Kauder DR. Trauma in the geriatric patient. *Arch Surg*. 1992;127(6):701-706.

Sgroi SM. Pediatric gonorrhea and child sexual abuse: the venereal disease connection. *Sex Transm Dis*. 1982;9(3):154-156.

Simmelink K. Lessons learned from three elderly sexual assault survivors. *J Emerg Nurs*.1996;22:619-621.

Tyra PA. Older women: victims of rape. *J Gerontol Nurs*. 1993;19(5):7-12.

Tyra PA. Helping elderly women survive rape using a crisis framework. *J Psychosoc Nurs Ment Health Surv*. 1996;34(12):20-25, 34-35.

U.S. Department of Justice, Bureau of Justice Statistics: *Age Patterns of Victims of Serious Crimes*. July 1997, NCJ 162031.

U.S. Department of Justice, Bureau of Justice Statistics: *Criminal Victimization in the U.S., 1995*. May 2000, NCJ 121129.

U.S. Department of Justice, Bureau of Justice Statistics: *Sex Offenses and Offenders*. Feb 1997, NCJ 163392.

Yurick AG, Speir BE, Robb SS, Ebert NJ. *The Aged Person and the Nursing Process*. 3rd ed. Norwalk, Conn: McGraw-Hill/Appleton & Lange; 1989.

Chapter 22

SEXUAL ASSAULT IN CORRECTIONAL SETTINGS

Thomas Ervin, RNC, FN, BSc
Sharon W. Cooper, MD, FAAP

The horrors experienced by many young inmates, particularly those who are convicted of nonviolent offenses, border on the unimaginable. Prison rape not only threatens the lives of those who fall prey to their aggressors, but it is potentially devastating to the human spirit. Shame, depression, and a shattering loss of self-esteem accompany the perpetual terror the victim thereafter must endure. (United States Supreme Court Justice Harry P. Blackmun, *Farmer v Brennan*, 1994)

The sentiment, or one should say judgment, expressed by those words is simple: a person who is incarcerated for a crime is no more or less likely than any other human being to suffer untold indignity and pain when sexually assaulted. Although the words by Justice Blackmun refer to a notorious case of sexual assault upon a male inmate by another male inmate, and the consequent cover-up of the situation by corrections personnel, they are equally true for instances of sexual assault upon female inmates (*Farmer v Brennan* 1994). It also is inconsequential whether the assault is carried out by fellow prisoners, by correctional staff, or as in the case of *Farmer v Brennan*, by the collusion of inmate and staff to perpetrate the occurrence and then subvert the justice systems' dealing with the acts. The effects are the same. The differences are akin to the difference in being shot with a .38-caliber revolver or a 9-mm automatic; relatively speaking, the effect is nearly identical.

OVERVIEW OF THE PROBLEM

Among the issues that must be addressed in discussing the problem of prison rape are the following:

1. Poor systems surveillance with resultant inaccurate epidemiology reports of the incidence and prevalence of prison rape

2. Inadequate laws to protect prisoners or to provide adequate reporting abilities by victims

3. Blatant indifference on the part of correctional staff to the victim impact of such sexual assaults

4. Insufficient facility capability to provide isolation and therefore protection for vulnerable inmates

5. High incidence of mentally impaired victims, for whom no special provisions are made and for whom adequate investigation of complaints is lacking

6. The problem of mixing juveniles into the adult prison population, placing them at extreme risk of exploitation, victimization, and subsequent mental health injury

7. Unavailability of counseling for victims of prisoner-on-prisoner sexual assault

8. Inadequate medical services for the sexually transmitted disease risk

9. Inadequate staff training programs on the topic of male and female prisoner-on-prisoner sexual abuse for both high-level corrections officials and front-line staff

10. Nonexistent standard operating procedures for response to prisoner-on-prisoner sexual assault

11. Inadequate numbers of guards and monitoring systems to ensure safety of the prison population

12. The need to consistently report sexual assault behind bars to local authorities and prosecutorial agencies for investigation and possible criminal prosecution

13. Lack of recognition and action to address the problem of racial tensions within prisons, which also contributes to violent sexual assaults of specific minority groups

14. Poor attention to the gang dynamics that exist in the prison systems and the need to prevent multiple-perpetrator sexual assaults

15. The common practice of merely transferring perpetrators to different units, where further abuse of a different group of potential victims is facilitated instead of taking appropriate disciplinary action

16. The practice of placing more than one prisoner per cell (double celling) without consideration of whether there has been a prior report or suspicion of a sexual assault involving one or more than one of the inmates

17. Poor public awareness of the serious and tragic nature of this type of crime, leading to misrepresentations of prison rape as a joke in the media

18. Poor recognition that prison rape is a contributing factor to prison homicides, violence against inmates and staff, and institutional riots and insurrections

19. Poor attention to the problem of custodial abuse of inmates

20. Inadequate federal laws to affect prison funding for the complex problem of prisoner sexual assault

Two of the only 16 existing epidemiological studies (Struckman-Johnson et al., 1996; Struckman-Johnson & Struckman-Johnson, 2000) that have attempted to assess the problem of prison rape reveal the following facts:

— From 22% to 25% of prisoners are victims of sexual pressuring, attempted sexual assault, or completed rapes

— Ten percent of prisoners are victims of a completed rape at least 1 time during the course of their incarceration

— Two thirds of those reporting sexual victimization have been repeatedly victimized on an average of 9 times during their incarceration—with some male prisoners experiencing up to 100 incidents of sexual assault per year

A bill introduced to the US Senate and House of Representatives titled "Prison Rape Reduction Act of 2002" seeks to address the issues in the sexual assaults perpetrated on incarcerated individuals at all levels. The following is an excerpt from that proposed bill.

Excerpt from Prison Rape Reduction Act of 2002 (12/25/01 draft)
SEC. 2. FINDINGS.

Congress finds that:

(1) there were 1,366,721 individuals incarcerated in Federal and State Prisons and 605,943 inmates in county and local jails at the end of 1999; 6.3 million individuals were under Federal and State jurisdiction on at least one occasion during 1999; more than 10 million separate admissions to and discharges from prisons and jails occurred during 1999;

(2) the best expert estimate of the number of individuals attacked at least one time during their incarceration is a national median number of 13.6%. In other words, at least 185,000 of the current inmates have been or will be sexually assaulted during time served and many will be assaulted repeatedly during their incarceration;

(3) due to lack of extensive research on inmate sexual assault it is difficult to truly gauge

the full extent of prison rape. The best estimate of the total number of current and former inmates who have been sexually assaulted in prison is _____;

(4) research in the field of youth corrections has shown that juveniles incarcerated with adults are five times more likely to report being sexually assaulted than those incarcerated in juvenile facilities; victims of sexual assault in adult facilities tend to be "younger, housed in higher security settings, and in the early part of their prison terms" in contrast to (sic) rest of the inmate population; the "prototype" of prison rape (victims) tend(s) to be the youngest inmates within a given institutional system, and corrections officers have been quoted saying that a young inmate's chances of avoiding rape are "...almost zero......He'll get raped within the first twenty-four to forty-eight hours. That's standard;" the American Correctional Association, and the American Jail Association—the professional associations representing the national correctional staff—call for juveniles to be detained in separate facilities from adults to guard against the risk of sexual assaults; that the suicide rate of juveniles in adult jails is 7.7 times higher than that of juvenile detention centers; youths transferred to adult court are more likely to re-offend than those sent to the juvenile justice system; and of those juveniles who committed crimes, the youths who had previously been tried as adults committed serious crimes at double the rate of those sent to juvenile court;

(5) the Supreme Court held, in Farmer v. Brennan, 511 U.S. 825 (1995) that prison officials who have been deliberately indifferent to the risk of sexual assault of prison inmates have violated the inmates' Constitutional rights;

(6) in light of Farmer, the current standards for prevention and treatment of sexual assault adopted by the Bureau of Prisons are inadequate as they include no procedures to ensure the standards are enforced;

(7) the oldest and largest correctional accrediting agency, the American Correctional Association, has established no standards for prevention or training in regards to sexual assault, neither in its accreditation review process, nor otherwise;

(8) most prison staff and prisoners are not adequately trained or prepared to prevent, report or treat inmate sexual assaults

(9) because of the cycle of victimization and stigmatization within the prison sub-culture, sexual assaults are infrequently reported and/or treated physically and mentally;

(10) the proliferation of sexual assault within prison walls is not only a violation of the Constitutional rights of incarcerated individuals, it is also a public health and safety threat because:

(A) the incidence of AIDS, HIV, Hepatitis C, and sexually transmitted diseases is at an all time high in prisons;

(B) once released, previously non-violent criminals who has(sic) been repeatedly raped, and thus physically and emotionally scarred for life, have a significantly higher propensity to commit violent acts against their communities; and

(C) the frequently interracial character of prison sexual assaults significantly exacerbates interracial tensions, both within prison and, upon release of perpetrators and victims from prison, in the community at large.

(11) despite the efforts of a small number of dedicated scholars and activists, insufficient data and research has been conducted or otherwise reported on the extent of prison sexual assaults;

(12) prison officials, National and State leaders, and the public at large, are unaware of the extent or epidemic character of brutality and horror that is the day-to-day life of a "target" prisoner; and

(13) when the question of prison rape is given priority attention prison officials can make an extraordinary difference in preventing and reducing the incidence of prison rape;

(14) the incidence of prison rape and sexual assault has a significant effect in interstate commerce in that:

(A) it increases substantially the cost incurred by Federal, State, and local jurisdictions to administer the prison systems of this Nation;

(B) it increases substantially the incidence and spread of AIDS, HIV, Hepatitis C, and sexually transmitted diseases, contributing to increased health and medical expenditures throughout the Nation; and

(C) it increases the risk of recidivism, violent crime, and interracial hostility and strife by individuals who are subjected to prison rape and sexual assault.

As obvious as the objectives of this proposed legislation may seem to some, they are not so clear to all. Some do not feel that inmates deserve to be protected from the vagaries of "jail justice" when they have crossed societal boundaries themselves. A common belief is that incarceration only happens to "the other person." At this writing, some 2 million individuals are behind bars in the United States, with approximately 1500 being added each week. It has been predicted by the Bureau of Justice Statistics (1999) that at our current rate 1 of every 20 Americans born in 1999 will spend some portion of their lives behind bars. On any given day of the year, 1 in every 150 persons is jailed (*Corrections in the US*, 2002). The rate of incarceration in the United States is 727 prisoners per 100,000 residents (McGuire & Pastore, 1999). This is in comparison to an incarceration rate in most European countries of only 100 per 100,000 people (Kuhn, 1999).

Seventy-one percent of those imprisoned are "inside" for nonviolent crimes (*Corrections in the US*, 2002). No one can reasonably condone the actions of those who do not conform to the basic tenets of society, those who violate laws on drugs or property rights. But the workings of the justice system are not intended to place perpetrators in situations that allow, or even encourage, victimization during incarceration leading an individual to reoffend upon release. No judge, legislature, or legal entity has ever declared rape a proper punishment for the commission of any crime.

The high number of prisoners reflects changes in public policy over the past 25 years there has been a trend toward longer sentences, stricter parole policies, mandatory minimum sentences, and most recently, the "three strikes" laws, which refer to the policy that a third felony conviction will result in a mandatory long-term sentence. This policy was thought to increase the removal of habitual offenders from the public arena, enhancing public safety.

Among both men and women it is thought that some 60,000 unwanted sexual acts occur daily behind bars (*Corrections in the US*, 2002). These are the acts of male inmates preying on other male inmates, female inmates accosting other female inmates, and both male and female staff in institutional facilities sexually assaulting, by force or coercion, inmates of both sexes. Female inmates are at extreme risk despite the fact that they are housed in an all-female prison. Although specific characteristics have been less well-defined, first-time offenders, young women, and women with mental disabilities are particularly vulnerable to sexual assault (*Betraying the Young*, 1998; *Rough Justice for Women Behind Bars*, 1999).

Although many statistics are maintained by the Federal Bureau of Prisons and the National Institute of Corrections, the incidence of prisoner-on-prisoner sexual assault is one aspect of data that is not formally tracked. This failure to document such a far-reaching occurrence within a correctional facility underlines the perception that a blatant indifference for this crime exists within the system. Documentation of such events usually reaches family and friends via letters from victims or statements taken from fellow prisoners after an assault and subsequent suicide takes place. The case of Rodney Hulin is particularly poignant and illustrative of the kind of circumstances that are so tragic regarding this form of abuse.

The Case of Rodney Hulin

Testimony before the United States Senate Committee on the Judiciary (Ms Linda Bruntmeyer, July 31, 2002):

"My name is Linda Bruntmeyer, and I am here today to tell you about my son, Rodney Hulin."

When Rodney was sixteen, he and his brother set a dumpster on fire in an alley in our neighborhood. The authorities decided to make an example of Rodney. Even though only about $500 in damage was caused by the fire, they sentenced him to eight years in an adult prison.

We were frightened for him from the start. At sixteen, Rodney was a small guy, only 5 foot 2 inches and about 125 pounds. And as a first-time offender, we knew he might be targeted by older, tougher, adult inmates.

Then our worst nightmares came true. Rodney wrote us a letter telling us he'd been raped. A medical examination had confirmed the rape. A doctor found tears in his rectum and ordered an HIV test, because, he told us, one-third of the prisoners there were HIV positive.

But that was only the beginning. Rodney knew if he went back into the general population, he would be in danger. He wrote to the authorities requesting to be moved to a safer place. He went through all the proper channels, but he was denied.

After the first rape, he was returned to the general population. There, he was repeatedly beaten and forced to perform oral sex and raped. He wrote for help again. In his grievance letter he wrote, "I have been sexually and physically assaulted several times, by several inmates. I am afraid to go to sleep, to shower, and just about everything else. I am afraid that when I am doing these things, I might die at any minute. Please sir, help me."

Still, officials told him that he did not meet "emergency grievance criteria." We all tried to get him to a safe place. I called the warden, trying to figure out what was going on.

He said Rodney needed to grow up. He said, "This happens everyday, learn to deal with it. It's no big deal."

We were desperate. Rodney started to violate rules so that he would be put in segregation. After he was finally put in segregation, we had about a ten minute phone conversation. He was crying. He said, "Mom, I'm emotionally and mentally destroyed."

That was the last time I heard his voice. On the night of January 26, 1996, my son hanged himself in his cell. He was seventeen and afraid, and ashamed, and hopeless. He laid in a coma for the next four months before he died."

This tragic testimony illustrates many of the previously cited problems that contribute to prison rape and the failure to protect the vulnerable population often introduced into the correctional system. This young man committed a minor offense, which resulted in what appears to be an overly harsh sentence. He was a youth and was integrated directly into an adult prison. It is well known that youths introduced into an adult system are at particular risk for violent beatings, sexual assault, and exploitation associated with becoming a sexual slave, sold by their "owners" who otherwise offer protection from gang assailants.

The consequences of these attacks are far reaching. It is not possible for an individual to undergo forced sex without subsequent trauma. This trauma may be equally physical and emotional, or as in those instances of coercion, mostly emotional or psychologic. Regardless of the type or extent of trauma sustained there will be consequences for the individual, for society, and for those professionals working with these special populations and the aftermath of their experiences.

The mental health ramifications of prison rape are extreme. The first risk factor for a poor mental health outcome rests on the fact that in the United States, there are more mentally ill inmates in prisons than in psychiatric hospitals (Chelala, 1999; Harrington, 1999; Torrey, 1999). Most correctional facilities have minimal mental health capability to address these already compromised inmates. When sexual assault occurs in one of its many forms, the resulting psychologic trauma is almost immeasurable. Posttraumatic stress disorder (PTSD), anxiety, depression, and the exacerbation of preexisting mental disorders take place (Dumond, 1992, 2000; Dumond & Dumond, 2002; Mariner, 2001). Inmates at risk for suicide become more unstable and are far more likely to attempt or succeed in committing suicide to avoid continuous trauma. Attention to these problems also requires funding and the development of a different practice philosophy at the highest levels in the correctional system.

The victim most often experiences anger, depression, loss of self-esteem and self worth, alteration of self-image, and a desire for revenge. A means to allow reclamation of the individual's identity and self-control will be manifested in some manner, whether it is internally focused or externally displayed. The immediate and long-term problems that can, and regrettably usually do, arise from such incidents may encompass any number of what are commonly referred to as societal ills.

Key Point:
The immediate and long-term problems that tend to arise from anger, depression, loss of self-esteem and self-worth, alteration of self-image, and the desire for revenge may include any number of societal ills.

Empirical evidence demonstrates that certain categories of inmates are especially vulnerable to sexual assault, including the following (Cotton & Groth, 1982, 1984; Dumond, 1992, 2000; Knowles, 1999):

— Inmates who are young and inexperienced

— Inmates who are short in stature, with small body habitus and who may be physically weak

— Prisoners who have mental illnesses or who have developmental disabilities

— Inmates who are not "street-wise" or who lack savvy

— Prisoners who are not gang affiliated

— Inmates who are homosexual, overtly effeminate, or transgendered

— Prisoners who have violated the "code of silence" or are seen as a "snitch"

— Inmates who are disliked either by the staff or by other inmates

— Inmates who have been prior sexual assault victims

The testimony regarding Rodney Hulin illustrates the fact that existing laws are inadequate to provide reporting of sexual assault to agencies with prosecution ability. It appears that inadequate staff training, regarding both the dynamics of prison rape and the high incidence of morbidity and mortality for victims, resulted in blatant disregard on the part of the prison staff for the plight of this youth. Despite receiving a medical confirmation of the rape and going to the proper channels to request being moved to a safer place, this youth was provided no protective custody.

The response of the warden in this case illustrates a lack of training and understanding of the extreme danger that this youth faced daily. His response could be considered criminal by many, since he acknowledged that a crime was being committed repetitively and he chose to ignore it, thereby abetting its occurrence. The youth's self-destructive efforts to be placed in segregation reveal his extreme desperation as he attempted to survive. The lack of mental health services for incarcerated victims of crimes adds insult to injury, and the final suicide of this youth was both tragic and preventable.

Our society and our justice system are predicated on fairness and equity. We do not hold the sons (or daughters) responsible for the sins of the fathers (or mothers). By extrapolation then, should we hold the perpetrator of a crime liable to a standard of retribution that far exceeds the letter or intent of the law in exacting justice far beyond equivalent measure to the illegal act?

ROLE OF THE MEDICAL PROFESSIONAL

For the medical professional, whether physician or nurse, there is the conundrum of providing medical interventions to a member of a population that one may find personally repugnant, justifiably so or not. To provide the unbiased, professional care called for in such a situation is not a choice. It is an obligation.

When it is difficult to cope with the nature of necessary service provisions, the medical professional must be just that—a medical professional. Society, through the exercise of the court, has rendered judgment. The medical professional need only render care.

INFECTIOUS DISEASE COMPLICATIONS IN PRISON RAPE

The National Institute of Corrections has published a comprehensive set of clinical practice guidelines for the prevention and detection of infectious diseases in the prison population. A significant amount of attention is devoted to the complications of close-quarter living and the general poor health of inmates (DeGroot, 2001; Reindollar, 1999). There is an excellent online document available for the management of HIV infection (http://www.nicic.org/pubs/bop-medical.htm) that represents the collaboration among the Centers for Disease Control and Prevention, the US Department of Health and Human Services, the National Institutes of Health, the American Corrections Association, the National Commission on Correctional Healthcare, and the National Institute for Occupational Safety and Health. The Federal Bureau of Prisons clinical guidelines for medical management address the concerns for the following issues:

— Viral hepatitis (A, B, C, and D)

— HIV infection

— Tuberculosis

— Sexually transmitted diseases

— Endocarditis prophylaxis

— Varicella

Some infections can cause an epidemic in a prison or jail and have the potential for serious consequences. Guidelines for the identification of infectious diseases include the recommendations cited in **Table 22-1**. Care must be taken both by other inmates and the prison staff who come into physical contact with the prisoners and risk possible body fluid contamination. The incidence of HIV/AIDS in the inmate population is not known, but a significant number of inmates become positive after a sexual assault. Obviously, gang rapes or sexual slavery makes a victim much more vulnerable.

ROLE OF SOCIAL SERVICES PROFESSIONALS AND PRISON STAFF

The focus and educational background needed to become a social services professional may enable professionals in these disciplines to be less judgmental about dealing with sexual assault in correctional settings. Perhaps the most complex difficulties fall on professionals working in corrections and law enforcement (including jailers, correctional officers, and on-site medical staffers, as well as attorneys for both prosecution and defense) who deal closely with the sexual victimization of incarcerated persons.

The correctional officer, whether a sheriff's jailer or state prison corrections agent, must cope with the reality of life behind bars. This reality is often harsher and more brutal than the layperson not working on a day-to-day basis in a correctional facility can comprehend. A rather basic paradigm among people working in prisons and jails reveals an entrenched mindset. This question is often asked of new employees in institutions: What is the difference between a minimum- and maximum-risk inmate? The answer is about 2 seconds. The implication is that one never knows exactly what to expect from inmates. It is not much of a leap from exercising necessary caution to constant paranoia and constant paranoia to disregard for the humanity of those incarcerated.

Under these conditions it can be seen why correctional personnel develop an attitude of disdain for the dangers one inmate may present to any other specific

Table 22-1. Process of identification of infectious diseases in the prison population	
INFECTTIOUS DISEASE	SCREEN, ASSESS, AND TEST INMATES
Tuberculosis (TB) infection and possible TB disease	— On initial incarceration before placed — Annually — When clinically indicated — To find evidence of spread surrounding a case of contagious TB disease
Human immunodeficiency virus (HIV) infection	— If history of risk behavior — If clinical indications — Before release — For surveillance purposes — After an exposure
Other infections transmittable by casual contact	— On intake and before being placed in the general population — Before assigned to the food service area — If clinical indications — With contact investigators

From Federal Bureau of Prisons Report on Infectious Disease Management, January 2001, p 3.

Key Point:
Some people in positions of authority or
power over others misuse such power, but this
is the exception—not the rule.

inmate. The overall control of the institution becomes paramount to the individual's needs. Sometimes institutionalization of sexual threats and coercion, either by direct perpetration or simply by "looking the other way," can become a control mechanism for staff. However, this is the exception, not the rule. Most correctional security personnel adhere to a high professional and personal ethic, one that any professional would do well to emulate. There are, however, medical and ancillary staffers, correctional officers, and jailers who brutalize inmates.

GANG-RELATED INCIDENTS

Hate crimes may be the incentive for prison rape. Numerous gangs exist behind bars and they are often racially based. The white supremacist movement has many adherents in the prison system. The Aryan Brotherhood and Aryan Circle represent two of the most violent gangs found in prison society. Other prison gangs include the Mexican Mafia, the Black Gangster Disciples, the White Knights, the Black Guerilla Family, and the Latin Kings, among others with a racially exclusive nature (Mariner, 2001).

SEXUAL PREDATORS

One of the most common, heinous misuses of power is the use of a known sexual predator, such as the infamous "booty bandit" Wayne Robertson, in the Eddie Dillard case, to intimidate, control, or punish other inmates for real or perceived transgressions of prison law (Arak, 1999). Should an inmate file a complaint, spit on, or "gas" (gassing consists of throwing a concoction of urine, feces, semen, and sometimes disease-infected blood on staff) an officer, or perhaps simply show disrespect, the offending inmate may be "celled up" with a much larger, aggressive, "nothing to lose," sexual predator. The consequence is obvious. This can make a very effective, unofficial disciplinary tool to control the inmate who is not "cooperative" or "programmed" as the officer believes he should be. Jailers may also use force or coercion against a male or female to obtain sexual favors. There are unfounded incidents as well. What of the female inmate who "likes" a particular male staff member who is either too moral or too professional to allow any relationship with the inmate? She may simply have two or more "witnesses" swear they saw the staff member do something improper. Often this can be enough to cost an officer or other male staff member his career or his own freedom. The same scenario may occur with a male inmate and a female staff member.

FROM VICTIM TO PREDATOR

Individuals who survive the single or multiple sexual assaults, in addition to having a very high incidence of PTSD and depression, may become violent themselves both as an act of immediate self-defense and in an effort to avoid further victimization. This transition from victim to perpetrator often follows the individual beyond the penal system confinement, contributing to the greater than 75% rate of return to incarceration for inmates. Nearly three fourths of US prisoners are held for nonviolent crimes, many of which are drug offenses. In fact, the number of prisoners incarcerated for drug crimes has increased sevenfold in the last 20 years. The transformation of these individuals into violent inmates is an example of the "hardening" process often described for those incarcerated for any length of time.

DISPOSITION OF CASES

Local law enforcement, prosecutors, defense attorneys, judges, and juries must sort through the prison rape case information and then make life-affecting decisions. At this point, the professionalism of all concerned becomes the predominant factor in justice being served.

In the case of Eddie Dillard (an inmate in a state prison who had kicked a female corrections officer) it was alleged that a number of officers conspired to "teach him a lesson" by placing him in a two-man cell ("celling him up") with another inmate nearly twice his size who had a reputation for raping smaller, susceptible inmates, earning him the nickname, "booty bandit." The confessed attacker in this instance, Wayne Robertson, freely admitted he had raped Dillard repeatedly. Robertson also testified in court that he understood this to be what the correctional officers expected him to do in order to "teach him (Dillard) how to do his time." Robertson freely admitted his actions in court by testifying "...rape is a vile act. I just took care of business...the cops needed me to show him what's what" (Court transcripts *Dillard v California Department of Corrections*, 2001). In this particular instance, a jury at trial exonerated the correctional officers involved of any wrongdoing.

The experiences of Stephen Donaldson indicate the extent of the problem of prison rape and the circumstances under which it often occurs. Donaldson was arrested for participating in a Quaker "pray-in" at the White House in the 1970s. The "pray-in" was a protest against the bombings in Cambodia during the Vietnam War. Mr. Donaldson was later acquitted of all charges leading to his arrest. He was, however, jailed at the time and brutally raped while in jail. He was a "target inmate" for the common reasons; he was young, middle-class, not gang affiliated or particularly street-wise, physically unimposing, and not part of the dominant racial group with which he was incarcerated. He has since been very active and an extremely competent and persuasive advocate for reform and intervention to curb or halt prison rape (Donaldson, 1993).

There is also the question of sexuality expressed in facilities for youthful offenders. The California Youth Authority (CYA) oversees 7000 plus individuals as young as age 12 years and as old as 25 years in its institutions and programs (California Youth Authority, 2002). The potential for forced sexual activity by older, more powerful inmates on their younger and weaker counterparts is great. As we all realize from reading the daily papers, the potential for sexual abuse by those in positions of trust or authority over youth is also enormous. A child in school or a parishioner in a church youth group is vulnerable. How much more vulnerable might a ward of the court "serving time" for criminal acts be to sexual predation?

Advocates of prison reform have written much on the inevitable consequences of incarcerating people and, in essence, denying that dimension of their humanity that pertains to sexuality. Is it reasonable to lock people up for years and not allow any sexual release other than autoeroticism? Is it unreasonable to lock people up who have shown they cannot or will not conform to societal norms, yet still provide them with the fullest degree of freedom of action possible, even to include the opportunity for recreational sexual expression? Questions such as these are beyond the scope of this text.

SUMMARY

It should be clear that the problems of sexual assault, and sexual activity in general, in correctional facilities are complex, fraught with peril for many, and in desperate need of workable solutions. Prison rape is a devastating event that victimizes prison members, sometimes transforming them into far more violent persons. It may also be a fatal event, either at the time of the assault or shortly afterward because of homicide or suicide, or even months to years later because of the transmission of HIV. The numerous stories of sadistic and often inhumane treatment caused by both inmates and custodial staff spearheads the necessity for establishing better procedures to investigate and punish this heinous crime. The recent research of the National Prison Rape Reduction Commission will play a key role in establishing standard operating procedures and providing a standard of care and law enforcement support badly needed for this extremely underreported serious crime.

REFERENCES

Arak, M. Booty Bandit. *Los Angeles Times.* October 24, 1999:3.

Betraying the Young: Human Rights Violations Against Children. New York, NY: Amnesty International;1998:1-6.

California Youth Authority. Demographics Summary Fact Sheet. Available at: http://www.cya.ca.gov. Accessed November 12, 2002.

Chelala C. More mentally ill people reported in US prisons. *British Med J.* 1999;319(7204):210.

Corrections in the US—The Picture Today. The Lionheart Foundation Web site. Available at: http://www.lionheart.org/corrections.html. Accessed November 12, 2002.

Cotton DJ, Groth AN. Inmate rape: prevention and intervention. *J Prison Jail Health.* 1982;2(1):47-57.

Cotton DJ, Groth AN. Sexual assault in correctional institutions: prevention and intervention. In: Stuart IR, ed. *Victims of Sexual Aggression: Treatment of Children, Women, and Men.* New York, NY: Van Nostrand Reinhold; 1984.

DeGroot AS. HIV incarcerated women: an epidemic behind the walls. *Corrections Today.* 2001;63(1):77-81,97.

Dillard v California Department of Corrections. 2001.

Donaldson S. *The Rape Crisis Behind Bars.* Vancouver, BC, Canada: University of British Columbia; 1993.

Dumond RW. The sexual assault of male inmates in incarcerated settings. *International Journal of Sociology of Law.* 1992;20(2):135-157.

Dumond RW. Inmate sexual assault: the plague which persists. *The Prison Journal.* 2000;80(4):407-414.

Dumond RW, Dumond DA. The treatment of sexual assault victims. In: Hensley C, ed. Prison Sex: Practice and Policy. Boulder, Colo: Lynne Rienner Publishers; 2002:67-88, 88-100.

Farmer v Brennan (92-7247), 511 US 825 (1994).

Federal Bureau of Prisons. *Report on Infectious Disease Management.* January, 2001:3.

Harrington SPM. New Bedlam: Jails—not psychiatric hospitals—now care for the indigent mentally ill. *Jail Suicide/Mental Health Update.* 1999;9(2):12-17.

Knowles GJ. Male prison rape: a search for causation and prevention. *The Howard Journal.* 1999;38(3):267-282.

Kuhn A. Incarceration rates across the world. *Overcrowded Times.* April 1999;10(2):1.

Mariner J. *No Escape: Male Rape in U.S. Prisons.* New York, NY: Human Rights Watch; 2001.

McGuire KP, Pastore AL. *Sourcebook of Criminal Justice Statistics 1998.* Washington DC: USGPO; 1999:79, 479, 487.

Prison Rape Reduction Act of 2002. Bill introduced on June 13, 2002 before US Congress, 12/25/01 draft. Available online at: http://www.hrw.org/reports/2001/prison/learn.html, http://www.spr.org/pdf/122501bill.pdf. Accessed November 12, 2002.

Reindollar RW. Hepatitis C and the correctional population (Emerging and reemerging issues in infectious disease-Hepatitis C: a meeting ground for the generalist and specialist.). *AJM.* December 27, 1999:1005.

Rough justice for women behind bars. New York, NY: Amnesty International; 1999.

Struckman-Johnson CJ, Struckman-Johnson DL, Rucker L, Bumby K, Donaldson S. Sexual coercion reported by men and women in prison. *J Sex Res.* 1996;33(1):67-76.

Struckman-Johnson CJ, Struckman-Johnson DL. Sexual coercion rates in seven Midwestern prison facilities for men. *The Prison Journal.* 2000;80(4): 379-390.

Testimony of Linda Bruntmeyer. Hearing of Rodney Hulin, United States Senate Committee on the Judiciary. July 31, 2002.

Torrey EF. How did so many mentally ill persons get into American's jails and prisons? *American Jails.* 1999;13(5):9-13.

Chapter 23

REVISED TRAUMA THEORY: UNDERSTANDING THE TRAUMATIC NATURE OF SEXUAL ASSAULT

Sandra L. Bloom, MD

INTRODUCTION

Sexual assault has immediate and long-term consequences that can be devastating for the physical, emotional, and relational health of the victim. This chapter addresses the current understanding of how exposure to the overwhelming stress of assault alters the psychobiology, personal adjustment, and systems of meaning for the victim. In addition, the consequences of these changes on physical health, mental health, social adjustment, revictimization, and ability to parent are outlined.

In the last three decades a large body of evidence-based knowledge has accumulated about the effects of overwhelming stress. Trauma theory represents a comprehensive biopsychosocial and philosophic model for understanding these effects. As understanding grows about the complex nature and impact of overwhelming experiences, the trauma of sexual assault is recognized as having an effect on every level of a person's adjustment. Posttraumatic stress disorder (PTSD) is a chronic and often disabling condition, and the prevalence of PTSD after rape is extraordinarily high. Even in the most conservative study, those with PTSD were two to four times more likely than those without PTSD to have other psychiatric disorders, particularly depression and somatization. Rape victims are far more likely to make suicide attempts and to develop substance abuse problems.

Evidence is accumulating about the nature and extent of psychobiologic changes secondary to sexual assault. The results of a growing body of studies on the physiologic effects of stress are disturbing, making clear that children's psychobiologic development and adult function can be profoundly affected by sexual assault. Victims of sexual abuse and assault often suffer from a multitude of physical disorders not directly related to whatever injuries they have suffered as a result of the assault. Compounding the problem is the reality of revictimization. One of the many horrors attending sexual assault is the tendency of victims to experience more than one sexual assault experience. Child sexual abuse survivors appear to be particularly vulnerable to revictimization experiences.

A victim is both helpless and powerless, and human beings generally choose to do anything to avoid feeling powerless. Consequently, a possible outcome for a person who has been victimized is to identify with the power of the perpetrator and to become someone who terrorizes and abuses others. Clear evidence shows that victimizers are more likely to have been victimized as children than people who do not victimize others.

A pernicious aspect of violence is its multigenerational impact. That violence in one generation often leads to violence in the next is now supported by considerable evidence. Parenting behavior can be profoundly affected by the impact of trauma.

The total estimated cost for child rape and other sexual abuse has been estimated to be $23 billion in lost productivity (Miller et al., 1993). The problem of sexual assault is so great and affects so many children and adults that there are not, nor will there ever be, enough mental health workers to address the sheer volume of people suffering from the multitude of problems secondary to exposure to violence. Therefore medical and social institutions must find ways to address the problem by creating environments that promote and sustain better physical, emotional, and relational health.

TRAUMA THEORY: UNDERSTANDING THE IMPACT OF SEXUAL ASSAULT

Until the 1970s when US servicemen returned from Vietnam and began sharing the overwhelming nature of their combat experiences and US women gathered in consciousness-raising groups to begin sharing their experiences of sexual assault, incest, and domestic violence, relatively little was known about the impact of the traumatic experience on the body, mind, social adjustment, and life philosophy of the victim. In the last three decades a large body of evidence-based knowledge has accumulated about the effects of overwhelming stress. Trauma theory represents a comprehensive biopsychosocial and philosophic model for understanding these effects. It also helps to understand how victims' bodies and minds respond normally to abnormal events and then become stuck, as a "state becomes a trait."

PSYCHOLOGIC TRAUMA DEFINED

To understand what trauma does, we must first understand what we mean by "trauma." There is much controversy over how we even define what a traumatic event is. The first studies of trauma survivors derived from work with disaster victims, combat veterans, and Holocaust survivors. In such cases the traumatic events are usually well defined and represent experiences of terror, exposure to atrocities, or the fear of imminent death. In fact, to obtain a formal diagnosis of "posttraumatic stress disorder" according to the DSM-IV, the victim must have experienced, witnessed, or been confronted with an event or events that involved actual or threatened death or serious injury, or threat to physical integrity of self or others (American Psychiatric Association [APA], 1994).

This certainly describes the situation of many victims of sexual assault, particularly stranger rape. However, child victims of sexual abuse and many victims of intimate partner rape are not in imminent fear of loss of life or even physical integrity. Yet sexual abuse and non–life-threatening rape are some of the most traumatizing of experiences. How can we explain this well-established clinical finding? The answer lies in the complexity of the interaction of the victim and the traumatic event.

According to Lenore Terr (1990), a child psychiatrist who did the first longitudinal study of traumatized children, "psychic trauma occurs when a sudden, unexpected, overwhelming intense emotional blow or a series of blows assaults the person from outside. Traumatic events are external, but they quickly become incorporated into the mind" (p. 8).

Complicating the question further, events occurring during and subsequent to the traumatic event can make a profound difference in how the victim experiences and interprets that event. The manner in which the victim's body and mind responded at the time of the trauma, and how his or her social support network reacted during and after the event play important roles in determining the ultimate outcome. It is also necessary to understand how the victim comprehends and interprets the events. An adolescent may be greatly relieved to be left alone in the house for a weekend, whereas a small child may experience the same event as overwhelmingly terrifying. Children lack the resources to cope with even minor threats and experience a threat to people they are attached to as a threat to themselves. Van der Kolk (1989) makes this point about the complicated nature of trauma when he writes, "Traumatization occurs when both internal and external resources are inadequate to cope with external threat" (p. 393). It is not only the trauma itself that does damage to the victim: it is also how the individual's mind and body react to the traumatic experience combined with the unique response of the individual's social group.

HEREDITY'S LEGACY: THE AUTONOMIC NERVOUS SYSTEM

A traumatic experience affects the entire person. The way we think, the way we learn, the way we remember things, the way we feel about ourselves, the way we feel about other people, and the way we make sense of the world are all profoundly altered by traumatic experience. All of these factors are rooted in the human experience.

Unlike other mammals, humans come into the world ill prepared to battle with natural enemies. Helpless for a prolonged period after birth, humans have few natural defenses. Like all mammals, humans are equipped to respond to emergencies with a "fight-or-flight" reaction via the autonomic nervous system. This state of extreme hyperarousal serves a protective function during an emergency, preparing the individual to respond automatically and aggressively to a perceived threat, preferentially steering toward action and away from the time-consuming effort of thought and language. However, prolonged hyperarousal leaves people physically and emotionally exhausted, burdened with hair-trigger tempers, irritable, and tending to perpetuate violence.

To protect against helplessness, humans developed a network of attachment relationships, living in extended kinship groups. The human capacity to manage overwhelming emotional states is shaped by experience with early childhood attachments and is maintained throughout life through attachment relationships. This development of extended social networks increases the likelihood that vulnerable offspring will be protected.

Heredity Off-Track

Although the fight-or-flight state of physiologic hyperarousal serves a vital survival purpose in times of danger, when hyperarousal stops being a state and turns into a trait, human beings lose their capacity to accurately assess and predict danger. A consequence may be avoidance and reenactment instead of adaptation and survival (Perry & Pate, 1993). The human need to rescue ourselves from this untenable physiologic state means that humans desperately seek to calm themselves down. If relief is not available from our fellow humans, people may turn to substances or behaviors that bring relief.

Very complex brains and powerful memories distinguish humans as extremely intelligent. Yet this very intelligence creates a vulnerability to the effects of trauma, such as flashbacks, body memories, posttraumatic nightmares, and behavioral reenactments. The dependence on language is also a critical factor. Experiences that took place before the age of language acquisition cannot be integrated into consciousness and a coherent sense of identity. Instead, the individual becomes haunted by an unresolved, and even unknown, past.

Traumatic experience disrupts attachment to the extent that the social world has failed to serve its protective function for the individual. Humans are particularly ill-suited to having the people to whom they are attached also be the people doing the violating. Emotions firmly secure individuals to one another, but trauma profoundly disrupts the ability to manage emotional experience. People lose the capacity to respond to situations with the appropriate emotion in appropriate measure and tend to overreact to events that should not provoke and underreact to events that should receive a more meaningful response. Any impaired ability to respond with the appropriate emotional signal impairs the capacity to create and maintain healthy relationships.

Key Point:
Trauma damages the victim in and of itself but also leads to damage through how the victim's mind and body react to the experience of trauma and through how the person's social group responds to the victim.

Finally, humans are physiologically designed to function best as an integrated whole. Out of that sense of wholeness and integrity emerges meaning, purpose, values, belief, identity, and wisdom. The fragmentation that accompanies traumatic experience degrades this integration and impedes maximum performance in various ways. Human brains function best when they are adequately stimulated but simultaneously protected from overwhelming stress. This explains the need for order, for safety, and for adequate protection. Without this balance between stimulation and soothing, humans cannot reason properly or make sense out of what has happened. Humans are meaning-making animals, requiring the ability to make sense of experiences, to order chaos, and to structure reality. Traumatic experience destroys the sense of meaning and therefore purpose. Individuals deteriorate into a repetitive cycle of reenactment, stagnation, and despair.

The Fight-or-Flight Response

The manifestation of the autonomic nervous system's response to stress is the fight-or-flight reaction. This massive response effects change in physiologic function that is so dramatic that in many ways, people are not the same when they are terrified as when they are calm. Attention becomes riveted on the potential threat, so the capacity for reasoning and exercising judgment is negatively influenced by the rising anxiety and fear.

People become less attentive to words and far more focused on threat-related signals in the environment—all of the nonverbal content of communication. As fear rises, they may lose language functions altogether, possibly mediated by the effect of rising levels of cortisol on the language centers of the brain (Van der Kolk, 1996a). Without language, people can take in vital information only in nonverbal form—through physical, emotional, and sensory experiences. As the level of arousal increases, "dissociation" may be triggered as an adaptive response to the hyperarousal, physiologically lowering heart rate and reducing anxiety and pain (Perry, 2001).

Each episode of danger connects to every other episode of danger in the human mind, so that the greater the danger exposure, the greater the sensitivity to danger. With each experience of fight-or-flight, the mind forms a network of connections triggered by every new threatening experience. When exposed to danger repeatedly, people become unusually sensitive, so that even minor threats can trigger an involuntary sequence of physical, emotional, and cognitive responses.

Childhood exposure to trauma, particularly repetitive exposure to interpersonal violence such as sexual assault, has even more dire consequences than adult exposure to a traumatic event for the first time. The expression of corticotropin-releasing factor (CRF), particularly during critical and sensitive moments in development, may have such a profound impact on the developing brain that the brain organizes itself around the traumatic event. Traumatized children are known to develop persistent physiologic hyperarousal and hyperactivity with increased muscle tone, increased startle response, profound sleep disturbances, affect regulation problems, and anxiety, all related to a use-dependent organization of brain stem nuclei involved in the stress response apparatus (Berry, 2000).

LEARNED HELPLESSNESS

Helplessness is a hallmark of a traumatic experience. If the factor of helplessness is removed, the context is changed, and a person may experience the same event as enjoyable or at least worthwhile. Consider the differences between being assaulted by a stranger in an alley and suffering the same injuries as a quarterback being bowled over by a player from the opposing team. If a person is able to master a situation of danger by successfully running away, winning the fight, or getting help, the experience of helplessness is also minimized. Conversely, repetitive exposure to helplessness is so toxic to emotional and physiologic stability that in the service of continued survival, persons are compelled to adapt to the helplessness itself, a phenomenon termed "learned helplessness."

Once an animal has learned to be helpless, it is likely that it will stay put, even when the opportunity for escape is clearly visible. For these animals, survival is now associated with staying where they are, behaviorally expressing the human sentiment of "things could always be worse." Change occurs only when there is active intervention that pulls the animal out of its cage. At first, the animal runs back in, having "learned to be helpless," but after sufficient trials, it finally catches on and relearns—or remembers—how to escape from the still-present danger. It is likely that the rehearsals of escape behavior also alter the animal's biochemistry so that change becomes possible. Although much of the maladaptive social behavior is reversed, these animals remain vulnerable to subsequent stress. As in human experience, animals show individual variation in their responses. Some animals are very resistant to developing "learned helplessness," while others are very vulnerable (Seligman, 1992).

People can learn to be helpless, too, and if people are subjected to a sufficient number of experiences teaching them that nothing they do will affect the outcome, they will then give up trying. This is an adaptive response, serving to conserve vital resources and buffering the vulnerable central nervous system against the negative impact of constant overstimulation. However, once the mechanism of learned helplessness is in place, it does not automatically reverse when escape becomes possible. Children who are repeatedly sexually assaulted learn that there is nothing they can do to adequately protect themselves or escape the situation and that, therefore, their only form of escape is within their own minds—a powerful incentive for dissociation. Later, even when escape is possible, their formerly adaptive response of coping can create a serious obstacle to positive change and may contribute to the dynamic of revictimization. Adults in situations of domestic violence may be exposed repetitively to marital rape and experience the same sense of helpless adaptation. Persons exposed to other forms of sexual assault may also freeze up and be unable to protect themselves when similar triggering circumstances are presented. In such ways, a formerly adaptive coping skill turns into a maladaptive syndrome.

THINKING UNDER STRESS—ACTION, NOT THOUGHT

The capacity to think clearly is severely impaired when individuals are under extreme stress. When danger is perceived, humans are physiologically geared to take action, not to deliberate and weigh alternative choices or to consider the potential outcome of actions. It is more important to respond almost reflexively to preserve life or to protect loved ones. When stressed, humans cannot think clearly, nor can they consider the long-range consequences of behavior. It is impossible to weigh all of the possible options before making a decision or to take the time to obtain all the necessary information that goes into making good decisions. Decisions tend to be based on impulse and on an experienced need to self-protect. As a consequence, such decisions are inflexible, oversimplified, directed toward action, and often very poorly constructed (Janis, 1982). It is not uncommon in such situations to see people demonstrate poor judgment and poor impulse control, which may even lead to violence. Many victims of repetitive exposure to violence have long-term problems with various aspects of thinking. An intolerance of mistakes, denial of personal difficulties, and anger as a problem-solving strategy are some of the problematic thought patterns that have been identified (Alford et al., 1988).

After prolonged exposure to stress, the brain can "reset" itself, and people may experience a state of chronic hyperarousal. In this state they may perceive danger everywhere, even when there is no real danger, because their bodies are signaling the arousal response automatically. As a result, their ability to think clearly and rationally can be chronically and erratically impaired. If this happens in childhood, children's capacities to study, to pay attention in the classroom, and to achieve academically may be severely compromised.

Key Point:
A state of chronic hyperarousal can be experienced after prolonged exposure to stress. The individual may see danger everywhere because the body is automatically signaling the arousal response. Thus, the person cannot think clearly and rationally and appears to be chronically and erratically impaired. Children who experience this hyperarousal state have great difficulty studying, paying attention in class, or achieving academically.

REMEMBERING UNDER STRESS

Exposure to trauma alters people's memory, producing extremes of remembering too much and recalling too little. Unlike other memories, traumatic memories appear to become etched in the mind, unaltered by the passage of time or by subsequent experience. In the last few years, a great deal of debate in the popular and academic press has occurred about whether or not people can "forget" traumatic events and then "remember" them years later, and about whether or not it is possible to "implant" false memories into someone's mind (Bowman, 1996a, 1996b; Brown et al., 1998; International Society of Traumatic Stress Studies [ISTSS], 1998). Much of the confusion about the topic springs from a fundamental ignorance or misunderstanding about the fact that there are several kinds of memory and that overwhelming stress affects the memory system in a way that other experiences do not (Armony & LeDoux, 1997; Cahill, 1997; McEwen & Magarinos, 1997; McNally, 1997; Roozendaal et al., 1997; Spiegel, 1997; Wolfe & Schlesinger, 1997).

Recent studies have demonstrated how dramatically traumatic experiences affect the brain. MRI studies of Vietnam veterans have demonstrated changes in right hippocampal volume in those with PTSD as compared to those without PTSD (Bremner et al., 1994). Other neuroimaging studies have shown similar alterations in women with PTSD who have experienced repeated childhood sexual abuse (Stein et al., 1997). Considerable research has supported the hypothesis that catecholamines influence memory storage processes: low doses of catecholamines enhance memory, while high doses impair memory (Cahill, 1997). The impact of stress hormones has been demonstrated in the amygdala, especially the right amygdala, indicating the importance of this structure in regulating memory storage, particularly for emotionally arousing events (Roozendaal et al., 1997). The hippocampal formation, so important to the human memory apparatus, appears to be particularly vulnerable to insults such as the effects of stress (McEwen & Magarinos, 1997). Data indicate the atrophic changes in the brain, particularly the hippocampus, appear to result from elevated glucocorticoid (such as cortisol) levels.

The result of all this is that the way of remembering things, processing new memories, and accessing old memories is radically changed when under stress. A growing body of evidence indicates that there are actually two different memory systems in the brain—one for verbal learning and remembering that is based on words, and another that is largely nonverbal (Van der Kolk, 1996b). The "normal" memory is the memory system based on language. Under normal conditions, the two kinds of memory function in an integrated way. Our verbal and nonverbal memories are thus usually intertwined and complexly interrelated. However, under conditions of extreme stress, our memory works in a different way.

The human verbally based memory system is particularly vulnerable to high levels of stress. When a person is overwhelmed with fear, he loses the capacity for speech and the capacity to put words to the experience, an occurrence commonly known as "speechless terror." According to recent studies, the part or parts of the brain involved in categorizing and retrieving information are compromised (Van der Kolk et al., 1997). Without words, the mind shifts to a mode of thinking characterized by visual, auditory, olfactory, and kinesthetic images; physical sensations; and strong feelings. This system of processing information is adequate under conditions of serious danger. It is a more rapid method for assimilating information, and by quickly providing data about the circumstances surrounding the danger and making rapid comparisons to previous experience, people may have a vastly increased possibility of survival in the face of threat.

However, the powerful images, feelings, and sensations do not just "go away" once the danger has passed. They are deeply imprinted, more strongly, in fact, than normal, everyday memories. The neuroscientist Joseph LeDoux has called this "emotional memory" and has shown that this kind of memory can be difficult or impossible to erase, although one can learn to override some responses (LeDoux, 1994). Many researchers studying various survivor groups have noted this "engraving" of trauma (Van der Kolk, 1996b). Problems may arise later because the memory of the events that occurred under severe stress is not put into words and is not remembered in the normal way. The normal integration between verbal and nonverbal experiences does not occur. Instead, the nonverbal memories remain "frozen in time" in the form of images, body sensations like smells, touch, tastes, facial expressions, voice tones, physical pain, and strong emotions.

A flashback is a sudden, intrusive re-experiencing of a fragment of one of those traumatic, unverbalized memories. Flashbacks are likely to occur when people are stressed or frightened, or when triggered by any association to the traumatic event. Their minds can become flooded with the images, emotions, and physical sensations associated with the original trauma. They feel like the traumatic experience is happening again, and they may have difficulty separating the past from the present. Often they do not recognize the experience they are having as a flashback but instead feel that they are "losing their minds" or having a "panic attack."

Trauma may result in "speechless terror," and the capacity to encode information in language is radically altered. As a result, the victim has developed what has become known as "amnesia" for the traumatic event—the memory is there, but there are no words attached to it, so it cannot be either talked about or even thought about. Instead, the memory presents itself as some form of flashback, nonverbal behavior, or a behavioral reenactment of a previous event. Even thinking of flashbacks as "memories" is inaccurate and misleading. When someone experiences a flashback, he does not remember the experience, but relives it. Often the flashback is forgotten as quickly as it happens because the two memory systems are so disconnected from each other.

Many times, the flashback occurs in the form of a physical symptom that is a reminder of the previous assault, as when a rape victim experiences sharp and penetrating pelvic pain that can then become a chronic pelvic pain syndrome. Symptoms such as these have come to be known as "body memories." Physical symptoms are not likely to be recognized by either the sufferer or health care professionals as related to a previous traumatic event. The physical symptom is experienced separated from any other reminders of the traumatic event, so the victim does not connect the pain in the present with the terrifying experience of the past. Her health care provider, lacking historical information, is not likely to consider this as a possibility in the differential diagnosis. This nonverbal memory may be the only memory a person has of the traumatic event, or at least of certain key portions of the event. She is likely to reject any interpretation of her physical symptoms as being related to a past trauma, in part because she hears such an explanation as a minimization of her pain, as if she were being told it is "all in her head," and in part because she is continuing to unconsciously protect herself against being flooded by the feelings connected to the past trauma.

Over time, as people try to limit situations that promote hyperarousal and flashbacks, limit relationships that trigger emotions, and employ behaviors designed to control emotional responses, they may become progressively numb to all emotions and feel depressed and alienated. In this state, it takes greater and greater stimulation to feel a sense of being alive. They will often engage in all kinds of risk-taking behaviors because that is the only way they feel "inside" themselves once again. If an experience cannot be remembered, one cannot learn from it. This is one of the most devastating aspects of prolonged stress.

The picture becomes even more complicated for children who are exposed to repeated experiences of unprotected stress. Their bodies, brains, and minds are still

Key Point:
Even when the danger has passed, the strong images, feelings, and sensations that have been aroused do not just go away. They persist, being more strongly felt than normal memories, and can be difficult or impossible to erase.

developing. We are only beginning to understand memory, traumatic memory, and how these memory systems develop and influence each other (Perry, 1993; Schwarz & Perry, 1994). Children who are traumatized also experience flashbacks that have no words. For healing to occur, people often need to put the experience into a narrative, give it words, and share it with themselves and others. Words allow one to put things into a time sequence—past, present, future, which finally allows a flashback to become a true memory instead of a haunting presence. Because a child's capacity for verbalization is just developing, his ability to put the traumatic experience into words is particularly difficult. In cases of childhood terror, language functions are often compromised. Instead, children frequently act out their memories in behavior instead of words (James, 1994). They show what happened even when they cannot tell. This automatic behavioral reliving of trauma is called "traumatic reenactment."

EMOTIONS AND TRAUMA—DISSOCIATION

Emotions can kill. It is possible to die of fright or to die of a broken heart. Every vital organ system is closely connected through the autonomic nervous system with the emotions. However, people rarely do die from emotional upsets. A fundamental reason for such rarity is the built-in "safety valve" called "dissociation."

Dissociation is defined as "a disruption in the usually integrated functions of consciousness, memory, identity, or perception of the environment" (APA, 1994). Dissociation provides a real advantage—it allows one to do more than one thing at a time. People can go on autopilot and automatically complete tasks previously learned well while being focused on something else.

Traumatized people make special use of this capacity as a way of buffering the central nervous system against life-threatening shock. Human beings can dissociate in a number of different ways.

One way to dissociate is so common that almost everyone does it—splitting off experience from feelings about that experience. So commonly do humans cut off feelings about what happened to them while still remembering facts about the event that it may not even be noticed that they do not feel the emotions that would normally be expected under the circumstances. In such cases, instead of seeing the emotional numbing that has occurred to the person, comments are made about "how well Jane is coping with her loss" or "how extraordinary it is that John never seems to get ruffled, even if someone is yelling at him." But Jane and John are not necessarily "coping well." They may be dissociated from their feelings, and their capacity for normal emotional interaction may be consequently diminished.

It is possible to cut off all emotions, but that usually happens only in extreme cases of repetitive and almost unendurable trauma, and is known as "emotional numbing." More commonly, people cut off or diminish specific emotional responses, based on the danger the emotion may present to continued functioning. Children experiencing trauma learn how to not feel: they learn to dissociate their emotions from their conscious experience and their nonverbal expression of that emotion. In doing so, they believe they can stay safer than if they show what they feel. That does not mean the emotion actually goes away. It does not.

As this process continues over time, the individual may increasingly shut off normal responses and dampen any emotional experience that could lead back to the traumatic memory. People may withdraw from relationships that could trigger memories, or curtail sensory and physical experiences that could remind them of the trauma. At the same time, the individual may be unconsciously compelled to reenact the traumatic experience through certain behavior. Such reenactment increases the likelihood that instead of managing to avoid repeated trauma, the person is likely to become revictimized.

Key Point:
In dissociation, people are able to function automatically while being focused on something completely different. When a person has experienced trauma, dissociation allows him to buffer the central nervous system against life-threatening shock.

As this process unfolds, the person is likely to become increasingly depressed. These avoidance symptoms, along with the intrusive symptoms such as flashbacks and nightmares, comprise two of the interacting and escalating aspects of PTSD set in the context of a more generalized physical hyperarousal. As these alternating symptoms come to dominate traumatized people's lives, they feel increasingly alienated from everything that gives their lives meaning—favorite activities, other people, a sense of direction and purpose, a sense of spirituality, a sense of community. It is not surprising that, for some people, slow self-destruction through addictions or fast self-destruction through suicide is often the final outcome of these syndromes. For other people, rage at others comes to dominate the picture, and these people are the ones who end up becoming significant threats to other people as well as to themselves.

For children who are traumatized, the responses to and consequences of trauma are amplified because the traumatic experiences interfere with the processes of normal development. For many children, in fact, traumatic experience becomes the norm rather than the exception, and they fail to develop a concept of what is normal or healthy. They do not learn how to think in a careful, quiet, and deliberate way. They do not learn how to have mutual, compassionate, and satisfying relationships. It should come as no surprise that these children often become maladjusted troublemakers who pose problems for teachers, schools, other children, and ultimately everyone.

ENDORPHINS AND STRESS—ADDICTION TO TRAUMA

The secretion of endorphins is an important part of the stress response. Endorphins provide relief from anxiety and distress. Both adults and children are elevated when social support is increased and lowered when social support is withdrawn. Not only do endorphins calm anxiety, improve mood, and decrease aggression, but they also are analgesics, chemically related to morphine and heroin. People who are exposed to repeated experiences of prolonged stress experience repeatedly high levels of circulating endorphins and are likely to develop what has been termed "stress-induced analgesia" (Glover, 1992). One hypothesis is that people can become "addicted" to their own internal endorphins and as a result only feel calm when they are under stress. When stress is relieved, they experience a withdrawal effect that leads to fearfulness, irritability, hyperarousal, and even violence, much like someone who is withdrawing from heroin (Ibarra et al., 1994; Volpicelli et al., 1999). This has been called "addiction to trauma" (Van der Kolk & Greenberg, 1987).

Key Point:
It has been hypothesized that some people become addicted to their own internal endorphins and only feel calm when they are under stress. Relieving stress for these individuals can lead to fearfulness, irritability, hyperarousal, or even violence.

This makes clear several perplexing symptoms. For example, stress-addicted children are likely to be those who cannot tolerate a calm atmosphere but must keep antagonizing everyone else until the stress level is high enough for them to achieve some degree of internal equilibrium again. These are children who as adults are unable to trust or be comforted by other people—in fact, other people have been the fundamental source of their distress. Instead, these children must fall back on whatever resources they can muster within themselves, resources that they can control, to achieve any kind of equilibrium. As adults, under stress, people who have been brutalized as children may again resort to behaviors that help induce some kind of alteration in the opioid system. These behaviors can include self-mutilation, risk-taking behavior, compulsive sexuality, involvement in violent activity, bingeing and purging, and drug addiction.

Violence is exciting and stressful. Repeated violent acting-out, gang behavior, fighting, bullying, and many forms of criminal activity have the additional side effect of producing high levels of stress in people who have grown addicted to such risk-taking behavior. This also helps to explain self-mutilation in its many forms. People who self-mutilate have learned that inflicting harm on the body will induce the release of endorphins that will provide some relief, at least temporarily (McCown et al., 1993).

TRAUMA-BONDING

Trauma-bonding refers to a relationship based on terror and the distortion of normal attachment behavior into something perverse and cruel (James, 1994). People who are terrorized, whether as adult or child victims of abuse, experience their abuser as being in total control of life and death. The perpetrator is the source not only of the pain and terror, but also of relief from that pain. He is the source of threat, but he is also the source of hope. Cognitively, the victim may want nothing more than to have a healthy relationship, but outside of conscious, cognitive awareness, what the victim has learned is how to relate to the perpetrator without being killed. This nonverbal awareness often determines who the person is chosen by or chooses to relate to, based on a need to repeat early childhood attachment behavior, even as adults. For victims of repetitive abuse, abusive relationships become the normative idea of what relationships are all about.

TRAUMATIC REENACTMENT

History repeats itself. People who have been traumatized develop what may begin as life-saving coping mechanisms, but these very mechanisms may lead to compulsive repetition. People often reenact what they cannot remember. People may cue each other to play roles in personal dramas, secretly hoping that someone will offer a different script, a different outcome to the drama, depending on how damaging the experiences have been. The only way that the nonverbal brain can "speak" is through behaviors. Traumatized people, through reenactment, are trying to repeatedly "tell their story" in very overt or highly disguised ways. They may use the language of physical symptoms or of deviant behavior.

Traumatized people are cut off from language, deprived of the power of words that gives meaning to their overwhelming experiences, trapped in speechless terror. Victims need the help, the words, the signals of caring others, but they must find some way to signal others about their distress in a language that has no words. Unfortunately, most of these "cries for help" fall on deaf ears. Instead, without hearing the meaning in the message, people judge, condemn, exclude, and alienate the person who is behaving in a self-destructive or antisocial way. The end result of this complex sequence of posttraumatic events is repetition, stagnation, rigidity, and a fear of change, all in the context of a deteriorating life. As emotional, physical, and social symptoms of distress pile up on each other, victims try desperately to extricate themselves by using the same protective devices that they used to cope with threat in the first place—dissociation, avoidance, aggression, destructive attachments, damaging behaviors, and substance addiction.

THE CONSEQUENCES OF TRAUMATIC EXPERIENCE

Children who are sexually assaulted demonstrate a number of adjustment problems (Berliner & Elliott, 1996). Sexually abused children are more likely to have sexual behaviors that pose problems for them at home and at school and that may lead to perpetrator behavior directed at other children (Hall et al., 1998). Children who have been both physically and sexually abused appear to be at highest risk of psychiatric disturbance, including PTSD, major depression, dysthymia, suicidality, self-mutilation, somatic complaints, poor self-esteem, anxiety disorders, sleep disturbances, substance abuse disorders, learning disabilities, conduct disorders, delinquency, aggression, increased health risk behaviors, and inappropriate sexual behavior (Ackerman et al., 1998; De Bellis et al., 1994).

As traumatized children make the transition into adolescence, adjustment problems continue. A community sample of 1490 adolescents, age 12 to 19 years, was analyzed to investigate the relationship between a history of sexual abuse and adolescent functioning. Both sexually abused girls and boys reported significantly more emotional problems, behavior problems, and suicidal thoughts and attempts than their nonabused counterparts. The results also indicated that the experience of sexual abuse carried far more consequences for boys than for girls with regard to the use of drugs and alcohol, aggressive/criminal behavior, truancy, and suicidal thoughts and behavior. Whereas 2.6% of the nonabused boys reported a former suicide attempt, the percentage of the sexually abused boys reporting a suicide attempt was 13 times higher (Garnefski & Arends, 1998).

Posttraumatic Stress Disorder

The prevalence of PTSD after rape is extraordinarily high. In a review of nine studies that investigated the prevalence of PTSD among victims of rape or other sexual violence, four studies indicated that the rate was greater than 70% (De Girolamo & McFarlane, 1996). The National Women's Study produced dramatic evidence of the mental health impact of rape by determining comparative rates of several mental health problems among rape victims and women who had never been victims of rape (Kilpatrick et al., 1992). Rape victims were three times more likely than women who had never been victims of crime to have ever had a major depressive episode and were 3.5 times more likely to be currently experiencing a major depressive episode. Rape victims were 4.1 times more likely to have contemplated suicide and 13 times more likely than people who were not rape victims to have actually made a suicide attempt. The fact that 13% of all rape victims had actually attempted suicide confirms the devastating and potentially life-threatening mental health impact of rape.

In a survey of over 2000 women asked about victimization experiences, rates of "nervous breakdowns," suicidal ideation, and suicide attempts were significantly higher for crime victims than for nonvictims. Victims of attempted rape, completed rape, and attempted sexual molestation had problems more frequently than did victims of attempted robbery, completed robbery, aggravated assault, or completed molestation. In this study, nearly one rape victim in five (19.2%) had attempted suicide, whereas only 2.2% of nonvictims had done so (Kessler et al., 1995). Most sexual assault victims' mental health problems came after their victimization (Kilpatrick et al., 1985).

There is a disturbingly high rate of comorbidity with PTSD, further complicating recovery for many survivors of sexual assault. Even in the most conservative study, those with PTSD were two to four times more likely than those without PTSD to have another psychiatric disorder, particularly somatization disorder (Solomon & Davidson, 1997). According to one study, somatization was found to be 90 times more likely in those with PTSD than in those without PTSD (Davidson et al., 1991).

In another study, people with one or more symptoms of PTSD were more likely than those without any mental disorder to experience poor social support, marital difficulties, and occupational problems, as well as greater impairment of income and more disability measures than even those with major depressive disorder. The people with PTSD symptoms were also more likely to have a number of chronic illnesses. Although these patients had a disproportionate utilization of the health care system, they were reluctant to seek mental health treatment, a finding that has been seen in many other studies as well (Solomon & Davidson, 1997). A partial listing of some of the most recent comorbid studies is daunting: panic disorder and social phobia, borderline personality disorder, somatiform disorders, obsessive-compulsive disorder, and anxiety disorders (Bleich et al., 1994; Ellason et al., 1996; Fierman et al., 1993; Herman et al., 1989; Orsillo et al., 1996; Perry et al., 1990; Pitman, 1993; Rogers et al., 1996; Saxe et al., 1994; Vasile et al., 1997).

Child sexual abuse has been found to be comorbid with many later psychiatric problems. A number of studies have found correlations between childhood sexual abuse and borderline personality disorders, panic disorder, suicide attempts, eating disorders, depression, bulimia and generalized anxiety, and increased risk for lifetime diagnoses of major depression, panic disorder, phobia, somatization

Key Point:
After rape, the prevalence of PTSD is extremely high, with rape victims also at risk for major depressive episodes and suicide.

disorder, chronic pain, and drug abuse (Angst et al., 1992; Bushnell et al., 1992; Connors & Morse, 1993; Herman et al., 1989; Leserman et al., 1996; Perry et al., 1990; Pollack et al., 1992; Walker et al., 1992). In a review of all post-1987 studies on the long-term consequences of sexual abuse, sexually abused subjects reported higher levels of general psychologic distress and higher rates of both major psychologic disorders and personality disorders than nonabused subjects (Polusny & Follette, 1995). In addition, child sexual abuse survivors report higher rates of substance abuse, binge eating, somatization, and suicidal behaviors than nonabused subjects. Adult survivors of child sexual abuse report poorer social and interpersonal relationship functioning; greater sexual dissatisfaction and dysfunction, including high-risk sexual behavior; and a greater tendency toward revictimization through adult sexual assault and physical partner violence.

There are at least 10 other trauma-related disorders, including brief reactive psychosis, dissociative identity disorder, dissociative amnesia, borderline personality disorder, somatization disorder, dream anxiety disorder, and antisocial personality disorder (Davidson, 1993). The connection between borderline personality disorder and trauma, particularly childhood trauma, has been studied extensively by a number of authors (Ellason et al., 1996; Herman et al., 1989; Perry et al., 1990; Sabo, 1997).

The clinical picture for sexual abuse survivors and other trauma victims who are exposed to repetitive trauma is particularly complicated. The most common clinical presentation encompasses seven clusters of symptoms best described as "complex PTSD" and includes alterations in regulating affective arousal, alterations in attention and consciousness, somatization, alterations in self-perception, alterations in perception of the perpetrator, alterations in relations to others, and alterations in systems of meaning. The presence of these symptom clusters has been demonstrated to differentiate adult victims of childhood interpersonal violence and abuse from adult-onset trauma syndromes associated with disasters (Herman, 1992; Van der Kolk et al., 1994).

Trauma and Substance Abuse

Another concurrent problem for victims of violence is the intimate connection between substance abuse and PTSD. People with PTSD are two to three times more likely to have a substance abuse disorder. Studies show that 27% to 35% of adult sexual abuse victims have a history of alcohol abuse and 21% a history of drug abuse (Green, 1993). In a subpopulation of female incest survivors who had been inpatients in psychiatric institutions, the numbers of substance abusers rose to 80% (Green, 1993). Battered women are 15 times more likely to abuse alcohol (Salasin & Rich, 1993). According to the National Women's Study, there was also substantial evidence that rape victims had higher rates of drug and alcohol consumption, and a greater likelihood of having drug and alcohol-related problems than nonvictims (Kilpatrick et al., 1992). Estimates are that as many as 75% of women in treatment for alcoholism have a history of sexual abuse (Bollerud, 1990). A history of childhood rape doubled the number of alcohol abuse symptoms that women experienced in adulthood, and there was a significant relationship between pathways connecting childhood rape to PTSD symptoms and PTSD symptoms to alcohol use (Epstein et al., 1998).

Sexual assault may have a great deal to do with the rising incidence of substance abuse among the adolescent population. In a 1995 Minnesota study of over 120,000 public school students in grades 6, 9, and 12, physical and sexual abuse were associated with an increased likelihood of the use of alcohol, marijuana, and almost all other drugs for both males and females. Use of multiple substances was highly elevated among victims of abuse, with the highest rates seen among students who reported both physical and sexual abuse. Abuse victims also reported initiating substance use earlier than their nonabused peers and gave more reasons for using, including coping with painful emotions and escaping from problems (Harrison et al., 1997).

SEXUAL ASSAULT AND NEUROBIOLOGIC CHANGES

Evidence is accumulating about the nature and extent of psychobiologic changes that are secondary to sexual assault. The results are disturbing, making it clear that children's psychobiologic development and adult function can be profoundly affected by sexual assault. In a longitudinal study of sexually abused girls, researchers have demonstrated that sexual abuse is associated with dysregulatory responses of the hypothalamic-pituitary axis, similar to changes seen in stressed animals. They have also noted elevated levels of urinary catecholamines, a twofold higher incidence of plasma antinuclear antibodies, and disproportionately high levels of illnesses and infections in the abused group (Putnam & Trickett, 1997). Other studies support the connection between the hypothalamic-pituitary axis and later problems in adulthood. It has been hypothesized that early adverse experiences result in an increased sensitivity to the effects of stress later in life and render an individual vulnerable to stress-related psychiatric disorders. This vulnerability may be mediated by persistent changes in corticotropin-releasing-factor–containing neurons, the hypothalamic-pituitary-adrenal axis, and the sympathetic nervous system (Heim & Nemeroff, 1999). Maltreated children with PTSD excreted significantly greater concentrations of urinary dopamine and norepinephrine over 24 hours than the control group of children with overanxious disorder (De Bellis et al., 1999).

Studies have demonstrated that abused children have reversed hemispheric asymmetry and greater left hemisphere coherence in contrast to nonabused children. These studies demonstrate that early abuse affects brain development in a number of ways and that the left hemisphere appears to be more vulnerable than the right (Teicher et al., 1997). Other researchers propose that childhood trauma alters limbic, mid-brain, and brain structures through "use dependent" modifications secondary to prolonged alarm reactions (Perry et al., 1995).

Sexually assaulted adults show profound psychobiologic changes as well. Women with a history of prior physical or sexual assault showed a significantly attenuated cortisol response to the acute stress of rape compared to women without such a history. In a study of female patients diagnosed with borderline personality disorder and a past history of sustained childhood abuse, psychobiologic indicators suggested that childhood exposure had negatively affected the serotonin system (Rinne et al., 2000).

Women who develop PTSD secondary to childhood sexual abuse show a much higher rate of neurologic "soft sign" scores, that is, subtle neurologic changes, than women who had also been sexually abused as children but did not have PTSD. These differences could not be explained by alcoholism or head injury. These subjects reported more neurodevelopmental problems and more childhood attention-deficit/hyperactivity disorder symptoms and had lower IQs, all of which were significantly correlated with neurologic soft signs (Gurvits et al., 2000). In fact, the list of biological abnormalities associated in PTSD is growing. Baseline heart rate and blood pressure are increased. The hypothalamic-pituitary axis is dysregulated, blood triiodothyronine level is increased, blood and urinary cortisol levels are decreased, and platelet alpha2-adrenergic receptor binding and platelet serotonin uptake are increased (Pitman, 1997). These findings are of particular significance to sexual assault victims, given the high rate of PTSD secondary to sexual assault.

THE HEALTH CONSEQUENCES OF TRAUMA

Victims of trauma often suffer from a multitude of physical disorders not directly related to whatever injuries they have suffered. The number of reports connecting PTSD with other physiologic conditions includes fibromyalgia, chronic pain, irritable bowel syndrome, asthma, peptic ulcer, other gastrointestinal illness, and chronic pelvic pain (Amir et al., 1997; Badura et al., 1997; Benedikt & Kolb, 1986; Davidson et al., 1991; Drossman, 1995; Geisser et al., 1996; Irwin et al., 1996;

Key Point:
The psychobiologic development of children and their later ability to function as adults are severely disturbed by sexual assault. Early adverse experiences raise the sensitivity to the effects of stress later in life and make a person more vulnerable to stress-related psychiatric disorders.

Walker et al., 1996; Walling et al., 1994). Child sexual abuse has been found to be comorbid with many later physical problems. A number of studies have found correlations between eating disorders, chemical dependency, irritable bowel syndrome, chronic pelvic pain, chronic pain, and drug abuse (Connors & Morse, 1993; Ellason et al., 1996; Irwin et al., 1996; Leserman et al., 1991; Reiter et al., 1991; Walker et al., 1992). There is now a science of stress-related disorders that details how stress negatively affects the body in a number of ways, producing short-term and long-term physical consequences (Sarno, 1998).

STRESS, MOODS, AND IMMUNITY

As the field of psychoneuroimmunology expands, a growing body of information discusses the relationship between stress, traumatic stress, and the immune system. Even mild stress has an impact on the immune system (Bachen et al., 1992; Brosschot et al., 1994). There is also evidence that interpersonal stressors have a different impact from nonsocial stressors. Subsequent analyses suggest that objective stressful events are related to larger immune changes than subjective self-reports of stress, that immune response varies with stressor duration, and that interpersonal events are related to different immune outcomes than nonsocial events (Herbert & Cohen, 1993). Factors such as stress, negative emotion, clinical depression, lack of social support, and repression/denial can negatively influence both cellular and humoral indicators of immune status and function. At least in the case of the less serious infectious diseases (colds, influenza, herpes), there is consistent and convincing evidence of links between stress and negative emotion, and disease onset and progression (Cohen & Herbert, 1996). The interaction between stress and immunity is complex, mediated by emotions. Thus concepts such as coping, control, helplessness, and hopelessness are required to understand the complex nature of the immune responses (Ursin, 1994).

In primates, there is a large body of evidence that disruptions in social relationships have many immunologic sequelae, particularly in the young monkey. There is evidence in infant monkeys that normal maternal care is important for the development and maintenance of normal immune function. The immune responses of adult monkeys are also affected by aggression within the group (Coe, 1993).

In two related studies, one of children in day care and another of children entering kindergarten, the development of respiratory illnesses was found to be related to stressful life events (Boyce et al., 1995). Another group evaluating adolescents found that there was a correlation between significant negative life events and lowered natural killer cell activity (Birmaher et al., 1994).

CHRONIC VIOLENCE AND HEALTH

Interest has grown in looking at the connection between women's experience of violence and subsequent health problems. A recent study by the Center for Disease Control surveyed almost 14,000 adults in a health maintenance organization, asking participants about their adverse childhood experiences, which were divided into categories that included physical, sexual, and emotional abuse, witnessing violence against one's mother, and living as a child with a household member who was either imprisoned, mentally ill, suicidal, or a substance abuser. There was a direct relationship between the number of categories of adverse childhood experience and adult diseases, including ischemic heart disease, cancer, chronic lung disease, skeletal fractures, and liver disease. The seven categories of adverse childhood experiences were strongly interrelated, and persons with multiple categories of childhood exposure were likely to have multiple health risk factors later in life (Felitti et al., 1998).

Although the correlation is often unrecognized, women who have been sexually abused and sexually assaulted routinely present to their gynecologists with a number of complaints. In a randomized survey of 1599 women, 31.5% of participants reported a diagnosis of gynecologic problems in the past 5 years. Those with problems were more likely to report childhood abuse, violent crime victimization, and spouse abuse (Plichta & Abraham, 1996).

Sexual abuse and assault take a heavy toll on sexual adjustment. A recent study examined the differential effects of child and adult sexual abuse on adult sexual functioning. Women who had a history of sexual abuse in childhood or adulthood experienced more sexual dissatisfaction than nonabused women and had higher numbers of unsafe sexual partners (Bartoi & Kinder, 1998). In a study looking at the relationship between sexual abuse of males and females and engagement in sadomasochistic sexual practices, self-reported sexual abuse was higher among the participants, and those who reported abuse were more likely to have visited a physician due to physical injuries secondary to the sexual activity. Furthermore, the higher the frequency of abuse, the poorer the body image of the abused male participants (Nordling et al., 2000).

Several other recent studies have found associations between childhood maltreatment and adverse adult health outcomes. A history of childhood maltreatment has been significantly associated with several adverse physical health outcomes. Maltreatment status was associated with perceived poorer overall health, greater physical and emotional functional disability, increased numbers of distressing physical symptoms, and a greater number of health risk behaviors. Women with multiple types of maltreatment showed the greatest health decrements for both self-reported symptoms and physician coded diagnoses (Walker et al., 1999). Women with a history of childhood sexual abuse may be particularly susceptible to the effects of heightened daily stress and may display this susceptibility in the report of physical symptoms (Thakkar & McCanne, 2000). Compared with nonvictims, victimized women reported more distress and less well-being, visited a physician twice as frequently, and had outpatient costs that were 2.5 times greater (Koss et al., 1991).

Key Point:
A significant relationship exists between a history of childhood maltreatment and adverse physical health outcomes.

SEXUAL ASSAULT AND REVICTIMIZATION

One of the many horrors that result from sexual assault is the tendency of victims to be revictimized. Child sexual abuse survivors appear to be particularly vulnerable to revictimization experiences. Victimization before age 14 years almost doubles the risk of later adolescent victimization. In a recent study, sexual victimization among university women was highest for those who had been first assaulted in early adolescence. Adolescent victims of rape or attempted rape, in particular, were 4.4 times more likely to be as seriously assaulted during their first year of college (Humphrey & White, 2000). Offering explanations for this phenomenon among adolescents, one group of investigators propose that revictimization appears to arise because the childhood and family factors that are associated with childhood sexual abuse are also associated with increased sexual risks during adolescence. Also, exposure to childhood sexual abuse may encourage early onset sexual activity, which places those exposed at greater sexual risk over the period of adolescence (Fergusson et al., 1997).

Prostitution

Prostitution can be thought of as a special case of revictimization for many sexually abused children and adults. Study after study shows a marked and dramatic relationship between prostitution and a previous history of sexual abuse. Running away from homes in which they are being abused provides children with distinct pathways into prostitution. Childhood sexual victimization nearly doubles the odds of entry into prostitution throughout the lives of women (McClanahan et al., 1999). In a study of 130 prostitutes working in San Francisco, 57% reported that they had been sexually assaulted as children (Farley & Barkan, 1998). Children who were sexually abused are 27.7 times more likely to be arrested for prostitution as an adult than are nonvictims (Widom & Kuhns, 1996).

Victim to Victimizer Behavior

When the effects of trauma are understood, it becomes possible to grasp how someone could be victimized and become a victimizer as a result. A victim is both helpless and powerless, and as we have seen, helplessness is a noxious human experience that people seek to avoid. Once victimized, a possible outcome for the victim is to assume the power of the perpetrator by becoming someone who terrorizes and abuses others. Such behavior can reduce anxiety while providing a certain excitement, and the combination of these two effects can become habit-forming.

These effects can also be profoundly culturally influenced. The traditional definition of masculinity does not allow for helplessness—a man cannot be a victim and still be considered masculine. In contrast, the traditional definition of femininity not only allows for, but also encourages, powerlessness and therefore the open possibility of victimization. It should come as no surprise, therefore, that boys and men would accommodate more easily to the victimizer role and women, the victim role. We must contend with the reality that normative standards about the acceptability of the sexual assault of women remain confused. In a 1993 national study of 1700 sixth to ninth graders, a majority of the boys considered rape "acceptable" under certain conditions and many of the girls agreed (Wallis, 1995). According to several sources, 51% to 60% of college men report that they would rape a woman if they were certain that they could get away with it. One out of 12 college men surveyed had committed acts that met the legal definition of rape; 84% of these men said what they did was definitely not rape (Warshaw, 1988).

The strong connection between child abuse, particularly child sexual abuse, and later committing a sexual offense is still being studied. The neglect of this important topic can probably be attributed to, or is at least consistent with, the neglect of the sexual abuse of boys and adult men. Most sexual abuse of adult men is happening in prisons, while boys are frequently abused at home and in other settings with trusted caregivers.

Childhood victimization is a significant predictor of the number of lifetime symptoms of antisocial personality disorder and of a diagnosis of antisocial personality disorder (Luntz & Widom, 1994). In one study, 595 men were evaluated for childhood sexual and physical abuse and perpetration history. Eleven percent of the men reported sexual abuse alone, 17% reported physical abuse alone, and 17% reported both sexual and physical abuse. Of the 257 men in the sample who reported some form of childhood abuse, 38% reported some form of perpetration themselves, either sexual or physical; of the 126 perpetrators, 70% reported having been abused in childhood. Thus, most perpetrators were abused, but most abused men did not perpetrate (Lisak et al., 1996).

Another group of researchers studied children age 9 to 14 years who were sexual offenders. The sex offenders were found to exhibit a significant history of nonsexual antisocial behavior, physical abuse, and psychiatric comorbidity; 65% of the boys had been sexually abused (Shaw et al., 1993). The differences between those who victimize adults and those who victimize children have also been studied with respect to sexual abuse. While an estimated 22% of those who victimized children reported having been sexually abused, fewer than 6% of those who victimized adults reported such backgrounds.

In a study of serial rapists incarcerated in US prisons, 56.1% were judged to have at least one forced or exploitative abuse experience in boyhood, as compared to a study of 2972 college males reporting 7.3% experiencing boyhood sexual abuse. Also, the rapist sample revealed higher rates of a family member as an abuser compared to the college sample. Fifty-one percent reenacted their own abuse as a preadolescent with their earliest victims being girls they knew in the neighborhood, their sisters, or a girlfriend. When investigators looked at men on death row, they found a history of family violence in all of them, including severe physical and/or sexual abuse in 14 of 16 cases (Freedman & Hemenway, 2000).

However, like any complex problem, there is no one-to-one direct relationship between being victimized and becoming a victimizer. Most sexually abused people do not go on to victimize people. It is not yet clear why some children follow such a course and other children, similarly victimized, do not. Nor does one kind of victim experience necessarily predict the ways in which an offender will victimize others. Although information is accumulating about the numbers of sexual offenders who have been sexually abused, the degree to which they may also have been physically abused, emotionally abused, or neglected is unknown. When sexual offenders deny having been sexually abused, insufficient data are available to analyze their exposure to other traumatizing or abusive situations.

Key Point:
Most sexually abused individuals do not go on to victimize others. It is not yet known why some children do follow this course and others who have undergone the same degree of abuse do not.

Sexual Assault and Parenting

One of the most pernicious aspects of violence is its multigenerational impact. Violence in one generation often leads to violence in the next. Parenting behavior can be profoundly affected by the impact of trauma.

Main and Goldwyn (1984) have elaborated experimentally on John Bowlby's original formulation of childhood attachment. In studying mothers and their children, they have noted that a mother's apparent experience of her own mother as rejecting is systematically related to both her rejection of her own infant as observed in the laboratory and to systematic distortions in her own cognitive processes. These distortions, such as idealization of the rejecting parent, difficulty in remembering childhood, and an incoherence in discussing attachment, are each significantly related to the mother's rejection of her own infant. Distortions in representation of an abusing parent may play a positive role in the perpetuation of child abuse.

Marked differences have been noted in the ability of physically abusive and nonabusive mothers to be sensitive to the moods and signals of their children (Fontana & Robison, 1984). Abusive mothers spent less time looking at their children, were less focused in their attention on them, barraged them with words and actions that were unaffected by the child's response, were physically coercive, and spent more time issuing directives and orders than mothers from similar backgrounds who do not abuse their children. In a study in which abusive and nonabusive mothers were evaluated on their ability to respond empathically to a crying child, the high-risk mothers were less empathic and more hostile in response to a crying child (Milner et al., 1995).

Mothers who were abusive to their children have been found to be more dissociative about their own history, tending to idealize their own childhoods more, to avoid dealing with the implications of the past, and to be inconsistent in their childhood descriptions as compared to mothers who broke the cycle of abuse (Egeland & Susman-Stillman, 1996). This finding has been supported in other studies, indicating that mothers with dissociative disorders can have significant difficulties in parenting compared to nondissociative inpatient mothers and a control group. They tend to show more abusiveness toward the child, have problems using constructive parenting skills, use more hurtful forms of discipline, demonstrate difficulties in showing affection, exhibit problematic attachment behaviors, are subject to cognitive distortions, have difficulties with the regulation of anger, and are inadequate in the ability to employ actions to promote the developmental growth of the child (Benjamin et al., 1996). Mothers with a history of child sexual abuse were significantly more anxious about intimate aspects of parenting than the comparison group. They also reported significantly more overall stress as parents. The index group recalled that their own parents were significantly less caring and that their fathers were more controlling than the comparison group. Mothers with a history of child sexual abuse who attend mental health services are often worried that their normal parenting behaviors may be inappropriate or seen as such by other people. These anxieties seem associated with their history of childhood sexual abuse (Douglas, 2000).

Girls whose mothers were sexually abused were 3.6 times more likely to be sexually victimized. Maternal sexual abuse history combined with maternal drug use placed daughters at the most elevated risk. Maternal sexual abuse history indicates a strong potential for the intergenerational transmission of child sexual abuse (Whiffen et al., 2000). Another study examined characteristics of mothers of boys who were involved in sexual abuse either as victims, perpetrators, or both. Depression, child abuse histories, and current attributions were investigated for 80 mothers of boys in three abuse referral groups—victimized perpetrators, nonvictimized perpetrators, and victims only—in comparison with a group of boys showing externalizing behaviors. Sexual victimization in their own childhood was reported by 55% of mothers of perpetrators and 30% of mothers of victims. High rates of spouse abuse were reported by both mothers of perpetrators (72%) and mothers of victims (50%) (New et al., 1999).

When researchers looked at maltreated children and their mothers, PTSD was significantly overrepresented in the children of mothers diagnosed with PTSD. The onset of maltreatment was significantly earlier among children whose mothers meet PTSD criteria than among other maltreated children (Famularo et al., 1994). These findings among mothers have been supported by findings of impaired parenting skills in fathers as well. In a sample of 1200 male Vietnam veterans and 376 of their partners, male veterans with current PTSD showed markedly elevated levels of severe and diffuse problems in marital and family adjustment, in parenting skills, and in violent behavior (Jordan et al., 1992). It is hypothesized that part of the problem for these parents is the prolonged hyperarousal that accompanies stress in those previously exposed to trauma. In laboratory experiments comparing the effects of stressors on mothers with a history of maltreatment and those without such a history, the mothers who had been physically abused in childhood tended to get more aroused and stay aroused longer after even a relatively mild stressor than mothers in the control group (Casanova et al., 1992, 1994).

Studies have supported the close connection between child abuse and domestic violence. In one study of abused children, 59.4% of the mothers exhibited behavior considered to be highly suggestive of current or previous victimization. In fact, in homes where domestic violence occurs, children are at 1500% greater risk of child abuse than the national average (National Victim Center, 1993). A review of child abuse studies reveals that one third of abused children will grow up to become abusive parents, one third will not, and another third are at risk. Abused mothers who were able to break the abusive cycle were significantly more likely to have received emotional support from a nonabusive adult during childhood, were more likely to have participated in therapy during some period of their lives, and were more likely to have had a nonabusive and more stable, emotionally supportive, and satisfying relationship with a mate. Abused mothers who reenacted their maltreatment with their own children experienced significantly more life stress and were more anxious, dependent, immature, and depressed (Egeland et al., 1988). Research has found that women who continued the cycle of child abuse reenacted their own abuse, identified with their abuser or with a nonprotective parent, had poor attachment with their own parents, used dissociation or other defensive behaviors to protect themselves from memories of their abuse, and had not been able to discuss their abuse to a supportive person (Green, 1998).

RESPONDING TO SEXUAL ASSAULT: CREATING SANCTUARY

Creating sanctuary refers to the process involved in creating safe environments that promote healing and sustain human growth, learning, and health (Bloom, 1997). The problem of sexual assault is so great and affects so many children and adults that it is no longer acceptable to pretend that all that is needed is to turn over these problems to mental health or health care professionals. There are not, nor will there ever be, professionals in sufficient numbers to address the sheer volume of people suffering from the multitude of problems that arise secondary to exposure to violence. Therefore all medical and social institutions must find ways to address the problem by creating environments that promote and sustain better physical, emotional, and relational health. To do this, it is helpful to start with a series of basic principles that arise naturally out of trauma theory.

The first fundamental attribute of creating sanctuary is changing the presenting question with which we verbally or implicitly confront another human being whose behavior we do not understand from "What's wrong with you?" to "What's happened to you?" Changing the position vis-à-vis other people in this way radically shifts the perspective, moving toward a position of compassion and understanding and away from blame and criticism. Rather than think of troubled or troubling people as "sick" or "bad," it is more useful to understand that psychologic injuries are comprehensible, treatable, and remedial, just as physical injuries are, even if the psychologically injured person must learn to live with some form of disability (Bloom, 2000). A recovery paradigm for the complex problems that accompany overwhelming trauma should provide the survivor with the single component often missing from treatment: hope.

The first and most essential assumption must be the human need for safety. The definition of safety, however, includes not just physical safety, but psychologic, social, and moral safety as well. Psychologic safety is the ability to be safe with oneself. Social safety is the ability to be safe in groups and with other people. Moral safety involves the maintenance of a value system that does not contradict itself and is consistent with healthy human development as well as physical, psychologic, and social safety. An environment cannot be truly safe unless all of these levels of safety are addressed. A focus on physical safety alone results in living in an armed fortress, paranoid and alienated from others.

The impact of traumatic experience directly leads to specific implications for any environment that is to be health-promoting. Exposure to helplessness means that interventions designed to help people overcome traumatizing experiences must focus on mastery and empowerment while avoiding further experiences of helplessness. The prolonged hyperarousal and the loss of the ability to manage emotional states appropriately that accompany traumatic exposure implies the need to understand that many behaviors that are socially objectionable and even destructive are also individuals' only method of coping with overwhelming and uncontrollable emotions. If they are to stop using these coping skills, they must be offered better substitutes—most importantly, healthy and sustaining human relationships.

Since quality thinking under stress is almost impossible, in formulating intervention strategies every effort should be made to reduce stress whenever good decisions are sought. The growing sources of social stress inflicted on individuals and families at home, in the workplace, and in the community must be assessed and the kinds of buffers that can be put into place to help attenuate the effects of these stressors evaluated.

The memory problems resulting from overwhelming stress imply that environments designed to intervene in the lives of suffering people must provide an abundance of opportunities for people to talk about their experiences. It means that programs focusing on nonverbal expression (including art, music, movement, and drama, as well as sports) are vital adjuncts to healing efforts and should be funded, not eliminated, in the schools and in the community. It means that the arts can play a central role in community healing, serving as a "bridge across the black hole of trauma" (S. L. Bloom, unpublished, 1996).

When the potent impact that trauma has on the emotions of survivors is recognized, the apparent need is to develop techniques for helping people manage their emotions more effectively. Systems are required that build and reinforce the acquisition of what Goleman (1998) has termed "emotional intelligence." Many of the maladaptive symptoms that plague our social environment result from the individual's attempt to manage overwhelming emotions that are effective in the short run but detrimental in the long-term. If we fail to protect children from overwhelming stress, then we can count on creating life-long adjustment problems that take a toll on the individual, the family, and society as a whole. If we expect people to give up their self-destructive addiction to substances and damaging behavior, then we must be willing to substitute supportive human relationships.

Key Point:
Intervention strategies are needed to help people "detoxify" from their addiction to trauma. Environments must be established that insist on safety.

The recognition of the importance of addiction to trauma implies that intervention strategies must focus on helping people to "detoxify" from this behavioral form of addiction by providing environments that insist on the establishment and maintenance of safety. People who have been traumatized need opportunities to learn how to create relationships that are not based on terror and the abuse of power, even though abusive power feels "normal" and "right." In such cases, people often need direct relationship coaching and the experience of engaging in relationships that are not abusive and do not permit or tolerate abusive and punitive behavior.

People who have been sexually assaulted or traumatized significantly in any way must face incomprehensible losses and to do so, they must be able to grieve. Today's society has difficulty with grief. Rather than help a grieving person find ways to work through their suffering and loss, we are more likely to advise them to "get over it," "put it out of your mind," or "forget about it"—all injunctions to not resolve the loss. This is particularly true when the losses that people sustain are not about the actual death of a significant other. Trauma survivors must grieve, and the consequences for not grieving are enormous. Unresolved grief prevents recovery from both the psychologic and the physical problems that result from exposure to a traumatic experience.

The process of recovery from trauma is a painful one. To heal, survivors must open up the old wounds, remember and reconstruct the past, resolve the accompanying painful emotions, and reconnect to their internal world and the world around them. To do so requires a vision of possibilities. It requires a clear recognition that recovery is possible, that there is a new life to be found after trauma, and that people are free to change and grow regardless of how trapped, imprisoned, or violated they were in the past. For the demoralized and depleted trauma survivor, other people must advance this vision of freedom.

SUMMARY

The sexual assault of children and adults in the United States is a pressing public health problem of extraordinary proportions. At least 20% of American women and 10% of American men are sexually assaulted before they reach adulthood, and one out of every eight adult women will be the victim of forcible rape in her lifetime. Trauma theory provides a comprehensive psychobiologic model for understanding the immediate, short-term, and long-term impact of traumatic stress in the lives of men, women, and children and for understanding why the outcome of exposure to trauma is so complex and multisystemic. The impact of sexual assault on neurobiology, mental health, physical health, and social adjustment, including the

Davidson JRT, Hughes D, Blazer D, George LK. Post-traumatic stress disorder in the community: an epidemiological study. *Psychological Med.* 1991;21:713-721.

De Bellis MD, Baum AS, Birmaher B, et al. Developmental traumatology, part I: biological stress systems. *Biol Psychiatry.* 1999;45:1259-1270.

De Bellis MD, Lefter L, Trickett PK, Putnam FW. Urinary catecholamine excretion in sexually abused girls. *J Am Acad Child Adolesc Psychiatry.* 1994;33:320-327.

De Girolamo G, McFarlane AC. Epidemiology of post-traumatic stress disorder among victims of intentional violence: a review of the literature. In: Mak FL, Nadelson CC, eds. *International Review of Psychiatry.* Vol 2. Washington, DC: American Psychiatric Press; 1996.

DeMause L. The history of child assault. *J Psychohistory.* 1990;18:1-24.

Douglas AR. Reported anxieties concerning intimate parenting in women sexually abused as children. *Child Abuse Negl.* 2000;24:425-434.

Drossman DA. Sexual and physical abuse and gastrointestinal illness. *Scan J Gastroenterol.* 1995;208(suppl):90-96.

Egeland B, Jacobvitz D, Sroufe LA. Breaking the cycle of abuse. *Child Dev.* 1988;59:1080-1088.

Egeland B, Susman-Stillman A. Dissociation as a mediator of child abuse across generations. *Child Abuse Negl.* 1996;20:1123-1132.

Ellason JW, Ross CA, Sainton K, Mayran LW. Axis I and II comorbidity and childhood trauma history in chemical dependency. *Bull Menninger Clin.* 1996;60:39-51.

Epstein JN, Saunders BE, Kilpatrick DG, Resnick HS. PTSD as a mediator between childhood rape and alcohol use in adult women. *Child Abuse Negl.* 1998;22:223-234.

Famularo R, Fenton T, Kinscherff R, Ayoub C, Barnum R. Maternal and child post-traumatic stress disorder in cases of child maltreatment. *Child Abuse Negl.* 1994;18:27-36.

Farley M, Barkan H. Prostitution, violence, and post-traumatic stress disorder. *Women and Health.* 1998;27:37-49.

Felitti VJ, Anda RF, Nordenberg D, Williamson DF, Spitz AM, Edwards V, Koss MP, Marks JS. Relationship of childhood abuse and household dysfunction to many of the leading causes of death in adults. The Adverse Childhood Experiences (ACE) Study. *Am J Prev Med.* 1998;14:245-258.

Fergusson DM, Horwood LJ, Lynskey MT. Childhood sexual abuse, adolescent sexual behaviors and sexual revictimization. *Child Abuse Negl.* 1997;21:789-803.

Fierman EJ, Hunt MF, Pratt LA, Warshaw MG, Yonkers KA, Peterson LG, Epstein-Kaye TM, Norton HS. Trauma and post-traumatic stress disorder in subjects with anxiety disorders. *Am J Psychiatry.* 1993;150:1872-1874.

Fontana VJ, Robison E. Observing child abuse. *J Pediatr.* 1984;5:655-660.

Freedman D, Hemenway D. Precursors of lethal violence: a death row sample. *Soc Sci Med.* 2000;50:1757-1770.

Garnefski N, Arends E. Sexual abuse and adolescent maladjustment: differences between male and female victims. *J Adolesc.* 1998;21:99-107.

Geisser ME, Roth RS, Bachman JE, Eckert TA. The relationship between symptoms of post-traumatic stress disorder and pain, affective disturbance and disability among patients with accident and non-accident related pain. *Pain.* 1996;66:207-214.

Glover H. Emotional numbing: a possible endorphin-mediated phenomenon associated with post-traumatic stress disorders and other allied psychopathologic states. *J Trauma Stress.* 1992;5:643-675.

Goleman D. *Working with Emotional Intelligence.* New York, NY: Bantam Books; 1998.

Green A. Childhood sexual and physical abuse. In: Wilson JP, Raphael B, eds. *International Handbook of Traumatic Stress Syndromes.* New York, NY: Plenum Press; 1993.

Green AH. Factors contributing to the generational transmission of child maltreatment. *J Am Acad Child Adolesc Psychiatry.* 1998;37:1334-1336.

Gurvits TV, Gilbertson MW, Lasko NB, et al. Neurologic soft signs in chronic post-traumatic stress disorder. *Arch Gen Psychiatry.* 2000;57:181-186.

Hall DK, Mathews F, Pearce J. Factors associated with sexual behavior problems in young sexually abused children. *Child Abuse Negl.* 1998;22:1045-1063.

Harrison PA, Fulkerson JA, Beebe TJ. Multiple substance use among adolescent physical and sexual abuse victims. *Child Abuse Negl.* 1997;21:529-539.

Heim C, Nemeroff CB. The impact of early adverse experiences on brain systems involved in the pathophysiology of anxiety and affective disorders. *Biol Psychiatry.* 1999;46:1509-1522.

Herbert TB, Cohen S. Stress and immunity in humans: a meta-analytic review. *Psychosom Med.* 1993;55:364-379.

Herman JL. *Trauma and Recovery.* New York, NY: Basic Books; 1992.

Herman JL, Perry JC, Van der Kolk BA. Childhood trauma in borderline personality disorder. *Am J Psychiatry.* 1989;146:490- 495.

Humphrey JA, White JW. Women's vulnerability to sexual assault from adolescence to young adulthood. *J Adolesc Health.* 2000; 27:419-424.

Ibarra P, Bruehl SP, McCubbin JA, et al. An unusual reaction to opioid blockade with naltrexone in a case of post-traumatic stress disorder. *J Trauma Stress.* 1994;7:303-309.

International Society of Traumatic Stress Studies (ISTSS). Childhood Trauma Remembered: *A Report on the Current Scientific Knowledge Base and Its Applications.* Northbrook, Ill: International Society of Traumatic Stress Studies; 1998.

Irwin C, Falsetti SA, Lydiard RB, Ballenger JC, Brock CD, Brener W. Comorbidity of post-traumatic stress disorder and irritable bowel syndrome. *J Clin Psychiatry.* 1996;57:576-578.

James B. *Handbook for Treatment of Attachment-Trauma Problems in Children.* New York, NY: Lexington Books; 1994.

Janis IL. Decision making under stress. In: Goldberger L, Breznitz S, eds. *Handbook of Stress: Theoretical and Clinical Aspects.* New York, NY: Free Press; 1982:69-87.

Jordan BK, Marmar CR, Fairbank JA, et al. Problems in families of male Vietnam veterans with post-traumatic stress disorder. *J Consult Clin Psychol.* 1992;60:916-926.

Kessler R, Sonnega A, Broment E, Hughes M, Nelson CB. Post-traumatic stress disorder in the National Comorbidity Survey. *Arch Gen Psychiatry*. 1995;52:1048-1060.

Kilpatrick DG, Best CL, Veronen LJ, Amick AE, Villeponteaux LA, Ruff GA. Mental health correlates of criminal victimization: a random community survey. *J Consult Clin Psychol*. 1985;53:866-873.

Kilpatrick DG, Edmunds C, Seymour A. *Rape in America: A Report to the Nation*. Arlington, Va: National Center for Victims of Crime; Charleston, SC: Medical University of South Carolina, Crime Victims Research and Treatment Center; 1992.

Koss MP, Koss PG, Woodruff WJ. Deleterious effects of criminal victimization on women's health and medical utilization. *Arch Intern Med*. 1991;151:342-347.

LeDoux JE. Emotion, memory, and the brain. *Sci Am*. 1994;270:50-57.

Leserman J, Drossman DA, Li Z, Toomey TC, Nachman G, Glogau L. Sexual and physical abuse history in gastroenterology practice: how types of abuse impact health status. *Psychosom Med*. 1996;58:4-15.

Lisak D, Hopper J, Song P. Factors in the cycle of violence: gender rigidity and emotional constriction. *J Trauma Stress*. 1996;9:721-743.

Luntz BK, Widom CS. Antisocial personality disorder in abused and neglected children grown up. *Am J Psychiatry*. 1994;151:670-674.

Main M, Goldwyn R. Predicting rejection of her infant from mother's representation of her own experience: implications for the abused-abusing intergenerational cycle. *Child Abuse Negl*. 1984;8:203-217.

McClanahan SF, McClelland GM, Abram KM, Teplin LA. Pathways into prostitution among female jail detainees and their implications for mental health services. *Psychiatr Serv*. 1999;50:1606-1613.

McCown W, Galina ZH, Johnson JL, DeSimone PA, Posa J. Borderline personality disorder and laboratory-induced cold pressor pain: evidence of stress-induced analgesia. *J Psychopatho Behav Assess*. 1993;15:87-95.

McEwen BS, Magarinos AM. Stress effects on morphology and function of the hippocampus. In: Yehuda R, McFarlane AC, eds. *Psychobiology of Post-traumatic Stress Disorder*. New York: New York Academy of Sciences; 1997;821:271-284.

McNally RJ. Implicit and explicit memory for trauma-related information in PTSD. In: Yehuda R, McFarlane AC, eds. *Psychobiology of Post-traumatic Stress Disorder*. New York: New York Academy of Sciences; 1997;821:219-224.

Miller TR, Cohen MA, Rossman SB. Victim costs of violent crime and resulting injuries. *Health Aff*. 1993;12:186-197.

Milner JS, Halsey LB, Fultz J. Empathic responsiveness and affective reactivity to infant stimuli in high- and low-risk for physical child abuse mothers. *Child Abuse Negl*. 1995;19:767-780.

National Victim Center. *Crime and Victimization in America: Statistical Overview*. Arlington, VA: National Victim Center; 1993.

New MJC, Stevenson J, Skuse D. Characteristics of mothers of boys who sexually abuse. *Child Maltreat*. 1999;4:21-31.

Nordling N, Sandnabba NK, Santtila P. The prevalence and effects of self-reported childhood sexual abuse among sadomasochistically oriented males and females. *J Child Sex Abuse*. 2000;9:53-63.

Orsillo SM, Weathers FW, Litz BT, Steinberg HR, Huska JA, Keane TM. Current and lifetime psychiatric disorders among veterans with war zone-related post-traumatic stress disorder. *J Nerv Ment Dis.* 1996;184:307-313.

Perry BD. Neurodevelopment and the neurophysiology of trauma, I: conceptual considerations for clinical work with maltreated children. *The Advisor: Am Professional Soc Abuse Child.* 1993;6:14-18.

Perry, BD. The neurodevelopmental impact of violence in childhood. In: Schetky D, Benedek E, eds. *Textbook of Child and Adolescent Forensic Psychiatry.* Washington, DC: American Psychiatric Press, Inc.; 2001; 221-238.

Perry BD, Pate JE. Neurodevelopment and the psychobiological roots of post-traumatic stress disorder. In: Koziol LF, Stout CE, eds. *The Neuropsychology of Mental Disorders: A Practical Guide.* Springfield, Ill: Charles C Thomas; 1993.

Perry BD, Pollard RA, Blakley TL, et al. Childhood trauma, the neurobiology of adaptation and use-dependent development of the brain: how "states" become "traits". *Infant Ment Health.* 1995;16:271-291.

Perry JC, Herman JL, Van der Kolk BA, Hoke LA. Psychotherapy and psychological trauma in borderline personality disorder. *Psychiatr Ann.* 1990;20:33-43.

Pitman RK. Post-traumatic obsessive-compulsive disorder: a case study. *Compre Psychiatry.* 1993;34:102-107.

Pitman RK. Overview of biological themes in PTSD. *Ann NY Acad Sci.* 1997;821:1-9.

Plichta SB, Abraham C. Violence and gynecologic health in women <50 years old. *Am J Obstetet Gynecol.* 1996;174:903-907.

Pollack MH, Otto MW, Rosenbaum JF, Sachs GS. Personality disorders in patients with panic disorder: association with childhood anxiety disorders, early trauma, comorbidity, and chronicity. *Compre Psychiatry.* 1992;33:78-83.

Polusny MA, Follette VM. Long-term correlates of child sexual abuse: theory and review of the empirical literature. *Appl Prev Psychol.* 1995;4:143-166.

Putnam FW, Trickett PK. Psychobiological effects of sexual abuse: a longitudinal study. *Ann N Y Acad Sci.* 1997;821:150-159.

Reiter RC, Shakerin LR, Gambone JC, Milburn AK. Correlation between sexual abuse and somatization in women with somatic and nonsomatic chronic pelvic pain. *Am J Obstet Gynecol.* 1991;165:104-109.

Rinne T, Westenberg HGM, Den Boer JA, Van den Brink W. Serotonergic blunting to meta-chlorophenylpiperazine (m-CPP) highly correlates with sustained childhood abuse in impulsive and autoaggressive female borderline patients. *Biol Psychiatry.* 2000;47:548-556.

Rogers MP, Weinshenker NJ, Warshaw MG, et al. Prevalence of somatoform disorders in a large sample of patients with anxiety disorders. *Psychosomatics.* 1996;37:17-22.

Roozendaal B, Quirarte GL, McGaugh JL. Stress-activated hormonal systems and the regulation of memory storage. In: Yehuda R, McFarlane AC, eds. *Psychobiology of Post-traumatic Stress Disorder.* New York: New York Academy of Sciences; 1997;821:247-258.

Sabo AN. Etiological significance of associations between childhood trauma and borderline personality disorder: conceptual and clinical implications. *J Pers Disord.* 1997;11:50-70.

Salasin SE, Rich RF. Mental health policy for victims of violence: the case against women. In: Wilson JP, Raphael B, eds. *International Handbook of Traumatic Stress Syndromes*. New York, NY: Plenum Press; 1993.

Sarno JE. *The Mindbody Prescription: Healing the Body, Healing the Pain*. New York, NY: Warner Books; 1998.

Saxe GN, Chinman G, Berkowitz R, et al. Somatization in patients with dissociative disorders. *Am J Psychiatry*. 1994;151:1329-1334.

Schwarz ED, Perry BD. The post-traumatic response in children and adolescents. In: Tomb DA, ed. *Psychiatric Clinics of North America: Post-Traumatic Stress Disorder*. Philadelphia, Pa: WB Saunders;1994;17:311-326.

Seligman MEP. *Helplessness: On Development, Depression, and Death*. New York, NY: WH Freeman; 1992.

Shaw JA, Campo-Bowen AE, Applegate B, et al. Young boys who commit serious sexual offenses: demographics, psychometrics, and phenomenology. *Bull Am Acad Psychiatry Law*. 1993;21:399-408.

Solomon SD, Davidson JRT. Trauma: prevalence, impairment, service use, and cost. *J Clin Psychiatry*. 1997;58:5-11.

Spiegel D. Trauma, dissociation and memory. In: Yehuda R, McFarlane AC, eds. *Psychobiology of Post-traumatic Stress Disorder*. New York: New York Academy of Sciences; 1997;821:225-237.

Stein B, Koverola C, Hanna C, Torchia MG, McClarty B. Hippocampal volume in women victimized by childhood sexual abuse. *Psychological Med*. 1997;27:951-959.

Teicher MH, Yutaka I, Glod CA, et al. Preliminary evidence for abnormal cortical development in physically and sexually abused children using EEG coherence and MRI. *Ann N Y Acad Sci*. 1997;821:160-175.

Terr L. *Too Scared to Cry: Psychic Trauma in Childhood*. New York, NY: Harper & Row; 1990:8.

Thakkar RR, McCanne TR. The effects of daily stressors on physical health in women with and without a childhood history of sexual abuse. *Child Abuse Negl*. 2000;24:209-221.

Ursin H. Stress, distress, and immunity. *Ann N Y Acad Sci*. 1994;741:204-221.

Van der Kolk BA. The compulsion to repeat the trauma: reenactment, revictimization, and masochism. In: *Psychiatric Clinics of North America: Treatment of Victims of Sexual Abuse*. Philadelphia, Pa: WB Saunders; 1989;12:389-411.

Van der Kolk BA. The body keeps the score: approaches to the psychobiology of post-traumatic stress disorder. In: Van der Kolk BA, McFarlane C, Weisaeth L. *Traumatic Stress: The Effects of Overwhelming Experience on Mind, Body and Society*. New York, NY: Guilford Press; 1996a.

Van der Kolk BA. Trauma and memory. In: Van der Kolk BA, McFarlane C, Weisaeth L, eds. *Traumatic Stress: The Effects of Overwhelming Experience on Mind, Body and Society*. New York, NY: Guilford Press; 1996b.

Van der Kolk BA, Burbridge JA, Suzuki J. The psychobiology of traumatic memory: clinical implications of neuroimaging studies. In: Yehuda R, McFarlane AC, eds. *Psychobiology of Post-traumatic Stress Disorder*. New York: New York Academy of Sciences; 1997;821:99-113.

Van der Kolk BA, Greenberg MS. The psychobiology of the trauma response: hyperarousal, constriction, and addiction to traumatic reexposure. In: Van der Kolk BA, ed. *Psychological Trauma.* Washington, DC: American Psychiatric Press; 1987:63-88.

Van der Kolk BA, Roth S, Pelcovitz D, Mandel FS. Disorders of extreme stress: results from the DSMIV field trials for PTSD. Paper presented at: 1994 Eli Lilly Lecture to the Royal College of Psychiatrists; February 2, 1994; London.

Vasile RG, Goldenberg I, Reich J, Goisman RM, Lavori PW, Keller MB. Panic disorder versus panic disorder with major depression: defining and understanding differences in psychiatric morbidity. *Depression Anxiety.* 1997;5:12-20.

Volpicelli J, Balaraman G, Hahn J, Wallace H, Bux D. The role of uncontrollable trauma in the development of PTSD and alcohol addiction. *Alcohol Res Health.* 1999;23:256-262.

Walker EA, Gelfand AN, Gelfand MD, Green C, Katon WJ. Chronic pelvic pain and gynecological symptoms in women with irritable bowel syndrome. *J Psychosom Obstet Gynaecol.* 1996;17:39-46.

Walker EA, Gelfand AN, Katon WJ, et al. Adult health status of women with histories of childhood abuse and neglect. *Am J Med.* 1999;107:332-339.

Walker EA, Katon WJ, Hansom J, et al. Medical and psychiatric symptoms in women with childhood sexual abuse. *Psychosom Med.* 1992;54:658-664.

Walling MK, O'Hara MW, Reiter RC, Milburn AK, Lilly G, Vincent SD. Abuse history and chronic pain in women, II: a multivariate analysis of abuse and psychological morbidity. *Obstet Gynecol.* 1994;84:200-206.

Wallis S. Discipline and civility must be restored to America's public schools. *USA Today Magazine.* 1995;124:32-35.

Warshaw R. *I Never Called It Rape: The MS. Report on Recognizing, Fighting and Surviving Date and Acquaintance Rape.* New York, NY: Harper and Row; 1988.

Whiffen VE, Thompson JM, Aube JA. Mediators of the link between childhood sexual abuse and adult depressive symptoms. *J Interpers Violence.* 2000;15:1100-1120.

Widom CS, Kuhns JB. Childhood victimization and subsequent risk for promiscuity, prostitution, and teenage pregnancy: a prospective study. *Am J Public Health.* 1996;86:1607-1612.

Wolfe J, Schlesinger LK. Performance of PTSD patients on standard tests of memory. In: Yehuda R, McFarlane AC, eds. *Psychobiology of Post-traumatic Stress Disorder.* New York: New York Academy of Sciences; 1997;821:208-218.

Chapter 24

SOCIAL SUPPORTS

Jeffrey R. Jaeger, MD
Ann E. Gaulin, MS, MFT

Rape and sexual assault, crimes of rage, control, violation, and dominance, often leave survivors with deep scars and unique needs. In 1974 two Boston College professors, Ann Burgess and Lynda Holmstrom, analyzing data collected from 80 rape survivors who came for treatment to the Boston City Hospital Emergency Department, discovered predictable reactions to sexual assault. Burgess and Holmstrom (1974) described the "rape trauma syndrome," characterized by specific somatic, emotional, and long-term psychologic reactions to an acute fear for one's life. Later, comparing their findings to research being done in Veterans Administration hospitals after the Vietnam War, it was discovered that rape trauma syndrome was comparable to what was being described by government researchers as "posttraumatic stress disorder." Burgess and Holmstrom argued that intervention must take into account this syndrome and where the survivor is in his or her recovery. If and when a survivor chooses to reach out and tell his or her story, the nature and extent of the support provided can play a critical role in the survivor's ability to modulate symptoms and recover from the trauma.

Key Point:
The rape trauma syndrome is characterized by somatic, emotional, and long-term psychologic reactions to an acute fear for one's life. It was described three decades ago and is comparable to aspects of posttraumatic stress disorder (PTSD).

This chapter will discuss the recent history of the "social" response to sexual assault, varying types of social support that can benefit the survivor at different stages of recovery, principles of program development, and components of coordinated community responses to sexual assault.

HISTORY

Rape is a uniquely human act. It is at once a very personal violation, yet at the same time, a form of violence with complex historical social sanctions. Mythology and literature abound in rationalizations and mischaracterizations of forced sexual activity. Laws founded in misogynist cultures protected perpetrators and blamed victims. Early laws in many cultures considered rape a form of property theft, thereby identifying women as a form of male property. Worldwide, it is probably correct to say that for most women, sexual assault and other forms of physical violence are still silently condoned or ignored, and systems of justice or "support" have remained informal at best (Brownmiller, 1975; Horos, 1974).

While there are vestiges of this "tradition" left in the American social system, our response to sexual assault has made major progress in the last 30 years. In the 1960s the civil rights movement helped usher in a resurgence of the women's movement. In this environment, women began to speak out about their histories and experiences with sexual assault. In 1969 the unacceptable treatment of a young girl who was raped led to the formation of the nation's first community-based rape crisis center, Bay Area Women Against Rape, in Berkeley, California. In 1973 the National Organization of Women (NOW) initiated "Rape Task Forces" in many communities, and by 1974 there were 136 NOW-affiliated anti-rape projects in 39 states (Warner, 1980; Webster, 1989).

Today, national organizations such as the Rape Abuse & Incest National Network (RAINN) claim over 850 rape crisis centers as registered members in 49 states.

These centers for victims of sexual violence offer a range of services from 24-hour hotlines with referral services to sophisticated, coordinated, community networks. Such efforts vary widely based on available resources and local interest. Because of the current diversity of community-based programs, it is impossible to give national statistics regarding how many sexual assault survivors have made use of formal social supports after a sexual assault. However, in Philadelphia, for example, a city of approximately one and a half million people, annual statistics of Women Organized Against Rape, Philadelphia's rape crisis center, indicate that over 4,000 women, men, and children used some aspect of their services during 2000.

NATURE OF SOCIAL SUPPORTS
SOCIAL SERVICES
While there is considerable overlap among the activities and missions of various types of agencies, it is reasonable to discuss these systems independently, because resources and grass-roots support may come from many different arenas in this field.

Rape Crisis Centers
Rape crisis centers are traditionally nonprofit, community-based organizations staffed by paid professional counselors and volunteers. Services are usually free and offered to adult and child survivors of both genders. Rape crisis centers traditionally offer a 24-hour hotline, hospital and court accompaniment, short-term crisis counseling services, and a strong advocacy-based organizational system within the community.

Within the last 10 to 15 years, rape crisis centers have begun to organize on a state level to form coalitions (see Appendix). These state coalitions usually distribute state and federal funding, monitor quality of services, and help establish guidelines for community education and training about sexual violence.

Key Point:
Rape crisis centers represent a community response that works to bring together multiple agencies and disciplines to best serve those who are sexually assaulted.

In many communities, rape crisis centers have been the glue that brings together different individuals and agencies with an interest in victim services. Some rape crisis centers, usually in urban settings, have partnered with researchers in investigating effective treatment modalities to reduce or eliminate symptoms of posttraumatic stress disorder in sexual assault survivors (Foa et al., 1999). The common coexistence of domestic violence and sexual assault within a relationship has resulted in some collaborative efforts between rape crisis centers and domestic violence agencies to provide longer-term and more effective counseling and treatment to these clients. Many rape crisis centers have also established partnerships with district attorneys, police, hospitals, and other agencies to provide more comprehensive services to individuals and families with increasingly more complex problems. By partnering with systems already established in the community, rape crisis centers have been better able to advocate for the establishment of protocols to meet survivors' needs.

Domestic Violence Programs
Survivors of sexual assault and abuse and survivors of domestic violence share many symptoms as well as needs. Thus it is natural that in many communities, especially rural ones, services for survivors of sexual assault and domestic violence are provided by the same nonprofit agencies. Domestic violence agencies also usually provide 24-hour hotlines with paid staff or volunteers. Often, they provide shelter for women and their children who need a safe environment to escape violence in their homes. Legal advocacy as well as emergency department and court accompaniment are similarly provided.

Counseling for survivors of domestic violence has traditionally focused on safety planning, empowerment, and restoration of self-esteem. Since many clients of domestic violence agencies receive services while still in the abusive environment, this focus on situational safety is necessary and critical to survival. The goals of counseling sexual assault survivors are the treatment and prevention of the debilitating effects of posttraumatic stress disorder. As more domestic violence survivors are encouraged to access services for sexual assault and more is learned about the biologic and psychologic effects of trauma, collaboration in providing counseling increases.

Victim Assistance Programs

Victim assistance programs, often funded through a prosecuting attorney's office, provide services for all victims of violent, interpersonal crime. Their main function is to offer court accompaniment and victim compensation services to survivors who report their assaults to the police department. Much of their funding comes from states' victim compensation funds collected from adjudicated offenders. Assistance in filing monetary claims to the state usually depends on the survivor making a police report about his or her assault.

HEALTHCARE SYSTEM

Acute Care

Survivors of sexual assault interact with the healthcare system at various points in their recovery. In the acute postassault setting, the medical provider's chief role is to assess and treat the victim's acute medical needs and collect evidence (Hampton, 1995). In addition, medical personnel play an important role as social supports for victims, both in the acute setting and throughout recovery.

The initial evaluation and examination of a victim of sexual assault, while necessary, are both traumatic and invasive. In the acute setting, usually an emergency department, medical personnel can employ strategies that begin the healing process or at least prevent repeat traumatization. Members of the medical team must ensure a safe, private environment for history-taking and examination, a responsibility that falls as much on the institution as on the physician or nurse (American Medical Association, 1995). The responsibility for calling a friend, family member, or rape crisis counselor may also belong to the medical acute-care provider.

Assisting with the restoration of a sense of order and predictability is an important role the healthcare provider must play during the acute evaluation. While carrying out an evaluation, the patient's safety must be emphasized (Hampton, 1995). Taking care to inform the patient in advance of what will happen during the examination and how long it might last, and then asking the patient's permission to begin the examination, will help restore the victim's sense of control over what is happening to his or her body (AMA, 1995).

Evidence collection and physical evaluation are time consuming and can be frustrating. The frustration can become evident to the patient, worsening his or her sense of isolation and repeating the trauma. Healthcare institutions have a responsibility to their staff and to survivors to adequately train and support staff involved in the care of sexual assault victims. Although it may seem peripheral to the care and social support of the victim, the creation and maintenance of a caring healthcare environment is crucial to allowing healthcare providers to fulfill their dual roles as support personnel and guarantors of safety and health.

Key Point:
The healthcare system and its providers have a responsibility to render acute care and a sensitive response to those who have been sexually assaulted, in a manner that recognizes the very real concerns related to safety and health.

Sexual Assault Nurse Examiner and Sexual Assault Response Team Programs

Often a victim's first contact with a "support" system after an assault occurs in an emergency department, where standard practice includes triage. Seriously ill patients are cared for first, and others wait to be assessed. In a high-volume emergency department, noncritically ill patients may wait hours to be evaluated. This strategy usually leads to nothing more serious than a decrease in customer satisfaction, but, in the case of a victim of sexual assault, such a wait can result in deterioration of evidence and delay in delivering support services. Even a trip to the bathroom may result in the loss of potentially invaluable evidence. In addition, the necessary examination protocols (see Chapters 4 and 15) require a level of aptitude and expertise often lacking among emergency department nurses and physicians. Standard medical training does not adequately prepare doctors and nurses to conduct medicolegal examinations, nor are these professionals routinely able to provide expert testimony.

Key Point:
SANE and SART programs seek to lessen the traumatizing nature of rape examinations as much as possible, and to increase effective collection and preservation of forensic evidence related to the assault.

To better meet the acute medical, legal, and support needs of sexual assault survivors, several communities have established sexual assault nurse examiner (SANE) and sexual assault response team (SART) programs. SANE programs provide 24-hour availability of personnel who can offer immediate, comprehensive, and compassionate evaluation and treatment of sexual assault victims. Program goals are to lessen the traumatizing nature of the rape examination, to reduce repeated questioning and examination of the victim, and to increase effective collection and preservation of evidence. The SANE practitioner (who can be a nurse, nurse practitioner, physician assistant, or other healthcare provider) is called immediately when a sexual assault victim is identified, whether by law enforcement personnel, rescue personnel, or emergency department staff. He or she is responsible for completing the entire evidentiary examination, including leading the team interview; conducting assessments of sexually transmitted disease (STD) and pregnancy as well as their prevention strategies; and performing the colposcopy evaluation with photographs. The SANE practitioner also ensures appropriate referrals for support and care, which often take lower priority when the responsibility for this is left to busy emergency department personnel (Selig, 2000). In a study of 100 rape kits (sealed packets of evidence and documentation collected at the time of victim presentation to an emergency department) submitted in Minnesota in 1996-1997, Ledray and Simmelink (1997) found that evidence collected by SANE personnel was of significantly higher quality than that collected by other personnel. Most notably, none of the kits submitted by SANE personnel contained serious errors or breaches of the chain of evidence, whereas 18% of the kits collected by non-SANE personnel were not admissible in court because of such errors.

A SART team might include SANE staff, law enforcement personnel, and rape crisis center staff or volunteers. It is also activated immediately upon identification of a sexual assault victim. Early involvement of law enforcement personnel reduces repeated questioning of the victim, because the medical history obtained by the SANE practitioner can link with the questioning by law enforcement personnel. A rape crisis center volunteer can provide necessary early support while navigating the criminal justice system and can establish an early link with the victim should he or she wish to pursue a relationship with the agency later.

Many communities have arranged to have representatives of the SART partner agencies located at one site. Such "co-location" facilitates better interagency cooperation and communication, and can further reduce the trauma of survivors who are spared having to travel between multiple sites to pursue post-assault follow-up. The International Association of Forensic Nurses (1999) has published standards of practice and educational guidelines for SANE programs and the US Department of Justice Office for Victims of Crimes has published a manual to assist individuals and communities interested in SANE/SART program development (Ledray, 1999).

Postacute Care Medical Support

Because only a minority of sexual assault survivors report their assault or make contact with established rape crisis centers or other social support, nonacute care medical providers are likely to provide post assault care and support for most survivors. The unique confidential relationship between a healthcare provider and the patient makes the provider-patient relationship a natural place for survivors to turn for support (Kimerling & Calhoun, 1994). It is also reasonable to expect all medical providers to have the basic skill set required to assess, evaluate, and treat the psychosocial complications of sexual assault. Healthcare providers should be familiar with the phases of the rape trauma syndrome (Burgess & Holmstrom, 1974) and should be comfortable treating depression, which affects most survivors after a rape. Most importantly, healthcare providers should provide a "safe," nonjudgmental setting where survivors can feel comfortable discussing their experience, their feelings, and their fears. Healthcare providers should have access to referral information should a patient decide in the postacute care setting to pursue professional post–sexual assault counseling (Petter & Whitehill, 1998).

CHURCHES AND RELIGIOUS GROUPS

Many people turn to religion for comfort and healing. Historically, sexual assault survivors have not always found consolation in organized religion or faith-based agencies. Often, organized religion has echoed the societal prejudices regarding the myths around sexual assault and the victim's culpability in his or her assault. However, in recent years, the voice for change has increasingly come from established religious groups. Churches and other religious groups have approached rape crisis centers for education regarding sexual abuse issues. Pastors, priests, nuns, and rabbis are now reaching out for special training in counseling their worshippers who have disclosed sexual abuse issues. Moreover, they are learning assessment skills to refer their members to mental health care providers as they learn of the longer-term effects of severe trauma.

Many rape crisis centers are finding that collaboration with community churches can be mutually helpful. Contact with established religious groups allows rape crisis centers to access an audience that may not have heard their message. By providing special workshops and training to church-sponsored groups, rape crisis centers are increasing awareness of sexual abuse issues and increasing access to services for survivors. Posttraumatic stress disorder and its impact on victims and their families are now being taught at many seminaries and pastoral colleges. It is hoped that with further collaboration, a survivor's choice to pursue healing through his or her faith will no longer mean that he or she forgoes helpful counseling.

OTHER SOCIAL SUPPORTS

Only approximately one in five victims of sexual assault is seen by a healthcare provider in the acute postassault period, and only approximately one in three agrees to report the assault to the police (Tjaden & Thoennes, 1998). In fact, most victims of sexual assault do not seek services from any established support system, including physicians, mental health care professionals, rape crisis centers, or victim assistance programs (Kimerling & Calhoun, 1994). It is hoped that ongoing public education and outreach will lead more victims to break the silence and to avail themselves of services. Improving access to and availability of services may also bring more survivors to a place where professionals can assist with the healing process. In the current setting, it is worthwhile to assess the role that traditional social supports can play in the lives of sexual assault victims.

Key Point:
Sexual assault is frequently not reported to either healthcare providers or law enforcement; therefore, official statistics are known to be underestimates of the true incidence and prevalence of sexual violence in our communities.

Most survivors of sexual assault turn to someone in their informal support network immediately after an assault. In their initial report of interviews with female survivors of rape, Burgess and Holmstrom (1974) reported that 48 of 92 women interviewed made special trips home after an assault, and an additional 25 reported turning to close friends for support. Evidence suggests that this form of social support is, not surprisingly, very important to recovery. Studies have indicated that social support reliably moderated psychologic distress after sexual assault (Linden, 1999). Kimerling and Calhoun (1994) demonstrated that the extent of informal social support, as determined by the number of people with whom the survivor felt she could confide, was a moderating factor in the severity of physical symptoms and perceived health up to 1 year after the assault.

Other studies have shown that the reaction of those close to the survivor can affect recovery. Silverman (1978) asserted that sexual assault traumatizes family members and significant others as well as the victim, and that how they cope with trauma influences how they interact with the victim. Interactions characterized as maladaptive include overprotection, or encouraging the victim to keep the assault secret. Adaptive responses include empathy and allowing the victim to express fears without fear of criticism (Silverman, 1978). The response of a significant other is obviously of primary importance in the recovery of sexual assault victims. Holmstrom and Burgess (1979), in a study of male partners of female sexual assault victims, postulated that what characterized a supportive partner was responding to his or her own concerns as a secondary issue, while partners who focused primarily on their own sense of victimization were considered less supportive. (Holmstrom & Burgess, 1979). Popiel and Susskind (1985) attempted to quantify victims' perception of the amount and quality of support received from various sources. In their interviews of 25 sexual assault victims performed 3 months after their assaults, they found that girlfriends, husbands or boyfriends, and police received the highest mean ratings of supportiveness; physicians, surprisingly, were rated the lowest. They also found that victims of "attempted" rapes had just as many problems with adjustment 3 months after the assault as those who identified their assault as "completed," yet had received much less support in that period, indicating that "support" is at least partially related to society's perception of the stressfulness of the assault.

Key Point:
The response of informal support networks (including family, friends, and significant others) is very important to a survivor of sexual assault or attempted assault, and can affect the recovery process.

PROGRAM DEVELOPMENT

The steps needed to establish or improve a community's response to sexual assault will vary greatly depending on the size of the community, the presence and organization of existing victims' rights or advocacy organizations, and the level of knowledge of the healthcare community regarding sexual assault. While no community is fortunate enough to have all the pieces in place, several principles for development and improvement are universal.

FIRST STEPS

Involve Multiple Disciplines

Early involvement of participants from any interested community agencies or departments will facilitate communication and cooperation as a program evolves and progresses. Competing agendas and distinct mandates may produce discord while the multidisciplinary, team-oriented program is in the planning stages. However, protocols initiated by a single agency may falter when introduced because police, healthcare, or other agencies find them unfeasible.

Development of a task force, with clearly defined goals, must be an initial step for any community interested in starting or improving their support services for survivors of sexual assault. Members will vary, but may include hospital administrators, emergency department nurses, rape crisis center leaders, and law enforcement representatives. Representation from the judiciary is important as well. Meetings should be regular and group leaders should ensure that all voices are heard in order to maintain continued engagement from all parties.

Special attempts must be made to recruit representatives from underserved minority communities and sexual minorities. Sexual assault victims from such communities have distinct issues and needs that are often overlooked both by the larger institutions involved in victim care and by the advocacy community.

Recruit Top-Level Support

Endorsement of goals and projects by respected leaders can help to ensure community support. The governor, mayor, chief of police, or other visible official can, with little effort on his or her part, play an effective role in securing funding and keeping the needs of the project "on the table" when decisions are made regarding the allocation of resources. Other members of administration may be more willing to promote the needs of the agency or program when their superiors have been publicly and visibly involved from the outset of a project.

Use Existing Personnel and Space

Significant reduction in costs can be achieved by assigning tasks to existing agencies and personnel. Smith et al. (1998) describe how they were able to avoid incurring "on-call" costs in their SART program by training psychiatric nurses, already on 24-hour call schedules, as SANE nurses. With appropriate training and medical oversight, these nurses learned to do pelvic examinations, STD counseling and prevention, and evidentiary examinations without additional costs to the program. In Grand Rapids, Michigan, unused space at the YWCA was converted to a sexual assault evaluation center when local hospitals were unable to dedicate space or staffing to the project (Rossman & Dunnuck, 1999). Obviously the caseload of a community will dictate the feasibility of such solutions, but creativity is necessary when funding and space are scarce.

Coordination of Services

As localities make decisions regarding how best to respond to sexual assault, it is helpful to look objectively at what attributes of sexual assault support systems have proven successful. A pair of studies examined communities that have developed successful coordinated community programs. Campbell (1998) first demonstrated that coordination of social services across multiple disciplines (medical, legal, counseling/advocacy) was predictive of a relatively positive victim experience with the social support system. In the follow-up study, Campbell and Ahrens (1998) tried to determine what specific elements of the coordinated response were most associated with a positive victim experience.

In interviews with advocates, medical and legal personnel, and survivors, they discovered that, compared with communities in which there was a low level of interagency coordination, communities with a high level of coordination were more likely to have a greater number of coordinated service programs. This refers to independent agencies and programs with separate missions who collaborate in victim services. These coordinated service programs included SARTs, drug and alcohol programs, churches, domestic violence shelters, and victim assistance programs. These collaborations were able to avoid the fragmentation of care and secondary traumatization that characterized the low-coordination communities. For example, one community observed that women at a drug and alcohol treatment center were very likely to have experienced sexual assault and, as a result, arranged for clients to receive counseling for both substance abuse and sexual assault without having to leave the facility.

Both the high- and low-coordination communities had systems in place for interagency training. In most communities, rape crisis center staff provided training for medical and legal personnel. However, the high-coordination communities were more likely to have reciprocal training. That is, their rape crisis center staff received training from other community personnel, such as police, child welfare agencies, and domestic violence agencies. Service providers in the high-coordination communities were more likely to have short, repeated, regular training sessions, as compared with longer, one-time training sessions in the low-coordination communities.

The authors conclude that well-coordinated programs seem to operate from a victim-centered focus as opposed to an agency- or service-centered focus. They propose that an examination and possible rejection of traditional models of service delivery may be a necessary step to develop the coordinated community response. Communities and advocates alike must acknowledge the profound and unique effect rape has on victims. This acknowledgment can then be translated into novel methods of care delivery and outreach (Campbell & Ahrens, 1998).

RISK REDUCTION AND EDUCATION

Rape crisis centers have traditionally focused their efforts on providing assistance to victims of sexual assault. However, education and prevention must also be a part of

Key Point:
Some very basic steps can establish or improve effective community responses to sexual assault, including:

1. *involve the multiple agencies and disciplines necessary to develop and effective services*
2. *invite respected leaders to participate and lend support to the effort*
3. *optimize efforts by using existing personnel and resources as building blocks*
4. *prioritize the coordination of services as they unfold and are developed*

Key Point:
The current thinking is that the ideal
prevention strategies target sexual stereotypes
and attitudes towards interpersonal violence,
especially among boys and young men.

the social support/social services picture if the number of new victims is to decrease. Historically, educational programs about rape and sexual assault have sought out potential victims and attempted to educate them regarding prevention. Experience has shown, however, that efforts to target women as victims have not done much to change the rates of assault and abuse. The current trend is to target prevention efforts at the attitudes and stereotypes of men in particular and society as a whole. Recent efforts to target young boys at the elementary and middle school levels have been endorsed by many rape crisis centers. High schools and colleges have developed innovative prevention strategies targeted at boys and young men as well (Foubert, 2000). Special programs to change sexual stereotypes and interpersonal violence have attracted an increasing number of men to the task as instructors. Traditionally women-oriented agencies, many rape crisis centers now employ males, especially in their training and education programs. Male role models are desperately needed in assisting with anti-violence education and modeling appropriate behavior for children and adolescents of both genders.

Outreach to parents has also been helpful in reducing the risks for sexual abuse of children. Moreover, as the authors' clinical experience has demonstrated, services to the family of sexual assault survivors greatly increases the chance of successful recovery. Therefore outreach to families is now recognized as an essential component of the rape crisis center's mission. Although family systems sometimes contain the very elements that stigmatize sexual assault survivors, such as sexism and victim-blaming, community education about myths and stereotypes can help reduce the negative impact a potentially nonsupportive family may have on a survivor. Support groups for parents and caregivers of sexually abused children are now common within the clinical and counseling components of many rape crisis centers, as are groups for partners and spouses of survivors. By structuring groups to address the psycho-educational needs of the survivor's family, rape crisis centers are increasing the likelihood of recovery for the survivor.

FUNDING

The greatest limitation to the implementation of ideal support systems for survivors of sexual assault is often funding. SANE training and equipment require much more than healthcare systems are accustomed to budgeting for the care of a specific category of patients. Rare communities have dedicated the resources necessary to allow their social support agencies to carry out their missions. In this setting, many rape crisis centers are no longer depending totally on federal antiviolence funds distributed by state coalitions or state and local governments. Many have begun to explore private and corporate foundations interested in funding targeted social service projects. Many foundations are looking for evidence of community collaborations in reducing urban violence, and rape crisis centers have been among the beneficiaries of these grants. Hiring staff with the experience and talent to navigate the process of grant application must be a necessary early step for agencies and rape crisis centers who hope to be sustained by these means.

ONE CITY'S EXPERIENCE: PHILADELPHIA'S PARTNERSHIP FOR QUALITY SERVICES

Philadelphia's rape crisis center, Women Organized Against Rape (WOAR), started in 1972 when Jody Pinto, a local artist, organized women to support other women as they made their way through confusing, frightening, and frustrating healthcare and legal systems. During the late 1970s and early 1980s, WOAR, like many other rape crisis centers, operated independently from other social service agencies. The mission of WOAR and other rape crisis centers was, in part, to stand against the sexism still present in many agencies then in place to "help" crime victims. However, as social consciousness grew within society and culture, it became evident that staying "outside the system" was not an entirely effective posture. An increasing number of activists came to believe that to effect system change, it was necessary to join with existing systems and foster change from within—or at least shoulder to shoulder. During the mid 1980s the Philadelphia Department of Health fiscally promoted a formal partnership among several groups and agencies to better deliver services to sexual assault victims. The partners included several hospitals, the police department, the sex crimes unit, the rape crisis center, and the district attorney's office. Procedures and protocols on appropriately sensitive treatment of sexual assault survivors were developed, and cross-training between agencies began.

Over 20 years later, this partnership continues to exist. The city government supplies limited funding for evidence collection supplies (rape kits), and while the basic partners have remained the same, there have been additions to the collaborative network. Forensic nursing personnel as well as sexual assault teams from local universities have become involved and have used this collaborative framework to improve service delivery to the growing number of trauma survivors in the Philadelphia area.

During the past few years experience has informed the partnership that survivors with special needs were not being properly served by the existing service agencies. WOAR conducted outreach to Philadelphia's large Hispanic population and through neighborhood assessments, began a formal partnership with several of the churches serving the Spanish-speaking immigrant population. Bicultural and bilingual counselors were hired to travel to the various Philadelphia churches primarily serving this population to offer sexual abuse counseling within their structures.

As with the Hispanic population of the city, the disabled population had not been fully represented in the existing coalition of services. WOAR entered a partnership with several members of the group Speaking For Ourselves, a consumer association for people with disabilities. Through cross-training endeavors, both groups have learned about each other. The groups have partnered to offer individualized training sessions for parents and caregivers of those with disabilities.

Partnership has not been without its problems. Funding concerns have limited the willingness and availability of many potential participants. Differences in attitudes regarding the care of victims have arisen. Nevertheless, every group and agency within this partnership has much to bring in terms of caring for victims and educating others about sexual assault and trauma. Each addition to the existing network informs the other members of the network and facilitates the growth and improvement of the city's ability to care for survivors of sexual assault.

CONCLUSION

Sexual assault remains one of the most traumatic events that can befall a person. The violation goes beyond the physical, encompassing emotional and spiritual violation as well. From the minute of the assault onward, the victim may never again view the world as a safe place. But when the physical and sexual abuse and assault ends, the "victim" begins the transformation to "survivor." Through both formal and informal means, an enlightened and caring society can assist with this transformation. Rape crisis centers, SANE and SART staff, healthcare providers, and family, friends, and church can play a powerful role in helping the healing process. Continued efforts at prevention by any and all agencies concerned can help to create a world where there are fewer and fewer victims of sexual assault until the services of these agencies are no longer needed.

APPENDIX: STATE COALITIONS

Alabama Coalition Against Rape
334-264-0123

Alaska Network on Domestic Violence and Sexual Assault
907-586-3650

Arizona Sexual Assault Network (AzSAN)
602-258-1195

Arkansas Coalition Against Sexual Assault
870-741-1328

California Coalition Against Sexual Assault (CALCASA)
510-839-8825

Colorado Coalition Against Sexual Assault
303-861-7033

Connecticut Sexual Assault Crisis Services
860-282-9881

Delaware: CONTACT Delaware, Inc.
302-761-9800

Florida Council Against Sexual Violence
850-297-2000

Georgia Network to End Sexual Abuse
404-659-6482

Hawaii Coalition Against Sexual Assault
808-733-9038

Hawaii Sex Abuse Treatment Center
808-535-7600

Idaho Coalition Against Sexual and Domestic Violence
208-384-0419

Illinois Coalition Against Sexual Assault
217-753-4117

Indiana Coalition Against Sexual Assault
317-568-4001

Iowa Coalition Against Sexual Assault (ICASA)
515-244-7424

Kansas Coalition Against Sexual and Domestic Violence
785-232-9784

Kentucky Association of Sexual Assault Programs
502-226-2704

Louisiana Foundation Against Sexual Assault
504-747-8815

Maine Coalition Against Sexual Assault
207-626-0034

Maryland Coalition Against Sexual Assault
410-974-4507

Massachusetts Coalition of Rape Crisis Services
508-721-9711

Michigan Coalition Against Domestic and Sexual Violence
517-347-7000

Minnesota Coalition Against Sexual Assault
612-872-7734

Mississippi Coalition Against Sexual Assault
601-987-9011

Missouri Coalition Against Sexual Assault
573-636-8776

Montana Coalition Against Domestic Violence and Sexual Assault
406-443-7794

Nebraska Domestic Violence Sexual Assault Coalition
402-476-6256

Nevada Coalition Against Sexual Violence
702-914-6878

New Hampshire Coalition Against Domestic and Sexual Violence
603-224-8893

New Jersey Coalition Against Sexual Assault
609-631-4450

New Mexico Coalition of Sexual Assault Programs
505-883-8020

New York State Coalition Against Sexual Assault
518-482-4222

North Carolina Coalition Against Sexual Assault (NCCASA)
919-676-7611

North Dakota Council on Abused Women's Services
701-255-6240

Ohio Coalition Against Sexual Assault
614-268-3322

Oklahoma Coalition Against Domestic Violence and Sexual Assault
405-848-1815

Oregon Coalition Against Domestic and Sexual Violence
503-365-9644

Pennsylvania Coalition Against Rape
717-728-9740

Rhode Island: The Sexual Assault and Trauma Resource Center
401-421-4100

South Carolina Coalition Against Domestic Violence and Sexual Assault
803-256-2900

South Dakota Coalition Against Sexual Violence and Domestic Violence
605-945-0869

Tennessee Coalition Against Sexual Assault
615-259-9055

Texas Association Against Sexual Assault
512-445-1049

Utah Coalition Against Sexual Assault (CAUSE)
801-322-1500

Vermont Network Against Domestic Violence and Sexual Assault
802-223-1302

Virginians Aligned Against Sexual Assault
804-979-9002

Washington Coalition of Sexual Assault Programs
360-754-7583

West Virginia Foundation for Rape Information and Services
304-366-9500

Wisconsin Coalition Against Sexual Assault
608-257-1516

Wyoming Coalition Against Violence and Sexual Assault
307-755-5481

National Sexual Violence Resource Center
123 N. Enola Drive
Enola, PA 17025
877-739-3895

Rape Abuse and Incest National Network
635-B Pennsylvania Avenue SE
Washington, DC 20003
800-656-HOPE
www.rainn.org

REFERENCES

American Medical Association. *Strategies for the Treatment and Prevention of Sexual Assault.* Chicago, Ill: American Medical Association; 1995.

Brownmiller S. *Against Our Will: Men, Women and Rape.* New York, NY: Simon and Schuster; 1975.

Burgess AW, Holmstrom LL. Rape trauma syndrome. *Am J Psychol.* 1974;131:981-986.

Campbell R. The community response to rape: victims' experience with the legal, medical, and mental health systems. *Am J Community Psychol.* 1998;26:355-379.

Campbell R, Ahrens CE. Innovative community services for rape victims: an application of multiple case study methodology. *Am J Community Psychol.* 1998;26:537-571.

Foa EB, Dancu CV, Hembree EA, Jaycox LH, Meadows EA, Street GP. A comparison of exposure therapy, stress inoculation training, and their combination for reducing posttraumatic stress disorder in female assault victims. *J Consult Clin Psychol.* 1999;67:194-200.

Foubert JD. The longitudinal effects of a rape-prevention program on fraternity men's attitudes, behavioral intent, and behavior. *J Am Coll Health.* 2000;48:158-163.

Hampton HL. Care of the woman who has been raped. *N Engl J Med.* 1995;332:234-237.

Holmstrom LL, Burgess AW. Rape: husbands' and boyfriends' initial reactions. *Fam Coord.* 1979;28:321-330.

Horos C. *Rape.* New Canaan, Conn: Tobey Publishing; 1974.

International Association of Forensic Nurses. *Sexual Assault Nurse Examination Guidelines.* Pittman, NJ: IAFN; 1999.

Kimerling R, Calhoun KS. Somatic symptoms, social support, and treatment seeking among sexual assault victims. *J Consul Clin Psychol.* 1994;62:333-340.

Ledray L. *SANE Development and Operation Guide.* Washington, DC: US Deptartment of Justice Office for Victims of Crime; 1999.

Ledray LE, Simmelink K. Efficacy of SANE evidence collection. *J Emerg Nurs.* 1997;23:75-77.

Linden JA. Sexual assault. *Emerg Med Clin North Am.* 1999;17:685-697.

Petter LM, Whitehill DL. Management of female sexual assault. *Am Fam Physician.* 1998;58:920-926.

Popiel D, Susskind E. The impact of rape: social support as a moderator of stress. *Am J Community Psychol.* 1985;13:645-676.

Rossman L, Dunnuck C. A community sexual assault program based in an urban YWCA: The Grand Rapids experience. *J Emerg Nurs.* 1999;25:424-427.

Selig C. Sexual assault nurse examiner and sexual assault response team (SANE/SART) Program. *Nurs Clin North Am.* 2000;35:311-319.

Silverman, D. Sharing the crisis of rape: counseling the mates and families of victims. *Am J Orthopsychiatry.* 1978;48:166-173.

Smith K, Holmseth J, Macgregor M, Letourneau M. Sexual assault response team: overcoming obstacles to program development. *J Emerg Nurs.* 1998;24:365-367.

Tjaden P, Thoennes N. *Prevalence, Incidence, and Consequences of Violence Against Women: Findings from the National Violence Against Women Survey.* Washington, DC: US Department of Justice, Office of Justice Programs; 1998 Nov. Report No. NCJ 172837.

Warner, C. *Rape and Sexual Assault: Management and Intervention.* Germantown, Md: Aspen Systems Corp; 1980.

Webster L. *Sexual Assault and Child Sexual Abuse: A National Directory of Victim Survivor Services and Prevention Programs.* Phoenix, Ariz: The Oryx Press; 1989.

Chapter 25

MOVING BEYOND A DON'T-ASK–DON'T-TELL APPROACH TO ABUSE AND ASSAULT

Janice B. Asher, MD

In 1979, Stark et al. (1979) authored a landmark study that for the first time shifted the view of interpersonal violence from a purely personal issue to a social problem with enormous medical implications. The American Medical Association (AMA) and the Centers for Disease Control and Prevention (CDC) have called interpersonal violence an epidemic (AMA, 1992; CDC, 1998). Nonetheless, the rate of detection of violence and its sequelae by clinicians remains appallingly low. In one study, medical practitioners identified fewer than 3% of physically abused pregnant women, even though the injuries were often visible (Wilson, 1996). In another recent large study, only 13% of women seen in hospital emergency rooms for abuse-related injuries were asked any questions about abuse (Abbott et al., 1995).

What are the reasons for lack of detection? Why are doctors not asking? Why are patients not telling? In this chapter, we will explore some of the reasons for this missed opportunity for the healthcare community to assess and even prevent relationship violence—physical, sexual, and emotional. We will also offer some strategies for removing the barriers and moving toward meaningful remedies.

DON'T ASK: ACKNOWLEDGED BARRIERS

Clinicians perceive many barriers to routinely screening for or asking relevant questions pertaining to violence (AMA Council on Scientific Affairs, 1992; Sugg & Inui, 1992). The barriers that clinicians readily acknowledge include:

—I haven't been trained to do this.
—I don't have time to do this.
—It isn't my job; it isn't a medical problem.
—I'm not a domestic violence expert.
—This doesn't happen in the patient population that I see.
—This is a personal problem and isn't my business.
—If it's so bad, why doesn't she leave?
—What's the point? She'll just go back to him or find another abuser.

"I HAVEN'T BEEN TRAINED TO DO THIS"

A majority of physicians have had no formal training in abuse assessment, and they cite this lack of training as the main reason for not routinely screening for abuse (Chambliss et al., 1995; Cohen et al., 1997; Horan et al., 1998; Parsons et al., 1995). Fortunately, relationship violence is increasingly viewed in the context of a public health epidemic; thus its importance as part of medical and nursing school curricula, as well as residency and postgraduate training programs, has been recognized (Alpert et al., 1997). Appropriate assessment of abuse and assault is now considered "standard of care" by the AMA and the CDC. The CDC has also recommended that healthcare providers be trained and has published guidelines for developing training programs (Short et al., 1998). In studies where training

Key Point:
Interpersonal violence is not detected in the majority of cases because of acknowledged or unacknowledged barriers limiting the effectiveness of clinicians.

programs have been offered, the incidence of violence assessment significantly increases (Harwell et al., 1998).

Even as physicians come to view relationship violence in all its forms as a problem with significant and pervasive healthcare implications, screening for violence remains inadequate. Results of a recent study indicate that over 60% of obstetrician-gynecologists do not routinely screen pregnant patients for violence, even though domestic violence is more common than preeclampsia, gestational diabetes, and placenta previa (Gazmararian et al., 1996). Similarly, over 70% of gynecologists do not routinely screen their gynecologic patients (Horan et al., 1998). Routine screening still needs to be increased.

"I Don't Have Time"

In the current medical practice milieu, clinicians are expected to make appropriate assessments and treatment plans during appointments that are often only 15 minutes long. Clinicians often complain that screening for abuse is "just one more thing" they are expected to "add on" to the patient visit. Although such a response is understandable, it is short-sighted. Clinicians are, in fact, spending large amounts of time with victims of abuse for issues that are violence-related but that are not identified as such. If they do not recognize that symptoms are related to or caused by abuse, then the diagnosis and treatment plan are doomed to failure and may even make the patient's situation more dangerous.

Another consideration that is particularly pertinent to the abused patient is that time constraints may make the clinician feel pressured to rapidly make an appropriate diagnosis and formulate a treatment plan. Such pressure may, in turn, lead to controlling behavior on the part of the clinician that may be seen as mirroring the controlling behavior of the abusive partner (Warshaw, 1996).

Abused women have more emergency room visits than do nonabused women. In addition, they have more hospitalizations and primary care physician visits than do nonabused women (Kernic et al., 2000). Over 50% of abused women, particularly those with a history of sexual abuse, have somatic complaints (Sutherland et al., 1998). These include headache, dizziness, shortness of breath, palpitations, chest pain, abdominal pain, pelvic pain, back pain, muscular pain, sleep disturbances, fatigue, and eating disorders (Badura et al., 1997; Golding, 1999; Lampe et al., 2000; Schoen et al., 2000). Clearly, each of these symptoms involves a lengthy history, an examination, and medical, or even surgical, work-up. If, on the other hand, such symptoms are known to exist in the context of abuse, the evaluation may be much more focused and efficient, as well as likely to lead to an improved outcome for the patient.

Physicians who fear that assessing for relationship violence will take too much time must realize how much unrecognized time is taken with symptoms related to abuse. Appropriate violence assessment in such cases is much more likely to save time and expense. In a study of patients enrolled in a large health plan, women who were victims of relationship violence cost the health plan 92% more than did nonabused female patients (Wisner et al., 1999).

"It's Not My Job; It's Not a Medical Problem"

Many clinicians claim that, because domestic violence is a social problem rather than a medical disease, it falls outside the realm of what should be included in medical care. A frequent comment is, "This is not why I went to medical school." This attitude is reminiscent of the view held by the medical community years ago when patients were not screened for tobacco or alcohol use. Both of those habits were considered to be social customs and were therefore not "medical" issues, unless the patient developed a medical illness as a result of tobacco or alcohol use. Physicians now routinely screen all patients for tobacco and alcohol use and know that physician encouragement influences smoking cessation and other healthy lifestyle changes.

Clinicians must appreciate that domestic violence assessment is indeed their job. The AMA has gone so far as to say that a physician may be held liable for injuries sustained in a domestic violence situation if that physician has made no assessment of prior similarly inflicted injuries (AMA Council on Ethical and Judicial Affairs, 1992).

Realistically, taking on an issue that does not fit the traditional medical model of curing disease and repairing injury is difficult in a practical sense: clinicians are not reimbursed to spend time with a patient examining complex contextual, preventive, and protective factors (Warshaw, 1996). Domestic violence cannot be put on a billing diagnosis if the patient is on the abusive partner's insurance plan. However, as already discussed, enormous amounts of time and resources are spent with victims of abuse. Understanding symptoms and injuries that exist in the context of abuse is simply good medicine.

"I'm Not a Domestic Violence Expert"

In fact, no physician is a domestic violence expert. It is reassuring that doctors do not need to be "specialists." Familiar models can be adapted to facilitate domestic violence assessment and referral. For example, when a gynecologist hears a harsh, diastolic heart murmur, he or she feels comfortable referring the patient to a cardiologist. The gynecologist knows to explain to the patient that there is a problem that requires further evaluation and treatment. The gynecologist will then give the patient a referral. He or she may even personally contact the consultant or arrange for a staff member to do so.

Similarly, after assessing for violence, clinicians may then refer patients to appropriate and available experts, including social workers, advocates, mental health workers, and other institutional and community resources. Because violence is not a medical issue per se, but rather a complex social problem with medical consequences, a team approach is not only viable, but also necessary. Addressing violence does not lend itself readily to the traditional medical model of clinician-driven treatment of disease. Whereas physicians (and to a lesser extent, other clinicians) have been trained to work autonomously to cure disease, this model does not serve either the clinician or the patient in the context of relationship violence (Alpert et al., 1997; Warshaw, 1996). Rather than viewing abuse as a disease to be "cured," it must be seen for what it is: a public health problem to be approached in a collaborative manner.

"Abuse Doesn't Happen in My Patient Population"

There is a common perception that abuse is not an issue in some patient populations (Cohen et al., 1997). Particularly if the couple is affluent or the abusive partner is well-known and well-respected in the community, the abusive partner is more likely to be believed. In such a scenario, the abused partner may be thought to be manipulative, lying, or disturbed. Alternatively, incidents of partner and child abuse may be more likely to viewed as accidents (Warshaw, 1996). In one study, 50% of clinicians surveyed believed that the prevalence of domestic violence in their practice was 1% or less (Sugg et al., 1999).

Key Point:
Abuse must be viewed as a public health problem that requires a collaborative effort to resolve.

There are also stereotypes for poor women or women of certain ethnic or cultural groups that lead to the notion that violence against such women is to be expected, or even that such violence is "normal." Although poverty, for example, is certainly a stressor and is a risk factor for domestic violence, it is not a cause of or excuse for violence.

"This Is a Personal Problem and Is Not My Business"

One of the ironies associated with the lack of routine violence screening is that clinicians often state that they do not wish to offend a patient by asking such personal questions (Sugg & Inui, 1992). Yet in recent years, with the explosion in sexually transmitted infections and, in particular, with the specter of human immunodeficiency virus (HIV) infection, clinicians have all learned to become comfortable taking detailed and extremely personal sexual histories from patients. When questioned in a nonjudgmental way, patients do not feel offended by questions about their personal safety. In studies of both battered and nonbattered women, 75% of both groups of women reported wanting healthcare providers to ask about domestic violence (Friedman et al., 1998; McNutt et al., 1999).

Until the latter part of the 20th century, what went on "behind closed doors" was considered to be a private family matter, even if it was child or spousal abuse. Now it is frequently assumed that if a patient wishes to discuss the painful issue of relationship violence, then the patient will raise the issue himself or herself. Such an attitude is particularly unfortunate with regard to abuse, because victims of abuse are more likely to disclose abuse to their health care providers than they are to anyone else, including friends, clergy, or family members—but only when asked (McFarlane et al., 1991; Norton et al., 1995; McLeer et al., 1989).

"Why Doesn't She Just Leave?"
There are many valid reasons why victims do not leave abusive relationships. Because they are more likely to sustain severe, even life-threatening injuries at the time they attempt to leave than at any other time, leaving may simply be too dangerous for them and/or for their children.

Another barrier to leaving the abuser is the lack of any safe, affordable place to go. In most areas, the shelter systems are overutilized and underfunded. At best, they represent extremely temporary stopgap measures. Even in affluent families, the victim of abuse, usually the woman, may have no access whatsoever to financial resources. Her partner may give her an "allowance" that is not sufficient for the family's needs and that is intended to ensure that she will not be able to put money away. The credit cards and all their assets may be in his name. It is not uncommon for divorce proceedings to be characterized by prolonged custody battles that are carried out by the abusive partner with the sole intention of impoverishing the victim.

An abused woman may be too overwhelmed by her situation and may even blame herself for the abuse. She may have previously told someone about her situation and received a response that left her feeling responsible for the behavior. Finally, there are many social and cultural constraints to leaving a long-term relationship. She may hear from her family members that she shouldn't "break up the family" (even though the abuse has already done precisely that), that her children "need a father," that he's "a good provider," or that everyone has "marriage problems."

"What's the Point?"
Some clinicians believe that even if a woman does leave, she will just get involved with another abuser. Most women who leave abusive partners do not, in fact, enter into subsequent violent relationships. Those individuals who do follow a pattern for repeatedly being victimized are generally those who have been severely traumatized as children and are engaging in a pattern of "traumatic reenactment." (See Chapter 23, Revised Trauma Theory: Understanding the Traumatic Nature of Sexual Assault).

Won't she just go back to him anyway? As we will discuss later, in the section on a model for behavioral change, leaving an abusive relationship is a process, not an event (Mayer & Liebschutz, 1998). Just as successful smoking cessation is usually preceded by several unsuccessful attempts, successful separation from an abusive partner is often preceded by several unsuccessful attempts at separation.

Don't Ask: Unacknowledged Barriers
In addition to the acknowledged barriers of moving beyond a don't-ask–don't-tell model for violence disclosure in a medical setting, there are also many more subtle or unacknowledged barriers. It is difficult, and potentially even painful, to go beyond the traditional medical paradigm to confront personal feelings and social beliefs (Warshaw, 1993).

Unacknowledged barriers to violence assessment include the following:

—The issue of relationship violence is too close for comfort with regard to clinicians' own personal histories as well as their sense of safety in their own communities (Sisley et al., 1999).
—Medical training itself may be viewed as an abusive experience.
—Victims of abuse may be difficult and unlikable patients.
—Physicians don't want to open a Pandora's box (Sugg & Inui, 1992).

TOO CLOSE FOR COMFORT

There are both societal and personal issues at play in the feeling that relationship violence is a subject too close for comfort. With regard to societal issues, everyone is brought up to accept cultural paradigms. Paradigms foster acceptance of ideas such as men "wear the pants in the family" and "rule the roost." Obnoxious, destructive, and even violent behavior by young males is often met with the response "boys will be boys." People learn that men are supposed to be sexually assertive and women are not. Confronting these stereotypes is difficult. Clinicians may need to call into question basic assumptions that they have held for their entire lives. Nonetheless, moving beyond stereotypes may help clinicians understand and assist patients, and themselves, to develop effective, meaningful coping strategies.

At a personal level, hearing about abuse is upsetting and even frightening. It may be difficult to be caring and compassionate while at the same time remaining neutral and dispassionate enough to avoid feeling personally and professionally overwhelmed. This is the nature of "secondary trauma" (See Chapter 26, Caring for the Caregiver).

The issue of relationship violence may also attack the core of a physician's personal experience (Matthews, 1997). It is frightening to contemplate living in a world where things like this happen "for no good reason." In a study of first-year medical students, 38% reported being victims of violence as children or as an adult (Cullinane et al., 1997). If previously abused medical students have not explored or resolved their own experiences, confronting similar experiences in their patients may be overwhelming. They may find it too painful to hear the patient's story or even to acknowledge the truth and validity of that story. Physicians function "within a system that devalues feelings..." (Warshaw, 1993). However, acknowledgment of their own histories can then be used as a foundation to model the support and advocacy discussions needed with patients (Alpert et al., 1997; Matthews, 1997).

MEDICAL TRAINING AS AN ABUSIVE EXPERIENCE

Medical training is physically punishing, emotionally draining, and socially isolating. It is often abusive and humiliating and we may feel anxious, exhausted, overwhelmed, depressed, and traumatized. . . . As we slowly begin to reorient our identities in terms of its values, we find ourselves internalizing its constructs and judging ourselves by its terms. . . . These kinds of parallels between medical training and battering relationships are double edged. They are precisely what can, if acknowledged, form a bridge between our experiences while, if avoided and denied, will recreate the problems [resulting from abuse]. (Warshaw, 1993, page 78)

The model of medical education often seems to be derived from fraternity "hazing" rituals, complete with intimidation, sleep deprivation, and a rigid hierarchical structure. For students and residents to survive in such a setting, they learn to be "tough" themselves and, in turn, expect the same from others, thereby perpetuating the structure. By emulating and ultimately becoming those in power, clinicians, originally the harassed students and residents, now identify with the power structure. In this context, they are likely to lack compassion and empathy.

Medical school teachers and mentors are in a position to change this draconian model of education and training by displaying compassion and empathy to trainees.

In addition to being positive role models, we can use our authority to ensure that trainees learn and employ violence assessment tools. There is abundant evidence that when violence assessment is mandatory, when there are institutional policies and protocols, when universal violence screening is a quality improvement issue, and when there are negative consequences for clinicians who do not appropriately screen, the assessment and violence detection rate markedly increases (Larkin et al., 2000; McLeer et al., 1989).

Sexual and Gender-Based Harassment

Another manifestation of abuse in medicine involves sexual harassment, particularly that aimed at female medical students and residents. In one study, 47.7% of female physicians reported gender-based harassment, and 36.9% reported sexual harassment. Gender-based harassment was described as occurring to females in a male-dominated setting or specialty and was not associated with a physical or sexual component, as opposed to sexual harassment. Frank et al. (1998) indicate the highest rates for both types were among medical students and younger physicians. The authors go on to state, "Present thought characterizes sexual harassment as primarily a manifestation of power, rather than sexual attraction. The profession of medicine, particularly in academic settings, may be especially prone to harassment because of the importance of hierarchy. This may account for the higher prevalence of harassment found in training environments. . . ." (Frank et al., 1998, page 356).

Sequelae of harassment include fatigue, depression, and a sense of isolation that make it difficult to endure hearing about similar experiences from patients. If physicians blame themselves for the harassment, which is a common response, then physicians may, in turn, be more likely to blame patients for their own ordeals. If physicians deny that the behavior experienced was, in fact, harassment, then they may, in turn, be more likely to deny that patients are experiencing abuse at all.

Key Point:
Sexual and gender-based harassment can produce fatigue, depression, and a sense of isolation. Clinicians must not tolerate this behavior. Furthermore, they must maintain an attitude of compassion and empathy for the victim as well as students and colleagues.

The medical profession, medical students, and patients deserve to function within an environment that does not tolerate sexual and gender-based harassment. There must be clearly stated institutional policies as well as appropriate, enforced sanctions and punishments for transgressors. Furthermore, clinicians must be compassionate and empathetic, not only toward patients who are victims of abuse and assault, but also toward students and colleagues.

VICTIMS OF ABUSE AS DIFFICULT PATIENTS

Clinicians simply do not like to see some patients. They inwardly groan when they see those patients' names on appointment lists. This scenario may be particularly true for some abused patients. Patients in abusive relationships seem to have a long list of somatic complaints with no discernible medical cause. They seem depressed, and they make clinicians feel depressed, but they do not want treatment. They may be substance abusers who go in and out of treatment programs but never seem to make headway. Even if physicians know the symptoms are caused by abuse, feelings toward the patients may be problematic. Physicians want victims to be "angels" and perpetrators to be "monsters," but reality is usually far less distinct. The patient may be a drug addict, be manipulative, or seem totally resistant to heartfelt and time-consuming efforts in her behalf. Her partner may appear likable, sympathetic, and caring. By acknowledging these feelings about "difficult" patients, physicians can take steps to move beyond these prejudices and obstacles.

PANDORA'S BOX

"When I see a patient who has appendicitis, I know that I can fix the problem. When I see a patient who's being abused, I feel like I'm about to fall into a deep hole. It's like opening Pandora's Box" (A surgical colleague's attitude toward medical assessment of violence).

In addition to being time-consuming and disturbing, the diagnosis of relationship violence may itself create problems (Warshaw, 1996). For example, a psychiatric referral may mean that the patient will be labeled as "mentally ill," a diagnosis that may be later used against her in a custody dispute. If a patient discloses that her partner is also abusing the children, the clinician may feel compelled as a mandated reporter to report the child abuse. If the batterer finds out that his partner has disclosed the abuse, she may be in even greater danger. If the patient reports that in addition to her partner abusing her, she is also hurting her children, the clinician is mandated to file a report against the patient. This is particularly disturbing, because the clinician has asked questions about abuse out of a desire to protect the patient!

Clinicians are justifiably concerned about a lack of time, lack of comfort, and a sense of powerlessness to assist the victims of such complex personal and social problems (Sugg & Inui, 1992). There are no easy solutions to these dilemmas. Fortunately, domestic violence advocacy organizations and child protective service agencies are becoming more aware of the intersection of domestic violence and child abuse and are beginning to deal with these complicated issues in a more coordinated fashion.

DON'T TELL—BARRIERS TO DISCLOSURE BY THE VICTIM

Why don't victims of abuse more readily tell clinicians what is happening to them? The number one reason that they cite is fear of retaliation by the abusive partner if they disclose the abuse (Rodriguez et al., 1996). A victim may have been told that he will kill her if she tells anyone, that he will hurt the children or take them away, that he will have her "locked up in a mental institution" because no one will believe her, or that he will have her deported. Clinicians need to recognize that the objective likelihood of these outcomes is not related to the subjective magnitude of the victim's fear.

Another reason that victims do not disclose the violence is shame. A universally employed tactic of abusers is to blame the victim—to make the abuse appear to be the natural consequence of her behavior. It is, in fact, easy to understand why victims of abuse actually want to believe that the abuse is their fault: if they have done something to precipitate the violence, then they can do something to prevent its recurrence. (Of course, this is not the case. The cause of, as well as the responsibility for, the violence rests with the perpetrator.)

Although abused women cite fear of retribution by the abuser as the main reason for not disclosing violence, they also frequently mention insensitive responses by their health care providers. For example, questions such as "Why don't you just leave?" or "What did you do to cause him to act like this?" increase the shame and sense of worthlessness that a victim of abuse feels. Such responses easily lead to a sense of hopelessness because the abuse is seen as a matter of "individual psychopathology" (Warshaw, 1993). The victim is then even less likely to mention the subject again.

Because a discussion about abuse is so difficult, it is easy to avoid the subject altogether. Physicians rationalize that they are not violence specialists, that they do not have time, that it is not their job, or that the patient is bringing this misery on herself (Warshaw, 1993). They bury their own experiences of personal abuse and cultural stereotypes and employ coping mechanisms such as denial, victim blaming, and "pathologizing" of the patient.

TREATING VICTIMS WITHOUT FEELING HOPELESS

Physicians and other clinicians are action-oriented. They want to "do something" so that patients will "get better." Viewing chronic lifestyles and behaviors, such as smoking or unhealthy dietary habits, as acute illnesses that need to be "cured" is inappropriate and futile. Applying a "fix-it" approach to patients who are in abusive and assaultive relationships causes what is inappropriate to become dangerous in

Key Point:
Victims of abuse face barriers that keep them from telling the clinician what is happening. Among these are fear of retaliation, shame, and insensitivity of the clinician.

Table 25-1. Stages of Behavior Change

Stage 1: Precontemplation

The patient does not perceive a problem. Her partner's violence is "no big deal" or is "no different from what happens in any other family." During this stage, the clinician can provide information: violence is common, it is not the victim's fault, it is dangerous for the victim and for children who witness the violence, and there are resources to help. The patient can be offered written material about violence, safety planning, and local resources. She can be offered a referral to a social worker or domestic violence counselor.

Stage 2: Contemplation

The patient perceives a problem and is considering change. However, although she may be more open to both information and offers of help, she probably feels intensely ambivalent about the risks versus the rewards of leaving the relationship. As a result, many patients remain in this stage for many years. During this stage, stressing the rewards of leaving, expressing optimism about the possibility of change, and supporting safety measures while the patient is considering change may be of great benefit. It is helpful to remind the patient that the abuse is not her fault and that help is available. Specifically, in addition to discussing safety strategies, she should be offered referrals to social service and advocacy resources.

Stage 3: Preparation

The patient is actively planning change. She has already taken some measures to prepare for ending the relationship. It is crucial to help her understand the potential danger for herself and her children when she does actually leave and even afterward. At this time, in addition to referrals to other experts, an exit strategy is essential. The patient should be urged to consider a plan that includes identifying people she can stay with, planning ways to save and hide money, making copies of all important papers and documents, etc.

Stage 4: Action

The patient has ended the relationship. She needs to appreciate that she is still vulnerable to violent assaults. Safety strategies must be emphasized. The clinician should support her decision while explaining that "relapse" is common; victims of abuse, for many reasons, often return to the abuser. However, this behavior is not "going around in circles." Instead, it is a return to a prior stage of change and is much more likely to result in a more successful move forward later. This knowledge and attitude are important for the clinician as well. Without this understanding, clinicians can easily feel overwhelmed by frustration and anger with the patient now perceived as "wasting our time."

Stage 5: Maintenance

The patient has maintained the successful behavior change for several months. Even at this time, she is not free from assaultive and abusive behavior from the partner. He may stalk her; he may engage in a prolonged custody battle to further exhaust, intimidate, and impoverish her; or he may engage the children in spying behavior against her. In addition, many emotional, financial, psychologic, cultural, and familial pressures may occur that do not support the changes she has made. For example, her partner may urge her to come back, promising that he will never hurt her again. She may feel pressure from her children or other family members to "keep the family together." She may feel emotionally and financially overwhelmed. The clinician must support her healthy behavioral changes while helping her avoid feeling demoralized if she returns to the relationship.

that a sense of outrage and urgency propels clinicians into wanting to exclaim, "You've got to get out now!" Because a person in an abusive relationship is at greatest risk for being seriously injured or even killed when he or she tries to leave, urging the victim to leave without having a well-thought out safety plan is irresponsible. Furthermore, such a response leaves a victim who is not planning on ending an abusive relationship feeling even more isolated and worthless.

STAGES OF BEHAVIOR CHANGE

The Transtheoretical Model (TTM) of Change, or Stages of Behavioral Change Model, as first described by Prochaska et al., (1994) takes into account stages of attitude that precede behavioral change. By understanding these different stages, clinicians can appreciate how to help patients who are either unwilling or unable to leave violent relationships. In so doing, the clinician can help the patient and not become frustrated or angry about the patient's "noncompliance" in leaving an abusive relationship. In addition, the patient does not feel like a "failure" for being unable to comply (**Table 25-1**).

CONCLUSIONS

Abusive relationships are typically complex and have societal, economic, psychologic, familial, and cultural components. A clinician's attempt to deal with the medical ramifications of abuse without some awareness of these complexities and interrelationships is likely to end in failure for both clinician and patient. By understanding stages of change in behavior modification, clinicians are in a much better position to assist the abused patient in attaining a greater level of safety for herself and her children and to take steps toward a life of health and self-determination.

In dealing with patients who have been victims of assault and abuse, clinicians do not need to be police officers, mental health professionals, or social workers. Clinicians have a vital role to play in contributing to the amelioration of this public health epidemic. In so doing, caregiver frustration and anger toward patients can be diminished as the satisfaction of helping patients live healthier, self-directed lives is reclaimed (Zimmerman et al., 2000).

Key Point:
Understanding the stages required to change a behavior will help the clinician see how to best help patients who cannot or will not leave abusive relationships.

REFERENCES

Abbott J, Johnson R, Koziol-McLain J, Lowenstein SR. Domestic violence against women: incidence and prevalence in an emergency department population. *JAMA.* 1995;273:1763-1767.

Alpert EJ, Sege RD, Bradshaw YS. Interpersonal violence and the education of physicians. *Acad Med.* 1997;72:S41-S50.

American Medical Association. Council on Ethical and Judicial Affairs. Physicians and domestic violence, ethical considerations. *JAMA.* 1992;267:113-116.

American Medical Association. Council on Scientific Affairs. Violence against women: relevance for medical practitioners. *JAMA.* 1992;267:3184-3189.

Badura AS, Reiter RC, Altmaier EM, Rhomberg A, Elas D. Dissociation, somatization, substance abuse and coping in women with chronic pelvic pain. *Obstet Gynecol.* 1997;90:405-410.

Centers for Disease Control and Prevention. *MMWR.* 1998;47(RR-1):1-128.

Chambliss LR, Bay RC, Jones RF III. Domestic violence: an educational imperative? *Am J Obstet Gynecol.* 1995;172:1035-1038.

Cohen S, De Vos E, Newberger E. Barriers to physician identification and treatment of family violence: lessons from five communities. *Acad Med.* 1997;72:S19-S25.

Cullinane PM, Alpert EJ, Freund KM. First-year medical students' knowledge of, attitudes toward, and personal histories of family violence. *Acad Med.* 1997;72:48-50.

Frank E, Brogan D, Schiffman M. Prevalence and correlates of harassment among US women physicians. *Arch Intern Med.* 1998;158:352-358.

Friedman LS, Samet JH, Roberts MS, Hudlin M, Hans P. Inquiry about victimization experiences with clinicians and health services. *J Gen Intern Med.* 1998;13:549-555.

Gazmararian JA, Lazorick S, Spitz AM, Ballard TJ, Saltzman LE, Marks JS. Prevalence of violence against pregnant women: a review of the literature. *JAMA.* 1996;275:1915-1920.

Golding JM. Sexual assault history and headache: five general population studies. *J Nerv Ment Dis.* 1999;187:624-629.

Harwell TS, Casten RJ, Armstrong KA, Dempsey S, Coons HL, Davis M. Results of a domestic violence training program offered to the staff of urban community health centers. *Am J Prev Med.* 1998;15(3):235-242.

Horan DL, Chapin J, Klein L, Schmidt LA, Schulkin J. Domestic violence screening practices of obstetrician-gynecologists. *Obstet Gynecol.* 1998;92:785-789.

Kernic MA, Wolf ME, Holt VL. Rates and relative risk of hospital admission among women in violent intimate partner relationships. *Am J Pub Health.* 2000;90:1416-1420.

Lampe A, Solder E, Ennemoser A, Schubert C, Rumpold G, Sollner W. Chronic pelvic pain and previous sexual abuse. *Obstet Gynecol.* 2000;96:929-933.

Larkin GL, Rolniak S, Hyman KB, MacLeod BA, Savage R. Effect of an administrative intervention on rates of screening for domestic violence in an urban emergency department. *Am J Public Health.* 2000;90:1444-1448.

Matthews MB. Ensuring students' well-being as they learn to support victims of violence. *Acad Med.* 1997;72:46-47.

Mayer L. The severely abused woman in obstetric and gynecologic care: guidelines for recognition and management. *J Reprod Med.* 1995;40:13-18.

Mayer L, Liebschutz J. Domestic violence in the pregnant patient: obstetric and behavioral interventions. *Obstet Gynecol Surv.* 1998;53:627-635.

McFarlane J, Chrisoffel K, Bateman L, et al. Assessing for abuse: self reports versus nurse interview. *Public Health Nurs.* 1991;1:245-250.

McLeer SV, Anwar RA, Herman S, Maquiling K. Education is not enough: a systems failure in protecting battered women. *Ann Emerg Med.* 1989;18:651-653.

McNutt LA, Carlson BE, Gagen D, Winterbauer N. Reproductive violence screening in primary care: perspectives and experiences of patients and battered women. *J Am Med Women's Assoc.* 1999;54(2):85-90.

Norton LB, Peipert JF, Zierler S, et al. Battering in pregnancy: an assessment of two screening methods. *Obstet Gynecol.* 1995;85:321-325.

Parsons LH, Zaccaro D, Wells B, Stovall TG. Methods of and attitudes toward screening obstetrics and gynecology patients for domestic violence. *Am J Obstet Gynecol.* 1995;173:381-387.

Prochaska JO, Redding CA, Harlow LL, Rossi JS, Velicer WF. The transtheoretical model of change and HIV prevention: a review. *Health Educ Q.* 1994;21:471-486.

Rodriguez MA, Quiroga SS, Bauer HM. Breaking the silence: battered women's perspectives on medical care. *Arch Fam Med.* 1996;5:153-158.

Schoen C, Davis K, Collins KS, Greenberg L, Des Roches C, Abrams M. *The Commonwealth Fund Survey of the Health of Adolescent Girls 1997.* New York, NY: The Commonwealth Fund; 2000.

Short LM, Johnson D, Osattin A. Recommended components of health care provider training on intimate partner violence. *Am J Prev Med.* 1998;14:283-288.

Sisley A, Jacobs LM, Poole G, Campbell S, Esposito T. Violence in America: a public health crisis-domestic violence. *J Trauma.* 1999;46:1105-1112.

Stark E, Flitcraft A, Frazier W. Medicine and patriarchal violence: the social construction of a "private event." *Int J Health Serv.* 1979;9:461-493.

Sugg NK, Inui T. Primary care physicians' response to domestic violence, opening Pandora's box. *JAMA.* 1992;267:65-68.

Sugg NK, Thompson RS, Thompson DC, Maiuro R, Rivara FP. Domestic violence and primary care: attitudes, practices and beliefs. *Arch Fam Med.* 1999;8:301-306.

Sutherland C, Bybee D, Sullivan C. The long-term effects of battering on women's health. *Womens Health.* 1998;41:41-70.

Warshaw C. Domestic violence: challenges to medical practice. *J Women Health.* 1993;2:73-79.

Warshaw C. Domestic violence: changing theory, changing practice. *J Am Med Women's Assoc.* 1996;51:87-100.

Wilson LM, Reid AJ, Midmer DK, Biringer A, Carroll JC, Stewart DE. Antenatal psychosocial risk factors associated with adverse postpartum family outcomes. *Can Med Assoc J.* 1996;154:785-796.

Wisner CL, Gilmer TP, Saltzman LE, Zink TM. Intimate partner violence against women: do victims cost health plans more? *J Fam Prac.* 1999;48:439-443.

Zimmerman GL, Olsen CG, Bosworth MF. A "stages of change" approach to helping patients change behavior. *Am Fam Physician.* 2000;61:1406-1416.

CARING FOR THE CAREGIVER: AVOIDING AND TREATING VICARIOUS TRAUMATIZATION

Sandra L. Bloom, MD

Vicarious traumatization is a term that describes the cumulative transformative effect on the helper of working with survivors of traumatic life events. The symptoms can appear much like those of posttraumatic stress disorder (PTSD), but also encompass changes in frame of reference, identity, sense of safety, ability to trust, self-esteem, intimacy, and a sense of control. The presence of vicarious traumatization has been noted in many groups of helping professionals who have close contact with people who have experienced traumatic events. Caregivers are at even higher risk if they have a history of trauma in their own backgrounds and if they extend themselves beyond the boundaries of good self-care or professional conduct.

The actual causes of vicarious traumatization have not yet been established, but this article proposes a broad view of causality that includes the biologically based notion of emotional contagion; the psychological impact of losing positive illusions; the professional prohibition against using normal social obstacles to defend against emotional contagion and the loss of positive illusions; organizational dysfunction that contributes to excessive vulnerability on the part of the caregiver; and conflicts inherent in the ideologic framework of present-day caregiving. These conflicts include the desacralization of healing, the commodification of healthcare, short-comings of the medical model, a bias toward individualism, and the presence of individual violence embedded within a context of cultural violence.

Individual steps can be taken to address the individual and organizational aspects of vicarious traumatization. These steps begin with a self-assessment of the presence of vicarious traumatization and an evaluation of present and possible strategies to address vicarious traumatization framed within an ecological model. Ultimately, it will be the responsibility of every caregiving and service organization to develop some "universal precautions" effective in protecting helpers against the impact of violence, even in its indirect form.

Key Point:
The symptoms of vicarious traumatization resemble those of PTSD, but also encompass changes in frame of reference, identify, sense of safety, ability to trust, self-esteem, intimacy, and sense of control.

WHAT IS IT?

As a social species, human beings are sociobiologically connected to each other. Witnessing another person's suffering is so traumatic that torturers frequently force their victim to observe the torture of another in order to elicit information. It has long been recognized that emergency workers, physicians, nurses, police officers, firemen, journalists, clergy, social service workers, colleagues, family members, and other witnesses and bystanders to disasters and other trauma can experience secondary symptoms themselves.

Currently the terms that are used most frequently to describe these symptoms are secondary traumatic stress, compassion fatigue, and vicarious traumatization. Although there are some differences, these terms will be used interchangeably in this chapter. Secondary traumatic stress is defined as the natural, consequent behavior and emotions that result from knowledge about a traumatizing event experienced by another and the stress resulting from helping or wanting to help a traumatized or suffering person. The symptoms are almost identical to those of PTSD (Catherall, 1995). Compassion fatigue is described as the natural, predictable, treatable, and preventable unwanted consequence of working with suffering people (Figley, 1995). Vicarious traumatization is defined as the cumulative transformative effect on the helper of working with survivors of traumatic life events, both positive and negative (McCann & Pearlman, 1990).

There is a relationship between terms used to describe this reaction to dealing with people exposed to trauma and the more traditional terms of "burnout" and "countertransference." The more familiar term, "burnout" refers to a collection of symptoms associated with emotional exhaustion and generally attributed to increased work load and institutional stress, described by a process that includes gradual exposure to job strain, erosion of idealism, and a lack of achievement (Pines & Arenson, 1988). Burnout may then be the result of repetitive or chronic exposure to vicarious traumatization that is unrecognized and unsupported by the organizational setting. In contrast, "countertransference" is a far broader term, referring to all reactions to a client and the material he or she brings. Countertransference reactions are specific to the particular client and are tied to interactions with that client. In this case, vicarious traumatization can be seen as a specific form of countertransference experience, differentiated from other countertransference reactions in that vicarious traumatization can continue to affect our lives and our work long after interactions with the other person have ceased (Stamm, 1997).

Various authors have described the signs and symptoms of secondary traumatic stress and vicarious traumatization. Secondary traumatic stress in a helper of someone who has been traumatized closely resembles PTSD and includes symptoms of hyperarousal, emotional numbing, avoidance, and intrusive experiences. Vicarious traumatization symptoms include typical symptoms of posttraumatic stress but also encompass symptoms indicative of a disrupted frame of reference, including disruptions in identity, worldview, and spirituality, and impacts on psychologic need areas.

Key Point:
With disturbance of the frame of reference, beliefs about other people and the world are affected, including beliefs about causality and higher purpose. Caregivers then see the world as a far more dangerous place and may come to see other people as malevolent and evil, untrustworthy, exploitative, or alienating. Maintaining a sense of hope and belief in the goodness of humanity is progressively more difficult.

When a person's frame of reference is disturbed, beliefs about other people and the world are affected as well as beliefs about causality and higher purpose (Rosenbloom et al., 1995). Caregivers may begin to see the world as a far more dangerous place than they did before their exposure to trauma, and if the trauma has been interpersonal, they may come to see other people as malevolent and evil, untrustworthy, exploitative, or alienating. It may become increasingly difficult to retain a sense of hope and belief in the goodness of humanity.

The psychologic need areas that can be affected by vicarious traumatization include safety, trust, esteem, intimacy, and control (Rosenbloom et al., 1995). A loss of a secure sense of safety can manifest as increased fearfulness, a heightened sense of personal vulnerability, excessive security concerns, behavior directed at increasing security, and increasing fear for the lives and safety of loved ones. The capacity to trust, particularly after interpersonal violence, may become so impaired that a belief develops that no one can be trusted. Likewise, trust in one's own judgment and perceptions can also be negatively altered. It may become very difficult, in the face of secondary exposure to traumatic events, to maintain a sense of self-esteem, particularly around areas of competence. It also may be increasingly difficult to maintain a sense of esteem about others, leading to a pervasive suspiciousness of other people's motivations and behavior. Problems with intimacy may develop, leading to difficulties in spending time alone; self-medication with food, alcohol, or drugs; or engaging in compulsive behaviors like shopping, exercise, or sex. Problems with intimacy may lead to isolating from others and withdrawing from relationships, including family, friends, and professional colleagues. Control issues may become so central that the more control the caregiver feels has been lost, the more control he or she tries to exert over self and others. Equally possible may be efforts to narrow or restrict the scope of one's world in the hope of avoiding anything that may be experienced as being outside of one's control.

The concept of vicarious traumatization emphasizes the positive as well as the negative impact of bearing witness to traumatic events. Disruptions in world view, identity, and key psychologic needs provide an opportunity for radical transformations that may lead to growth and higher consciousness rather than degradation and constriction. As caregivers, it is our responsibility to make choices in our own personal, professional, and organizational lives that support positive, rather than negative, transformative changes.

WHO GETS IT?

Although the concept of secondary traumatic stress is less than two decades old, there is a growing body of studies detailing the existence of many different survivor groups. For example, counselors with high domestic violence caseloads have been shown to have classical symptoms of vicarious traumatization. Specific challenges of this kind of work include difficulties with confidentiality, fear for the safety of their clients, and feelings of isolation and powerlessness (Iliffe & Steed, 2000).

People who treat victims of sexual abuse are known to experience vicarious traumatization. A study compared the rates of vicarious traumatization of clinicians working with sexual abuse victims with those working with cancer victims and found that those clinicians working with sexual abuse victims were more negatively affected (Cunningham, 1996). It has been recognized that therapists working with sexual abuse survivors may experience a grief process themselves as they come to terms with their own exposure to the sexual abuse of children (Cunningham, 1999). In addition, there are reports of negative transformations of worldview and increased fears about the safety of children (Simonds, 1996). In a study of counselors working with sexual violence survivors, the counselors who had a higher percentage of survivors in their caseload reported more disrupted beliefs, more symptoms of PTSD, and more self-reported vicarious trauma, irrespective of their own trauma histories (Schauben & Frazier, 1995).

Vicarious traumatization affects investigators of sexual abuse as well as therapists. In a study looking at the impact of secondary traumatic stress on child protective service workers, the results indicated that secondary traumatic stress symptoms were common among those surveyed and were more likely to occur in those who had worked at the job the longest, had worked longer hours, were female, and who had a history of experiencing or witnessing trauma (Meyers, 1996). In another study, among the "veterans" in child protective services (2 years or more), 62% scored in the high range on an emotional exhaustion scale, considered by some to be the heart of burnout (Anderson, 2000).

Several studies have looked at the impact that working with sex offenders has on counselors. Similar to other findings, the rate of vicarious traumatization appears to be related to years of experience in clinical practice, the counselor's own trauma history, and particular work settings (Kostouros, 1998).

Hospital personnel are known to be vulnerable to the effects of secondary traumatic stress. Several papers have reported on the impact of exposure to trauma on nursing professionals (Alexander & Atcheson, 1998; Crothers, 1995; Lyon, 1993; Schwam, 1998). A recent review article documents the emotional needs of both parents whose children are hospitalized and staff members who work on pediatric intensive care and neonatal intensive care units (Peebles-Klieger, 2000). In a study looking at the effects of exposure to multiple acquired immunodeficiency syndrome (AIDS)-

related deaths on group therapy, group members exerted a traumatizing effect on group therapists, who experienced death images, survivor guilt, psychic numbing, suspicion of counterfeit nurturance, and a struggle for meaning (Gabriel, 1994). In another study of healthcare workers, physicians, nurses, social workers, and support staff recruited from 20 publicly funded human immunodeficiency virus (HIV) programs who were given measures of stress, coping, empathy, burnout, and secondary traumatic stress, the four groups experienced moderate levels of burnout and low levels of secondary traumatic stress (Garrett, 1999).

In a study of vicarious traumatization among law enforcement professionals, patrol officers and detectives from homicide and child sexual abuse were studied. The study found that dissociation and maladaptive coping predicted pathology and distress. It was also noted that a personal history of child abuse made it more likely that the individual would work in units with high exposure to trauma and would be more vulnerable to dissociative and anxiety disorders (Hallett, 1996).

A summary of risk factors indicates that having a past history of traumatic experience is a substantial risk factor for developing vicarious traumatization. Caregivers who extend themselves beyond the limits of customary service delivery by overworking, ignoring healthy boundaries, or taking on too many trauma survivors in their caseload are also at risk. Less experience as a therapist can put someone at risk, but so can too much experience, presumably because of the excess of exposure to traumatic material. Having a high percentage of traumatized children, particularly sexually abused children, in one's caseload is a risk, as is working with a high number of patients suffering from dissociative disorders. Experiencing too many negative clinical outcomes is also a risk factor.

There also appear to be protective factors that help alleviate or protect against the development of vicarious traumatization. These protective factors are similar to those that have been uncovered in the studies of people who are resilient under stress (Williams & Sommer, 1995). Good social support is key. Strong ethical principles of practice, knowledge of theory, ongoing training, the development of competence in practice strategies and techniques, and awareness of the potential of vicarious traumatization and the need to take deliberate steps to minimize the impact all serve as protective factors.

WHAT CAUSES IT?

Trying to describe what causes vicarious traumatization is like trying to describe what causes PTSD. The reasons for why some patients develop PTSD following a traumatic event and others do not may turn out to be very similar to the reasons why some people develop vicarious traumatization and others do not. Like PTSD, vicarious traumatization can be viewed as a "normal reaction to abnormal stress," or as a picture of adaptive coping skills gone wrong. Similar to any discussion of the causality of PTSD, there are biologic, psychologic, social, and moral, spiritual, and philosophical components of the individual that interact with the professional and sociopolitical context of the individual's life space to produce the final outcome.

BIOLOGIC CAUSALITY: EMOTIONAL CONTAGION

Listening to victims of trauma can produce a noxious physiologic and psychologic state in the listener that is strongly defended against. Therefore members of victims' social groups are likely to take measures to prevent the victims from sharing their experience and thereby spreading the contagious effect. This presents powerful negative consequences for the victims, because the tendency to avoid disclosure of emotions is associated with increased risks for physical illness, greater physiologic work, and impaired information processing (Harber & Pennebaker, 1992). One theory is that stress, in activating the complex human stress response, produces many kinds of powerful neurochemicals, including cortisol, an immune system

Key Points:
Risk factors for vicarious traumatization include:
— *Having a past history of traumatic experience*
— *Overwork*
— *Ignoring health boundaries*
— *Taking on too much*
— *Lack of experience as a therapist*
— *Too much experience as a therapist*
— *Dealing with large numbers of traumatized children, especially sexually abused children*
— *Working with large numbers of patients who suffer from dissociative disorders*
— *Having too many negative clinical outcomes*

suppressor. It is thought that the chronic inhibition of negative emotions produces increasing work for the autonomic nervous system, and this increased load functions as a chronic stressor with the result that biologic survival systems that should only be "on" under emergency conditions are reset to be "on" all the time (Pennebaker, 1997).

Likewise, the benefits of emotional expression have been known since ancient times. The word *catharsis* derives from the Greek, meaning purification or cleansing. People who are traumatized are often overwhelmed by their emotions, particularly in the acutely traumatized state. Suppressing emotional states is bad for their health. Caregiving relationships help surface those emotions, often long buried, and the helper is the one who is most likely to be exposed to the overwhelming nature of the victim's emotional states. Good caregiving requires that the caregiver respond to this state of emotional contagion in certain limited and prescribed ways, and respond by containing, rather than expressing, the caregiver's own physiologic states of hyperarousal, fear, anger, and grief.

PSYCHOLOGIC CAUSALITY: LOSS OF POSITIVE ILLUSIONS

Working with victims of violence and interpersonal trauma is so difficult because it changes caregivers who are willing to listen. Confrontation with the magnitude of interpersonal violence shatters our own protective assumptions as we let in the reality of "It really happened." As we wrestle with this reality, we come to recognize that "It could happen to me" and feel all the vulnerability that goes along with that recognition. For some, their own past history of interpersonal violence or child abuse is a personal reality because "It did happen to me" and all the unwanted reminders of an unresolved past are triggered by the patients' stories. The recurring sense of helplessness that victims feel may also affect the helpers, bringing with it a sense of hopelessness, expressed as "There's nothing I can do."

A central focus of the concept of vicarious traumatization is a disturbed frame of reference. Trauma shatters the basic assumptions, the frame of reference of the victim. Positive illusions about oneself, other people, and the world are destroyed. Exposure to traumatized people can destroy clinicians' positive illusions when they are confronted repeatedly with the terrible things that have happened to their patients, often at the hands of other people. The maintenance of positive illusions depends on consensual validation—on other people maintaining the same illusions. Therefore, the greatest conflict, and the one most likely to produce symptoms of vicarious traumatization, would revolve around cases of family violence including child abuse, spousal abuse, rape, and particularly child sexual abuse. The reality of family violence threatens one of our most cherished cultural notions—the family as a safe place.

SOCIAL CAUSALITY: INABILITY TO USE NORMAL SOCIAL OBSTACLES

Traumatic experiences shatter basic personal and cultural assumptions about the primary way we order reality. Suddenly there is no safety, the world no longer makes sense, other people cannot be trusted, the future is no longer predictable, and, because of dissociation, the past is no longer known (Janoff-Bulman, 1992). After the trauma, one of the most perplexing experiences for the individual victim is that the world goes on as before. Other people outside of the trauma envelope appear relatively oblivious to the traumatic event. For the victim, personal reality is no longer congruent with cultural reality. The individual spontaneously attempts to realign the two realities, and early on he or she may attempt to talk about the experience and to share the overwhelming affect states. The need to talk, to confess, and to release stored tension is powerful and important for health.

The culture, however, actively inhibits the individual's responses. People normally use certain defensive maneuvers to protect themselves from the overwhelming nature of trauma victims' stories and experience. Listeners will switch the topic away from the trauma and attempt to press their own perspective on the victim.

Key Point:
The greatest conflict and the one most likely to predict symptoms involves cases of family violence (child abuse, spousal abuse, rape, and child sexual abuse in particular). The reality of family violence threatens one of the caregiver's most cherished cultural ideas: that the family is a safe place.

They often exaggerate the victim's personal responsibility or even avoid contact with the victim altogether. In mounting these social obstacles to meaning-making, the listeners avoid having their own cognitive schemas disrupted, and they avoid the hyperarousal that is frequently an accompaniment of emotional contagion (Coates et al., 1979; Harber & Pennebaker, 1992). The price for the individual victim, however, is a high one. Individuals cannot make meaning out of the traumatic event without a cultural context and the consensual validation that accompanies it; yet the cognitive imperative demands a resolution of the conflict and a restablization of the sense of personal reality. The only viable solution is further dissociation.

Since the Vietnam War, there has been an increasing recognition of many forms of violent perpetration and the effects this exposure to violence has on children and adults. Good caregivers are carefully trained to avoid using the kinds of social defenses that other people use against the impact of this increased recognition. Instead, clinicians and other caregivers are taught to screen for violence, to carefully listen, to avoid giving in to their own inclinations to distance themselves, and to empathize with the experience and emotions of others. The inability to use the social barriers available to other people makes helping professionals more likely to experience vicarious traumatization.

ORGANIZATIONAL CAUSALITY: SICK SYSTEMS

There are also organizational contributors to the development of vicarious traumatization. Organizational settings that refuse to accept the severity and pervasiveness of traumatic experience in the population they are serving will thereby refuse to provide the social support that is required for caregivers if they are to do adequate work.

Like dysfunctional families, dysfunctional systems often look very similar to each other. In such systems, there is an ongoing culture of crisis, where long-term and preventive solutions are never formulated because time and resources are spent simply "putting out fires" every day. Democratic processes within the organization are given over to authoritarian decision making with the establishment of rigid hierarchies, a culture of shaming, blaming, and judgmentalism. Conflicts are never really addressed or resolved. Instead, order is maintained through isolation, splitting, overcontrol, manipulation, and deceitful practices. Mistrust grows and people avoid relationships with each other and individualism increases. There is little humor in the environment because positive emotion is discouraged, while negative emotional expression is tolerated or even encouraged. If this situation is not rectified, a culture of toughness and meanness develops in which the threat of some form of violence is used to control others and may become actual violence if the threat is not sufficient to keep members in line. Despite this, the system denies that any real problems exist, tolerates a high level of hypocrisy in its daily functioning, and actively discourages any confrontation with reality (Bloom 1997; Bloom & Reichert, 1998).

These kinds of dysfunctional systems can be significant contributors to the development of vicarious traumatization and may even be a fundamental cause. In the caregiver context, the helper can at least feel capable of providing some meaningful assistance to the victim. But the caregiver, embedded in a situation of powerlessness and lack of social support, may find that all efforts to bring this assistance to bear are foiled by the institutional setting within which he or she is practicing. For many helpers, the stress they experience as a result of the systems within which they work is far greater, more pervasive, and more disabling than anything that happens in the consulting room or office with their clients.

MORAL, SPIRITUAL, AND PHILOSOPHICAL CAUSALITY: THEORETICAL CONFLICTS

Finally, there are profound conflicts inherent in the ideologic framework of present-day caregiving that also play a role in making caregivers more vulnerable to the

Key Point:
Dysfunctional systems resemble dysfunctional families, having some or all of the following characteristics:

— An ongoing culture of crisis, where long-term and preventive solutions are not formulated because all time and resources are spent on "putting out fires"

—The replacement of democratic processes with authoritarian decision making and rigid hierarchies

—A culture of shaming, blaming, and judgmentalism

—Maintenance of order through isolation, splitting, overcontrol, manipulation, and deceitful practices, leading to mistrust and avoidance

—Little humor, with positive emotions discouraged and negative emotions tolerated or encouraged

—Eventual development of a culture of toughness and meanness or actual violence

—Denial that any real problems exist

—A high degree of hypocrisy in daily functioning

—Active discouragement of confronting reality

effects of vicarious traumatization (Bloom, 1995). The effects of these conflicts are not direct, but instead comprise a background "noise." They include the desacralization of healing, the commodification of health care, the shortcomings of the medical model, a bias toward individualism, and the issue of individual violence embedded within a context of cultural violence.

As a result, the culture has set up a pressure-cooker environment that serves no one well except, perhaps, profiteers. Demands to carry increasing caseloads with an attendant increase in paperwork combined with significant decreases in staffing and resources have made many healthcare settings unbearable. Under such conditions, it is increasingly difficult for caregivers to find the time or psychic energy to provide the level of compassion that victims of violence require if they are to take the first steps in recovery. Instead, caregivers must decide daily who they are going to hurt—themselves and their own family by not living up to the financial expectations of the companies that employ them, their patients who continue to expect a healing response, or the institutions whose survival is ever more critically dependent on their fast-paced performance. Placed in such untenable moral dilemmas that they feel powerless to affect, healthcare professionals succumb to both physical fatigue and compassion fatigue.

There are also shortcomings inherent in the traditional "medical model" of caregiving. In this model, the patient is largely passive, waiting for cure, or at least alleviation of symptoms, to be delivered by a medical practitioner. The model of sickness that is a part of the medical model places the locus of the problem within the individual who is defective in some way. In contrast, the trauma therapist rapidly learns that one of the keys to recovery for the victim is empowerment, not passivity, and that further experiences of helplessness are often damaging.

The trauma model is more clearly informed by an injury model than a sickness model, implying that previously healthy individuals were injured by a force or person outside of themselves, thus making the site of the injury not a defect within the person, but a problem of relationship and context. An injury model sets the injured party squarely within a social context within which the injury occurred or was not prevented from occurring. It also implies that there is a dual responsibility for recovery, shared by the injured party and by society. The role of the caregiver is very different in the sickness versus the injury model, leaving the caregiver vulnerable to various role strains and stresses:

— How do I keep my patient safe when only my patient has the power to keep herself safe?
— What is the best way to "empower" people?
— What is my responsibility and what is not my responsibility?
— When do my interventions promote recovery and when do they inhibit discourage recovery?
— If this person is suffering from an injury that is a result of a social, fixable problem, what is my role in preventing further injury to this person and to others?

If they attempt to stay politically disengaged, or "scientifically neutral," caregivers may find themselves medicalizing or pathologizing disorders that are actually a result not of a medical problem, but of a social, political, or economic problem. In doing so, they may find themselves part of an oppressive system rather than countering that system.

If instead, caregivers stand up and powerfully bear witness to the violence they have observed, they are likely to be labeled as outcasts, troublemakers, lacking in scientific rigor, and subverters of the system. It is an impossible dilemma. Caregivers, schooled in individualism, tend not to turn to others in any organized fashion in order to protect themselves and therefore must contain the overwhelming emotions to which they have been exposed.

WHAT CAN BE DONE ABOUT IT?

Caregivers must develop their own personal and professional strategies for bringing about change in key areas that will help reduce or prevent the further evolution of a process that could lead to burnout.

Prevention strategies are focused on both individual and environmental approaches. Individual approaches encompass the personal physical, psychologic, and social health of the helper, as well as the professional life of the helper, while environmental responses are divided between the organizational or work setting and societal strategies. Such strategies may be viewed in an ecologic framework, including such elements as follows:

PERSONAL-PHYSICAL
— Engage in self-care behaviors, including proper diet and sleep
— Undertake physical activity, such as exercise and yoga

PERSONAL-PSYCHOLOGIC
— Identify triggers that may cause you to experience vicarious traumatization
— Obtain therapy if personal issues and past traumas get in the way
— Know your own limitations
— Keep the boundaries set for yourself and others
— Know your own level of tolerance
— Engage in recreational activities, including listening to music, reading, spending time in nature
— Modify your work schedule to fit your personal life

PERSONAL-SOCIAL
— Engage in social activities outside of work
— Garner emotional support from colleagues
— Garner emotional support from family and friends

PERSONAL-MORAL
— Adopt a philosophical or religious outlook and be reminded that you cannot take responsibility for the client's healing but rather must act as a midwife, guide, coach, or mentor
— Clarify your own sense of meaning and purpose in life
— Connect with the larger sociopolitical framework and develop social activism skills

PROFESSIONAL
— Become knowledgeable about the effects of trauma on self and others
— Attempt to monitor or diversify case load
— Seek consultation on difficult cases
— Get supervision from someone who understands the dynamics and treatment of PTSD
— Take breaks during workday
— Recognize that you are not alone in facing the stress of working with traumatized clients—normalize your reactions
— Use a team for support
— Maintain collegial on-the-job support, thus limiting the sense of isolation
— Understand dynamics of traumatic reenactment

ORGANIZATIONAL/WORK SETTING
— Accept stressors as real and legitimate, impacting individuals and the group as a whole
— Work in a team
— Create a culture to counteract the effects of trauma
— Establish a clear value system within your organization
— Develop clarity about job tasks and personnel guidelines

— Obtain supervisory/management support
— Maximize collegiality
— Encourage democratic processes in decision making and conflict resolution
  (S. L. Bloom, unpublished data)
— Emphasize a leveled hierarchy
— View problem as affecting the entire group, not just an individual
— Remember the general approach to the problem is to seek solutions, not
  assign blame
— Expect a high level of tolerance for individual disturbance
— Communicate openly and effectively
— Expect a high degree of cohesion
— Expect considerable flexibility of roles
— Join with others to deal with organizational bullies
— Eliminate any subculture of violence and abuse

SOCIETAL
— General public and professional education
— Community involvement
— Coalition building
— Legislative reform
— Social action

A summary of what a caregiver can do about vicarious traumatization includes *anticipating* vicarious traumatization and protecting oneself through awareness of the problem, *addressing* the signs of vicarious traumatization through self-care, and *transforming the pain* by creating meaning, infusing meaning into current activities, challenging negative beliefs, and participating in community building (Saakvitne et al., 2000).

CONCLUSION: DEVELOPING ORGANIZATIONAL UNIVERSAL PRECAUTIONS

Anyone trained in a medical setting can recall learning about how to maintain "universal precautions" against the spread of infection. For most infections such precautions necessitate the use of gloves, gowns, masks, and frequent scrubbing of exposed body parts and other surfaces. Unfortunately, developing universal precautions against the spread of the effects of violence requires the employment of practices that are not necessarily as obvious or as easy to implement, but that are nonetheless necessary if we are to promote health and not spread disease.

It is clear that secondary traumatic stress is a predictable outcome of significant exposure to traumatized people. Therefore any caregiving environment should anticipate the occurrence of vicarious traumatization and establish built-in "hygienic" practices that can serve as antidotes to the spread of the "infection" within the organization. From what we know about individuals and groups under stress, certain characteristics stand out.

Clear, considerate, empathic communication and the promotion of social support are primary objectives for any organization that hopes to reduce the occurrence of compassion fatigue. The ability to express oneself emotionally is vital to continued well-being. This can only occur in an environment that (1) recognizes that the occurrence of secondary stress is a normal reaction to an abnormal situation and (2) condones the need for continuous positive social support as the normative standard of behavior for each individual and for the group as a whole. Likewise, each individual must establish a plan for self-care that includes adequate breaks, exercise, relaxation, and socialization. The studies of resiliency indicate that people do best if they can use their own initiative and creativity to solve problems with a maximum degree of autonomy, rather than being required to adhere to stringent and inflexible rules that are not always relevant to the situation. They must have appropriate and clear boundaries between themselves and suffering others while still maintaining a deep sense of commitment to a set of higher beliefs and standards. One of the most under appreciated and yet most important factors that contributes to creating a stress-reducing environment is a sense of humor and the shared laughter that often emerges as "gallows humor" in highly stressful environments. A health-promoting organization is one in which the democratic processes of decision making and conflict resolution are routine, issues of meaning and purpose are central, and there exists a culture of active nonviolence.

Medical care has come under close and often brutal scrutiny in the last few decades, and caregivers have repeatedly been found wanting in the qualities that most people value highly—compassion, emotional warmth, kindness, concern. It is possible that as the amount of violence has increased in our environment, the people "in the trenches"—nurses, physicians, and other healthcare workers—have caught the infection of violence through vicarious traumatization, because of the close contact with an infectious agent not recognized soon enough for its virulence. Public health workers have a professional, social, and moral responsibility to urge colleagues and patients to restructure the social environment so that the pathogen of violence finds less fertile ground to reproduce. At the same time, healthcare workers must also develop institutional universal precautions against an infection that makes them the carriers of the virulent disease called *violence*. Every episode of violence—physical, emotional, sexual, or social—must be viewed as a potentially lethal pathogen whose impact must be minimized if the environment is to become healthy. This requires providing support, concern, and care not only for patients, but among caregivers as well.

REFERENCES

Alexander DA, Atcheson SF. Psychiatric aspects of trauma care: survey of nurses and doctors. *Psychiatr Bull.* 1998;22:132-136.

Anderson DG. Coping strategies and burnout among veteran child protection workers. *Child Abuse Negl.* 2000;24:839-848.

Bloom SL. The germ theory of trauma: the impossibility of ethical neutrality. In: Stamm BH, ed. *Secondary Traumatic Stress: Self-Care Issues for Clinicians, Researchers, and Educators.* Lutherville, Md: Sidran Press; 1995:257-276.

Bloom SL. Creating Sanctuary: *Toward the Evolution of Sane Societies.* New York, NY: Routledge; 1997.

Bloom SL, Reichert M. *Bearing Witness: Violence and Collective Responsibility,* Binghamton, NY: Haworth Press; 1998.

Catherall DR. Coping with secondary traumatic stress: the importance of the therapist's professional peer group. In: Stamm BH, ed. *Secondary Traumatic Stress: Self-Care Issues for Clinicians, Researchers, & Educators.* Lutherville, Md: Sidran Press; 1995:80-92.

Coates D, Wortman CB, Abben A. Reactions to victims. In: Frieze IH, Bar-Tal D, Carroll JS, eds. *New Approaches to Social Problems.* San Francisco, Calif: Jossey-Bass; 1979.

Crothers D. Vicarious traumatization in the work with survivors of childhood trauma. *J Psychosoc Nurs Ment Health Serv.* 1995;33:9-13.

Cunningham M. *Vicarious Traumatization: Impact of Trauma Work on the Clinician* [dissertation]. Garden City, NY: Adelphia University School of Social Work; 1996.

Cunningham M. The impact of sexual abuse treatment on the social work clinician. *Child Adolesc Soc Work J.* 1999;16:277-290.

Figley CR. Compassion fatigue: Toward a new understanding of the costs of caring. In: Stamm BH, ed. *Secondary Traumatic Stress: Self-Care Issues for Clinicians, Researchers, & Educators.* Lutherville, Md: Sidran Press; 1995:3-28.

Gabriel MA. Group therapists and AIDS groups: an exploration of traumatic stress reactions. *Group.* 1994;18:167-176.

Garrett C. *Stress, Coping, Empathy, Secondary Traumatic Stress and Burnout in Healthcare Providers Working with HIV-Infected Individuals* [dissertation]. New York: New York University; 1999.

Hallett SJ. *Trauma and Coping in Homicide and Child Sexual Abuse Detectives* [dissertation]. San Diego: California School of Professional Psychology; 1996.

Harber KD, Pennebaker JW. Overcoming traumatic memories. In: Christianson SA, ed. *The Handbook of Emotion and Memory: Research and Theory.* Hillsdale, NJ: Lawrence Erlbaum Associates; 1992:359-387.

Iliffe G, Steed LG. Exploring the counselor's experience of working with perpetrators and survivors of domestic violence. *J Interpers Violence.* 2000;15:393-412.

Janoff-Bulman R. *Shattered Assumptions: Towards a New Psychology of Trauma.* New York, NY: The Free Press; 1992.

Kostouros PA. *Vicarious Traumatization Among Sex Offenders* [master's thesis]. Victoria, British Columbia: University of Victoria; 1998.

Lyon E. Hospital staff reactions to accounts by survivors of childhood abuse. *Am J Orthopsychiatry.* 1993;63:410-416.

McCann IL, Pearlman LA. Vicarious traumatization: a framework for understanding the psychological effects of working with victims. *J Traumatic Stress.* 1990;3:131-147.

Meyers TW. *The Relationship Between Family of Origin Functioning, Trauma History, Exposure to Children's Traumata and Secondary Traumatic Stress Symptoms in Child Protective Service Workers* [dissertation]. Tallahassee: Florida State University; 1996.

Peebles-Klieger MJ. Pediatric and neonatal intensive care hospitalization as traumatic stressor: implications for intervention. *Bull Menninger Clin.* 2000;64:257-280.

Pennebaker JW. *Opening Up: The Healing Power of Expressing Emotions.* New York, NY: Guilford; 1997.

Pines AM, Arenson E. *Career Burnout: Causes and Cures.* New York, NY: Free Press; 1988.

Rosenbloom DJ, Pratt AC, Pearlman LA. Helpers' responses to trauma work: Understanding and intervening in an organization. In: Stamm BH, ed. *Secondary Traumatic Stress: Self-Care Issues for Clinicians, Researchers, and Educators.* Lutherville, Md: Sidran Press; 1995:65-79.

Saakvitne W, Gamble S, Pearlman LA, Lev BT. *Risking Connection: A Training Curriculum for Working with Survivors of Childhood Abuse.* Lutherville, Md: Sidran Press; 2000:168.

Schauben LJ, Frazier PA. Vicarious trauma: the effects on female counselors of working with sexual violence survivors. *Psychol Women Q.* 1995;19:49-64.

Schwam K. The phenomenon of compassion fatigue in perioperative nursing. *AORN J.* 1998;68:642-648.

Simonds SL. *Vicarious Traumatization in Therapists Treating Adult Survivors of Childhood Sexual Abuse* [dissertation]. Santa Barbara, Calif: The Fielding Institute; 1996.

Stamm BH. Work-related secondary traumatic stress. *PTSD Res Q.* 1997;8:1-3.

Williams MB, Sommer JF. Self-care and the vulnerable therapist. In: Stamm BH, ed. *Secondary Traumatic Stress: Self-Care Issues for Clinicians, Researchers, and Educators.* Lutherville, Md: Sidran Press; 1995:230-246.

SANE-SART History and Role Development

Linda E. Ledray, RN, PhD, SANE-A, FAAN

Although the violence of rape has occurred throughout history, a concerted effort to better understand the issue and to better meet the needs of survivors did not begin until the early 1970s, when rape crisis centers were initiated across the United States (Brownmiller, 1975). The development of sexual assault nurse examiner (SANE) programs also began in the early 1970s, although different terminology was used to describe the role during the early years (Ledray & Chaignot, 1980).

SANE program development was facilitated by the landmark Violence Against Women Act (VAWA) of 1994. This bill was introduced by Senator Joseph Biden and signed into law on September 13, 1994, as Title IV of the Violent Crime Control and Law Enforcement Act of 1994. In addition to doubling the federal penalties for repeat offenders and requiring that date rape be treated the same as stranger rape, this act made $800 million available for training and program development over a 6-year period, with $26 million appropriated for the first year. This was an important recognition of the need for improving services for crime victims. VAWA funding in recent years has facilitated the continued development of sexual assault programs in the United States.

The Need For SANE Programs

Violence has a significant impact on the physical and psychosocial health of millions of Americans every year. Because women are so often the victims of violence, women who come to emergency departments (EDs) for even minor trauma must be thoroughly evaluated. ED staff must be aware of the types of injuries most likely to result from violence. The potential victim must be asked about the cause of the trauma to determine if it is the result of rape, requiring further evaluation.

In recent years healthcare facilities have begun to recognize their responsibility to have trained staff available to provide this specialized service for victims of sexual assault. Treating injuries alone is not sufficient. In 2000, Coney Island Hospital was fined $46,000 by state regulators after a rape victim came to the medical facility and a sexual assault evidentiary examination was not performed accurately. The victim waited 3 hours before being examined and then potentially significant evidence, including her underwear and vaginal swabs, was lost. The Department of Health investigation also found that the hospital failed to provide complete care, including medication to prevent pregnancy. The authorities believed that had correct evidence collection and chain-of-custody occurred, the evidence may have been useful to secure a conviction against the serial sex offender charged with her rape. As a result, New York passed the Sexual Assault Reform Act, requiring New York state medical facilities to develop specialized sexual assault examiner evidence collection programs in 2001 (Chivers, 2000).

It was not until 1992 that the guidelines of the Joint Commission on the Accreditation of Health Care Organizations (JCAHO) first required emergency and ambulatory care facilities to have protocols on rape, sexual molestation, and domestic abuse (Bobak, 1992). By 1997 the guidelines also required health care facilities to develop and train their staffs to use criteria to identify possible victims of physical assault, rape or other sexual molestation, domestic abuse, and abuse or neglect of older adults and children (JCAHO, 1997). Although JCAHO does not yet require that specially trained forensic examiners or SANEs be available to do the evaluation, JCAHO sometimes asks if they are available. It is no longer optional for medical facilities to identify and provide appropriate and complete services to victims of rape and abuse. The SANE role continues to develop as an important component of the emergency medical response to survivors of sexual assault. Perhaps one day it will be a requirement to have a SANE or forensic examiner available to the ED to obtain Level One Trauma status.

The impetus to develop SANE programs began with nurses, other medical professionals, counselors, and advocates working with rape victims in hospitals, clinics, and other settings across the country. It was obvious to these individuals that the services to victims of sexual assault were inadequate and not equal to the same high standard of care as services provided to other ED clients (Holloway & Swan, 1993; O'Brien, 1996). When rape victims came to the ED for care, they often had to wait as long as 4 to 12 hours in a busy, public area. Their wounds were seen as less serious than those of other trauma victims, and they competed unsuccessfully for staff time with critically ill patients (Holloway & Swan, 1993; Sandrick, 1996; Speck & Aiken, 1995). Often they were not allowed to eat, drink, or urinate while they waited, for fear of destroying evidence (Thomas & Zachritz: 1993). Physicians and nurses often were not sufficiently trained to do mediolegal examinations, and many were lacking in expert witness testimony ability (Lynch, 1996). Even when they had been trained, staff often did not complete a sufficient number of examinations to maintain their level of proficiency (Lenehan, 1991; Tobias, 1990; Yorker, 1996). When the victim's medical needs were met, his or her emotional needs all too often were overlooked, or the survivor was blamed for the rape by the ED staff (Kiffe, 1996; Speck & Aiken, 1995).

Typically, the rape survivor was faced with a time-consuming, cumbersome succession of examiners, some with only a few hours of orientation and little experience. ED services were inconsistent and problematic. Often, the only physician available to do the vaginal examination after the rape was male (Lenehan, 1991). Although approximately half of rape victims were unconcerned with the gender of the examiner, the other half found this extremely problematic. Male victims also prefer to be examined by a woman, because they usually have been raped by a man and experience the same generalized fear and anger toward men that female victims experience (Ledray, 1996).

As the result of nurses specializing in this area, research became available on the complex needs of this population. Nurses and other professionals realized the importance of providing the best ED and follow-up care possible (Lenehan, 1991). For 75% of these victims, the initial ED contact was the only known contact they had with medical or professional support staff (Ledray, 1992). Nurses were aware that, before the implementation of the SANE model, they were credited with only assisting the physician with the examination, but in reality they were doing everything except the pelvic speculum examination (DiNitto et al., 1986; Ledray, 1992). It was clear to these nurses that it was time to reevaluate the system and to consider a new approach that would better meet the needs of sexual assault victims.

HISTORY OF SANE PROGRAM DEVELOPMENT

As a result of identifying the goal of better meeting the needs of this underserved population, the first SANE programs were established in Memphis, Tennessee, in 1976, in Minneapolis, Minnesota, in 1977, and in Amarillo, Texas, in 1979 (Antognoli-Toland, 1985; Ledray, 1993; Ledray & Chaignot, 1980; Speck & Aiken, 1995). Unfortunately, these nurses worked in isolation until the late 1980s.

In 1991 Gail Lenehan, editor of the Journal of Emergency Nursing, recognized the importance of this new role for nurses and published the first list of 20 SANE programs to facilitate communication and sharing of information among programs (Emergency Nurses Association [ENA], 1991). In 1992, Lenehan implemented "The Sexual Assault Nurse Examiner" column in each issue for the same purpose. This proved to be extremely important for professional development.

The publication of this initial list of programs led to 72 individuals from 31 programs across the United States and Canada coming together for the first time in 1992 at a meeting hosted by the Sexual Assault Resource Service and the University of Minnesota School of Nursing in Minneapolis, Minnesota. The International Association of Forensic Nurses (IAFN) was formed at that meeting (Ledray, 1996). Membership in IAFN surpassed the 1000 mark in 1996, and in October 2001 was more than 2000 (Lynch, 1996).

Initial SANE development was slow, with only three programs operating by the end of the 1970s; today development is progressing much more rapidly. By October 2001 there were over 600 SANE programs registered at www.sane-sart.com, the SANE-SART Web site funded by the Office for Victims of Crime (OVC) operated by the Minneapolis-based Sexual Assault Resource Service. This number is expected to increase much more rapidly in years to come.

After years of effort on the part of SANEs, the American Nurses' Association (ANA) officially recognized forensic nursing as a new specialty of nursing in 1995 (Lynch, 1996). SANE is the largest subspecialty of forensic nursing. At the October 1996 IAFN annual meeting, Geri Marullo, Executive Director of the ANA, predicted that within 10 years the JCAHO would require every hospital to have a forensic nurse available (Marullo, 1996).

WHAT IS A SANE? SAFE? FE?

At the 1996 IAFN annual meeting, the SANE Council voted on the terminology to be used to define this new position in the standards. The overwhelming decision was to use the title Sexual Assault Nurse Examiner, or SANE. A SANE is a registered nurse who has advanced education in the forensic examination of sexual assault victims. Programs that use physicians to conduct the evidentiary examination have chosen to use the more generic term Sexual Assault Forensic Examiner (SAFE) or Forensic Examiner (FE).

SANE SCOPE OF PRACTICE

A SANE provides 24-hour on-call services for male and female victims of sexual assault or abuse. Most programs provide services only for adult and adolescent survivors, but an increasing number are obtaining the additional training recommended by IAFN to provide services for child victims.

MEDICAL CARE

The purpose of the SANE examination of the sexual assault survivor is specifically to assess, document, and collect forensic evidence. In addition, prophylactic treatment of sexually transmitted diseases (STDs) and prevention of pregnancy are provided by the SANE following a preestablished medical protocol or with the approval of a consulting physician or advanced practice nurse. Although the SANE may treat minor injuries, such as washing and bandaging minor cuts or abrasions, further evaluation and care of any major physical trauma is referred to the ED or a designated medical facility.

The SANE conducts a limited medical examination, not a routine physical examination, and it is important that this is explained clearly to the client. Obvious pathology or suspicious findings that may be observed are reported to the client with a suggestion for follow-up care and referral. Evaluation and diagnosis of medical pathology are beyond the scope of the SANE's practice.

Key Point:
A Sexual Assault Nurse Examiner (SANE) is a registered nurse who has advanced education in the forensic examination of sexual assault victims. Programs that use physicians to conduct the evidentiary examination have chosen to use the more generic term Sexual Assault Forensic Examiner (SAFE) or Forensic Examiner (FE).

REPORTING

The SANE provides the rape survivor with information to ensure that the survivor can anticipate what may happen next, make choices about reporting and deciding who to tell, and obtain necessary support after she leaving the SANE facility. This usually includes a discussion between the victim and the SANE about reporting to law enforcement. If the survivor has made a choice not to report, she will need to discuss why she may be hesitant to report. The SANE ensures that the victim makes the decision about reporting based on factual information rather than on fear. In most cases the SANE will encourage the survivor to report the crime, and if a rape crisis center advocate is not available during the examination, the SANE will make referrals to advocacy agencies that can provide the support necessary to help the survivor through the criminal justice process.

EMOTIONAL SUPPORT AND CRISIS INTERVENTION

The SANE will also provide emotional support and crisis intervention, working with the rape crisis center advocate when one is available. The SANE will make an initial assessment of the survivor's psychologic functioning sufficient to determine if he or she is oriented to person, place, and time; is suicidal; or is in need of further referral for follow-up support, evaluation, or treatment beyond that of advocacy.

EDUCATION, TRAINING, RESEARCH, AND PROGRAM EVALUATION

In addition, the SANE, as a specialist in sexual assault, is active in training other health care and community agency professionals to provide services to sexual assault victims. Recognizing the importance of evidence-based clinical practice, the more established SANE programs also conduct ongoing program evaluation and periodic research studies to evaluate the impact, treatment needs, outcomes, and services provided to sexual assault victims.

SANE STANDARDS OF PRACTICE

At the 1996 annual meeting of IAFN, the SANE Council voted and adopted the first SANE Standards of Practice (IAFN, 1996). The standards include goals of SANEs; definition of the practice area; conceptual framework of SANE practice; components of evaluation and documentation; forensic evaluation components; and SANE minimum qualifications.

HOW A MODEL SANE PROGRAM OPERATES

A SANE is usually available on call, typically off premises, 24 hours a day, 7 days a week. The on-call SANE is paged immediately whenever a sexual assault or abuse survivor enters the community's response system. If the protocol indicates a rape advocate should be called, the staff or SANE will also page the advocate on call.

HOSPITAL-BASED SANE PROGRAMS

If the SANE program is hospital-based, victims may enter the system by the following:

1. Calling local law enforcement, who will provide transportation to the hospital emergency department or SANE examination clinic.

2. Going directly to the hospital emergency department or hospital clinic.

3. Calling the designated crisis line for assistance.

During the time it takes for the SANE to respond (usually no more than 1 hour), the ED or clinic staff evaluate and treat any urgent or life-threatening injuries. If treatment is medically necessary, the ED staff will treat the client, always considering the forensic implications and documenting any life-saving and stabilizing medical procedures. If clothes or objects are removed from the victim by the ED staff, forensic procedures for handling and storage of the physical evidence should be used as much as possible, including taking pictures of the victim for forensic purposes.

Whenever possible the SANE, rather than the ED staff, should take forensic photographs. If medical necessity dictates treatment before the arrival of the SANE, ED staff will need to take photographs following established forensic procedures.

When the ED staff determines that the victim does not require immediate medical care, the survivor is made comfortable in a private room near the ED. This area should enhance the victim's sense of safety and security, and should provide comfort and quiet while she or he awaits the arrival of the SANE and advocate. A soundproof room with comfortable furniture, preferably a sofa that accommodates lying down, a telephone, and a locked door are preferred. Family members who accompany the victim, with the victim's permission, should be allowed to wait in the room as well. If there was no oral sex, the victim may be offered something to eat or drink while waiting.

If the victim chooses to file a police report but has not done so yet, the triage nurse calls the police to take the initial report at the hospital. If the victim is upset and gives permission, a hospital chaplain or social worker should be called to wait with the victim until the SANE, advocate, or counselor arrives.

COMMUNITY-BASED SANE PROGRAMS

If the SANE program is community based, victims may enter the system by the following:

1. Calling the local law enforcement agency where they will be triaged for injuries and, if only minor injuries or no injuries are present, will be transported to the community-based SANE facility.

2. Going to the ED of a local hospital, where staff will check for injuries, and if only minor injuries or no injury present, will arrange transportation to the community-based SANE program.

3. Going directly to the community-based SANE program facility during office hours.

4. Calling the designated crisis line for assistance and receiving a referral to the community-based SANE program.

Community Response and Responsibilities

In responding to a sexual assault victim in the community, law enforcement is charged with initiating the investigation of the crime and determining if the client has serious injuries necessitating ED evaluation or care. If moderate to severe injury is detected, the victim is evaluated by paramedics and transported to the hospital ED. This includes fewer than 4% of rape victims, because rape seldom involves serious injury (Ledray, 1999a).

As in hospital-based SANE programs, when no injuries are suspected, the client is transported from the crime scene to the community SANE facility, where she is met by the SANE within one hour. If the victim goes directly to a hospital ED, the staff will evaluate the victim for life-threatening injuries requiring immediate treatment. When these are present, the ED staff will admit the victim to the ED and notify the on-call SANE to come to the hospital ED. The ED staff will evaluate and treat the injuries, always considering the forensic implications and documenting any life-saving and stabilizing medical procedures. Clothing or objects removed from the client are handled and labeled to maintain the proper chain of evidence. Photographs of the injuries may be taken for forensic purposes by the ED staff. After the patient is stabilized medically, the SANE will collect the forensic evidence in the designated ED area.

When the ED staff determines that the patient does not require urgent or life-saving medical care, the survivor is not admitted to the hospital. Instead, law enforcement personnel provide transportation to the community-based SANE program facility for further evaluation and examination.

Key Point:
Access to a community-based SANE program is by the following:

1. *The victim calling local law enforcement agencies, where he or she will be checked for injuries and, if only minor or no injuries are present, will be transported to the community-based SANE facility.*

2. *The victim going to the ED of a local hospital, where the staff will check for injuries and, if only minor or no injuries are present, will arrange transportation to the community-based SANE facility.*

3. *The victim going directly to the community-based SANE program facility during office hours.*

4. *The victim calling the designated crisis line for assistance and receiving a referral to the community-based SANE facility.*

SANE Responsibilities

Once the SANE arrives, she is responsible for completing the entire sexual assault evidentiary examination, including:

— Crisis intervention, including helping the survivor decide whether or not to report the crime

— Sexually transmitted disease prevention

— Pregnancy risk evaluation and emergency contraception

— Collection of forensic evidence

— Referrals for additional support and care

These are addressed in detail elsewhere in this book.

When the Victim Is Uncertain About Reporting. If the survivor has not yet decided whether or not to report the assault, the SANE will discuss any fears and concerns and provide the information necessary to make an informed decision. If the victim decides not to report at that time, but is unsure about reporting at a future date, the SANE should explain available options and the limitations of making a delayed report. The SANE will also offer to complete an evidentiary examination kit that can be held in a locked refrigerator for a specified time (usually one month or according to state statutes if any exist), in case the victim chooses to report later.

Mandatory Reporting. In states with mandatory reporting laws for felony crimes or child abuse, the SANE must follow established protocol regarding reporting after explaining the process and her responsibilities to the victim, or to the victim's family when a child is involved and a parent is present.

When the Victim Does Not Want to Report. If the victim decides not to report and an evidentiary examination is not completed, the SANE should still offer medications to prevent STDs, evaluate the risk of pregnancy, and offer pregnancy prevention. The SANE also makes referrals for follow-up medical care and counseling, and provides the victim with written follow-up information.

When a Report Is Made. When the victim decides to report or to consider reporting at a later date, a complete evidentiary examination is conducted following the SANE agency protocol. In most agencies the complete examination is conducted within 72 hours of the sexual assault, sometimes even longer.

After obtaining a signed consent, the SANE will conduct a complete examination, including the collection of evidence in a rape kit; assess and document injuries; provide prophylactic care for STDs; evaluate pregnancy risk and offer preventive care; initiate crisis intervention; and provide referral for follow-up medical and psychologic care.

Discharge. If the victim is alone, the SANE should discuss whom to call and where to go from the hospital. Every effort must be made to find a place for the victim to go where she or he will feel safe and will not be alone. When necessary, arrangements may be made for shelter placement. If the victim is intoxicated or does not want to leave until morning, arrangements may be made for a place to sleep in a specified area of the hospital when this type of space is available. In many facilities this will be an ED holding room or crisis center. If necessary, a community referral can be made to better meet the victim's long-term housing needs.

SANE TRAINING
STATE LEVEL CERTIFICATION

In the absence of national certification, the development of state certification or licensure was driven by the desire to establish credibility when the SANE is required to testify in court. State-level certification is being considered in several states. Massachusetts developed a statewide sexual assault training program under the auspices of the Public Health Department for both nurse and physician certification. They require recertification every 2 years based on competency (Massachusetts Nurses Association, 1995). Texas established multidisciplinary criteria for a state level certification out of the Attorney General's Office (J. Ferrell, personal communication, October 3, 1998).

NATIONAL CERTIFICATION

There is currently no national SANE certification. However, the IAFN recognizes the importance of establishing national level certification for SANEs to ensure both consistency in practice and credibility in the courtroom. National certification through IAFN will begin in 2002.

As a first step toward national certification, the SANE council of IAFN adopted recommendations for SANE training curriculum (IAFN, 1998; Ledray, 1999b). They are available through IAFN. Existing basic SANE training programs based on these recommendations consist of 40 or more hours of didactic instruction.

Some programs also specify a designated number of clinical hours after completing the classroom training. The range when required is from an additional 40 hours to as many as 96 hours of clinical experience (Antognoli-Toland, 1985; Kettleson, 1995). Most programs do not have a set number of required clinical hours, but rather train until the trainee is observed by an experienced forensic examiner to demonstrate competence, using a competency checklist for each clinical skill (Gaffney, 1997; Ledray, 1999a). Additional clinical hours usually include:

— Normal vaginal speculum and bi-manual examination experience

— Normal well-child examinations

— Courtroom observation

— Adult or child evidentiary examination observations

In addition to initial training, most SANE programs require specific criteria for maintaining certification. Although no two programs are the same, the most common requirements include a combination of the following:

— Completion of a specific number of examinations per year

— Attendance at staff meetings

— SANE relevant literature reviews

— IAFN or other forensic conference attendance

— Externships with physicians, nurse practitioners, or SANEs

— Continuing to take call and be actively involved in the SANE

SANE TRAINING COMPONENTS PROGRAM

SANE didactic training typically includes the following components:

Programmatic

— Role of the SANE and forensic nursing history

— Program goals, objectives, vision, and mission

— Review of program policies and procedures

— Working with the media

— Facilities familiarization

— SANE program evaluation research

— Training program evaluation

Medical

— STD statistics, symptoms, and treatment options

— Pregnancy risk evaluation, prevention, testing options, and termination options

— The normal genitalia (pelvic and anal)

— Normal growth and development in adults, adolescents, and children

— Techniques for drawing blood

— Physical assessment, injury identification, and criteria for a medical referral to physicians

— Using the colposcope and obtaining 35 mm and/or video pictures (if available)

— Follow-up resources and needs of the rape victim

Legal

— Local state rape laws and the police report and investigation process

— Role of local law enforcement officers

— Understanding and obtaining informed consent

— Maintaining confidentiality

— Role of the local prosecuting attorney

— Local court process

— Establishing credentials as an expert witness

Forensic Practices and Procedures

— The types of evidence collected in rape cases and the utilization of evidence

— Determining what specimens to collect

— Maintaining chain of evidence

— Evidentiary examination timing and protocol

— Nongenital pattern injury

— Genital injury

— Photographing injuries

— Procedure for collecting, labeling, storing, and processing laboratory specimens

— Medicolegal interviewing

— Documentation and record keeping

— Testifying in court as an expert and factual witness

Psychologic

— The emotional needs of the rape victim and how to meet them

— Crisis intervention with the rape victim

— Suicide risk evaluation

— Role of local rape crisis center advocate

— Typical fears about reporting and what it means to report in the local community

— Follow-up resources and needs of the rape victim

SANE TRAINING TRENDS
More and more universities across the country are developing and offering university-based forensic nursing courses, and SANE continuing education training

is being developed and offered at an increasing number of universities across the country. Several forensic nursing courses offered at the university level qualify for university credit and offer advanced degrees in forensic nursing. These include Fitchberg University in Massachusetts and Beth-El College of Nursing, Colorado Springs, Colorado. Other institutions, such as Seton Hall University School of Nursing, Rutgers University, and Columbia University, offer SANE continuing education training programs. Mount Royal College in Calgary, British Columbia, offers forensic nursing courses via the Internet that can be taken from any computer, anywhere in the world, for credit through their institution.

SART: A COMMUNITY APPROACH

No SANE program can operate in isolation. To be optimally effective and to provide the best service possible to victims of sexual assault, the SANE must function as a part of a team of individuals from community organizations, organized either formally as a Sexual Assault Response Team (SART) or informally as collaborators.

Communities that have chosen to organize formally have developed different concepts of a SART. These concepts vary: in some communities a team of individuals responds together and interviews the victim jointly at the time of the sexual assault examination. In other communities individuals work independently on a day-to-day basis, but communicate regularly, possibly daily, and meet weekly or monthly to discuss mutual cases and solve mutual problems to make the system function more smoothly.

WHO IS ON A SART?

SART members typically include a SANE, a law enforcement officer, a detective, a prosecutor, a rape crisis center advocate or counselor, and ED medical personnel. The makeup of the SART varies from area to area, depending on community needs and resources. Ideally, the team will include representatives from the community who can best help the victims. The SART may also include school counselors, battered women advocates, counselors who work with prostitutes, and any combination of representatives of programs in the community who are concerned about the problem of sexual assault. The team membership may change over time depending on the needs of the clients and the goals of the SART team.

TWO SART MODELS
Joint Interview SART Model

In communities using this model, multiple members of the SART respond to the ED together to conduct the sexual assault examination interview. This team usually includes law enforcement, the SANE, and a rape advocate. They are all present during the victim's initial statement so that the account of the assault must be given only once. This SART model is based on the belief that interviewing the victim is traumatic and causes additional psychologic "harm" to the victim. It is believed that conducting only one interview thus helps prevent further harm to the victim.

The single interview is also preferred because it helps prevent confusion between professionals recording information. Because they are all hearing the victim's account of the assault at the same time, they are more likely to record the same information. As a result, problems in explaining different accounts of the details of the sexual assault are reduced.

In this model, when a rape victim who has not made a police report comes to the ED, law enforcement is called immediately to determine if a crime has been committed. The SANE and advocate may also be called to help facilitate the victim's admission to the SART system. With the advocate present to provide support, the SANE and police conduct an in-depth interview of the victim after briefly conferring to coordinate questioning and reduce repetition. In California the

Key Point:
To be optimally effective and to provide the best possible service, the SANE must function as part of a team, which may be organized formally as a Sexual Assault Response Team (SART) or informally. These vary from a team of individuals who respond together and jointly interview the victim at the time of the sexual assault examination to individuals who work independently on a day-to-day basis but who communicate regularly, possibly daily, and meet weekly or monthly to discuss mutual cases and solve mutual problems to make the system work more smoothly. Team members typically include the SANE, law enforcement officer, detective, prosecutor, rape crisis center advocate or counselor, and ED medical personnel. The makeup varies depending on the resources and needs of the various communities. Other possible members include school counselors, battered women advocates, counselors who work with prostitutes, and any combination of representatives of programs in the community that address the problem of sexual assault. The membership may change with time as needs and goals change.

penal code gives the victim the right to have any two individuals of her choice present for support during police questioning. The advocate may be one of these two. Once the interview is completed the police officer will wait outside the examination room while the SANE collects the evidence. The evidence is then turned over to law enforcement. With the victim's permission, the advocate may remain in the examination room to provide support during the evidentiary examination. When the examination is completed the SANE will make any necessary arrangements for follow-up medical care, and the advocate will make arrangements to contact the victim for follow-up supportive counseling and legal advocacy.

Members of the joint interview model SART may meet regularly to discuss cases, or they may communicate informally after each initial ED experience.

Joint Interview SART Model Limitations
Although the coordinated effort has some advantages, there are also some limitations to this approach. If the victim is not sure whether to report the assault, there may be additional pressure to do so in areas where the protocol requires law enforcement personnel to be called to the hospital to determine if a crime has been committed. Calling law enforcement may be necessary to authorize payment for the examination before the SANE becomes involved. The advocate will support the victim in whatever decision she makes, even if the decision is to not report.

If the victim decides not to report, however, the victim may have limited access to healthcare for STD and pregnancy risk evaluation and prevention. If the victim decides not to report, hospital care then is not paid for by the crime victim fund. When the police determine that a crime was committed, they authorize reimbursement for the SANE examination, which includes STD and pregnancy prevention. They will, however, usually require that a police report is made. In areas where payment is authorized through another agency, reporting is not necessarily a requirement for payment for services.

In addition, while repetition of the account of the sexual assault is an unpleasant experience that most victims want to avoid, the assumption that it "harms" them and is truly traumatic is only an assumption. Research of treatment efficacy has shown that repetition of the account of the assault in detail may have a beneficial, desensitizing, healing affect (Foa et al., 1999).

Cooperative SART Model
Other parts of the country have modified the initial SART model to meet the needs of their community while trying to maintain the team concept that the SART model fosters. In many of these areas, the team members meet regularly and communicate routinely about cases, but they do not actually respond at the same time. They function cooperatively, not conjointly.

In the cooperative SART model, when law enforcement personnel are called to the scene of a sexual assault, they protect the client from further harm, protect the crime scene evidence, and take a limited statement from the victim to determine if a sex crime was committed. In rural areas where there is a greater distance required for transport, they may call the hospital or rape center responsible for paging the SANE and rape advocate on call. In urban areas the SANE and advocate are usually paged when the victim arrives at the medical facility.

When the police and victim arrive at the hospital, the triage nurse decides whether the victim needs immediate medical evaluation by a physician or can be directed immediately to the SANE area for forensic examination. The SANE stays with the victim during any necessary medical evaluation, and until he or she is cleared medically and transferred to the SANE examination area.

The police officer is not present during the SANE interview or the forensic examination, and may not even wait at the hospital. Rather, the SANE calls the police when the examination is completed, and they then return for the victim. After discussing the examination findings with the SANE, the police also may take possession of the evidence at that time and provide the survivor with a safe ride home.

If the victim comes to the hospital before contacting the police, with the victim's permission, the SANE may call the police to come to the hospital to take the initial report. Usually, the SANE waits until the evidentiary examination is completed to make this call. The advocate stays with the victim and, with the victim's permission, remains present during the police interview.

The rape center advocate may bring a victim to the hospital or may be paged at the same time the SANE is paged. The advocate also may contact the victim later to provide follow-up advocacy and counseling. The rape center advocate usually goes with the sexual assault victim to meet with the sex crimes detective and prosecutor as well.

Most areas have a standing SART meeting to discuss broader concerns and to communicate informally about specific cases. At this meeting the SART usually focuses on broader policy issues, rather than specific cases as seen in case review sessions. The team members attending policy meetings are the directors or managers of the involved agencies. As the primary decision makers of each agency present at the meeting, they can resolve issues as a group.

Cooperative SART Model Limitations

When the victim must describe the assault to the police, the SANE, and the advocate at different times, the memory and the completeness of each account may vary somewhat. When these discrepancies occur, they must be addressed if the case goes to court. In many states sexual assault advocates who have completed the required training cannot be subpoenaed to testify in court; however, both the SANE and law enforcement will be called to testify. Separate interviews require more effort on the part of all team members to ensure that they meet or communicate over the phone to discuss cases, issues, and concerns.

For a SANE-SART program to be optimally successful, all agencies involved must work together to meet the multiple needs of the rape victim and to prosecute the offender. Regardless of how the SART model operates, who is included on the team, and what name is used to describe the team, the result must be a coordinated community response with the needs of the victim in the forefront, not the needs of the team.

EVIDENCE OF SANE EFFICACY

BETTER COLLABORATION WITH LAW ENFORCEMENT

SANE programs, working collaboratively as a part of a SART, can ensure police obtain records of examinations in a timely fashion and can interpret the findings for them when necessary. As a part of the initial consent for the evidentiary examination, SANE programs often also obtain consent to share information with law enforcement agencies and to communicate with them. Many SANEs routinely ask for the name, address, and phone number of friends or relatives with whom the survivor might decide to stay, and through whom they may be contacted later. This information often is helpful to the police (Ledray, 1992). Police report they prefer to work with a few forensically trained nurses because it makes their job easier in many ways (Yorker, 1996).

HIGHER REPORTING RATES

In EDs without a SANE program, survivors sometimes encounter busy, insensitive physicians, nurses, or police, and may decide it is not worth the effort to report and follow through with prosecution (Frank, 1996). By providing the rape survivor with additional assistance, resources, and support, SANEs facilitate follow-through with the legal process (Frank, 1996; Ledray, 1992). This support results in an increase in reporting by victims (Arndt, 1988). In one program 38% of 337 rape survivors were uncertain about reporting when they first came to the hospital ED. After

Key Point:
Communities that have SANE programs can experience the following benefits:
— Better collaboration with law enforcement
— Higher reporting rates
— Shorter examination times
— Better forensic evidence collection
— Improved prosecution

working through their fears and concerns with a knowledgeable SANE, an additional 12% decided to report, and the police were called to the ED. An additional 23% agreed to have an evidentiary examination completed because they thought they would report at a later time. Only 3% of the 337 survivors in this study did not report (Ledray, 1999a).

Fazlollah (2001), an investigative reporter working with a team of reporters, discovered law enforcement officers in a large Eastern city had downgraded and wrongly classified more than 2000 reports of rape to "service calls" over a 5-year period. Victims were presumed to be not credible, were subjected to polygraph examinations, and had their cases dropped with no notice or recourse. Working with community advocacy groups, the new police commissioner for this city assigned 45 new detectives to sex crimes investigations and reopened 2000 rape cases. While the investigation is still under way, 46 arrests have already been made from cases dating back to 1995. The number of reported sexual assaults also increased by 50% in each of the next two years after the discovery. Fazlollah (2001) cautions that whenever a community's "unfounded rate" for sexual assault cases is more than the national average of 10%, and the reported rate of sexual assaults is less than the national average of 75 reports per 100,000 population, there is cause for concern. He went on to state that cities with SANE programs were more likely to have significantly higher reporting rates and that the same percentage of cases were prosecuted. He believes this suggests that more difficult cases were being successfully prosecuted, possibly as a result of better evidence collection. He recommended further comparison of cities with and without SANE programs (Fazlollah, 2001).

SHORTER EXAMINATION TIME

Not only does a SANE program shorten the survivor's wait before the examination begins, but SANEs also shorten the time a survivor must spend in the ED. A Canadian study found that, although specially trained physicians and nurses could complete an evidentiary examination equally well, the average time for the examination was shorter for the SANE than for the physician. There were more frequent interruptions for the physician in the busy ED where the physician was needed to attend to other patients (Stermac & Stirpe, 2002). Unlike the ED physician who may be called away during the rape examination to see a more urgent ED case, the SANE is able to stay with the survivor until the entire examination is completed.

BETTER FORENSIC EVIDENCE COLLECTION

Just as with any specialized clinical skill, competent forensic evidence collection is the result of both training and experience. Unfortunately, forensic principles are rarely taught in medical or nursing schools. When physicians and nurses who work in EDs are taught the basic forensic principles of evidence collection, few have the opportunity to conduct sufficient rape examinations to develop or maintain this proficiency. A primary advantage of the SANE program is that, with a limited number of dedicated nurses completing all of the evidentiary examinations in a given hospital or regional area, they are able to complete an adequate number of examinations to develop and maintain this proficiency.

As a result of periodic meetings with the prosecuting attorneys about the use of evidence in the courtroom, the quality of evidence collected has evolved over the years of the SANE program operation, and today is more complete and helpful in obtaining a conviction. For instance, one program now routinely collects an extra tube of blood that can be held and run for drug or alcohol analysis if the assailant claims the victim was so drunk that she does not remember giving consent or that she exchanged sex for drugs (Ledray, 1992).

Results of research data collected by SANE programs on the incidence of injury to rape victims or of finding sperm after a rape have also been helpful to county attorneys needing to explain that the lack of injuries or the absence of sperm does not mean the woman was not raped (Ledray, 1992).

In a study comparing 24 sexual assault evidence kits collected by SANEs to 73 evidence kits collected by non–SANE-trained physicians and nurses, the SANE kits were better documented, more complete, and always maintained proper chain of evidence (Ledray & Simmelink, 1997). Of the kits collected by non-SANEs, 48% did not maintain proper chain of custody. Thirteen (18%) of the kits completed by non-SANEs either had no indication of who had collected the evidence, or it was illegible, making the evidence available useless. One hundred percent of the kits collected by SANEs maintained proper chain-of-custody.

IMPROVED PROSECUTION

The role of the SANE does not end with the initial collection of evidence. Courtroom testimony is also important. Concerns about SANE credibility are unfounded. Several county attorneys who were initially concerned later found that the SANE was an extremely credible witness in court as a result of extensive experience and expertise in conducting the sexual assault examination. SANEs are also often more accessible and more willing than clinicians in private practice to adjust their schedules to testify, because court testimony is an expected part of their chosen position (Ledray & Barry, 1998). Prosecuting attorneys have come to trust the competence of the SANE as a witness if the case goes to trial (Yorker, 1996). The testimony of the SANE is backed up by solid credentials and impressive numbers of victims seen (Lenehan, 1991). A common concern of physicians turning over the examination to the SANE is that they will still be called to testify in court. Physicians may be called to testify about injuries that they treat. However, in thousands of cases evaluated in one midwestern city, there was no case in which the testimony of the SANE about the evidence collected was insufficient and the ED physician was required to testify (Ledray & Simmelink, 1997).

The Santa Cruz County Attorney believes that having the SANE collect evidence and be available to testify in court has resulted in more guilty pleas (Arndt, 1988). One SANE program reported a 100% conviction rate for over 3 years in cases that went to court and in which the SANE testifies (O'Brien, 1996). Another SANE program has a 96% conviction rate in cases in which the SANE did the examination (Smith, 1996). In New York City the prosecutor reported that an assailant continued to deny he had any sexual contact with the rape victim until he was confronted with the evidence collected by the SANE. He pled guilty to the maximum charge and accepted a 15-year prison sentence (Chivers, 2000).

SUMMARY

Although the initial growth of the SANE-SART concept was slow, it is anticipated that the development will continue to be rapid in this decade. The concept has proven effective in improving both the quality of service provided to the rape victim and the quality of forensic evidence collected. Ensuring optimal care for survivors of rape is no longer optional for medical facilities, and the SANE-SART model is clearly the most effective method for providing this care.

REFERENCES

Antognoli-Toland P. Comprehensive program for examination of sexual assault victims by nurses: a hospital-based project in Texas. *J Emerg Nurs.* 1985;11:132-136.

Arndt S. Nurses help Santa Cruz sexual assault survivors. *Calif Nurse.* 1988;84(8):4-5.

Bobak IM. Violence against women. *Maternity and Gynecologic Care.* St. Louis, Mo: Mosby; 1992.

Brownmiller, Susan. Against our will. *Men, Women, and Rape.* New York, NY: Simon and Schuster; 1975; 472.

Chivers CJ. In sex crimes, evidence depends on game of chance in hospitals. *New York Times.* August 6, 2000; Metropolitan Desk:1-6.

DiNitto D, Martin PY, Norton DB, Maxwell SM. After rape: who should examine rape survivors. *Am J Nurs*. 1986;86:538-540.

Fazlollah M. The Philadelphia story: from cover up to collaboration. Paper presented at: First National SART Training Conference; May 26, 2001; San Antonio, Tex.

Foa EB, Davidson J, Frances A, Culpepper L, Ross R, Ross D. The expert consensus guideline series: treatment of post-traumatic stress disorder. *J Clin Psychiatry*. 1999;60:4-76.

Frank C. The new way to catch rapists. *Redbook*. December 1996:104-105, 118, 120.

Gaffney D. Sharing our caring: Development of a Sexual Assault Nurse Examiner Team. Columbia University School of Nursing–Forensic Nursing Specialty. June, 1997. Unpublished paper.

Grell, K. ENA Sexual assault nurse examiner resource list. *J Emerg Nurs*. 1991;17:31A-35A.

Holloway M, Swan A. A&E management of sexual assault. *Nurs Stand*. 1993;7(45):31-35.

International Asscociation of Forensic Nurses (IAFN): SANE Standards of Practice; 1996.

Joint Commission on Accreditation of Health Care Organizations (JCAHO). *Comprehensive Accreditation Manual for Hospitals: The Official Handbook*. Oakbrook Terrace, Ill: JCAHO; 1997.

Kettleson D. Nurses trained to take evidence [Unit News/District News]. *District News* [District of East Hawaii]. June 1995:1.

Kiffe B. Perceptions: Responsibility Attributions of Rape Victims [master's thesis]. Minneapolis, Minn: Augsburg College; 1996.

Ledray LE. Sexual assault nurse clinician: a fifteen-year experience in Minneapolis. *J Emerg Nurs*. 1992;18:217-220.

Ledray LE. Sexual assault nurse clinician: An emerging area of nursing expertise. In: Andrist LC, ed. *Clinical Issues in Perinatal and Women's Health Nursing*. Vol. 4, No. 2. JB Lippincott Co: Philadelphia, Pa; 1993.

Ledray LE. The sexual assault resource service: a new model of care. *Minn Med*. 1996;79(3):43-45.

Ledray LE. IAFN Sixth Annual Scientific Assembly highlights [Sexual Assault: Clinical Issues]. *J Emerg Nurs*. 1999a;25:63-64.

Ledray LE. *Sexual Assault Nurse Examiner (SANE) Development and Operation Guide*. Washington, DC: Office of Victims of Crime, US Department of Justice; 1999b.

Ledray LE, Barry L. SANE expert and factual testimony [Sexual Assault: Clinical Issues]. *J Emerg Nurs*. 1998; 24:284-287.

Ledray LE, Chaignot MJ. Services to sexual assault victims in Hennepin County. *Evaluation and Change*. 1980;(special issue):131-134.

Ledray LE, Simmelink K. Efficacy of SANE evidence collection: a Minnesota study [Sexual Assault: Clinical Issues]. *J Emerg Nurs*. 1997;23:182-186.

Lenehan GP. A SANE way to care for rape victims. *J Emerg Nurs*. 1991;17:1-2.

Lynch VA. President's report: goals of the IAFN. Paper presented at: Fourth Annual Scientific Assembly of Forensic Nurses; November 1-5, 1996; Kansas City, Mo.

Marullo G. Utility of the colposcope in the sexual assault examination. Paper presented at: Fourth Annual Scientific Assembly of Forensic Nurses; November 1-5, 1996; Kansas City, Mo.

Massachusetts Nurses Association. (December 1995) MNA Collaborates with DPH to Train Sexual Assault Nurse Examiners.

O'Brien C. Sexual assault nurse examiner (SANE) program coordinator. *J Emerg Nurs.* 1996;22(6):532-533.

Sandrick KJ. Medicine and law. tightening the chain of evidence. *Hosp Health Netw.* 1996;70(11):64, 66.

Smith HG. SART: special team helps net convictions. *Press-Telegram.* June 5, 1996.

Speck P, Aiken M. 20 years of community nursing service. Memphis Sexual Assault Resource Center. *Tenn Nurse.* 1995;58(2):15-18.

Stermac LE, Stirpe TS. Efficacy of a two-year-old sexual assault nurse examiner program in a Canadian hospital. *J Emerg Nurs.* 2002;28(1):18-23

Thomas M, Zachritz H. Tulsa sexual assault nurse examiners (SANE) program. *J Okla State Med Assoc.* 1993;86(6):284-286.

Tobias G. Rape examinations by GPs. *Practitioner.* 1990;234:874, 877.

Yorker BC. Nurses in Georgia care for survivors of sexual assault. *Georgia Nurs.* 1996;56:5-6.

ROLE OF EMS PREHOSPITAL CARE PROVIDERS

Rena Rovere, MS, FNP

Care of rape victims begins in the prehospital phase with emergency medical services and/or police personnel. Prehospital care providers should be trained in providing safety, security, and support. Victims are more likely to cooperate with the many complex medical and legal procedures that follow a sexual assault if the victims' first contacts are supportive and positive.

Those who come in contact with assault or abuse victims should have an understanding of the principles and application of forensic science to emergency medical services. As the first responders at the sexual assault crime scene, prehospital care providers must assess injuries and treat them appropriately. It is also important for prehospital care providers to protect potential evidence during medical evaluation and interventions and work closely with law enforcement personnel.

Because severe trauma in rape victims is rare, the physical needs of survivors are often limited (Linden, 1999). Triage to an appropriate facility should be based on extent of injuries and the facility's forensic examination capabilities. Most victims should be brought to a health care facility with the capabilities of providing a thorough forensic evaluation of the injuries and expert evidence collection beyond a standard medical evaluation (Ciancone, 2000; Landis, 1997). Prehospital care providers should seek facilities that perform a large number of forensic examinations.

Most states require healthcare facilities to report sexual assaults to law enforcement. A multidisciplinary team approach including everyone who comes into contact with the victim will lead to the best possible outcome for the victim.

PSYCHOLOGY OF VICTIMS

Nearly 80% of sexual assault victims know their attackers (Baden & Roach, 2001; Linden, 1999; Tjaden, 1998). Sexual assault victims' perceptions of violation and loss of control are often enormous. The rape trauma syndrome is a cluster of various symptoms that may present in survivors as a response to a life-threatening situation. Victims of rape may have a wide range of emotional demeanors and behaviors (Burgess, 2000; Burgess & Holmstrom, 1974; Crowley, 1999). The symptoms after a rape have been compared to a victim of war demonstrating "battle shock" or, as Burgess describes, the acute phase of disorganization (Burgess, 2000; Burgess & Holmstrom, 1974). Victims of domestic violence/sexual assault may exhibit responses similar to "prisoners of war," specifically appearing withdrawn, flat, or muted (McRae, 2001).

Prehospital care providers should focus on helping victims maintain a sense of control and safety after an assault. Often it is best to be willing to listen while saying very little and provide physical support and safety to victims (Ehrman, 1998). It is appropriate to reassure victims that they are safe. Statements such as, "Things will be all right now," should be avoided. Rather, victims should be supported in the here and now. It is important to assure victims of their current safety.

Key Point:
Not only do prehospital providers need to assess injuries and provide appropriate treatment, but they are responsible for protecting potential evidence during medical evaluations and interventions and for working closely with law enforcement personnel.

Key Point:
Prehospital providers should help victims maintain a sense of control and safety after an assault. One of the most important steps in the emotional support and healing process is to return control to the victim.

Victims deserve not to be judged, regardless of their circumstances, appearance, risky lifestyle, race, or class (Burgess & Holmstrom, 1974). A victim is never responsible for a sexual assault. Responsibility for the rape rests completely with the assailant.

Victims may express outward emotions of confusion, anger, anxiety, fear, laughing, hysteria, and crying. Although a guarded or controlled emotional expression may be demonstrated as a subdued affect, such expression does not mean that a crime was not serious in nature or that the crime victim is not upset (Burgess, 2000). Physical reactions may be minor complaints related to the nature of the assault, including complaints of aches, soreness, pain, or abdominal discomfort. Additional manifest-ations of the rape trauma syndrome that may occur at any time include self-blame, guilt, powerlessness, vengefulness, resignation, or despair (Burgess, 2000; Burgess & Holmstrom, 1974).

One of the most important steps in the emotional support and healing process is to return control to victims. Compassionate care begins with verbal and nonverbal communication. It is important to use the victim's name and introduce yourself and your role. It may be helpful to sit at eye level and speak with a low voice, using a calm, soothing tone. It is appropriate to express admiration for the victim's courage in reaching out for help.

Prehospital personnel must remember that victims have suffered a life-threatening experience and that they need reassurance that they are safe (Bullock, 1998). It is important to ask permission to touch rape victims, even to take their blood pressure or assess injuries. After a physical violation, any touching may be perceived as unacceptable.

Efforts must be made to ensure privacy of the victim's communication and their confidentiality. Victims may feel inhibited about disclosing the abuse/assault. It may be helpful to seek a private setting, such as the back of the ambulance. The victims' permission is sought to ask a few limited questions to enable a focused assessment for injuries. It is important to victims that you maintain confidentiality regarding identity, history, and examination findings. It may be helpful to make a pledge that information provided by victims will only be discussed with healthcare workers or law enforcement directly involved in their care.

Prehospital personnel must explain various options and respect victims' decisions. Prehospital care providers may be the only contact victims have with healthcare or legal systems for many reasons, such as the victim changing his or her mind about seeking further assistance; declining transport to a medical facility; or, in certain states, exercising the option to report the crime to authorities or declining to report; or experiencing other fears related to retribution or the response of family or significant others. Victims are presented with choices, resource information, or referral numbers to local rape crisis centers and Crime Victim's Boards for Comp-ensation. Victims may refuse care other than in the prehospital setting, so that providing information and resources at that time can be a critical intervention.

FORENSIC EVIDENCE

Because trace evidence can be lost from the scene of a crime, the role of prehospital care providers with respect to evidence preservation can be crucial. In the case of sexual assault, victims themselves are a major part of the "crime scene." Accord-ingly, it is important to preserve possible evidence found on victims' skin, clothing, wounds, or body fluids such as urine or blood.

Physical assessment should be focused on complaints or injuries. It is important to gather only the information needed to provide appropriate medical care and to ensure the safety of the victim. Detailed questioning about the assault is usually not helpful in determining the healthcare needs of the victim and may provide conflicting information with that which is gathered later or may dissuade the victim from recounting details repeatedly.

It is best to begin with the objective assessment and documentation of behavior, outward appearance, clothing, and injuries. It is sometimes difficult to find the best descriptors of victims' emotional demeanor or behavior. Nevertheless, it is important to try to document victims' actions and behaviors with words that would permit a reviewer of your document to be able to visualize the victims' demeanor. Some objective descriptions of victims' behaviors are as follows:

Key Point:
The objective assessment begins with the assessment and documentation of behavior, outward appearance, clothing, and injuries.

— Crying, sobbing uncontrollably

— Tearful, weeping

— Poor eye contact

— Looks away from providers

— Sitting slumped

— Sitting on edge of seat

— Head bent

— Fetal position, knees pulled to chest

— Fists clenched, tense

— Chewing finger nails

— Legs jumping; restless

— Throwing things

— Speaking loudly

— Words slurred, or incomprehensible

— Arms wrapped around body

Although documenting the exact location of the event is usually not pertinent to providing victim care, prehospital care providers should document what is visible on arrival beginning with victim location, especially if that location is different from the location of the event.

PRESERVE CRIME SCENE EVIDENCE REGARDING CLOTHING
Document the clothing condition identified at initial contact with the victim, as follows:

— Items ripped or torn

— Soiled

— Wet

— Missing buttons

— Partially clothed

— Missing shoes or items of clothing

— Clothing inside out

— Inappropriate clothing for climate conditions

It is important to preserve victims' clothing. A basic principle of forensic science is to get possible evidence dry and to keep it dry (Lynch, 1997). Prehospital care providers should document any modifications to clothing that were made after an assault, such as clothing put on backwards, grooming, or debris removed. It is necessary to collect as evidence victims' clothing worn at the time of an assault. Therefore it is important to ensure that victims wear or bring to the hospital the clothing worn during the assault. If victims are no longer wearing the clothing, but can provide the location, each item of clothing is placed in a separate bag, preferably paper, not plastic, to permit continued air drying and to avoid cross contamination of possible trace evidence. Victims should be instructed to bring a change of clothing, including underwear, following the medical evaluation and forensic examination.

PRESERVE CRIME SCENE EVIDENCE REGARDING WOUNDS
Although trauma in sexual assault is usually minor, victims may have physical injuries such as tissue tears, ecchymosis, abrasions, redness, and swelling (Linden, 1999; Riggs, 2000). These may be subtle findings that are difficult to observe. Most rapists use only enough force to gain cooperation (Atabaki, 1999; Burgess & Holmstrom, 1974). Some of the methods of assault used in committing rape include slapping, punching, grabbing, strangling, hair pulling, biting, restraints, or physical weight or force to overpower victims.

The medicolegal terms used to describe injuries are primarily categorized in terms of their forensic definition. Contusions are characterized as areas of tenderness, with or without swelling or redness from the impact of blunt forces against the body, and may be the result of being slapped, punched, or impacted with an object. Fingernails can cause abrasions and scratches, as superficial tissue tears, which may be recognized as a pattern. The forensic definition of a laceration is blunt force trauma to tissue that occurs from crushing impact and may result in an open wound with irregular edges or margins. Sharp force injuries are incised wounds from penetration with a sharp object that cuts tissue. The wound characteristics are smooth, clean tissue margins or edges, which are consistent with a sharp object such as broken glass, a knife, or paper cut (Crowley, 1999). A brief description of the wound without categorization, "a 2-3 cm linear open wound with sharp edges" would describe a wound adequately.

The prehospital assessment should focus on areas of discomfort, tenderness or pain, without disturbing or removing the clothing when possible. When any two objects come into contact with each other, there is a transfer from one object to the other, or Locard's exchange principle (Baden & Roach, 2001).

Care and description of wounds after sexual assault should be approached different-ly than that after nonassault and may contribute an important role in preserving possible evidence related to wounds. Wounds should be described objectively in terms of the anatomical location, such as inside the upper left arm. A description of wounds must be documented; Approximate size, amount of bleeding, deformity, swelling, and tissue color surrounding are necessary facts to include.

The first aid related to these wounds must be limited to preserving life and limb. A principle of forensic science is that anything biological has potential DNA evidence (Baden & Roach, 2001). Therefore, prehospital care providers should not clean wounds, especially bite marks that may contain identifying DNA evidence in the assailant's saliva. Prehospital care providers should wrap wounds that are bleed-ing and should splint deformities. However, the application of cold compresses to tissue swelling, such as a contusion, might be postponed so that skin changes or soft tissue swelling would not be affected by vasoconstriction until visualized and photo-documented at the medical facility.

PRESERVE CRIME SCENE EVIDENCE REGARDING BODY FLUIDS

If sexual assault victims need to empty their bladders before transport, they must be instructed not to wipe their genitals after urination and to collect urine samples in jars or leak-proof containers. The specimen is handled as follows: (1) label contain-ers with victims' name, date, and time collected; (2) place containers in biohazard bags; and (3) turn bags over to hospital staff. Important evidence of a possible drug-facilitated rape may be lost if urine is not obtained as soon as possible after an assault (Li, 1999; Lynch, 1997).

Victims must be instructed not to change any sanitary device—tampon, napkin, or panty liner—after an assault until forensic evidence collection at the medical facility takes place. Discarded sanitary devices should be collected if possible.

Victims should not eat, drink, or take anything by mouth if there was an oral assault within the last 6 to 8 hours because of possible loss of evidence (Crowley, 1999).

Key Point:
A chain of custody is a written trail of ownership or possession of potential evidence.

A "chain of custody" should be clearly documented for each item of clothing, body fluid, or debris collected by prehospital providers from victims. A chain of custody is a written trail of ownership or possession of potential evidence. Another principle of forensic science is to avoid cross-contamination by securing each item separately, listing the items collected, and documenting the individual who received the items as part of the chain of custody (Crowley, 1999).

Documentation of assault victims' care differs in several ways from other noncriminal cases. There is greater significance to document legibly, clearly, and objectively the prehospital care provider's observations of the behavior, or emotional state of victims, without bias to the lifestyle. Such documentation may become important related to seemingly insignificant observations, relatively minor complaints, subtle findings of injury, and items of clothing or debris.

Clear, objective documentation of data is important. Objective data are characterized as what one is able to visualize, hear, feel, or sense in terms of observation (e.g., crying, pants on inside out, zipper broken, button missing, scratches on neck).

Subjective documentation is characterized as information related by victims regarding history, degree of pain, or level of discomfort. Chief complaints should be documented when possible in "quotes" from the victim. If complaints are obtained from parties other than the victim, the source of the information should be documented as such. Victims' exact complaints are what they are able to relate that is pertinent to medical care and treatment. Often law enforcement requests transport. Prehospital care providers should clarify who initiated calls for transport.

Information about perpetrators or assailants may be documented but should not be solicited or questioned, because it is not pertinent to prehospital medical assessment, treatment, and stabilization.

Key Point:
Objective documentation comprises those things that one can visualize, hear, feel, or sense in terms of observation. Subjective documentation comprises information related by the victim regarding history, degree of pain, or level of discomfort.

Transporting Victims to Hospitals

Transport to a medical facility should not be delayed. The greatest amount of forensic evidence can usually be collected within hours of an assault (Lynch, 1997; Riggs, 2000; Ryan, 2000). Prehospital care providers should inform victims that they will have choices related to examinations, permission to photograph, collection of evidence for DNA screening, and medical treatment prophylaxis options. Victims should have control over which facility is sought for care. Victims should be advised of options based on the following:

1. Forensic examiners (sexual assault nurse examiners [SANE] programs)

2. Forensic equipment capabilities

3. Sexual assault response team (SART) support services (rape crisis counselor, social worker, and/ or law enforcement) (Selig, 2000)

4. Support of close friend or significant other

Sexual assault forensic examiners are usually hospital employees specially educated and prepared in history taking, forensic interviewing, evidence collection, injury identification, and documentation. SANE personnel are registered nurses or advanced practice nurses, such as nurse practitioners, who have additional education, training, and supplementary skills in the principles and application of forensic science. Physician assistants, as well as emergency medicine or gynecologic physicians, are other medical professionals likely to have received similar training.

Some of the forensic tools available are as follows:

1. Standardized sexual assault evidence collection kit

2. Colposcope, a binocular microscope able to magnify minor tissue trauma

3. Photographic capability to document tissue trauma

4. Rulers

5. Ultraviolet light sources (Wood's lamp)

6. Chemical markers (toluidine blue dye)

7. Body diagrams

8. Other forensic techniques in evidence collection and injury identification

Prehospital care providers can help victims maintain a sense of control, provide safety after an assault, and express pride for having the strength and courage to begin the process. Each victim deserves dignity, respect, and the right to confidentiality. It is important to strive to recognize potential evidence related to debris, clothing, skin, wounds, or body fluids. The principles of forensic science are applied to preserve evidence and transport it in order to maintain the chain of custody. Prehospital care records are best when documented objectively, clearly, and nonjudgmentally. Through a multidisciplinary team approach in caring for the sexual assault survivor the best outcome for the victim can be achieved.

REFERENCES

Atabaki S. Medical evaluation of the sexually abused child: lessons from a decade of research. *Pediatrics.* 1999;104:178-186.

Baden M, Roach M. *Dead Reckoning, the New Science of Catching Killers.* New York, NY: Simon & Schuster; 2001.

Bullock K. Domestic violence and EMS personnel [letter]. *Ann Emerg Med.* 1998;31:286.

Burgess AW. *Violence Through a Forensic Lens.* Prussia, Pa: Nursing Spectrum Publishing; 2000.

Burgess AW, Holmstrom LL. Rape trauma syndrome. *Am J Psychiatry.* 1974;131:981-986.

Ciancone AC. Sexual assault nurse examiner programs in the United States. *Ann Emerg Med.* 2000;35:353-357.

Crowley SR. *Sexual Assault, the Medical-Legal Examination.* Stamford, Conn: Appleton & Lange; 1999.

Ehrman WG. Approach to assessing adolescents on serious or sensitive issues. *Pediatr Clin North Am.* 1998;45:189-204.

Landis JM. Victims of violence: the role and training of EMS personnel. *Ann Emerg Med.* 1997;30:204-206.

Li J. Gamma-hydroxybutyrate intoxication and overdose. *Ann Emerg Med.* 1999;33:476.

Linden JA. Sexual assault. *Emerg Med Clin North Am.* 1999;17:685-695.

Lynch VA. *Clinical Forensic Nursing: A New Perspective in Trauma.* Bearhawk Consulting Group, Co. & Publishing; 1997.

McRae AL. Alcohol and substance abuse. *Med Clinic North Am.* 2001;85:779-801.

Riggs N. Analysis of 1,076 cases of sexual assault. *Ann Emerg Med.* 2000;35:358-362.

Ryan MT. Clinical forensic medicine. *Ann Emerg Med.* 2000;36:271-273.

Selig C. Sexual assault nurse examiner and sexual assault response team (SANE/ SART) program. *Nurs Clin North Am.* 2000;35:311-319.

Tjaden P. *Prevalence, Incidence, and Consequence of Violence Against Women: Findings from the National Violence Against Women Survey.* Washinton, DC: National Institute for Justice; 1998 Nov: 1-16. NCJ172837.

ADDITIONAL READING/RESOURCE

Bechtel K. Evaluation of the adolescent rape victim. *Pediatr Clin North Am.* 1999;46:809-823.

Ferris LE. The sensitivity of forensic tests for rape. *Med Law.* 1998;17:333-350.

Hazelwood RR, Burgess AW. *Practical Aspects of Rape Investigation: A Multidisciplinary Approach.* 2nd ed. New York, NY: Elsevier; 1995.

Oster NS. Critical incident stress challenges for the emergency workplace. *Emerg Med Clin North Am*. 2000;18:339-353.

Weiss SJ. EMT domestic violence knowledge and the results of an educational intervention. *Am J Emerg Med*. 2000;18:168-171.

Chapter

LAW ENFORCEMENT ISSUES

Patsy Rauton Lightle

Investigating sexual assault is a demanding task. No single group of individuals is immune to the possibility of sexual assault. When sexual abuse involves a child or the elderly, the investigative tasks become even more complex due to difficulties with language, cognitive skills, and physical and mental impairment that can hinder the interview process. It is imperative that law enforcement personnel be cognizant of the indicators of sexual abuse and understand that some techniques have proved useful in these investigations. The processes and techniques described in this chapter are largely based on the author's field experience and subsequent design of several protocols, including the South Carolina Law Enforcement Division's protocols and kits for Adult Sexual Assault Evidence Collection, Child Sexual Assault Evidence Collection, Chronic Sexual Assault Evidence Collection, Suspect Evidence Collection, and the Child Postmortem Evidence Collection. In addition, a few basic textbooks provide general background information, (Fisher et al., 1987; Henry, 1979; Kinnee, 1994; Wicklander & Zulawski, 1993).

It is crucial that an investigator with the training and experience necessary to support successful prosecution be assigned to conduct the thorough and methodical investigation of sexual abuse crimes. The law enforcement officer must have a basic understanding and knowledge of sexual offenses and feel comfortable seeking outside expert advice when needed. In all cases the safety and well-being of the victim should be the first priority. Attention to details is a must. The case should be worked and closely monitored with prosecution as the final goal.

Key Point:
The investigator assigned to the case must be thorough and methodical, have a basic understanding of sexual offenses, and be comfortable seeking other experts' advice when needed.

PROCESSING THE SCENE AND COLLECTING EVIDENCE

Law enforcement personnel are usually the first responders once the crime is reported. The steps in the investigative process should be followed carefully; many of these are the same steps taken for any criminal assault. These steps are as follows:

Key Point:
The steps for a sexual assault investigation are often the same as would be taken in any criminal assault.

1. Record exact time and location of the assault. 911 tapes and law enforcement dispatch tapes can be useful to confirm this information for court purposes.

2. While traveling to the scene, carefully note fleeing persons, vehicles, witnesses, etc.

3. If the first notification of the assault is received in person, detain this person for investigation and written statement. If unable to detain the person, obtain enough information to locate him or her at a later time. When a third party reports the assault, document identification information for follow-up interview(s). This person will be a crucial witness.

4. Record exact time of the arrival and notify communications that you are on the scene. Do not use a telephone at the crime scene to report your arrival. Use your mobile radio, hand-held radio, or agency-issued cell phone, but never a telephone at the scene. The suspect may have picked up the telephone at the scene to call someone or held it as he or she disconnected the telephone cord from the wall jack. The smooth surface of the telephone would be an excellent source for the suspect's fingerprints. The use of the same telephone by a law

enforcement officer at the scene contaminates the print by adding additional fingerprint ridge detail or by smearing the suspect's fingerprint, thereby causing that print to be unsuitable for comparison.

5. If the victim is injured, request Emergency Medical Services (EMS) and provide first aid. Do not move seriously injured people unless it is to protect them from additional harm. Be sure to document if the emergency medical technician (EMT) moves or touches anything within the crime scene. Document what, when, and why the alterations were made and if any medications were given to the victim. Emergency medical staff or a law enforcement officer will take the victim to a licensed health care facility where a sexual assault evidence collection protocol is performed. This protocol provides a standardized and coordinated approach to the collection of information and forensic evidence, as well as treatment for injuries and prevention of sexually transmitted diseases and pregnancy. The victim will need to take an additional set of clothing because the clothing he or she is wearing will be collected for forensic evidence processing.

6. An initial incident report detailing information to support a crime should be taken. Record the names and addresses of all persons present when you arrive. Record the names of all officers present with you at the time of arrival, as well as officers who come later to assist.

7. Only one officer should enter the scene.

8. Isolate a large area around the assault scene to prevent loss of evidence. Establish a perimeter and secure it using crime scene tape, ropes, cones, barricades, etc. and at least one officer to provide security until evidence collection and documentation by the forensic crime scene unit and lead investigator are completed.

9. Consider the weather conditions for crimes occurring outside and protect the scene. Document weather conditions, persons present, and any nearby vehicle information, including license number, make, model, and color. Avoid discussion of the crime; the suspect may appear as a neighbor or an onlooker.

10. Once the scene is secured and the victim is safe and located away from the scene, a complete, thorough background investigation should be conducted. A crime scene log-in or sign-in sheet is kept at all crime scenes. The officer in charge of security for the crime scene can also be in charge of the sign-in sheet. It includes the name, agency, and telephone number of all individuals who enter and depart from the scene. The security officer ensures that only authorized individuals enter through one designated entrance to the scene. Cross-contamination occurs when individuals are allowed to use more than one entrance into the building. In addition, it is extremely difficult to account for everyone who enters and departs from the scene when more than one entrance is used.

11. Isolate and separate witnesses or suspect(s). Do not permit any conversation among them. Hold witnesses and suspects for investigators.

12. Do not allow anyone to smoke in the crime scene area. People, including officers, are often nervous or excited at the scene and need to smoke a cigarette or chew gum, unaware that the cigarette butt or gum they throw down or put in an ashtray will contaminate the scene. An officer's cigarette butt will be tested for saliva, secretor status, and DNA, adding "evidence" to the scene that is not involved with the crime. A secretor secretes his or her blood type in body fluids such as saliva, semen, vaginal fluids, and sweat. For example, should a suspect smoke a cigarette at the crime scene, this would be collected as evidence. The forensic analyst analyzes the cigarette for saliva and determines the blood type of the person who smoked the cigarette. The same analysis can be performed with

chewing gum, bite marks, etc. The chewing gum is analyzed for saliva, secretor status, DNA, and dental impression and also contaminates the scene. The collection and analysis of irrelevant material wastes resources and time on the investigation. Additionally, do not allow anyone to use the toilet or the sink at the scene. The toilet handle may have the suspect's fingerprints on it, the sink and hand towel may have been used by the suspect to "clean up," and in some cases, evidence has been flushed or stuffed down the toilet.

The crime scene should be photographed and sketched before the scene is searched and before evidence is seized. Photographs should be taken of the entire location where the assault took place. If it is a house, for example, every room is photographed from different angles, along with the exterior of the house, including entry points; broken windows; evidence such as bloodstains, hairs, etc.; the surrounding yard; and neighbor's houses and bystanders. The forensic photographer should document the date, time, weather/light conditions, type of film and camera, and must initial each roll of film.

Key Point:
Photographs, sketches, searches, and processing for fingerprints are important components of the investigation.

The investigator will note the surrounding area of the house and identify the point of entry of the suspect by looking for unlocked doors, forced entry, open windows, position of curtains or blinds, strewn papers, furniture that is in disarray or has been moved, etc. Some assailants vacuum the scene before leaving to remove any evidence of his or her person but fail to remove the vacuum bag from the vacuum cleaner. This is collected as evidence and taken to the forensic laboratory for trace analysis.

A sketch is made using measurements from fixed points such as doors, walls, stairs, etc.; it is not drawn to scale. A legend is helpful to identify the items in the sketch. Once the sketch is completed and initialed, a thorough search of the crime scene is performed after obtaining a valid search warrant or consent to search by the owner. All physical evidence is photographed and placed in a separate paper bag—not plastic—sealed with evidence tape, labeled, and initialed. Do not allow two items to come into contact with each other as evidence can transfer from one to the other. For example, wet blood from a pair of panties can contaminate a victim's bra if they are allowed to come into contact. Hair and fibers can also be easily transferred from one item to another.

The crime scene is also processed for fingerprints. Most prints at a scene are latent, or hidden, fingerprints. There are various methods for "lifting" these prints. These prints should be photographed with an identifying marker and documented as to location, date, and time. Two other types of prints that may be found at the scene are patent prints and etched prints. The patent print is a visible print usually made by the fingertips, which are impregnated with body oil, blood, or dirt, or when the surface is soft and pliable such as putty or wax. These fingerprints are simply photographed and need nothing more to enhance their ridge detail. An etched print occurs when a person handles an object, usually metal, and a chemical reaction from that person's body fluid on the fingers etches a print on the object. These prints look just like those "lifted" with powder and are easily identifiable by a fingerprint examiner. These prints are then compared to known fingerprint standards of the suspect(s). If applicable, a blood spatter expert must photograph and measure bloodstain patterns to reconstruct the scene before blood samples are collected. A good rule of thumb to remember is that, with every crime, the suspect leaves identifiable evidence behind at the scene or takes something of the victim with him. This theory justifies the necessity for a thorough and methodical crime scene search.

If the assault occurred outdoors, the investigator has a responsibility to choose the method for the search for evidence. There are five accepted methods, with the grid method and strip method being the best for outdoor searches that encompass a large area. An alternate light source is used by law enforcement to process evidence for body fluids, hairs, fibers, and fingerprints. This is especially valuable when the assault occurs outdoors. If the assault occurs in a wooded area, the alternate light source, using a battery pack or generator, can be mobilized to locate seminal stains on objects such as leaves and grass. Most law enforcement agencies have an alternate light source or access to such in their state.

When the assault occurs in a vehicle, the make, model, year, license number, vehicle identification number (VIN), and color should be documented. The vehicle should be moved if possible to a forensic or law enforcement garage for processing. If a vehicle is involved in another way, such as transporting the suspect and/or victim, then the investigator should check the engine to see if it is cold, warm, or hot to the touch to corroborate the victim's statement that the vehicle was used and, possibly, the time the assault occurred.

A copy of the photographs, the crime scene sketch, an inventory of evidence seized, and the logbook are given to the investigator for court purposes. The inventory of evidence seized includes: a description of the evidence, the name of the officer who collected it, the location, date, and time collected, and a checkmark indicating that the evidence was photographed in its original position and location before collection.

A good investigator knows he or she must do the following:

— collect evidence from the crime scene

— understand and use the forensic evidence from the medical examination

— conduct interviews of the victim, victim's family, and friends

— canvass the neighborhood

— conduct background investigations

— locate a suspect

— interview or interrogate the suspect

— make an arrest

— successfully bring the suspect to court for a conviction

THE INTERVIEW PROCESS

A sexual assault investigator should be skilled in interviews and interrogations, able to interpret verbal and physical behavior, and skilled in obtaining information that indicates guilt or innocence.

Interviewing the victim of sexual assault is one of the most important measures law enforcement officers take in conducting an investigation. Interviewing is an essential aspect of the investigation because it secures information from the victim, witnesses, friends, parents, spouse, and other involved parties. Appropriate and productive interviewing involves close personal contact between law enforcement and the public. The reputation of the law enforcement agency as well as the effectiveness of the law enforcement officer may depend on how well the officer conducted the interview.

The purpose of the interview is to obtain information leading to the arrest and conviction of the assailant. Although uncommon, the suspect may be at the scene when the first officer arrives. Should this happen, the officer should take accurate notes, arrest the suspect if evidence is present to indicate guilt, and determine if the suspect is armed. It is important to search for and seize any weapon and record the number, description, and location of the weapon seized. The officer should also secure any evidence found on the suspect and document any spontaneous statements. The first officer should tell the suspect he or she is under arrest, use the

Key Point:
A good investigator collects evidence, uses forensic evidence from the medical examination, interviews all parties involved, canvasses the neighborhood, conducts background checks, locates the suspect, conducts interviews or interrogations of the suspect, makes the arrest, and is successful in bringing the suspect to court for a conviction.

Key Point:
The goal of the interview is to obtain information that will lead to an arrest and conviction of the assailant.

"Miranda" warning as appropriate, and not allow any conversation between the suspect and other parties. Do not interview or interrogate the suspect. Isolate the suspect from other witnesses, and if he or she is arrested inside the crime scene area, remove him or her as soon as possible. Do not allow the suspect to return to the crime scene should he or she be arrested outside of the crime scene area. The suspect's return would then contaminate the crime scene. Do not allow the suspect to wash his or her hands, change clothes, smoke, or use the toilet because evidence will be lost. Do not leave the suspect alone, and observe and document his or her behavior. The first officer should note the suspect's mental and physical condition, noting such signs as nervousness, the potential influence of drugs, torn and/or stained clothes, glass, leaves, or fibers in his or her hair, and injuries to his or her skin. The suspect is transported to a secure facility as soon as possible, where a "Suspect Evidence Collection Kit and Protocol" will be performed.

An investigator skilled in interviewing will then interview the suspect. The investigator must ensure that the suspect is interviewed in a manner that maximizes the potential for uncovering the truth. The investigator obtains a criminal history or background check on the suspect to see if he or she has had any past arrests and/or convictions. The officer should build a rapport when interviewing the suspect. Time must be spent getting to know as much about the suspect as possible before interviewing him, making inquiry into the suspect's employment history, education, means of transportation, past prison time, relatives, leisure activities, and relatives with whom he or she associates. In addition, basic information is obtained, including full name, nickname(s), alias, gender, race, date of birth, Social Security number, height, weight, build (e.g., small, medium, thin, average, stocky, obese), hair color, hair length, facial hair, eye color, glasses, contacts, scars, tattoos, teeth, unusual physical features, detection of body odor, speech impediment, language/accent, mental or physical impairments, emotional condition, address that includes the name and number of people living at the address, and marital status. The body of the suspect will be inspected during the collection of the "Suspect Evidence Collection Kit" for injuries, bruises, wounds, scars, and bite marks. The officer will ask the suspect how he or she obtained the injuries and document and photograph all injuries and marks.

Interview strategy includes acknowledging that the offender has a problem and that the investigator is concerned with helping him. Other strategies include de-emphasizing the criminal nature of the perpetrator; avoiding threatening words, tone, or actions; interpreting the suspect's body language; listening sympathetically; and asking open-ended questions. The investigator allows the suspect to make a full statement and then follows with more probing questions. This statement is reduced to writing, and the suspect is asked to sign it. All alibi statements and changes in the statement should be documented. When handwritten notes have been involved, as in stalking cases, a handwriting exemplar is requested of the suspect. Some of the defenses an officer might expect from the suspect include denial, minimization of his or her behavior, justification for his or her actions including suggestions that the actions were beneficial for the victim or that he or she was under undue stress, and fabrication of events to explain his or her behavior.

Key Point:
An interview is a structured conversation presented in a nonaccusatory manner referencing the interviewee's involvement in the crime. An interrogation is a conversation in which the person being interviewed is accused of being involved in the crime and is closely regulated legally.

There is a difference between an interview and an interrogation. An interview is a structured conversation presented in a nonaccusatory manner referencing the interviewee's involvement in the crime. An interrogation is a conversation in which the person being interviewed is accused of being involved in the crime. Law closely regulates interrogations. A qualified, trained investigator adhering to departmental/agency policy on interrogation techniques will proceed with the interrogation. The investigator will use the Miranda warning when it applies. The officer may have the suspect re-enact the crime and show events that led up to, during, and after the assault. The suspect may show the location and aid in finding evidence. When this occurs, it is important that an officer located in another vehicle videotape or photograph the event.

There are many determining factors in deciding who interviews the victim. The victim's age, his or her mental and/or physical impairments, and the availability of a forensic interviewer versus a specially trained investigator with good interview skills will play an important part in selecting the interviewer. Sensitivity and experience on the part of the person performing the interview may determine the successful apprehension and conviction of the assailant. The victim will be asked basic questions such as the following:

— Did the victim know the suspect?

— If not, describe his or her race, height, weight, color of hair, hair length, facial hair, glasses, body odor, scars, tattoo or other physical markings, and clothing.

— Does the victim know the suspect's name, address, family, friends, daily routine, hobbies, work history, and present occupation?

— What does the victim remember of the assault?

It is important to thank the victim for doing his or her best to help the investigator gather information to help identify the assailant. The investigator, as well as a psychological profiler, is interested in the victim's recall of the type of restraint (if any) that was used, conversation that the assailant had with the victim, instruments used to draw or write on the victim's body, any physical or mental torture, photographs or videos taken of the victim, and sexual preference and dysfunction exhibited by the assailant. It is important that the investigator follow up with the victim on a regular basis in the event additional details of the assault are remembered and to assure the victim that law enforcement is continuing its investigation and has not forgotten about the victim or the case. An investigator should never promise a victim that he or she will apprehend the assailant but should provide assurance that everything will be done to apprehend the assailant.

The investigator also needs to interview the victim's family and friends. A neighborhood canvass is another important step. The investigator will show identification and explain the purpose of the canvass. Most law enforcement agencies have a standard neighborhood canvass questionnaire. The questionnaire may be revised according to the circumstances of the case. Basic questions on a questionnaire include the neighbor's name, address, date of birth, employment, work address, and telephone number. The investigator will also ask the name and age of residents, whether they were aware of the crime, when they first learned of the crime, whether they know the victim. If they know that victim, the investigator will go on to ask for the date, time, and location that they last saw or talked to the victim, whether they were present at the crime scene, and what they have heard about the crime. The investigator takes a statement if the neighbor has any knowledge of the crime.

SEARCH WARRANTS

The importance of search warrants cannot be overemphasized. Search warrants are a significantly underutilized investigative tool. The ability to obtain sufficient information or probable cause to support a search warrant is important, and developing probable cause begins at the investigation's onset. An officer should keep a log of information obtained daily that helps to validate the charges to be filed. These should be as detailed as possible when describing a person, place, or object. If it is a person, all the basic personal traits such as race, gender, height, weight, eye color, hair color, hair length, build, and physical marks such as tattoos or scars should be noted. If it is a place of residence or business, etc., the address, description of building, landmarks, and neighboring houses or buildings are documented. All outbuildings on the property are included because they may be used to conceal evidence. A map and/or aerial photographs aid in the correct identification of a place to be searched. The description should be detailed enough so that the officer who has never been to the particular location can locate it by following the portrait set forth in the search warrant. After obtaining probable cause, a search is made of the suspect's house, car, office, storage shed, garage, lockers, etc.

A legal search can provide material regarding additional suspects and/or victims and corroborate the victim's statements. For example, a child may state she was in the yellow house on the corner of the street, on a bed, and in a blue room with horses in it. This description would sound like a child's fantasy to a jury. When an officer obtains this statement, an affidavit should be drafted addressing the facts developed from the interview to include information in support of the presence of certain items. The list of items to be seized should be detailed enough to include evidence that could lead to further investigation. This affidavit will be presented to a judge who will determine if it supports sufficient probable cause for the issuance of a search warrant. The officer executes the search warrant by proceeding to the yellow house in the neighborhood, photographing the house, and searching it. Inside the yellow house the officer should find the blue room and photograph it. Finally, as the officer enters the room he observes a wallpaper border that has a horse design on it. This logically explains what the child meant by "in a room with horses" and corroborates the child's story. It also corroborates the child's story that she was on the bed in the blue room, which would place her in a position to see the ceiling and the wallpaper border. The wallpaper is photographed and the bedspread seized for forensic purposes. Remember that physical evidence goes beyond blood, hair, semen, and saliva, including colors, wallpaper, photos, books, television shows, or a certain song. An officer can help corroborate a victim's statement by broadening the definition of "physical evidence."

CORROBORATING EVIDENCE

Corroborating evidence is evidence that confirms a victim's statement. It strengthens the prosecutor's case, especially in a child sexual assault, and it reduces the child's stress by supporting his or her testimony. It also makes it difficult for the defense attorney to attack the child's allegations on memory and suggestibility grounds, and ensures justice. Investigators frequently have no physical evidence because they consider only blood, semen, hair, and saliva. In child sexual assault cases, this type of evidence is not often found, so other physical corroborating evidence should be sought. For instance, if the child claims she was abused during a particular television show, obtain a TV Guide for the day and time that the show aired in the area. Document and save this material for court purposes to corroborate the victim's testimony. Other examples of less commonly used physical evidence include the following:

Key Point:
Corroborating evidence supports the victim's statement, strengthens the prosecutor's case, reduces the child's stress by supporting testimony, and makes it difficult for the defense attorney to attack the child's credibility.

— If the child claims the abuse occurred during school hours, a check with the child's school attendance records could verify his or her absence at the time of the assault.

— If the child states she heard a particular song playing on the radio during the abuse, obtaining a copy of the play list from the radio station could be helpful.

To aid officers in searching for corroborating evidence, a multidisciplinary team should go over the victim's statement sentence by sentence and word for word. After each sentence, ask yourself: is there anything that can be corroborated? If the child's interview and statements were audio taped or videotaped, the officer will have to arrange to have it transcribed before meeting with the multidisciplinary team. The suspect's statement should be treated the same way. An officer's thorough investigation enhances the credibility of the victim, increases the likelihood of a guilty plea, and eliminates the possibility that the victim is traumatized again by testifying in front of the abuser and a jury.

BITE MARKS

Bite marks are valuable evidence and have been overlooked and missed for years as an essential part of a criminal investigation. Bite marks are latent or patent images left on a victim or subject. Bite marks are photographed to document these latent images, creating a permanent record of photographic evidence of the crime. Persons who have been bitten can be the attacker or the victim of the attacker. For the most part, bite marks have been found on persons involved in crimes related to sexual abuse. In some cases it is possible to match the bite mark to the dental impression of the person suspected of having committed the crime. Likewise, bite mark evidence could prove that the suspect did not create the bite mark, thereby eliminating him or her as a suspect.

Bite marks can be used much like fingerprints. Their individual morphologic characteristics and relationship with each other in the dental arch leave a distinct mark on the victim. The bite mark may appear as a semicircle or oval mark on the body depending on the nature of the bite and the presence or absence of clothing on the victim. Additional bite marks may be seen on the child's body in different stages of healing indicating chronic abuse.

Bite marks are found on various areas of a victim's body but most often on the chest, face, abdomen, and extremities. Bite marks may be covered with blood but will almost always be covered with saliva. Saliva contains nucleated squamous epithelial cells, which are valuable in DNA analysis. Be sure the bite mark is swabbed to collect the saliva before the photographs are taken.

The odontologist, or forensic dentist, relies on bite mark evidence photography to serve as a permanent record of the bite mark. The photography should be performed as soon as possible after the assault and the follow-up photos should be taken in 3 days and 10 days. If needed, reflective ultraviolet photography of the bite mark may be performed at later dates to show any latent images that may exist. This can be done even if the bite mark is still barely visible on the skin. By using ultraviolet lighting with photography, bite marks have shown up as long as 4 months after the assault because of the collection of blood underneath the skin as a result of bruising.

A forensic odontologist or a dentist trained by a forensic odontologist should take the photographs. These professionals are familiar with approaching a child, elder, or special needs victim of suspected abuse. They will work with the victim in the presence of a trusted relative or guardian, inform the victim of the procedure to reduce anxiety, and allow the victim to become accustomed to the photographer. When photographing the size of a bite mark, the use of a ruler certified and approved by the American Board of Forensic Odontology is advisable. Photographs and impressions should be taken from the suspect. Impressions from the victim are collected as needed.

OTHER CONSIDERATIONS

Investigators should be familiar with their state laws regarding issues such as criminal sexual conduct, privacy and wiretapping, emergency protective custody, termination of parental rights, obscenity, sexual exploitation with a minor/elder, mandated reporting statutes, and penalties for failure to report.

Case management is of vital importance to every law enforcement officer and to successful prosecution. The investigation of criminal sexual assault generates a tremendous amount of paperwork, and the ability of the investigator to collect, document, organize and process the information is critical. The ultimate goal of any criminal investigation is to identify the assailant, prevent him from harming any more citizens, and successfully provide information to the prosecution for conviction. The time to start preparing for court is when the investigator initially arrives on the scene. Proper documentation, collection, and organization of evidence is essential. Case management is now an integral part of an investigation because it controls the workload, flow of information, and paper flow. Being able to manage this process assists in developing a better case and provides the prosecution with all the necessary documents for court preparation and prosecution. Sometimes a year or so elapses before the case is tried in court, and the quality of case management determines the officer's ability to testify in a confident and convincing manner despite the passage of significant time.

When an investigator is preparing a case file for court, the following information should be in the case file:

1. Cover sheet

2. Brief synopsis that includes a chronology of events

3. Offense report with all supplemental reports

4. Arrest reports

5. Follow-up reports, statements, arrest and/or search warrants

6. Forensic laboratory reports as applicable, including DNA, trace, latent prints, question documents, polygraph results, toxicology findings, evidence, evidence forms, and chain of custody

7. Background sheets

8. Criminal histories

9. Medical information

10. Victim and Suspect Sexual Assault Evidence Collection Protocols

11. Photographs

12. Sketches

13. Videotapes, audio tapes

14. List of witnesses with their address and telephone number and their involvement in the case

The investigator should set up a meeting with the appointed prosecutor to provide this information in an orderly fashion. It is the responsibility of the investigator to understand the results of the victim's sexual assault evidence collection protocol and examination. It is important to note that law enforcement is extremely dependent on the nurse or physician who collects the evidence. The forensic laboratory can only examine what is collected at the sexual assault examination. Improper collection and preservation of the evidence could potentially destroy the case, which is why law enforcement and the medical professional must work closely together. In addition, law enforcement officers are not taught a medical terminology course at police academies when becoming a certified police officer. The evidence and information collected at the licensed healthcare facility may be properly collected, but if the investigator does not have a full understanding of the medical indicators, crucial evidence is missed and not compared to the victim's statements and/or the suspect's standards. For example, the result of the examination could be motile sperm versus non-intact sperm, indicating the length of time the semen was deposited and the time the victim was presented at the health care facility. The investigator should be told of these results, and medical personnel should take the time and effort to explain to the officer the difference and importance of motility of the sperm.

Key Point:
Law enforcement personnel are extremely dependent on the medical professional who collects the evidence and interprets it. Thus the medical and law enforcement professions must work closely together to build a case.

503

Another example is extensive bruising on the victim that should be noted by the medical staff and bleeding time tests performed to rule out a bleeding dyscrasia or disorder in the victim. If a bleeding disorder is not eliminated, then the bruises on the victim that he or she stated were caused by the assailant during the assault will simply be explained away by the defense as the victim being someone who simply bruises easily. The medical staff should draw a tube of blood and perform three tests that rule out any bleeding disorders. These three tests are a complete blood count (CBC), a prothrombin time (PT), and a partial thromboplastin time (PTT). The medical staff should inform the investigator that these tests were performed, explain why they were performed, and offer an explanation of the results. The investigation will be comprehensive when the investigator is aided by the medical information. It is then the investigator's responsibility to convey and explain the importance of the medical and forensic information to the prosecutor if the prosecutor is not familiar with sexual assault cases. Working closely with the prosecutor can help the prosecution to be performed effectively in the courtroom and all necessary information to be conveyed to the jury. Finally, the investigator is responsible for being well prepared for giving testimony in court. Suggestions are as follows:

— Know your case, your victim, the circumstances, and the connection of the evidence between the suspect and the victim.

— Look professional, be courteous, and speak distinctly.

— Respond to questions with brief answers, and address your answers to the jury and judge.

— If you don't understand a question, be comfortable enough to politely ask them to repeat the question. Asking the defense or prosecution to repeat the question also allows the officer a bit more time to think about the question and formulate an answer.

It cannot be overemphasized that the investigator should be well prepared for court. The investigator must describe the details and steps taken in the investigation. The only successful means of doing this is to review all investigative reports, photographs, sketches, forensic reports, and statements and to meet with the involved parties near the time of the court appearance.

CONCLUSION

Abuse is not a subject that has recently surfaced. In the 1800s the famous case of Mary Ellen was reported (National Association of Counsel for Children, 2002). She was an adopted child who was repeatedly abused by her mother and the abuse was reported to a social worker. The social worker was shocked by the abuse she observed when she checked on Mary Ellen and reported the abuse to law enforcement. Law enforcement in turn told the social worker it was a family problem and there was nothing that could be done. The social worker did not give up. Knowing it was a crime to treat animals inhumanely, the social worker disguised Mary Ellen by wrapping her in a blanket and the case was tried under the inhumane treatment of animals. Today, social intervention, law enforcement, and the judicial system have come a long way to bring about justice for victims of sexual abuse. Every state has adopted "Megan's Law," which requires child sex offenders to register their address and changes of address with local law enforcement agencies (Sex Offender Registration, Child Abuse and Neglect State Statute Series, 1998). Every agency that deals with victims of sexual assault should be armed with knowledge, compassion, experience, and case management to continue the fight to protect the innocent, convict the guilty, and make this world a safer place in which to live.

REFERENCES

American Prosecutors Research Institute (APRI). *Sex Offender Registration, Child Abuse and Neglect State Statute Series 1998.* Alexandria, Va: APRI's National Center for Prosecution of Child Abuse, Vol. 111, no. 17.

Fisher AJ, Svensson A, Wendel O. *Techniques of Crime Scene Investigation.* New York, NY: Elsevier Science Publishing Co., Inc.; 1987.

Henry JB. *Clinical Diagnosis and Management.* Philadelphia, Pa: W.B. Saunders Company; 1979.

Kinnee KR. *Practical Investigation Techniques.* Boca Raton, Fla: CRC Press; 1994.

National Association of Counsel for Children 2002. Children and the law: child maltreatment. NACC Web site. Available at: http://nacchildlaw.org/childrenlaw/childmaltreatment.html. Accessed October 16, 2002.

Wicklander DE, Zulawski DE. *Practical Aspects of Interview and Interrogation.* Boca Raton, Fla: CRC Press; 1993.

The Role of Police as First Responders

Maureen S. Rush, MS
Jeanne L. Stanley, PhD

In the latter part of the 20th century, there was a heightened societal awareness of the devastating nature of sexual assaults. With this new awareness, many communities implemented significant reforms in police procedures and services for sexual assault victims. Improvements included the creation of training programs for police and specific units dedicated to providing services to sexual assault victims. After implementing these initial changes, however, the reform movement lost momentum. Very few advances in police procedures and services for sexual assault victims are ongoing, and there is little ability to evaluate the effectiveness of existing programs.

Many programs created in the late 1970s and early 1980s that remain today are based on outdated research. Although the research existing when the programs began was instrumental in bringing about an awareness of issues confronting sexual assault victims, such research failed to address a complete understanding of the varied circumstances of, reactions to, and outcomes for sexual assault victims (Resick, 1993).

This chapter provides first responders, specifically police personnel, with an understanding of their role in responding to a sexual assault case. This role focuses on both providing empathetic care and services to victims of sexual assault and to ensuring the proper performance of investigative work to support the criminal prosecutions of such cases. Areas addressed include the specifics of necessary preparation; victim contact; medical examinations; investigative interviews; criminal prosecution; victim reactions; and ongoing contact and victim support.

Preparation for First Responders

Preparation through education and training is the first responder's key to providing comprehensive services to sexual assault victims. In some communities, police departments have developed specialized investigative units trained to address the unique issues associated with sexual assault crimes. In all communities, however, first responders need to have access to both initial and continuing education designed to address sexual assault issues. First responders require education about the broad range of victim reactions to sexual assaults; the various methods of empathetic questioning; the most up-to-date forensic procedures; and the many myths, stereotypes, and assumptions about victims of sexual assault. Training should also include the various ways victims present themselves after a sexual assault as well as the importance of avoiding value judgments regarding the impact of sexual assaults on victims.

A first responder must understand that from a legal standpoint, stranger rape and acquaintance rape are equally important and are therefore given equal weight throughout the investigation and prosecution. To that end, many states have enacted legislation specifically addressing the prosecution of perpetrators in spousal sexual assault cases. Finally, continuing education is needed to inform first responders of changes and modifications in laws regarding sexual assault, rape, spousal sexual assault and child sexual abuse (Avner, 1990).

To gain a more complete understanding of the complicated circumstances of sexual assault victims, first responders must be educated and trained regarding issues such as race, ethnic background, age, gender, religion, economic status, disabilities, and sexual identity. Such education and training are designed to decrease misinterpretations of victim reactions and increase opportunities to assist victims.

First responders must also be educated about, and establish relationships with, available community resources and social services for sexual assault victims. Most communities have access to local and/or national rape crisis/sexual assault centers and related service providers or hotlines. Familiarity with such services allows the first responder to make appropriate and useful recommendations focusing on the specific needs of each victim. For example, knowing which shelters are able to provide support for both victims and their children after a spousal sexual assault can make the resources offered more appropriate for each victim. It is also useful to establish relationships with service providers who address the unique issues facing male victims as well as lesbian, gay, bisexual, and transgender victims of sexual assault. Knowing which referral sites have multilingual counselors or interpreters is also helpful.

VICTIM CONTACT

The first responder to the scene of a sexual assault is often a police officer. First responders' actions can have a tremendous impact on victims' perceptions. Victims' initial contact with first responders often creates an indelible perception about the entire justice system (Avner, 1990). Tempkin (1997) found that victims' best perceptions toward police occur when the police are empathetic, compassionate, professional, and nonjudgmental. To ensure the best outcome for victim care and criminal prosecution, police must begin by learning what is beneficial in interactions with victims.

Victims' initial contact with police is usually through a police or 911 dispatcher. Even this potentially brief interaction can affect victims' perception of the justice system. The actions of police dispatchers can have a significant impact on the immediate care and long-term well-being of victims. Police dispatchers begin by assessing the safety of victims. They investigate whether victims are still in immediate danger and whether immediate medical attention is needed at the scene. Police dispatchers also provide important information regarding victim care to responding police personnel. For instance, if victims are minors, police dispatchers may deploy to the scene additional personnel specifically trained to address the needs of minors.

Police dispatchers also play a role in collecting information used in criminal prosecutions. They obtain basic data regarding victims' names, ages, and current location. Such information may also include time-sensitive or "flash" information that relates to the time and location of the assault, descriptions of the assailant(s), any vehicle that may be applicable, other physical identifiers, and direction of the assailant's flight. Police dispatchers immediately broadcast this information to all available patrol and detective units in the field. Officers, in turn, survey their patrol areas for such perpetrators. If the victim knows his or her assailant, the police dispatcher may also ask for specific locations where such assailants are often found (e.g., bars or restaurants).

Police dispatchers may also give specific directions to victims to preserve important prosecution evidence and assist the forensic components of investigations. They may instruct victims not to shower or bathe, wash or discard clothing or bed linens, disturb the contents of any rooms occupied by perpetrators, or reenter vehicles that

Key Point:
Police as first responders need both initial and ongoing education and training to provide essential support and services to victims of sexual assault.

Key Point:
Victims' perceptions of police first responders are enhanced when police are empathetic, compassionate, professional, and nonjudgmental.

may have been occupied by offenders. To preserve crime scenes, police dispatchers should also instruct victims, if deemed safe, to remain at their current location until police arrive. Dispatchers should remain on the phone with victims until police arrive to ensure victims' physical safety and to provide psychologic support.

Unless victims require immediate medical services, police officers generally provide the initial on-scene contact with sexual assault victims. The police officers' approach to victims can significantly affect the outcome of the encounter. Confidentiality should be maintained in addressing both the physical and psychologic needs of sexual assault victims. This includes the use of unmarked police cars and plainclothes officers to maintain victims' privacy from family, neighbors, and friends. Because perpetrators sometimes threaten further violence if victims seek police aid, a "low profile" approach may help to address victims' fear of reprisal by such perpetrators. It may also aid in an investigation should the perpetrator actually return to the scene of the crime.

During initial meetings with victims, police should be aware of other situational factors that are important to victims. For example, police may need to arrange support services for any children present during a sexual assault and childcare while victims are engaged in medical examinations and police interviews. Officers can determine if the presence of victims' family members or friends is helpful or harmful to victims. It may or may not be helpful to have family members or friends accompany victims to medical examinations for emotional support or to act as interpreters for non-English-speaking victims. When language barriers exist and interpreters are not available, family or friends may be enlisted to assist in gathering necessary information about the assault. This may, however, limit the amount of personal information victims discuss, or it may introduce subjective or inaccurate translations. Police must determine whether trained interpreters would be more helpful. By considering such situational factors during initial meetings with victims, police are better able to address the needs of victims and obtain the most accurate information regarding sexual assaults.

If a suspect is apprehended, either immediately at the scene or within a short period of time after the assault, police on the scene will take victims to the apprehension location in order to identify assailants. Because officers must ask victims to view suspects, it is important to be mindful of victims' vulnerabilities. Officers on the scene should inform the victim in advance what steps will take place, the sequence of these steps, and what the victim's role will be in the process. By doing this, police not only assist victims through the process, but they also ensure valid identification of perpetrators.

Several important factors that may impact officers' ability to fulfill these roles should be taken into consideration during the initial interview with a sexual assault victim. First, the psychologic and physical status of victims may hinder officers' ability to gather detailed and accurate information. Although basic "flash" information must be gathered immediately, assigned investigators may be able to obtain a more detailed description of assaults after victims have an opportunity to recover from the initial crisis. A particularly sensitive approach in these cases may also help victims regain their sense of physical safety rather than making them feel overwhelmed with many questions when they already feel vulnerable.

Victims of sexual assault may request to speak with a same-gender officer. Research shows the importance of having female officers present during initial contacts in cases involving female victims (Temkin, 1997). However, male and female officers, if properly trained, may be equally effective in their response.

When emergency medical services (EMS) personnel are the first responders to a sexual assault scene, the interaction between police and EMS personnel is critical in relaying important information quickly and accurately. Police officers should

Key Point:
A sensitive approach that allows the victim to guide the interview may help victims regain their sense of physical safety and control.

Key Point:
First responders should provide up-to-date, appropriate resource information to victims, because victims may decide not to seek further interventions.

interview EMS personnel to obtain information that they have gathered from the victim. All of this information should be included in the final police reports. Accuracy is important in that it will eventually affect the criminal prosecution. Police officers must understand the role of EMS personnel in the medical care of victims and be alert to the need for immediate transport for definitive medical care.

The first police responder on the scene must take copious notes about the scene, the condition of the victim, and any statements given by the victim. For example, if the victim has torn clothing, is bleeding, bruised, or has any other physical injuries from the attack, the officer must document all this information on the initial investigative report. It is also imperative that all irregularities at the scene be detailed. For instance, the phone cord may have been pulled from the wall, furniture may have been overturned, or other signs of a struggle may be present. Detailed information at the initial scene may strengthen the case for the prosecution phase.

Not all victims will want the services of the police, nor will all victims want to follow through on the prosecution of the case. It is therefore important that police and EMS personnel have written resources and referral information to give to victims who decide they do not want the police to intervene. This material may be the only source of intervention and may benefit victims long after the initial crisis has passed. Included should be a basic description of the legal and medical issues and procedures following a sexual assault, such as medical examinations, police interviews, police investigations, and interactions with the justice system. Other basic resource and referral information that may benefit sexual assault victims includes the location and description of sexual assault and rape crisis agencies and programs that provide services for the prevention and treatment of sexually transmitted diseases, HIV infection, and pregnancy.

Because many victims find it difficult to reach out for support, and even the smallest barrier may appear to a sexual assault victim to be an insurmountable obstacle, it is imperative that first responders disseminate simple, up-to-date, accurate, and accessible information. Accordingly, first responder groups need an ongoing systematic means for updating and disseminating resource and referral information to their personnel. Written information also must be easy to read, multilingual, socioculturally sensitive, and on a reading level accessible to most individuals. First response personnel may need to read the information to the survivor.

MEDICAL EXAMINATIONS

After initial meetings, the next step is often to prepare and transport victims to medical examinations. These evaluations may take place in designated hospital emergency centers with personnel trained for such cases and thus may require transport to a facility not near the homes of victims or the location of assaults.

Victims benefit from a brief explanation of the medical examination process. The medical examination is performed both to identify and treat victims' injuries and to retrieve forensic evidence (e.g., semen or hair samples). Victims should bring a change of clothing and shoes to the hospital, because their clothing will be kept for forensic purposes. Such evidence may subsequently be used in court and possibly for DNA testing. Victims should also be informed that personnel such as physicians, nurses, rape crisis volunteers, counselors, or social workers might be present during the examination or emergency department evaluation. It is important to let victims know that they may be asked intimate questions by medical staff, investigators, and ultimately officers of the court.

In most instances, unless victims are medically impaired, police rather than EMS transport victims to hospitals. Although initial transport may necessitate using marked police vehicles, subsequent transports, such as driving victims home or to police facilities, should involve unmarked police vehicles. In some jurisdictions, police and advocate groups work very closely in their initial responses to sexual assaults. In these instances, advocates may perform transports from hospitals to victims' homes or police facilities.

INVESTIGATIVE INTERVIEWS

Investigating officers conduct a detailed interview with the victim after the medical evaluation and treatment. The interview can take place immediately after the evaluation or at a later time. Victims may choose to postpone giving their statements so that they have some time to rest. However, some researchers believe that victims may be more at ease discussing the details of assaults within the first 24 hours after the assault and that since victims tend to lose memory of the details of the event as time passes, interviewers should take statements as soon as possible if victims are willing (MacDonald, 1995).

Interview techniques are of particular importance when taking statements from sexual assault victims. Allowing the victims to give their statements at their own pace and without interruption before asking additional clarification questions assists victims in maintaining a sense of control at a time when they feel as if very little is in their control.

Interview locations are also important for the well-being of victims. If victims are interviewed at police stations, it is preferable to use statement rooms that are comfortable and out of the bustle of main squad rooms. In some circumstances, it may be wise to give victims a choice regarding location of the interview. Some victims may feel more comfortable in their own or a friend's residence than in a police station. If interviews must be taken at medical facilities, interviewers may find it helpful to use private spaces or private patient rooms instead of sterile examination rooms.

Along with being aware of the needs and reactions of survivors, interviewers must be equally aware of the importance of gathering accurate and useful information about assaults. Overt accusations, or even subtle insinuations, regarding victims' veracity are unacceptable and are likely to dissuade victims from continuing interviews openly. Discrepancies in the victims' statements do not automatically mean that victims are not telling the truth. Some victims may omit certain information regarding how they met their assailant (e.g., at a bar) for fear of victim blaming and embarrassment.

Key Point:
Interviewers must be flexible, open, and aware of the victim's needs, as well as avoid subtle insinuations about the victim's veracity.

MacDonald (1995) recommends that police who interview victims of rape systematically apply routine interviewing procedures combined with a flexibility and openness toward the person to avoid preconceived explanations and foregone conclusions. Basic interviewing techniques are applicable even though such interviews are stressful for both victims and interviewing officers. For example, open-ended questions and closed-ended questions serve different but necessary purposes during interviews. Closed-ended questions assist in gathering specific information (i.e., when and where). Open-ended questions may be used to expand victims' responses (i.e., how did that occur?). Other fundamental interviewing skills include active listening and attending skills.

Despite the best attempts at being thorough, supportive, and attentive to victims' needs, some victims choose not to prosecute their assailants. Nevertheless, police should still follow normal procedures, including obtaining as much information about perpetrators as possible, such as modus operandi (MO) and other salient points. This information may help to solve other open sexual assault cases and may possibly prevent further sexual assaults.

CRIMINAL PROSECUTION

First responders operate on two levels. First, as already discussed, they provide critically important care and services to sexual assault victims. Second, they conduct investigations that may be the basis for criminal prosecutions and, consequently, may be scrutinized in the courts.

Every element of each first response may become part of the "discovery," or the evidence used to prosecute criminal cases. Because defendants are entitled to such information, defense attorneys may be entitled to review all statements, including "flash" information, given by victims to police and dispatchers; 911 radio tapes, which may have victims or friends providing descriptive information regarding attacks and perpetrators; first responders' initial reports; investigators' interviews and final investigative reports; and forensic evidence gathered at the scene and by examining medical personnel at the hospital. Trial preparation begins the moment first responders receive a victim's call for help.

Accordingly, first responders in the law enforcement community should apply the same criminal investigative guidelines to investigations of both known and stranger perpetrators. Any deviation from standard investigative techniques in the cases of spousal sexual assault may be exploited by a defense attorney and used to undermine the prosecution's case against the alleged perpetrator. It is also important to adhere to guidelines in such investigations because the perpetrator of a spousal sexual assault may be involved in other sexual assaults. MacDonald (1995) believes that "even if the victim knows the man who raped her, knowledge of his MO (modus operandi/method of operation) may help solve other rapes that he may have committed" (MacDonald, 1995, page 140).

Key Point:
The same criminal investigative procedures must be used whether or not the perpetrator is known to the victim, even in cases of spousal assault.

VICTIM REACTIONS

The role of the first responders in sexual assault cases is multidimensional. To provide needed care and services to victims and to perform a thorough investigation on which a criminal prosecution may be successfully based, first responders require a significant level of insight into the emotional state of victims.

Police education and training are necessary regarding the multifaceted aspects of victims' reactions to sexual assaults. It is insufficient to believe, as was once thought, that there are one or two correct theories and linear progressions regarding victims' responses to sexual assaults. Such preconceptions lead to stereotyping of "correct" reactions and often cause police to form negative impressions of victims who do not exhibit such "correct" reactions. Resick (1993) believes that the three major theories of rape reaction—Crisis Theory, Behavioral Theory, and Attribution Theory of Coping—each offer their own versions of victims' reactions. Yet one-dimensional perspectives do not address the complex and multifaceted range of reactions experienced by sexual assault victims. Such perspectives may offer police a general understanding of victims' reactions but limit a complete understanding of all possible reactions. Instead of looking for specific behavioral reactions after an assault, it is more useful to look for general overarching themes in the victim to better understand a victim's reaction to an assault.

Reactions differ from person to person in the degree, length, and sequence of emotional, behavioral, and analytical responses. Varying reactions may also affect the length of time taken by victims to contact police. Minutes, hours, days, months, and years may pass before victims are able or willing to approach police. Length of time is not an indicator of severity or "realness"; rather it reflects different reactions of the survivor to the incident.

Other factors add to the diverse range of reactions, such as victims' situational and psychologic circumstances before, during, and after the assault. Examples of situational differences include whether perpetrators were strangers, acquaintances, spouses, family members, same gender or opposite gender, or whether multiple perpetrators were involved. Differences in the circumstances of assaults may also involve the extent, if any, of physical injury and the level of violence experienced by victims.

Psychologic reactions can vary dramatically from person to person, ranging from appearing calm and controlled to intense expressions of emotions. Rape trauma syndrome (Burgess & Holmstrom, 1974) is often used in teaching personnel about victims' general reactions to sexual assault. Officers arriving at the scene of a recent assault are likely to experience victims in the acute phase of rape trauma syndrome, a period marked by disorganization and a broad range of emotions. The continuum of initial reactions can vary from victims' strongly expressive reactions, such as tenseness, crying, restlessness, and even smiling, to a more controlled style of expressing emotions in such forms as subdued affect, calmness, and composure (Burgess & Holmstrom, 1974). Emotional reactions are often related to the fear, anxiety, humiliation, self-blame, shame, and anger experienced by victims.

Physical outcomes related to attacks may include bruising, contusions, breaks, and bleeding. Genital disturbances may involve discharge, bleeding, cuts, and pain. Immediate behavioral reactions may involve disturbances in the ability to concentrate, form cohesive sentences, and focus on questions and statements.

Weeks and months following the trauma mark the beginning of the long-term reorganization process. Survivors may experience feelings of depression, restlessness, and exhaustion similar to symptoms of posttraumatic stress disorder (PTSD) (Kirkpatrick et al., 1992). Symptoms can include nightmares, flashbacks, disturbed eating and sleeping patterns, sexual dysfunction, and difficulty in social adjustments. Over time, the process of reorganizing victims' understanding of the world before and after trauma may occur and potentially lead to some degree of resolution and integration of the event into their life.

Ongoing Contact and Victim Support

It is important that first responders maintain ongoing contact with victims in order to keep victims informed and updated throughout the legal process. It is imperative that assigned investigators remain in contact with victims to ensure a successful conclusion for victims, which may not necessarily mean a conviction. A successful conclusion may be viewed as victims' ability to move on with their lives as they understand that their assault was indeed significant, and that it was recognized as such by police.

Conclusion

All crimes against people are personal and important to the victim; they deserve the full attention of first responders. However, there is no crime as personal to the victim as a sexual assault. Because this is such a violation of a person's body and psyche, it requires a higher level of sensitivity and diligence from first responders. All first responders, such as police and EMS, must also remember they are the gateway to the criminal justice system. As such, they must remember that during the criminal proceeding judges, prosecutors, defense attorneys, and juries may scrutinize all of their initial and long-term actions. In addition, they must be extremely aware that their approach will affect, either positively or negatively, the victim for the rest of the victim's life. Through effective and ongoing training, sensitivity, and professionalism, first responders can successfully fulfill all of their responsibilities to the survivor and to the criminal justice system.

References

Avner JI (Chairperson). *New York State Governor's Task Force on Rape and Sexual Assault Rape, Sexual Assault, and Child Sexual Abuse: Working Towards a More Responsive Society.* Albany, NY: New York State Division for Women; 1990.

Burgess A, Holmstrom L. Rape trauma syndrome. *Am J Psychiatry.* 1974; 131:981-986.

Kirkpatrick DG, Edmunds CN, Seymour AK. *Rape in America: A Report to the Nation.* Arlington, Va: National Victim Center; 1992.

MacDonald JM. *Police Response to Rape.* Springfield, Ill: Charles A. Thomas; 1995: 140.

Resick PA. The psychological impact of rape. *J Interpers Violence.* 1993;8:223-255.

Temkin J. Plus ça change: reporting rape in the 1990's. *Br J Criminology.* 1997;37:507-528.

Chapter 31

LEGAL ISSUES IN SEXUAL ASSAULT FROM A PROSECUTOR'S PERSPECTIVE

Mimi Rose, JD

The criminal justice system is an offender-based system that determines if a crime was committed, by whom, and, if the accused is found guilty, what sanction should be imposed. Theoretically the victim, any eyewitnesses, scientific or medical evidence, expert opinion, photographs, and physical evidence prove that a crime occurred and identify the perpetrator (Parrish, 1996). The proof must be substantial. The familiar quantity of belief—beyond a reasonable doubt—must be met (Goldner et al., 1995). In a criminal case, the government (representing the community) determines if a person will be prosecuted and what crimes are alleged to have been committed. What constitutes a crime is defined by statute, and the statutes are interpreted by judicial opinions. For example, in criminal codes there are words and phrases such as "force," "consent," "prompt complaint," and "excited utterance" (Myers, 1998a). In a criminal case, if a person is convicted, the sanction is primarily deprivation of individual liberty by probation, incarceration, or both, depending on several case-specific factors (Goldner et al., 1995).

In contrast, a civil lawsuit is initiated by one party (or person) filing a complaint against another party. In a civil lawsuit, the party found in the wrong (liable) is primarily required to pay money damages as restoration to the wronged party or is prohibited (enjoined) from or required to perform certain conduct. A civil case is initiated by a person filing legal documents claiming to have been injured in some way by another.

Personal injury can be both a crime and a civil matter. Thus, the victim of a sexual assault may be involved in both the criminal and the civil legal systems. In a criminal prosecution, the victim may be subpoenaed by the government to testify as a witness against the alleged perpetrator of criminal acts. The victim may also hire an attorney to bring a civil lawsuit for money damages if desired. In this chapter the criminal justice system is observed from a prosecutor's perspective, focusing on crimes of sexual assault and exploitation.

CRIMES OF SEXUAL ASSAULT

The criminal law is constantly changing to reflect shifting community values. Legislators are constantly revising, repealing, and creating new criminal statutes to be more reflective of contemporary thinking and values (Trost, 1998). The shifts in the criminal law regulating sexual conduct provide excellent examples.

Unlike standard medical practice, which is not geographically determined, the United States Constitution gives individual states the authority for each state to promulgate their own criminal laws and penalties. Although there is general uniformity about what constitutes criminal sexual acts from state to state, there are unique variations in each state's penal code (Myers, 1998a). Each state's laws must be consulted. For illustration purposes I will refer to the criminal laws of Pennsylvania.

Key Point:
Criminal laws and penalties are created by each state and reflect unique variations peculiar to that state. Therefore, it is necessary to study specific crimes, laws, and penalties for the state in which you are practicing.

Very generally, sexual offenses involve four types of conduct:

— Sexual intercourse

— "Deviate" sexual intercourse (oral or anal sex)

— Digital penetration or penetration of the genitals with an object

— Indecent contact, which involves touching of the genitals or other body parts for sexual gratification without penetration

If such conduct occurs under any of the following conditions, it is a crime:

1. The act occurs without the complainant's consent.

2. Force or threat of force is used. The force required to commit a sex offense is no longer limited to physical force. The law now recognizes that psychologic, moral or intellectual pressure of sufficient magnitude may be sufficient. Psychologic force has been legally upheld in many cases in which there is an unequal relationship, such as parent-child, teacher-pupil, clergy person–congregant, and doctor-patient.

3. The victim is unconscious or involuntarily intoxicated by drugs or alcohol, and this is known to the assailant.

4. The complainant suffers from a mental disability rendering her incapable of giving consent.

5. The complainant is less than age 13 years.

6. The complainant is less than age 16 years and the assailant is 4 or more years older.

The foregoing analysis can be stated simply as follows: Sexual contact is permissible between consenting adults. Sexual contact becomes a crime either when there is no consent or when one participant is not an adult. Both actual consent and legal capacity to consent to sexual contact is required for it to be lawful.

Key Point:
Sexual contact is permitted between consenting adults. It becomes criminal when there is no consent or one of the participants is not an adult. For sexual contact to be lawful, both actual consent and legal capacity to consent are required.

STATUTE OF LIMITATIONS

All crimes (except murder) have a statute of limitations that puts a limit on how much time a person has to report a crime to the police for purposes of arrest and prosecution (Goldner et al., 1995). The time limits vary for different crimes and from state to state. The statute of limitations may also differ depending on whether the crime is a felony or a misdemeanor. Generally, felonies are more serious offenses, and carry a longer possible sentence than misdemeanors. In Pennsylvania, for example, the statute of limitations for a sex crime committed against an adult is 5 years if it is classified as a felony and 2 years if it is a misdemeanor. If the victim is under age 18 years at the time of the offense, she must make a police report within 5 years beyond her 18th birthday if the crime is a felony. If the assault is a misdemeanor, she has 2 years after her 18th birthday to notify the authorities.

The different time requirements for children that allow a minor to reach adulthood before disclosing abuse to authorities is a recent change in the law. Historically, children had the same statute of limitations as adults, leading to the unrealistic and unfair result that a child molested at age 5 years would be forever precluded from holding the perpetrator criminally accountable unless she filed a police report before her 10th birthday. Changes in the law reflect our evolving understanding of sexual violence and abuse, and the needs and vulnerabilities of children (Palusci et al., 1999).

THE CRIMINAL JUSTICE PROCESS

Sexual assault may be reported to the police in several ways. If the victim is an adult, she may call 911, or if she seeks medical attention, hospital protocol may require law enforcement notification. If the victim is a child, sexual assaults frequently come to police attention through reports received by the county child welfare agency. In many counties, police investigators specialize in sex crimes and child abuse investigations (Pence & Wilson, 1992, 1994). In large urban jurisdictions, there are commonly specialized police units with several officers exclusively assigned to these sensitive complex cases (Lanning & Walsh, 1996).

Although law enforcement protocols vary from county to county, police usually take the victim for a medical examination for health reasons and for possible forensic evidence collection (Ells, 1998). Investigators interview the victim and any eyewitnesses, go where the assault occurred, take photographs, and collect evidence from the crime scene (Spaulding & Bigbee, 2001). Evidence collection often requires a search warrant if the evidence is believed to be within the perpetrator's control. If the suspect is known to the police, he or she is informed of the investigation and given the opportunity to make a statement. As a general rule, subject to important exceptions, suspects in police custody cannot be questioned without being advised of their right to refuse to give a statement and their right to have a lawyer present during police questioning, and without being warned that any statement could be used against them. The recitation of these rights is commonly known as Miranda warnings (Leo, 2001), named for the landmark legal case Miranda vs. Arizona.

If the assailant is a stranger to the victim but he or she had the opportunity to observe the assailant during the assault, the victim may be shown a series of photographs or a line-up of several individuals similar to the description of the assailant and be asked to identify the perpetrator. If the victim is unable to identify her assailant, circumstantial evidence or DNA obtained from forensic examination of the victim may be sufficient to prosecute. At the conclusion of evidence gathering and after all statements are taken, the police submit their investigation to the district attorney (also known as the prosecutor or states attorney). The district attorney or an assistant district attorney determines if there is enough evidence to arrest the suspect and with what crimes the suspect is to be charged based on the evidence. Some jurisdictions convene a grand jury comprising community members who make the determination if there is sufficient evidence to bring the accused to trial. The standard used by police and prosecutors to decide whether or not a suspect should be arrested for a crime is the finding of "probable cause" (Bulkley et al., 1996). Probable cause is found where a law enforcement officer believes that a crime probably has been committed and that the suspect is probably the perpetrator. (The difference between a probable cause finding to arrest and the much higher standard of proof "beyond a reasonable doubt" required for a criminal conviction is why every arrest does not result in a conviction.)

PRELIMINARY ARRAIGNMENT

After arrest, the preliminary arraignment begins the judicial process. The defendant (the name for the suspect after arrest) is fingerprinted, photographed, and computer-checked to determine if he or she has ever been arrested for other crimes. Bail is set. The dollar amount of bail is based on the nature of the offense, the defendant's prior criminal history, any ties to the geographical area, and any prior willful failure to appear at court hearings. This amount or a percentage of this amount is required to be paid by the defendant for release from custody before a trial. Bail is collateral to compel the defendant to appear at court dates. If the defendant fails to appear, bail is forfeited. The higher the risk of flight from trial, the higher the bail imposed. Community safety and victim safety are also factored into determining bail amount. It is important to understand that the purpose of bail and pretrial detention is not to punish the offender. An arrested person in the United States is cloaked with the presumption of innocence until proven guilty (Goldner et al., 1995).

Key Point:
Police and prosecutors use the standard of "probable cause" as the basis for making an arrest for a crime; this means a law enforcement officer believes that a crime probably has been committed and the suspect is probably the perpetrator.

APPOINTMENT OF COUNSEL

At the preliminary arraignment, the defendant is entitled to a lawyer. Depending on income, a person must either hire an attorney or, if income-eligible, the public defender's office is appointed to represent the accused.

At the preliminary arraignment, a person is given formal notice of the charges and notice of the next court hearing. In addition to monetary bail, conditions such as prohibiting contact with the victim, abstention from drugs or alcohol, house confinement, or electronic monitoring of the defendant may be imposed as conditions of release.

THE PRELIMINARY HEARING

In many states the next court proceeding in a sexual assault case is the preliminary hearing, usually held within a few weeks after an arrest (Goldner et al., 1995). At the preliminary hearing, a judge reviews the charges and hears brief testimony, usually from the victim, to determine if the legal requirements of the crime are met so that the case may ultimately go to a trial. The preliminary hearing is one of many legal safeguards to ensure the accused's right to fairness. Basically, this proceeding requires judicial review of the police and the prosecution's decision to arrest a suspect on given charges. At this hearing, the credibility of the witness is not decided, nor is any corroborating evidence required. It is necessary only for the victim to give a brief account of essential facts to determine if there is legally sufficient evidence to have the case go to trial.

Key Point:
The sexual assault victim's first encounter with the judicial system is during the preliminary hearing. This is the victim's first time to speak of the assault before a judge, a defense attorney, and the defendant in a courtroom open to the public by law.

The preliminary hearing is the sexual assault victim's first encounter with the judicial system. It is the first time the victim is asked to speak of the assault before a judge, a defense attorney, and the defendant in a courtroom open to the public by law. This difficult experience can be empowering or retraumatizing depending on several factors, including the sensitivity of the judge, prosecutor, and court staff. In some jurisdictions, sexual assault preliminary hearings are held in a designated courtroom with prosecutors who are victim-sensitive and competently trained in both the law and the dynamics of sexual assault to handle these cases. In some jurisdictions, the victim is not even required to testify at the preliminary hearing. Instead, testimony by the investigating police officer as to what the victim told him or her is sufficient evidence. Often, when a victim must appear, advocates are present in the courtroom to offer support and social service referrals.

The time between the preliminary hearing and the trial varies; it could take weeks or even months. This is the time for building a strong case. After the preliminary hearing, the case is assigned to the prosecutor who will take the case to trial (Heiman et al., 2001). Although it is highly desirable to have the same trained prosecutor handle a case from the preliminary hearing through trial, in larger jurisdictions this option, known as vertical prosecution, is sometimes not possible. It often happens that a case is assigned to two successive prosecutors. In these situations, the victim advocate can provide needed victim support and continuity.

The prosecutor is the director of the case (Myers, 1998a). Police reports, witness interviews, hospital records, etc., which tell of the events leading up to the assault and its aftermath, are the script. The incident is recreated for the jury by testimony from the witnesses and the production of physical and/or scientific evidence. Meeting with witnesses, finding additional witnesses or evidence not initially uncovered by the police, researching the law, and thinking about trial strategy occupy both the defense attorney and prosecutor in anticipation of a trial.

When an alleged sexual assault is committed by an unknown assailant, lack of consent by the victim is presumed, and the central issue is the identity of the assailant. These "stranger" sexual assaults often receive media coverage but, in fact, only a small percentage of sexual assault prosecutions occur between strangers.

Much more often, the alleged perpetrator is known to the victim either as an acquaintance, family member, or intimate partner. In these latter cases, consent is frequently raised by the defense.

What constitutes legal consent (Schulhofer, 1998)? Can someone consent to sexual activity up until a point and then say no? What does the law require of the victim as a valid expression of nonconsent? Is a verbal utterance of "no" sufficient, or must a person physically resist to constitute a rape? Can a person with a developmental disability consent? Does intoxication negate consent? Can a child give legal consent to engage in sexual activity with an adult? The answers to these questions depend on the facts and circumstances of each case as set forth in criminal statutes and as interpreted by judicial opinion. As already stated, the law is constantly evolving to reflect changing community attitudes about sexuality and gender-based violence (Panichas, 2001).

CORROBORATION

The law does not require corroboration to arrest or convict a person of sexual assault. The testimony of the victim, if believed, is sufficient. At the close of a case, the judge will instruct the jury that they may convict on the victim's word alone.

Because sexual assault seldom occurs in the presence of witnesses and often leaves no physical injury, the victim's account may be the only testimonial evidence available. Physical evidence collection is critical (Hazelwood & Lanning, 2001). In a sexual assault, it is important to document and photograph bruising and injury, torn clothing, or a room in disarray after a struggle and to collect physical evidence such as bed sheets, towels, and clothing for forensic testing. Forensic examination of the victim to determine the presence of sexual fluids, hairs, or blood is usually indicated (Brown, 1997). When forensic evidence is recovered, DNA testing is conducted by obtaining blood samples from the accused. (See also Chapters 15 and 16.)

A sexual assault trial often occurs several months after the incident. It is often difficult for a complainant to convey the emotional state and demeanor during a traumatic assault in a courtroom environment. It is extremely helpful for medical personnel to accurately document observable emotional states of a sexual assault victim. Accurate, timely documentation of statements from a victim witness is also important. If the defense claims that the victim consented to sexual activity, documentation of observable signs or statements conveying the victim's emotional state is often powerful corroboration of nonconsent.

Medical personnel are often necessary witnesses at a sexual assault trial (Myers, 1998b). A physician, nurse, or social worker can be subpoenaed by either the prosecution or the defense to testify as a fact witness or as an expert witness. A fact witness is a person who has seen or heard something that either the prosecution or the defense believes supports their theory of the case (Myers, 1998b). At trial, a fact witness is asked to testify about his or her observations (Myers, 1998b). Because the accuracy of memory can diminish over time, it is important that these observations be documented close in time to their occurrence. If required to testify, the health-care provider usually is allowed to bring any records to court and refer to those records during testimony.

THE EXPERT WITNESS

Generally, witnesses are not permitted to give opinions or impressions about what they have observed. As Sergeant Joe Friday, a popular TV detective from the 1950s would say, "The facts, ma'am, just the facts." It is the jury's function to draw opinions and conclusions about the credibility and weight of the evidence. However, there is an important exception to this general rule. If the subject matter is ruled by the judge to be beyond what a jury member would be expected to understand, and if it is determined to be generally accepted in the scientific, medical, or other professional community from which the witness belongs that the witness has the requisite education and experience concerning the subject matter at issue, then that witness may be qualified as an expert in a given field and permitted to give an opinion about the evidence (Myers, 1998b). In a sexual assault case, expert testimony is often given by physicians or sexual assault nurse examiners concerning the significance of physical findings or lack of physical findings from a forensic examination performed on an alleged sexual assault victim. For example, qualified medical personnel are frequently asked their opinion about whether the physical findings are consistent with the history given by the victim. Whereas the presence of trauma or sexually transmitted disease is obviously significant, it is often crucial that the expert explain why lack of injury could also be compatible with the alleged victim's history of assault. This lack of trauma testimony is often used by procedures when there is a delay in reporting a sexual assault—a common occurrence in child sexual abuse. In other cases, lack of trauma can be explained by the nature of the sexual assault. For example, in Pennsylvania the legal requirement for the crime of rape is penetration, however slight. It often is a necessary hardship for medical professionals to interrupt their work to come to court. Many times a physician's or nurse's ability to educate a jury makes all the difference between a just or unjust verdict.

THE TRIAL

A criminal trial places the burden on the state (or the commonwealth—the term used in a few states) to prove the legal elements of a crime beyond a reasonable doubt (Bulkley et al., 1996). There is no burden on the accused to prove anything whatsoever. The accused need not testify or offer any witnesses, although he may elect to offer defense witnesses. From the time of the arrest, the accused is cloaked with a presumption of innocence that is removed only if there is a conviction. The role of the defense is to attack the state's evidence. This may be accomplished by the defense attorney offering evidence, defense witnesses, or the defendant's testimony. Other than witnesses who are called by the defense to cast a doubt on the state's case, the state's evidence is put to the test through cross-examination.

SEXUAL ASSAULT OF MALES

Sexual assault of males presents unique issues in the investigation and prosecution of these crimes. Perpetrators of sex crimes on males can be male or female. Male-male sexual assaults often occur in the context of prison rape or in a homosexual dating relationship. Although these crimes may be quite violent, they can be difficult to prosecute because of the reluctance of males to report sexual victimization.

Adult males who have sexual contact with boys under the statutory age are prosecuted under the same laws that regulate heterosexual sexual conduct with minors. These boys typically are seduced into an emotional relationship with the perpetrator and groomed into a sexual relationship. Unlike father-daughter incest relationships, boy victims are often fatherless. Craving adult male attention, they look to have their emotional needs met outside the family in scholastic, athletic, religious, or other extracurricular activities, supervised by potential male mentors. Although relationships can be enormously beneficial to a developing child, when sexualized, the result can be emotionally devastating (Finkelhor & Browne, 1985). It is particularly difficult for a boy to disclose sexual molestation by an adult male (Holmes & Slap, 1998). Along with the pain and emotional turmoil of feeling betrayed by an important person in the boy's life, there may be great confusion and anxiety about sexual identity issues. Boys may initially minimize their participation in sexual activity. In these cases, exaggerated claims of force by the perpetrator can conceal a child's great anxiety about their sexuality. Consequently, boys disclose far more infrequently than girls. Interestingly, when a boy does disclose and testifies in a criminal trial, the conviction rate as compared to girls is much higher. Societal

Key Point:
Those who perpetrate sex crimes on males can be male or female. Male-male sexual assaults often occur in the context of prison rape or in a homosexual dating relationship. Although these crimes may be violent, they can be difficult to prosecute because males are reluctant to report sexual victimization.

attitudes that sexualize females from an early age but not males probably contribute to juries having less trouble believing allegations made by a young boy.

These attitudes also influence societal responses to boys who are sexually seduced by adult women. Films like "Summer of 42" and "Tea and Sympathy" romanticize a young boy's initiation into sexual manhood in the arms of an older woman. Mentally switching the gender of the perpetrator and the child helps to uncover unconscious gender bias in value judgments about these situations. Regardless of gender, molestation can have detrimental consequences for a developing child.

DOMESTIC VIOLENCE AND SEXUAL ASSAULT

Adult sexual assault is an act or series of acts that involve nonconsensual sexual contact. Domestic violence is broadly defined as the threat to inflict injury or the infliction of injury to a current or former intimate partner (American Academy of Pediatrics, 1999a). Domestic violence is often the relational context in which sexual assault occurs. Although law enforcement, prosecution, and victim services have become much more knowledgeable about sexual victimization and the dynamics of domestic violence, the interrelationship between the two must also be considered. For example, throughout the country there are specialized police units, typically one for domestic violence and one for sexual assault; prosecution departments, usually one for domestic violence and one for sexual assault; and specialized courtrooms to hear these sensitive cases, again one courtroom dedicated to domestic violence and one exclusively for hearing sexual assault cases (OVC Monograph NCJ, 1999). One can see the potential blind spots resulting from over-specialization. Many sexual assault victims are reluctant to participate in the prosecution of their perpetrator because of a history of domestic violence. Not surprisingly, when counties begin to integrate domestic violence and sexual assault interventions and services, the victims feel more understood, supported, and safe. In turn, they are more likely to participate in holding the offender accountable and ending the violence. (See also Chapter 14.)

The prosecution of sexual assault in the context of an intimate relationship is a relatively recent event (Futter & Mebane, 2001). Historically, one essential element of the crime of rape was that the perpetrator and the victim were not married. For hundreds of years, it was not a crime to rape one's spouse. Within the last 20 years, the laws have changed. In Pennsylvania, for example, the first legal change allowed for spousal rape prosecution if the victim spouse reported the assault within 90 days (compared to a 5-year reporting period for nonmarital sexual assault). Further, whereas nonmarital rape was classified as a felony of the first degree, spousal rape was designated a lesser crime: a second-degree felony. Within the last decade, many states have abolished the legal distinction between spousal and nonspousal sexual assault. However, these cases remain some of the most difficult to prosecute. Victims are often quite reluctant to disclose sexual violence by someone with whom they have had a previously consensual sexual relationship. Juries also seem to have difficulty understanding sexual violence in the context of an intimate relationship (Futter & Mebane, 2001). As law enforcement, legal and medical providers, and the community at large gain a better understanding of the interrelationship between different forms of violence and abuse, we will better see both the forest and the trees.

Key Point:

Many states have now abolished the legal distinction between spousal and nonspousal sexual assault, but these cases remain among the most difficult to prosecute.

JURY SELECTION

Sexual assault trials may be decided by a jury or a judge. In some states, only the defense may choose between having a case heard before a judge or jury. In other states, the prosecution may demand a jury trial even if the defense wants to waive the right to a trial by jury and have a judge determine the verdict. Theoretically, the jury selection process is designed to create a forum of 12 persons who can listen to a case in a fair, impartial, and unbiased manner. These 12 persons must also agree to apply the judge's instructions about the law to the evidence as it is presented. In all cases, it is critical for both sides to exclude persons with a fixed prejudice or bias against the victim or the alleged offender. Because sexual attitudes, including gender, sexual orientation, and morality, are usually deeply ingrained opinions determined by personal experience, education, and social class, jury selection becomes critically important. The outcome of a sexual assault trial could be decided on jury selection alone, regardless of the evidence.

ADMISSIBILITY OF EVIDENCE

For evidence to be admissible in a criminal trial it must be relevant, reliable, and material to the issues. The probative value must outweigh the prejudicial impact of the evidence. In sexual assault cases, the admissibility of evidence of a victim's prior or current sexual activity conduct with someone other than the accused is frequently a contested issue. Until a few decades ago, no laws protected sexual assault victims from defense character assassinations, which suggested to the jury that the victim was sexually active, promiscuous, or even a prostitute, and therefore immoral. These character attacks were frequently used to suggest that the victim consented to sexual activity with the defendant (Schulhofer, 1998). Through the efforts of sexual assault victim advocates, legislatures passed rape shield laws to prevent the introduction of a victim's sexual life if it has no relevancy but to put the victim on trial. In a sexual assault case, the accused may have prior criminal convictions for sexual assault or other crimes of interpersonal violence, which the prosecution would like known to the jury. This evidence of other crimes is admissible only in narrowly drawn exceptions to the general rule that other crimes evidence is inadmissible. Similar to the reasons precluding parading a victim's sex life, the purpose of this rule is to require the jury to decide if the defendant committed the crime based on proof, not prejudice created by prior criminal convictions. It should be emphasized, however, that prior convictions for crimes that support the defendant's commission of the crime on trial may be admissible if there is a common pattern that serves to prove intent or identity.

DEFENSES

The most common defenses in adult sexual assault cases are consent if the parties know each other and if there is corroboration of sexual contact, misidentification if the assailant is a stranger, and fabrication if there is no corroboration of sexual contact.

In sexual assault cases involving very young child victims, the most common defenses are claims of the suggestibility of the child to adult questioning. These defenses include claims of false allegations in the context of a custody dispute, nonsexual touch that is misinterpreted by the child (typically in the context of bathing or toileting), or allegations that the child is fantasizing that he or she experienced sexual contact after exposure to adult sexual activity from videotapes or parental observation. One of the most difficult problems with sexual assault cases involving preschool age children is their developmental immaturity with regard to providing testimony. Although there have been many advances in the law to facilitate the testimony of young children, these cases present difficult challenges.

In latency-age children and adolescents, common defenses to allegations of sexual abuse include the child's retaliation for strict parenting and discipline. If the alleged offender is a stepparent or the companion of a parent, the theory that the child falsely disclosed abuse to get the defendant out of the house is quite often the defense. Consent is rarely raised with young victims, because it is generally not a legal defense to child sexual abuse.

It is vitally important to our criminal justice system that law enforcement officers and prosecutors investigate sexual assault cases with great sensitivity and skill before arrest or trial. A prosecutor's job is not to seek convictions but to obtain justice. Although these goals are often the same, each case must be carefully evaluated.

Key Point:
For evidence to be considered admissible in a criminal trial, it must be relevant, reliable, and material to the issues at hand. The probative value must outweigh the prejudicial impact of the evidence.

Key Point:
In our criminal justice system, the law enforcement officers and prosecutors must investigate sexual assault cases with great sensitivity and skill before arrest or trial. The prosecutor's job is not to seek convictions, but to obtain justice.

At the conclusion of the trial, the fact finder (either judge or jury) reviews the evidence and arrives at a verdict (Bulkley et al., 1996; Goldner et al., 1995). There is usually more than one criminal charge for the fact finder to consider. The defendant may be acquitted or convicted of all charges, or convicted of some and acquitted of others. If a jury cannot reach a unanimous verdict after a long period of deliberations, the jury is declared deadlocked, and a mistrial (often referred to as a hung jury) is declared by the judge. A mistrial necessitates the case being tried again before another fact finder.

If a defendant is convicted of a sex crime, the penalty is determined by state law. Most states have sentencing guidelines that give a suggested sentence for the crime in mitigated, standard, and aggravated ranges. The mitigating or aggravating factors are decided by the sentencing judge. Although a judge may deviate from the guideline recommendations, the reasons must be substantial. By the implementation of sentencing guidelines, more judicial uniformity in sentencing is achieved. In some states, certain sex crimes, particularly when committed by an adult against a child, carry mandatory lengthy prison sentences. While treatment for sex offenders is available in prison facilities and outpatient clinics, the outcome of any treatment depends on many factors. All would agree that compulsive sexual behavior carries a great risk of recidivism.

CONCLUSION

Sexual assault raises many challenges for the criminal and civil legal systems in terms of proving allegations and deciding evidence within the framework of societal values and prejudices. Changes in the law reflect changing community attitudes about sexuality and gender-based violence, and improved technology to evaluate evidence. Medical providers are often called upon to serve as fact witnesses or to provide expert testimony in sexual assault cases. Careful documentation and evidence collection is therefore crucial.

REFERENCES

American Academy of Pediatrics. Committee on Child Abuse and Neglect. Guidelines for the evaluation of sexual abuse of children: Subject review. *Pediatrics.* 1999a;103:186-191.

Breaking the Cycle of Violence: Recommendations to Improve the Criminal Justice Response to Child Victims and Witnesses. OVC Monograph NCJ #176983, June 1999.

Brown ML. Dilemmas facing nurses who care for MSBP patients. *Pediatr Nurs.* 1997;23:416-418.

Bulkley JA, Feller JN, Stern P, Roe R. Child abuse and neglect laws and legal proceedings. In: Briere J, Berliner L, Bulkley JA, Jenny C, Reid T, eds. *The APSAC Handbook on Child Maltreatment.* Thousand Oaks, Calif: Sage Publications; 1996:271-296.

Ells M. Forming a multidisciplinary team to investigate child abuse. *Portable Guide to Investigating Child Abuse.* Washington, DC: US Department of Justice. 1998.

Finkelhor D, Browne A. The traumatic impact of child sexual abuse: A conceptualization. *Am J Orthopsychiatry.* 1985;55:530-541.

Futter S, Mebane WR, Jr. The effects of rape law reform on rape case processing. *Berkeley Women's Law J.* 2001.

Goldner JA, Dolgin CK, Manske SH. Legal issues. In: Monteleone J, ed. *Recognition of Child Abuse for the Mandated Reporter.* St. Louis, Mo: G.W. Medical Publishing; 1995:171-210.

Hazelwood RR, Lanning KV. Collateral materials in sexual crimes. In: Hazelwood RR, Burgess AW, eds. *Practical Aspects of Rape Investigation: A Multidisciplinary Approach.* 3rd ed. Boca Raton, Fla: CRC Press; 2001:221-232.

Heiman W, Ponterio A, Fairman G. Prosecuting rape cases: Trial preparation and trial tactic issues. In: Hazelwood RR, Burgess AW, eds. *Practical Aspects of Rape Investigation: A Multidisciplinary Approach.* 3rd ed. Boca Raton, Fla: CRC Press; 2001:347-364.

Holmes WC, Slap GB. Sexual abuse of boys: Definition, prevalence, correlates, sequelae, and management. *JAMA.* 1998;280:1855-1862.

Lanning KV, Walsh B. Criminal investigation of suspected child abuse. In: Briere J, Berliner L, Bulkley JA, Jenny C, Reid T, eds. *The APSAC Handbook on Child Maltreatment.* Thousand Oaks, Calif: Sage Publications; 1996:246-270.

Leo R. Interrogations and false confessions in rape cases. In: Hazelwood RR, Burgess AW, eds. *Practical Aspects of Rape Investigation: A Multidisciplinary Approach.* 3rd ed. Boca Raton, Fla: CRC Press; 2001:234-242.

Myers JEB. *Legal Issues in Child Abuse and Neglect Practice.* 2nd ed. Thousand Oaks, Calif: Sage Publications; 1998a.

Myers JEB. Expert testimony. In: JEB Myers ed. *Legal Issues in Child Abuse and Neglect Practice.* Thousand Oaks, Calif: Sage Publications; 1998b:221-281.

Palusci VJ, Cox EO, Cyrus TA, Heartwell SW, Vandervort FE, Pott ES. Medical assessment and legal outcome in child sexual abuse. *Arch Pediatr Adolesc Med.* 1999;153(4):388-392.

Panichas GE. Rape, autonomy, and consent. *Law & Society Review.* 2001;35(1).

Parrish R. Battered child syndrome: Investigating physical abuse and homicide. *Portable Guide to Investigating Child Abuse.* Washington, DC: US Department of Justice. 1996.

Pence D, Wilson C. *The role of law enforcement in the response to child abuse and neglect.* Washington, DC: US Department of Health and Human Services, National Center on Child Abuse and Neglect. 1992.

Pence D, Wilson C. *Team Investigation of Child Sexual Abuse: The Uneasy Alliance.* Thousand Oaks, Calif: Sage Publications; 1994.

Schulhofer SJ. *Unwanted Sex: The Culture of Intimidation and the Failure of Law.* Cambridge, Mass: Harvard University Press; 1998.

Spaulding RP, Bigbee PD. Physical evidence in sexual assault investigations. In: Hazelwood RR, Burgess AW, eds. *Practical Aspects of Rape Investigation: A Multidisciplinary Approach.* 3rd ed. Boca Raton, Fla: CRC Press; 2001:261-298.

Trost CT. Chilling child abuse reporting. Rethinking the CAPTA amendments. *Vanderbilt Law Rev.* 1998;51:189.

Hearing the Cry: Investigating and Prosecuting Adult Sexual Assault Cases

Tracy Bahm, JD
Duncan T. Brown, JD
Mary-Ann Burkhart, JD
Caren Harp, JD
Susan Bieber Kennedy, RN, JD
Lisa Kreeger, JD
Susan Kreston, JD

Millicent Shaw Phipps, JD
Laura L. Rogers, JD
Christina Shaw, JD
Cari Michele Steele, JD
Victor I. Vieth, JD
Dawn Doran Wilsey, JD

INTRODUCTION

Rape is an ugly word reflecting the heinous nature of the act itself. The emotional torture experienced by rape victims persists long after the pain and fear accompanying the attack are gone.

This emotional torture may be compounded when prosecutors choose not to file charges because proving the case is "too difficult." Although prosecutors are justified in devoting scarce resources to those cases with the best chance of success, the egregious harm sexual assault levies against its victims and society requires prosecutors to pause before dismissing these cases. In many cases, a difficult case can be proved with proper investigation and prosecution.

To this end, this chapter gives an overview of investigative strategies that should be employed in all cases. Several problematic legal issues that can often be dealt with in pretrial motions will be discussed. Finally, the chapter explores several types of problematic cases and presents trial strategies that may enable prosecutors to overcome the obstacles inherent in these cases.

INVESTIGATION OF SEXUAL ASSAULT CASES

CORROBORATING THE VICTIM'S STATEMENT

When a victim's statement stands alone, it is easier for the defense attorney to attack the allegation. To reduce the victim's stress, strengthen the government's case, and ensure justice, investigators and prosecutors must find and offer the jury evidence corroborating a victim's statements. The following rules will aid in the search for corroborating evidence.

Do not think too narrowly. In many cases, investigators fail to locate corroborating physical evidence because their definition of physical evidence is too narrow. Many investigators think of physical evidence only in terms of hair, fibers, blood, and semen. Because this type of physical evidence is not always present, an officer confined to this narrow definition will routinely come up empty-handed. Instead, an officer should think of physical evidence as any object or item that corroborates any aspect of the victim's report of abuse.

Search the victim's statement for clues. If the victim's statement is audio or video recorded, the statement should be transcribed. Working as a multidisciplinary team, investigators tear the statement apart sentence by sentence, word by word. After each line of the transcript, it should be considered whether there is anything in the sentence that can be corroborated. If the victim claims the defendant smelled of alcohol, is it possible to find a witness to document the defendant was drinking that evening? If the victim claims the defendant had a body odor, can that be corroborated? Perhaps the defendant had just had a workout and didn't have time to shower, or is simply someone who colleagues will acknowledge often has an unpleasant odor. If the victim describes a certain sexual sound the defendant made during the rape, a wife or previous girlfriend of the defendant should be located who can corroborate this claim.

Search for evidence that brings the crime to life. Clothing or other items should be seized to bring the crime home to the jury as a real event. Even in a fondling case that leaves no physical evidence on the clothing, the clothing may be relevant to show the small stature of the victim, the ease of reaching under the clothes or a myriad of other purposes. Grass stains, for example, may corroborate the victim's claim the assault took place outside. More importantly, the clothes will make the assault less abstract for the jury. When the jurors see and touch the clothes, it puts them at the scene of the crime and allows them to picture the victim's ordeal. This is why thousands of Americans flock to museums to be near Babe Ruth's bat, Judy Garland's ruby slippers, or remnants of the Titanic. Seeing the item connects us to an individual or an event in a powerful, personal way.

There is always a crime scene. The location of the victimization is a crime scene that must be inspected. Even if there is no reason to believe that blood, semen, or other evidence can be found at the site of the abuse, the crime scene must be photographed. The photographs will give the jury a picture of the victim's ordeal. If the assault took place in an abandoned farmhouse or rusty pickup, the pictures can rebut the defendant's claim of a consensual encounter. Is this the sort of scene where you would plan a romantic encounter, or is it the sort of scene where an assault without detection is the only goal? The photographs can also be used to aid the victim's testimony. For instance, the victim can use the photographs to point to locations in the house where various acts took place.

In addition to photographing the crime scene, it is necessary to determine the ease with which abuse could take place undetected. Is there a working lock on the victim's door? How far is the victim's room from other sleeping quarters in a house or hotel? How thick are the walls? Thick walls may explain a suspect's boldness in assaulting a victim while others are awake or nearby.

Use the suspect to corroborate the victim's statement. Even if the defendant is adamant in denying the assault, the suspect will often admit many of the important details surrounding the abuse. If the victim gave the police 100 pieces of information and you can show, through the defendant, that at least 90% of the information is accurate, this enhances the victim's credibility. Just as was done with the victim's statement, the interview with the suspect is transcribed and taken apart line by line. Claims made by the defendant are investigated to see if they are true. If the investigator finds wives and girlfriends who refute the defendant's claim of impotency, the prosecutor can now show the defendant to be a liar, and the jury may wonder what else the accused has lied about. Beyond this, a concerted effort is made to obtain an outright confession from the suspect.

INTERROGATION OF SUSPECT

If you ask most prosecutors who handle adult sexual assault cases to anticipate the most likely defense to be raised, they will tell you that the first tactic is the "not me" or SODDI (Some Other Dude Did It) defense. If there is DNA evidence or the belief that DNA evidence is available, the identity defense changes to the defense of consent. In other words, "Yes, I had sex with her, but she consented to it," which is not a crime. The case effectively becomes a he said–she said case, making it extremely difficult to successfully prosecute. Unfortunately, most people hold beliefs about rape that are myths. We think of a rape as something that happens when a man in a ski mask comes out of a dark alley with a weapon, drags a woman away, and rapes her. In reality, nonstrangers commit the vast majority of rapes. Weapons are seldom used. The violence used, if any, is usually just enough to facilitate the rape.

Generally, law enforcement officers know these tactics. They may feel that interrogation of the suspect is therefore not particularly valuable, because they believe that all that the suspect will say is that she consented. Officers do not think that an admission to having had sex is a "confession." Therefore, they rarely interrogate every suspect in a rape case. On the contrary, the initial interview or interrogation of a suspect can be crucial to the case. Getting the defendant locked into a particular story or version of events drastically improves the prosecutor's case. The more detail that the suspect gives, the better. If the suspect never gives a statement to police, he has the ability at trial to wait until after the state presents its case, and then to argue whatever defenses or versions of events best suit his case. If the defendant does not testify at trial, defense attorneys have even been known to argue, "It did not happen. But if it did, it was consensual." And juries have been known to acquit in those cases.

The tactics used in interrogation of suspected rapists can vary greatly. A seasoned law enforcement officer will understand the value of spending some time getting to know the suspect without showing any signs of having passed judgment on him. This enables the interviewer to evaluate what tactic is most likely to work with the particular suspect. According to Lisak & Ivan (1995) who have done extensive studies on rapists (both incarcerated and nonincarcerated), a common characteristic among rapists is that they lack empathy for their victims. Therefore, interviews that try to evoke sympathy or empathy for the victim will not work with rapists. Another common interrogation tactic that is not likely to work is the "good cop, bad cop" routine, where the suspect is supposed to be intimidated or frightened by the prospect of a long prison sentence. Many rapists do not view their behavior as inappropriate, let alone criminal behavior.

If the officer or detective is careful in his or her use of language and avoids calling the behavior "rape," there is some likelihood that the suspect will admit to the elements of the crime, not realizing that the elements constitute a rape. Making the suspect believe that you share his mindset about women (i.e., typical rape myths such as women provoke, want, and deserve rape) might lead him to confess to some, if not all, of the elements of the crime. This takes a great deal of patience on the part of a very well-trained police officer or detective. Another tactic that many officers find works well with sex offenders is the use of a ruse (telling them a valuable piece of evidence exists when indeed it does not).

A truly effective interrogation of a rape suspect will follow a thorough interview of the rape victim. This allows for the person conducting the interview of the suspect to challenge the suspect's version of events with facts known to the interviewer. For example, if the victim has scratch marks on her leg and early signs of bruising on her wrist, and the suspect claims the sex was consensual, he can be confronted with the facts and asked for an explanation of them. He might then resort to admitting the force used, even if he minimizes it. This should only be done, however, after the suspect has given his full version of events.

The bottom line on the issue of interviewing or interrogating rape suspects is that the interviewer must have a thorough understanding of the dynamics of rape. He or she must be disavowed of all rape myths and must be able to confront the suspect in

Key Point:
The bottom line in relation to interviewing or interrogating rape suspects is that the interviewer must have a thorough understanding of the dynamics of rape. He or she must be disavowed of all rape myths and must be able to confront the suspect in a nonconfrontational manner, allowing the suspect to share the most information possible.

a nonconfrontational manner to allow the suspect to share the most information possible. The interviewer needs to view the interview as potentially the most important piece of evidence at trial. He or she must be prepared to defend any and all tactics used and must be sure that the defendant's rights were protected at all times. However, he or she must also realize that no other person in the criminal justice system is situated to get the information from the suspect that they can get. It is crucial for the investigator to take as much time as necessary to do a thorough job.

When a prosecutor is preparing to try a rape case and knows that the defense is consent, he or she can arrange the case in a manner that helps to overcome the defense. The prosecutor will give the jury as much corroborating evidence as possible. The direct examination of the victim will be extremely thorough, using sensory perceptions to show the jury that she is not fabricating any part of the rape. All of this is greatly aided by a good interrogation of the rape suspect at the outset of the case.

RAPE KIT

Whether the victim of a sexual assault reports the incident to a crisis center, law enforcement officer, family, or friend, he or she is generally encouraged to seek medical attention and a rape examination. Books, magazine articles, and Internet sites also relay the need for physical assessment and testing of the rape survivor (Baumgarden, 2001; Schiro, 2002; Scarborough Hospital Sexual Assault Center, 2002).

It is important for the victim to get medical attention for several reasons. It is necessary to document and treat any physical injury. The victim may need testing and treatment for sexually transmitted diseases, AIDS, and hepatitis as well as pregnancy testing and follow-up. Finally, evidence may be collected from a victim's body and clothing. Forensic evidence from a victim's body should be collected within 72 hours of the assault, even if a victim is not interested in proceeding with a prosecution. After that period of time, evidence may be difficult to recover or may be unusable. A victim who is initially reluctant to involve police or hesitant to report the crime may change his or her mind, and evidence collection is vital. Some states mandate reporting of sexual offenses by medical or hospital personnel. For example, California Penal Code § 13823.11(a-g) states ". . . when conducting a physical examination of a sexual assault victim, law enforcement authorities shall be notified." In recent years, healthcare facilities have begun to recognize their responsibility to have trained staff available to provide specialized services for victims of sexual assault (Ledray, 2001).

In 1988, California was the first state to standardize their sexual assault protocol statewide. Although the use and contents of Sexual Assault Evidence Collection Protocols ("rape kits") are now common, variations exist state-to-state and even within a state. Rural and urban jurisdictions with different per capita incidents of sexual assaults will have variable experience with and exposure to the kits. Collection and processing of evidence is critical, while unfortunately, training is erratic. Training of personnel who handle and use the kits is essential, including how evidence is collected and how it is labeled, stored, and transferred from the collection site to the laboratory for examination and testing.

The kit is a box containing a detailed protocol and the medical equipment necessary to conduct a thorough forensic medical examination on a sexual assault victim. It may be used in the investigation of a rape involving a female or male, adult or child victim. The rape kit is used to collect trace evidence, such as hair, fibers or soil; suspect body fluids, such as semen, blood, saliva, and skin cells; and reference, or known, standards from the victim. It contains step-by-step instructions for collection of evidence. It should also instruct the health professional as to "chain of custody" issues, familiar to law enforcement and criminologists, but not a well-known concept in the medical arena. The evidence collection will include fingernail cuttings; head hair, pubic hair, saliva and blood samples; and oral, vaginal, and rectal swabs from the victim; pubic hair combings to detect foreign hair; dried secretion swabbings; photographs; and bite mark impressions.

The examination and evidence collection process may take 1 to 4 hours in a hospital emergency room, university health center, or clinic. What is crucial, from a victim's point of view, is that the physical examination and evidence collection are done simultaneously. Although the examination is intrusive and time consuming, as well as expensive, the survivor who voluntarily goes to or is taken to a hospital for a rape examination is subjected to the examination only once. Evidence collected is used by police in making an arrest and by prosecutors seeking a conviction of the alleged perpetrator.

In some jurisdictions, kits are distributed to facilities through programs funded by their state Legislature through Departments of Public Safety or Health. In Massachusetts, the District Attorney's Association (MDAA) was funded in 1999 through a S.T.O.P. Violence Against Women Act Grant to complete a study of the kits, making recommendations for improvements, which were incorporated into the next year's manufactured kits (Sexual Assault Evidence Kits, 2002). In some states, victims of sexual assault or their insurance must pay the hospital costs for processing the kit, which may be as high as $800.00. A Michigan Senator, Shirley Johnson, introduced a bill in fall 2001 to provide funding for the state Crime Victim Compensation Fund to cover the costs of rape kits (Hughes, 2001).

Federal programs and federal dollars must be considered in discussion of rape kits. Between fiscal years 1996 and 2000, federal funding was made available to state and local governments to carry out projects intended to develop or improve the capability to analyze DNA evidence through the Forensic DNA Laboratory Improvement Program (now known as the Crime Laboratory Improvement Program [CLIP]). For fiscal year 2001, approximately $253 million has been appropriated in the budget to include both CLIP and the Convicted Offender DNA Backlog Reduction Program (Tully et al., 2000). Currently, forensic laboratories across the country face a backlog of convicted offender DNA samples to analyze and enter into the federal database for DNA profiles. Because of shortages of laboratory personnel and equipment coupled with the increase in use of DNA evidence in criminal cases, laboratories have had to prioritize their analyses for the highest-profile cases, often leaving samples from cases without suspects unanalyzed. In the past, rape kits would be collected from victims, and in many cases, would not be tested unless a suspect was identified. DNA and other evidence potentially available to the prosecutor remained untested and of no use unless an offender was located. Only then could the forensic evidence from the victim be matched against a possible offender.

One of the prosecutor's greatest challenges regarding sexual assault evidence collection is ensuring that their jurisdiction has the requisite personnel, training, and supply of the kits.

DNA

Forensic science and criminal prosecutions have undergone a period of rapid change because of the evolution and use of DNA evidence. DNA has become part of our criminal justice vocabulary, and high-profile, live-TV criminal prosecution cases brought DNA to the public. Forensic DNA typing has become an integral part of the criminal justice system used by prosecutors to prove identity. Not since fingerprinting has a forensic technique so revolutionized the way crimes are prosecuted. In fact, DNA evidence is so influential that it has begun to overwhelm traditional forms of evidence such as eyewitness testimony. Even other forms of scientific evidence such as serology and trace evidence (hair and fibers) have found their conclusions challenged by the discriminating power of DNA testing. Forensic DNA testing evidence has also garnered much attention outside the courtroom.

Nearly every day, newspapers across the country contain articles relating a case solved with, a conviction obtained using, a prisoner exonerated by, or a new database containing DNA evidence. Juries have almost come to expect the prosecution to present evidence of a DNA match in certain cases, such as sexual assaults and homicides. Due to the convergence of these forces, an ever-increasing number of prosecutors are encountering DNA evidence in their typical casework because the prosecution must prove identification of the defendant in every case.

Although forensic DNA often receives the most public interest and legal scrutiny, DNA is used in many applications other than in forensics, such as paternity determinations; identification of remains in mass tragedies and war; determination of plant, animal, and microorganism origins; and in pharmaceutical, wildlife, and diagnostic laboratories. The use of DNA in other fields assists the prosecutor's use of such evidence by demonstrating acceptance of and reliance on DNA in scientific areas.

Key Point:
The biologic materials collected by police officers and analyzed by forensic laboratories most commonly are blood and seminal fluid. These materials are the most likely to be left at the scene of a murder or sexual assault and are also replete with genetic material.

The most common biologic materials that police officers collect and forensic laboratories test are blood and seminal fluid. Not only are these materials the most likely to be left at the scene of a murder or sexual assault, they are also replete with genetic material. With the development of polymerase chain reaction (PCR), which amplifies small pieces of DNA, and mitochondrial DNA (mtDNA) testing, which employs mitochondrial DNA rather than nuclear DNA, analysts are now able to yield profiles from other types of biologic samples. Forensic laboratories that use mtDNA testing are most likely to type bone, hair shafts (without a root), and teeth. This is because these parts of the body contain few cells, but plenty of mitochondria. DNA typing of saliva and sweat, which also contain few cells, is now possible only because of PCR-based typing technologies. Such advances as automated Short Tandem Repeat (STR) testing allow analysts to type smaller and smaller samples. In the future, cases involving DNA typing of samples of fecal material, vomit, urine, dandruff, and simple shed skin cells may also be used to develop admissible DNA evidence.

Defense attorneys faced with DNA evidence linking their clients to the crimes charged would often attack the validity of the evidence in an effort to prevent the jurors from ever seeing it. The appropriate time for such an attack is pretrial in an admissibility hearing. Jurisdictions in the United States generally follow 1 of 2 standards for determining the admissibility of new or novel scientific evidence. Generally, states that have adopted evidentiary rules similar to the Federal Rules of Evidence require that the proponents of new or novel scientific evidence prove by a preponderance of the evidence that the evidence is relevant and that the scientific procedures employed are reliable. In *Daubert v Merrell Dow Pharmaceutical, Inc.,* (1993), the Supreme Court provided a nonexclusive and nonexhaustive list of factors that judges should consider when determining reliability. These factors are (1) the testability of the theory or technique; (2) publication and peer review; (3) the known or potential error rate; (4) the existence of standards or protocols; and (5) general acceptance. All other states follow the standards announced in *Frye v United States* (1923) that, while similar, put greater emphasis on the scientific community's acceptance of the methodology. Prosecutors seeking to present DNA evidence in these jurisdictions must show that the procedures underlying the DNA evidence are generally accepted among members of the relevant scientific community. Some jurisdictions, however, employ a unique version of the Frye standard based on a state court's interpretation of the general acceptance test. For example, California follows the *Kelly-Frye* standard as described in *People v Kelly* (1976), which incorporates a third prong into the *Frye* standard relating to the particular laboratory's procedures.

The prosecutor faces some challenges in presenting DNA evidence in court, keeping in mind that DNA evidence is simply evidence for the jury's purpose, another form of proof by which the prosecutor will prove his or her case.

The prosecutor should avoid giving the fact-finder a molecular biology lesson, offering detailed explanations of testing techniques, using technical and confusing demonstrative exhibits, and expecting the judge or jury to be fluent in the many scientific terms and acronyms associated with DNA (such as "PCR," "STR," "RFLP," "VNTR," etc.). The prosecutor using DNA in court must be ready to present the state's case succinctly, meet objections, and prepare for the defense, just as he or she would do with any other evidence. Preparation is key.

When presenting any DNA evidence, a qualified and competent expert is the witness who will be called to offer a brief, basic explanation of DNA. This will include what DNA is, where it is found, what substances contain DNA, and the power of DNA with regard to identification. The prosecutor should also ask for a description of the nonforensic uses of DNA. The expert, most likely the scientist who performed laboratory testing of samples with DNA evidence, or the director or supervisor of the laboratory, will also explain the standards and protocols followed in the laboratory. This expert will also offer a brief, basic explanation of the testing process utilized when biologic evidence is presented for testing (the molecule is broken apart with heat, regions of interest are broken apart with heat, size fragments are recorded by laser, genetic locations are examined for size, the results are interpreted by the expert). The witness will define the essential terms (standard = known, sample = unknown). It is recommended that use of terms such as "allele," "locus," "primer," "nucleotide," "base pair," "heterozygote," and "homozygote" be avoided. It is simply not necessary for the judge or jury to try to understand the scientific terms. Anyone who has observed a jury in the midst of long, technical, and scientific recitations of complex matters can attest to the fact that "tuning out" occurs before cognitive recognition. The expert will also present the test results, which may include terms such as "match," "partial profile," "exclusion," "inconclusive," and "no result." It is helpful to use visual displays, such as charts or grids of test results, especially for partial profiles or when there are multiple test results. Demonstrative displays help demonstrate the profile rarity to the fact-finder. Autorads, electropherograms, and raw data should not be displayed, as they are unnecessary and confusing and may lead to misinterpretation. Finally, a brief, basic description of how statistics are calculated and used should be presented because statistical analysis enables the witness to talk about rarity or frequency within human populations. The prosecutor will have the witness explain a database, compare the suspect profile to the database frequency, and explain what a profile rarity means, using expressions of rarity "match," "source," "unique," and "rare"— all terms the jury or judge will recognize and comprehend.

To qualify an expert in DNA, the prosecutor will use much of the same techniques and questions typically used to qualify any other type of expert witness. The witness's education and training, forensic experience, nonforensic experience, publications, familiarity with professional literature, memberships and associations, and previous qualification as an expert will all be elucidated for the jury or judge. In addition, it will be necessary to build trust in the witness's laboratory by questioning the expert about issues such as the laboratory following national forensic standards, quality assurance and control, internal validation of testing procedures, proficiency testing, laboratory and personnel accreditation and peer review of the laboratory's work. Of course the prosecutor will review all of these questions with the expert in advance of the actual testimony so he or she is familiar with the expert and gains information from that expert.

Commonly encountered objections will include "the laboratory's testing techniques have not been shown to be reliable," "the laboratory expert is not a statistician," "the witness did not perform the tests," "the witness cannot testify about a database she/he did not create and which was not introduced into evidence," or "the witness's positive identification DNA testimony invades the province of the jury."

A knowledgeable and prepared prosecutor can overcome these objections if the witness is sufficiently qualified to testify as an expert in the field of forensic DNA analysis. For example, quite often in DNA cases, the analyst who conducted the DNA tests is not the same person who actually testifies. Defense attorneys have argued that the analyst performing the DNA profiling must testify as a result of hearsay, confrontation, or chain of custody issues. Appellate courts rarely accept such arguments for several reasons. Practically speaking, laboratories simply cannot afford to have their analysts away testifying all the time. This is precisely why laboratories typically designate 1 person as the "in-court" representative. In addition, the rules of evidence permit the expert to testify as to the validity of the testing procedures based on information provided by someone else. The defense can cross-examine the expert fully as to the basis for his or her opinion.

Cross-examination of the defense expert presents a challenge to the prosecutor that can actually be enjoyable. The type and discipline of the expert retained by the defense to assist in the evaluation of prosecution DNA typing results may vary significantly. The prosecutor must find out as much as possible about the expert before cross-examination and tailor the questioning to the background, qualifications and extent of opinion testimony offered by the particular expert. Resources for gaining this information include the prosecution expert, transcripts of prior testimony, Internet sites, and the American Prosecutors Research Institute DNA Forensics Program.

The prosecutor can support the technology used and the results obtained by the testing laboratory by using the expert presented by the defense. The prosecutor, to affirm the scientific acceptance and reliability of the DNA typing technique at issue, can use the defense witness who criticizes one or more of the procedures employed by the prosecution laboratory. The prosecutor must be prepared to question the expert on issues of bias, lack of forensic DNA typing experience, and the amount of income derived from expert testimony (*State v Love*, 1997).

An important advance in the forensic use of DNA testing has been the DNA database. Rather than linking only a known suspect to a known crime scene sample, databases facilitate breakthroughs without traditional investigation, called "cold hits." Crime scene samples can immediately match suspects. Crime scene samples can also match each other, revealing serial crimes and prompting coordinated investigations. Presently, every state has a DNA database enacting statute. In addition, the FBI has developed a Combined DNA Index System (CODIS) to link federal, state, and local databases into a nationwide network. Although the statutes that create these databases vary widely, most detail the convictions that require sample submission and the procedures employed to limit access and ensure privacy. Some even specify the DNA typing technology to be used. The range of defense challenges are as variable as the statutes themselves, including procedural and substantive due process, equal protection, ex post facto clauses, the First Amendment, unreasonable search and seizure, compelled self-incrimination, cruel and unusual punishment, the Ninth Amendment, privacy rights, and vagueness claims. Courts reviewing these many statutes have generally upheld them, as long as their requirements are administratively (not judicially) carried out.

Since forensic DNA testing first proved a prisoner's innocence in 1988, DNA has taken a prominent role in "post conviction" proceedings such as habeas corpus and new trial petitions; pardons and clemency hearings; and parole and probation hearings. To date, DNA evidence has corrected errors made by the judicial system in at least 81 cases, 10 of which were death penalty cases (H. Dao, telephone interview, March 2000; Death Penalty Information Center, telephone interview, March 2000). Prosecutors dealing with requests for post conviction DNA testing must balance competing interests: achieving finality in criminal adjudications and ensuring that innocent persons are not convicted and incarcerated. Allowing some access to postconviction DNA testing benefits not only the individual prisoners, but also the entire criminal justice system by instilling the public with confidence and ensuring that justice prevails. In response to this issue, some jurisdictions have opted for a proactive approach, reviewing convictions and offering free DNA testing to the prisoners. The postconviction DNA program of the San Diego County District Attorney's Office, for example, reviews cases in which (1) biologic evidence is available, (2) the prisoner has consistently maintained his innocence, (3) identification was an issue at trial, and (4) the state of the technology and evidence are such that testing could yield a result that would exonerate the defendant.

PRETRIAL MOTION PRACTICE IN SEXUAL ASSAULT CASES

THE RULES OF EVIDENCE

Navigating the rules of evidence is a perpetual challenge for prosecutors. Pressing the rules to the state's advantage through a skillful pretrial motion practice requires a thorough understanding of the theoretical underpinnings of the rules, how they have been applied in the past, and the facts of the case at bar. Strategic use of the evidentiary rules can mean the difference between conviction and acquittal in sexual assault prosecutions.

Preparation is the key to establishing relevance and admissibility of evidence. There are 5 general guidelines to preparation, as follows:

1. ***Know everything about the rule of evidence to be argued.*** Be versed in its theory and basic test for admissibility. An understanding of the historical context of a rule is the foundation for a cogent argument about its application in the current case.

2. ***Know every detail about the testimonial or physical evidence to be offered under the proposed rule and the purpose for its introduction.*** Knowledge of the details of testimony and specific characteristics of physical evidence (chain of custody, identifying marks, etc.) demonstrates thoughtful consideration of the relevance and admissibility issues and will increase the court's confidence in the state's position. The state must be certain of the purpose for introduction of the evidence, what the state intends to establish with it, and why the proffered evidence is the most probative evidence available on that point. Thorough knowledge of the evidence and its purpose will allow the prosecutor to concede to limitations on the evidence while still accomplishing the state's objective. Agreeing to certain limitations on controversial evidence can be another way to gain the court's confidence.

3. ***Know how the evidence and current facts relate to existing case law.*** Knowledge of the facts and evidence to be introduced, coupled with an understanding of the case law that supports the state's position are critical to establishing relevance and admissibility. Unfavorable case law should be distinguished on the facts. As a reminder, case law unfavorable to the state's position must be disclosed to the court. In addition to being mandated by the professional code of conduct, candor before the tribunal can dramatically enhance the credibility of an argument.

4. ***Lay a solid foundation for the evidence at the pretrial hearing.*** Do not pass over the details. They will be necessary later for argument.

5. ***File all motions and briefs of record.*** Formality demonstrates the importance of the evidence and the state's resolve in seeing it introduced.

Other Bad Acts

Rule 404(b) of the rules of evidence is sometimes overlooked by prosecutors, but it can be fertile ground for admissible evidence that corroborates the victim's testimony and strengthens the state's case. The rule provides that "Evidence of other

Key Point:
The 5 general guidelines to preparation are as follows:
1. *Know everything about the rule of evidence to be argued.*
2. *Know every detail about the testimonial or physical evidence to be offered under the proposed rule and the purpose for its introduction.*
3. *Know how the evidence and current facts relate to existing case law.*
4. *Lay a solid foundation for the evidence at the pretrial hearing.*
5. *File all motions and briefs of record.*

crimes, wrongs or acts is not admissible to prove the character of a person in order to show that he acted in conformity therewith. It may, however, be admissible for other purposes such as proof of motive, opportunity, intent, preparation, plan, knowledge, identity or absence of mistake or accident" (Strong et al., 1997). The list of other purposes is neither exhaustive, nor exclusive, and many of the purposes overlap (Strong et al., 1997). The following are suggestions of "other acts" evidence that may be relevant and admissible in sexual assault cases.

Motive. Motive is never an element of the offense charged, but it can be used to show that the defendant desired the result of the criminal conduct. In sexual assault cases, the state may use the testimony of other victims to show that the defendant desired sexual gratification through violence, control, humiliation, or other means.

Intent. Unlike motive, intent is an element of every offense charged and must be proven by the state. Motive and intent are similar, however, in that they both attempt to establish what was in the mind of the defendant at the time of the criminal conduct. Any evidence that demonstrates the defendant desired, pursued, and acted in a way that brought about the result of the criminal conduct should be proffered to establish intent.

Opportunity, Preparation, and Plan. These 3 purposes are very similar. Many sexual assaults, especially those committed by acquaintance rapists, have a "scripted" quality. The assault is often the product of a preconceived plan to gain the victim's confidence or trust, then isolate the victim, make her vulnerable, and place the defendant in control. Prior conduct with other witnesses establishing this "script" may be admissible to establish the defendant's opportunity, plan, or preparation.

Identity. Identification evidence is critical in cases in which the defendant is unknown to the victim. In these cases, other victims may be used to establish a pattern of conduct unique to the defendant. Such conduct may include the use of specific words and phrases by the defendant; the use of specific sex acts, positions, or implements; or specific conduct of the defendant or force upon the victim before, during, or after the assault. The uniqueness and repetitive pattern of these "other acts" may serve as a signature, and may be admissible to establish the identity of the defendant. In cases of acquaintance or date rape, the defense may attempt to block introduction of this evidence by admitting identity and claiming the conduct was consensual. In these cases, the aforementioned evidence should still be proffered for one of the other acceptable purposes such as motive, intent, plan, etc.

Knowledge and Absence of Mistake or Accident. Again, these purposes are similar to those already discussed and prosecutors can look to evidence of plan, preparation, intent, etc. to find evidence that establishes the knowledge and/or absence of mistake or accident.

State of Mind. Especially in acquaintance assaults, evidence of prior violence, threats, or the cycle of violence followed by "making up" may help the state establish the victim's fearful state of mind, thereby rebutting the consent defense. It may also help demonstrate the defendant's intent, motive, plan, etc.

Hearsay Exceptions

Hearsay exceptions are another important avenue prosecutors must explore to find relevant and admissible evidence to strengthen the state's case. Federal Rule of Evidence 803, adopted in most states, offers numerous exceptions to the general prohibition against out of court statements.

Present Sense Impression. Also known as the "unexcited utterance," this exception allows the state to introduce any statements made while the declarant perceived the event or condition, or immediately thereafter. These might include statements by responding officers to dispatchers or other officers as they observed the condition or behavior of the victim or defendant, similar statements by emergency medical personnel responding to the call, neighbors, or other witnesses.

Excited Utterance. Prosecutors generally have fairly wide latitude in the use of the excited utterance exception. Any statements relating to a startling event made while the declarant is still experiencing the effects of the event should be proffered under this exception. These can include 911 tapes or statements made to anyone by the victim after the attack, as long as the victim was still under the stress of the assault, without adequate time to reflect on the circumstances and fabricate the statement.

Statements Made for Medical Diagnosis and Treatment. Statements made for medical diagnosis and treatment include those made to emergency medical personnel, SANE and SART nurses, doctors, and other healthcare providers. This exception includes statements about the cause and source of the injuries or condition.

Other Evidentiary Considerations

The following are some other evidentiary options prosecutors may want to explore in the presentation of sexual assault cases.

Flight as Evidence of Guilt. Most jurisdictions allow introduction of evidence that establishes the defendant's guilty mind. This can include flight after the criminal act, failure to appear in court, change of physical appearance (hair style, hair color, facial hair, etc.), concealment of evidence, and attempts to intimidate or contact witnesses or the victim.

Context. Context evidence is the information that allows the jury to see the complete setting for the events, not just sporadic events in an evidentiary vacuum. It is said to "...complete the story of the crime on trial by placing it in the context of nearby and nearly contemporaneous happenings" (Strong et al., 1997). It is sometimes likened to what used to be "res gestae" evidence. In acquaintance assaults, this evidence helps establish the parameters of the relationship between the victim and the defendant.

RAPE SHIELD STATUTES

The fundamental purpose of rape shield statutes is to prevent the accused from introducing evidence at trial about the victim's sexual history. Rape shield statutes prevent the exploitation of the victim's sexual history, protect the victim's right to privacy, and exclude irrelevant evidence. These statutes are a relatively recent creation.

During the 1970s and 1980s, the criminal justice system made dramatic changes in the way it handled rape cases. These efforts were primarily to reduce the prejudices faced by rape complainants. The changes brought new concerns about possible constitutional violations. These statutes are continually challenged as unconstitutional, on their faces and as applied. In almost every circumstance, the resolution of these challenges has turned on the justification for the rules.

History

Common law rules generally deemed character evidence inadmissible. However, there were 2 exceptions to this general rule, one of which was that character evidence was allowed when the defendant was charged with forcible rape, regardless of the defense raised (Galvin, 1986). One rationale behind this rule was that it was "more probable that an unchaste woman would assent to such an act" (People v Collins, 1962). The other exception went to the credibility of the victim as a witness. "If the victim admits some form of previous sexual conduct it can be inferred that she is a woman of bad moral character. If she is an immoral person, then it can be inferred further that she is a person who would not have conscientious scruples about lying on the witness stand. . . . If a woman consents to sexual intercourse outside of marriage then she is a person who would also lie" (*Brown v*

State, 1973). This inference was not applicable to males nor to female witnesses in any context other than sexual crimes (Galvin, 1986).

Reformists of the women's movement, who began the fight to enact rape shield laws in the late 1960s, saw results by 1974 when the first rape shield statute was enacted in Michigan. In the following 4 years, more than 30 states had followed with similar statutes (Galvin, 1986). In 1978, Congress enacted the Privacy Protection for Rape Victims Act creating Federal Rule of Evidence 412, which deems evidence of an alleged victim's sexual history inadmissible. Congress stated that the purpose behind this rule was to end the "degrading and embarrassing disclosure of intimate details about" the victims in rape cases (124 Cong Rec, 1978). The hope of President Jimmy Carter was to encourage women to report rape, the least reported crime, and to foster communication and trust between victims and police investigators and prosecutors (124 Cong Rec, 1978).

The Supreme Court of the United States, in *Michigan v Lucas* (1991), deemed Michigan's rape shield statute "a valid legislative determination that rape victims deserve heightened protection against surprise, harassment, and unnecessary invasions of privacy." The Supreme Court, thereby, gave their implicit approval of rape shield statues.

The Four Models of Rape Shield Statutes

The Michigan Model

This category of rape shield statutes is followed by approximately half the nation and generally excludes all evidence of a victim's sexual history with few limited exceptions. These exceptions include evidence of the victim's "past sexual conduct with the actor" and "evidence of specific instances of sexual activity showing the source or origin of semen, pregnancy, or disease" (Mich Comp Laws Ann, 2001). Michigan's law states in pertinent part: "(1) Evidence of specific instances of the victim's sexual conduct, opinion evidence of the victim's sexual conduct, and reputation evidence of the victim's sexual conduct shall not be admitted . . . unless and only to the extent that the judge finds that the following proposed evidence is material to a fact at issue in the case and that its inflammatory or prejudicial nature does not outweigh its probative value: (a) Evidence of the victim's past sexual conduct with the actor. (b) Evidence of specific instances of sexual activity showing the source or origin of semen, pregnancy or disease. . . ." (§750.520j).

The Federal Model

Federal Rule 412 is similar to the Michigan Model in that both render evidence of a victim's sexual past inadmissible but for a few limited exceptions. The difference is a broad exception in Federal Rule 412. This exception covers instances in which the accused's constitutional rights would be violated if such evidence were not introduced. Federal Rule of Evidence 412 states in pertinent part: "(a) Notwithstanding any other provision of law, in a criminal case in which a person is accused of rape or of assault with intent to commit rape, reputation or opinion evidence of the past sexual behavior of an alleged victim of such rape or assault is not admissible. (b) . . . evidence of a victim's past sexual behavior other than reputation or opinion evidence is also not admissible, unless . . . (1) admitted in accordance with . . . (c)(1) and (c)(2) and is constitutionally required . . .; or (2) admitted in accordance with . . . (c) and is evidence of _ (A) past sexual behavior with persons other than the accused offered by the accused, upon the issue of whether the accused was . . . the source of semen or injury; or (B) past sexual behavior with the accused . . . ." (Privacy Protection for Rape Victims Act, 1978).

The Arkansas Model

The Arkansas Model does not automatically prohibit the introduction of evidence as do Michigan and the Federal Rules. Arkansas provides for an in-camera hearing where the judge can weigh the probative value of the introduction of evidence of the victim's sexual past against its prejudicial effects. The admissibility of the evidence depends on the judge's findings. Arkansas law states in pertinent part: "(b)

. . . opinion evidence, reputation evidence or evidence of specific instances of the victim's prior sexual conduct with the defendant or any other person . . . is not admissible by the defendant, either through direct examination of any defense witness or through cross-examination of the victim or other prosecution witness, to attack the credibility of the victim, to prove consent or any other defense . . . (c) Notwithstanding the prohibition in subsection (b), evidence directly pertaining to the act upon which the prosecution is based or evidence of the victim's prior sexual conduct with the defendant or any other person may be admitted at the trial if the relevancy of the evidence is determined in the following manner: (1) A written motion shall be filed by the defendant . . . stating that the defendant has an offer of relevant evidence prohibited by subsection (b). . . (2) A hearing on the motion shall be held in camera no later than (3) three days before the trial is scheduled to begin. . . (B) A written record shall be made of the in camera hearing. . . . (C) If, following the hearing, the court determines that the offered proof is relevant to a fact in issue, and that its probative value outweighs its inflammatory or prejudicial nature, the court shall make a written order stating that evidence, if any, may be introduced by the defendant and the nature of the questions to be permitted . . ." (Ark Code Ann, 2001).

The California Model
California's statute permits evidence of the victim's sexual history to be introduced for certain purposes. California and the states following this model allow evidence of the victim's prior sexual conduct so long as it is not used to show consent. This model also calls for a hearing to determine the relevancy and value of the evidence. California law states in pertinent part: "(1) A written motion shall be made by the defendant to the court and prosecutor stating that the defense has an offer of proof of the relevancy of evidence of the sexual conduct of the credibility of the complaining witness. (2) The written motion shall be accompanied by an affidavit in which the offer of proof shall be stated. (3) If the court finds that the offer of proof is sufficient, the court shall order a hearing out of the presence of the jury . . ." (California Evidence Code).

It is crucial to know and understand the relevant rape shield statute in your jurisdiction. These statutes set a guide to the type and degree of evidence needed to successfully prosecute a sexual assault case.

Constitutional Issues
Proponents of rape shield laws believe they shield victims of sexual assault from being revictimized during the court process (Price, 1996). Those opposed to the laws believe that such laws exclude important evidence and violate constitutional rights of the defendant (Price, 1996).

The constitution guarantees certain procedural and protective rights to all criminal defendants. Those rights include, among others, the ability to confront and cross-examine one's accuser and the ability to present a defense, as stated in Amendment 6 of the United States Constitution. Defendants often endorse the argument that rape shield statutes deny them these rights (Price, 1996). However, the United States Supreme Court has ruled that these rights have limitations (Fishman, 1995). In *Michigan v Lucas* (1991) the court stated that the right to confront and cross-examine can be limited if the evidence would tend to harass the victims, threaten their safety, or otherwise be prejudicial. The right to confront and cross-examine is therefore not absolute. Rape shield statutes that limit the admissibility of evidence do not on their face violate the constitution; however judges retain discretion on the breadth of the limitations imposed by rape shield statutes (Fishman, 1995).

Issues such as due process, equal protection, vagueness, and the protection against self-incrimination have also been used as grounds to constitutionally challenge rape shield laws (Fishman, 1995). Constitutional challenges to rape shield laws require courts to weigh the potential prejudice to the victim against the relevance and necessity of the evidence in providing a fair and accurate trial for the defendant (Fishman, 1995). Therefore, a close examination of the applicable rape shield

Key Point:
The US Constitution guarantees certain procedural and protective rights to all criminal defendants, including (1) the ability to confront and cross-examine one's accuser and (2) the ability to present a defense. Defendants often claim that the rape shield statutes deny them these rights. However, the US Supreme Court has ruled that these rights have limitations.

statute as well as a determination of the purpose for which the evidence is being offered is necessary.

As stated, there are 4 main variations of rape shield laws, each taking a different approach to the breadth of the exclusion and the purposes for which prior sexual activity is or is not admissible. There are several reasons for a defendant to attempt to introduce evidence of a complainant's prior sexual behavior (Fishman, 1995). Evidence that the victim previously consented to sexual activity or evidence that her behavior caused the defendant to reasonably believe she was consenting during the time in question could lead to the inference that the victim actually consented to sexual activity with the defendant during the incident in question (Fishman, 1995). It is exactly these inferences, however, that rape shield statutes seek to prevent. Without legislation prohibiting the introduction of prior sexual behavior, a defendant would be able to introduce such evidence and improperly damage the credibility of the victim in the eyes of some fact-finders. Such evidence is unfairly and improperly prejudicial and thus is excluded.

When the purpose of introducing such evidence is to demonstrate that the victim has a motive to lie or that the defendant was not the perpetrator, however, a closer analysis of the prejudicial effect of the evidence may be required. Evidence of prior sexual behavior may or may not be admissible for these purposes, depending on the breadth of rape shield statute in a given jurisdiction. Courts must carefully weigh the necessity against the prejudice of this information in order to maintain the spirit of rape shield statutes and prevent the accuser from being victimized and humiliated.

In summary, although rape shield statutes aim to prevent all evidence of a victim's sexual past from being admissible, jurisdictional variations create differing limitations on the exclusion of this evidence. Evidence of a victim's past sexual behavior may be admissible for very limited purposes. A thorough understanding of the applicable rape shield statute and interpretive case law is essential for investigators and prosecutors of sexual assault.

PROBLEMATIC CASES
DATE RAPE/ACQUAINTANCE RAPE
Perhaps the most difficult of sexual assault cases involves a victim and perpetrator on a "date" that turned into a sexual assault. In these cases, the perpetrators will often acknowledge sexual contact but contend it was consensual. The first thing an investigator should determine is whether the "date" was, in fact, a date. Perhaps the suspect simply invited the victim over to study or for other purposes. If the circumstances surrounding the event do not appear to be a date, it reduces the possibility of a consensual encounter. In investigating a case of this nature, the officer should take detailed notes of the victim's emotional behavior at the time of the outcry. Crying, shaking, wincing for pain, and other indicators corroborate the victim's claim that the defendant's conduct was not consensual but was, in fact, a rape. If the victim did not make a prompt report to the police, it is necessary to find out to whom she reported the rape shortly after the attack. Other witnesses may be able to provide the same evidence. The victim's and the perpetrator's clothes from the night of the attack are collected. There may be manifestations of the attack on the clothes of which even the victim was unaware. It should be determined if the victim suffered any injuries. Even if the victim did not report promptly and any injuries have healed, friends or other witnesses may have seen injuries such as a black eye. These witnesses should be found and interviewed.

The crime scene should be examined, photographed, and sketched out. Even if there is no direct evidence of the attack, the crime scene can be of assistance in innumerable ways. If the defendant claims the conduct was consensual and yet the act in question took place in an office or other room ill-equipped for a consensual encounter, this may highlight the absurdity of the defendant's claim. If the location of the crime scene makes it difficult for a victim's scream to be heard, this evidence would also be helpful. The suspect and victim's friends should be interviewed to see how the respective parties described the "date" to their friends. Even if the victim did not allege a rape, but simply refused to discuss the encounter with her friends, this can be evidence corroborating the encounter was not consensual. If the suspect's friends heard him bragging about the sexual encounter, this may corroborate that this was not a romantic encounter so much as an attempt by the suspect to pleasure himself at the expense of the woman unfortunate enough to be near him.

ALCOHOL-FACILITATED SEXUAL ASSAULTS

It has been recognized for decades that alcohol use contributes to criminal behavior. A 1958 study found alcohol was present in the victim, perpetrator, or both in 64% of homicide cases (Wolfgang, 1981). Another study found that 58% of men imprisoned for violent crimes were drinking alcohol before the offense (Mayfield, 1981). A study of rapes in Winnipeg, Canada between 1966 and 1975 found that either the offender or the victim or both consumed alcohol in 72% of the cases (Johnson et al., 1981).

Given the prevalence of alcohol in sexual assault cases, prosecutors must develop effective strategies to investigate and prosecute crimes involving this element. The alternative is to forego a large number of felony crimes under the umbrella excuse "too difficult to prove."

In a case of sexual assault in which both victim and perpetrator consumed alcohol while on a date, a defense attorney will typically argue that alcohol rendered the victim's memory unreliable and reduced her inhibitions against having sex with the defendant.

Alcohol and Memory

The effect alcohol has on memory varies greatly from individual to individual and depends on various factors, including the quantity of alcohol consumed and the time period over which the consumption occurred. Alcohol may impair the storage of actual memories (Browning et al., 1992). If a victim's memory is so impaired she cannot recall whether she consented to sexual activity, prosecution is problematic.

To say that alcohol may impair the storage or retrieval of memory, however, does not mean that alcohol causes a victim to insert a false memory or to be overconfident in the accuracy of what she does recall. Indeed, 1 study finds alcohol intoxication produces no significant overconfidence in the subjects' judgments as to the accuracy of their recall (Nelson et al., 1986). Accordingly, a victim strong in her assertion of nonconsensual sexual contact is not necessarily, or even probably, unreliable.

At every stage of the trial, a prosecutor must educate the jury that alcohol does not mean the victim's memory is untrustworthy. During voir dire, the jury should be directed to recall their own experiences with alcohol and the likelihood that they can retrieve many memories from occasions on which they consumed alcohol.

Potential jurors should be asked the following questions:

— Do you ever drink alcohol?

— After consuming alcohol, do you typically recall major events such as where you were and who you were with?

— Do you believe rape to be a traumatic experience? If so, do you consider it plausible that, drunk or sober, a rape victim will recall the trauma despite her best efforts to forget?

— Do you believe that when a woman drinks to excess and consents to some physical contact, she forfeits a right to say no to all sexual contact?

A victim must also educate the jury that her memory is reliable. To this end, proper trial preparation is paramount. A victim should not minimize her use of alcohol and, if she cannot recall the details of the evening, this should be conceded during direct examination.

If the victim cannot recall everything about the evening yet is confident of the pertinent facts, she should be asked to give the jury insight as to why she can recall some but not all of the evening. Ideally, the answer will be something like this: "Well, I was drinking a lot, and I can't remember the color of the room or things of that nature. But when I tell a man to stop touching me and he proceeds to remove my pants and cause me physical pain by inserting his penis into my vagina, that's something I can remember."

There is evidence that victims and witnesses are more likely to be accurate when recalling "central, salient" details of an event as opposed to peripheral details (Myers et al., 1996). There is also evidence that core features of stressful events are more readily recalled (Myers et al., 1996). One researcher found that "while memories of ordinary events disintegrate in clarity over time, some aspects of traumatic events appear to get fixed in the mind, unaltered by the passage of time or by the intervention of subsequent experience" (Van der Kolk & Fisler, 1996).

If a victim recalls peripheral events such as the time she left home, the time she returned, where she went, whom she saw or what she ate for dinner, other witnesses should be questioned to see if they can corroborate these details. This enables you to argue before the jury that if the victim remembers inconsequential events, she can certainly recall the ordeal of rape.

A prosecutor can emphasize this point in closing argument by conceding the obvious and mocking its relevance. The following hypothetical argument illustrates this point:

Defense counsel challenges the victim's credibility by contending that her use of alcohol makes her memory unreliable. Those of us who have used alcohol know that at some point our memories can be lost. This, however, is not a case of forgetting, it's a case of remembering. The victim in this case remembers being pushed, remembers her pants being pulled down, remembers the feel of the defendant's penis inside her vagina, and remembers saying "NO" to all of this. The victim no doubt wishes to forget that she was raped, but alcohol has never been so compassionate.

Alcohol and Reduced Inhibitions

Another common argument of defense attorneys is that the alcohol reduced the victim's inhibition against having sex. It is true that alcohol may reduce inhibitions and cause the drinker to do things she would not do sober. As an example, 1 alcoholic describes her first experience with alcohol as follows:

The first time I used alcohol I was thirteen. I drank 1-2 beers (Colt 45) with my friend Morreen, my boyfriend Bill, and several other friends. Morreen and I stood on our heads to get the effect quicker. I did a cheerleading jump off a 2½ foot wall and forgot to put my legs together to land on my feet and landed squarely on my tailbone, chipping it. I remember before the accident that I was full of energy, laughing and having fun. I think it made it easier to make out with my boyfriend (McGovern, 1996).

In response to this defense, a prosecutor may have 3 arguments at her disposal. First, if the victim said no to the sexual contact, then her inhibition against having sex with the perpetrator was not reduced. In many cases, it is a cruel insult to suggest that alcohol would certainly place the victim in bed with her perpetrator. Indeed, 1 study finds the incidence of female initiated sexual activity decreases with the use of alcohol (Harvey & Beckman, 1994).

Second, the effect of alcohol on reducing inhibitions also applies to the perpetrator. Alcohol may be a disinhibitor to a variety of sexually inappropriate practices. For instance, perpetrators of incest frequently use alcohol as a disinhibitor to their crimes and as a defense when their conduct is challenged (Liles & Childs, 1986). If the perpetrator was under the influence of alcohol, any inhibition against coercing sex may have been reduced. There is evidence that men may use alcohol as an excuse for aggression. In 1 study, men who falsely believed they had consumed alcohol showed greater sexual arousal to tape recordings of rape and sadism than to tapes of non violent, consensual intercourse (Briddell et al., 1994).

Third, the argument can be made that the perpetrator took advantage of the victim's intoxication. An unfortunate part of our culture is the belief that getting a woman drunk makes the possibility of becoming intimate with her easier. In a 1986 survey, 75% of college men report having used alcohol or drugs in an effort to obtain sex from an otherwise unwilling woman (Briddell et al., 1994).

The jury should be reminded of our cultural myths concerning alcohol and sex and this information should be used in cross-examination of the defendant. Typical questions to use are as follows:

— You bought the alcohol, didn't you?

— You encouraged the victim to continue to consume?

— You noticed the alcohol was affecting the victim?

— Did you begin the evening with the objective of having sex with the victim?

— Was having sex with the victim an idea you developed after you got her drunk?

If the defendant contends the encounter was a consensual, romantic experience, his conduct after the rape should be explored. Did he send the victim flowers? Did he call the victim again? In speaking to his friends, did the perpetrator describe the victim in caring or derogatory terms?

DRUG-FACILITATED SEXUAL ASSAULTS

Drug-facilitated sexual assaults are receiving increasing attention throughout the country. In these cases, perpetrators use drugs to subdue their victims before the sexual assault. Some of the most common places where these crimes occur are in clubs or bars, on college campuses, and in other party settings. However, it is not uncommon to see a drug-facilitated sexual assault occur during a casual date or other interaction. The drugs used are easily slipped into drinks and consumed by unsuspecting victims, producing an incapacitating effect.

Several drugs are reportedly used to facilitate sexual assaults. These include ethanol (alcohol), benzodiazepines, gammahydroxybutyrate (GHB), hallucinogens, opiates, and other miscellaneous drugs, including barbiturates, antihistamines, sedative antidepressants, muscle relaxants, scopolamine, and herbal sedatives. Ethanol (alcohol) is widely consumed in the United States and is often not considered a drug. The majority of drug-facilitated sexual assault cases the Federal Bureau of Investigation (FBI) handles include ethanol use or involvement, probably because it is easily obtained and other drugs are commonly mixed with it.

The category of drugs called benzodiazepines includes 1 of the most common and well-publicized date rape drugs, flunitrazepam (Rohypnol). Several other benzodiazepines are also used, such as triazolam (Halcion), alprozalam (Xanax), diazepam (Valium), and clonazepam (Klonopin), to name a few. Of these, only Rohypnol is banned in the United States. Rohypnol is a central nervous system depressant and is 10 times more potent than Valium. While it is illegal in the United States, it is legally available in more than 70 countries and is often smuggled into the United States from many different countries, especially Mexico and Columbia, through mail and delivery services, and by individuals who bring it across the border (Drug Enforcement Agency [DEA], 1995). The effects of Rohypnol can occur within 15 to 30 minutes after ingestion and last up to 8 hours or more, depending on the dosage (DEA, 1995). The drug's effects are increased when combined with alcohol and can sometimes be fatal (DEA, 1996).

Key Point:
The following are 3 arguments against the claim that alcohol reduces a victim's inhibitions against having sex:
1. If the victim said no to the sexual contact, her inhibition against having sex with the perpetrator was not reduced.
2. The effect of alcohol in reducing inhibitions also applies to the perpetrator. If the perpetrator was under the influence of alcohol, any inhibition against coercing sex may have been reduced.
3. It is possible that the perpetrator took advantage of the victim's intoxication.

Key Point:
In drug-facilitated sexual assaults, perpetrators use drugs to subdue their victims before the sexual assault. Some of the common locations for this are in clubs or bars, on college campuses, or in other party settings.

GHB is a central nervous system depressant. GHB is usually a street manufactured drug. It is often mixed with alcohol or fruit drinks to mask its salty or soapy taste. The effects occur within 15 to 30 minutes and last 3 to 6 hours, depending on the dosage (American Prosecutors Research Institute [APRI], 1999). When combined with alcohol or taken in large doses, GHB can result in coma and even death.

Hallucinogens are also used in drug-facilitated sexual assaults. These include ketamine (Special K), phencyclidine (PCP), marijuana, or others such as MDMA (Ecstasy), lysergic acid diethylamide (LSD), or scopolamine. Hallucinogens are popular date rape drugs because often the victim voluntarily ingests them to get the analgesic, sedative effects. They are fairly rapidly absorbed and some, like ecstasy, intensify the sensation of touch.

Opiates are strong central nervous system depressants that produce a sense of euphoria and well-being. Included in the opiate category are codeine, morphine, hydrocodone, hydromorphone, and meperidine. Opiates, like hallucinogens, may be voluntarily ingested by the victim to obtain the effects of the drug.

Key Point:

If a negative screening for the 2 most commonly identified drugs, Rohypnol and GHB, is obtained, this indicates that the investigation should consider the possibility of the use of other drugs that may have been used to produce an anesthetic effect.

Many other drugs or categories of drugs are used as date rape drugs. These include antihistamines, antidepressants, barbiturates, and muscle relaxants. Most drugs in these categories are legally available in this country. In addition, many over-the-counter drugs are included in this group. A negative screen for the 2 most commonly identified drugs, Rohypnol and GHB, should not be the end of the investigation, but rather an indication to investigate the possibility of the use of other drugs that may have been used to produce the same anesthetic effect.

Prosecuting a drug-facilitated sexual assault case is extremely challenging. The largest obstacle to overcome in such cases is a result of the very nature of the drugs themselves. Common symptoms that are reported by victims of drug-facilitated sexual assault are unconsciousness, drowsiness, confusion, dizziness, vomiting, and nausea. These symptoms directly mimic the symptoms of someone who is intoxicated. Very often the victim is given the drug during the evening, when the body's natural inclination is to rest. The victim may fall asleep because of the effects of the drug and remain sleeping throughout the night until the next morning when she would naturally arise.

Dissolving the drug in an alcoholic drink may increase the victim's symptoms. Victims often do not remember the attack itself but wake up only knowing that something is very wrong. They may have hazy memories of waking up for a few seconds during the assault and then losing consciousness again (Reno, 1999). Thus, their ability to recount and testify to the crime is very limited. The lack of memory of the actual assault on the part of the victim is the most obvious hurdle for the prosecutor to overcome. Although most can remember a fair amount of the details before the assault, many have extremely hazy, if any, memories of the actual assault. Most victims are in a semi-conscious or catatonic state. Certainly, these victims cannot consent to any type of sexual conduct in this state, but the real challenge for the prosecutor is proving that the crime occurred.

Consequently, the lack of physical evidence in a drug-facilitated sexual assault case becomes even more problematic. Often, victims are not even sure that a sexual assault occurred until days or even weeks later. Thus, there has been no rape kit or collection of other physical evidence preserved from the scene. Even if the victim makes a report fairly soon, Rohypnol and GHB are metabolized by the body very quickly. GHB is metabolized within 12 hours, and Rohypnol is generally metabolized within 48 hours (LeBeau, 1999). If the assault occurred within a recent time period, the victim should give a blood and/or urine sample and submit to a sexual assault examination. It is important to recognize that a urine sample may show traces of the drug several days after the attack. A urine sample collected the morning after the attack is the most effective way to detect the presence of drugs.

Blood samples are only effective if the exposure to the drug is in the hours before the sample is drawn. Also, the blood sample should be collected in a 10-mL gray topped tube, with additional blood drawn for other forensic testing. Usually, however, the victims do not report the attack until well after the time frame during which any drugs can be traced.

Thus, it is imperative that a thorough investigation be conducted in these types of cases. The interview of the victim is an important evidence-gathering tool. Officers must be encouraged to be extremely cautious about leading questions or other attempts to help fill in information. It will usually be frustrating for both the victim and the officer that the victim is unable to fill in more gaps in her memory, but all attempts must be made to make sure that what she can recollect is accurate information. From her account, the officer may be able to establish many pieces of the crime, such as a general timeline and the actual location of the crime.

Often, interviewing any other possible witnesses can lead to more clues than the victim herself may be able to give. For example: Who was she with before the incident? How did she appear? Was there any noticeable change in her demeanor? Who did she leave with? What was her condition when she left? Who saw her first afterward? What did she say? All of these questions may help fill in the missing information.

If the officer has been able to establish the physical scene of the crime, search warrants should be issued for both the crime scene and the defendant's home. It is important to look for any evidence of drugs, prescriptions, drug cooking equipment, etc. Many perpetrators find recipes for cooking GHB on the Internet. A search of the suspect's computer can prove enlightening. The officer should tag and test any open drink glasses or bottles for drug residue. It is important that the toxicologist screen for several of the most common drugs, not just Rohypnol and GHB. Many investigators opt for a "pretextual" phone call in states that allow such wiretapping. The victim and suspect are often acquainted with one another or have friends in common. The victim simply calls the suspect and attempts to elicit incriminating evidence about the attack. Finally, a search should look for any corroborating evidence that would normally be collected in a sexual assault, such as stained sheets, used condom, marks or scars on defendant that the victim can remember, etc.

The prosecutor must be prepared to go forward without a positive drug screen. The prosecutor should file any appropriate pretrial motions, such as rape shield, other acts evidence, and requests for reciprocal discovery in those jurisdictions that provide such. These motions are very important in this type of case. If it is possible to elicit testimony about other similar acts of the defendant, the victim's credibility can be bolstered. Similarly, if the defense is able to elicit testimony regarding the victim's sexual history, it can be very damning to the state's case. All pretrial motions should be carefully considered.

Because the victim will usually be unable to provide specific details of the case, experts play a critical role during trial. Toxicologists, pharmacologists, and chemists all may be proper experts. They can generally educate the jury about the date rape drug used during the crime and its properties. They can testify to the effects of date-rape drugs, some of which may be corroborated by witnesses who saw the beginning or ending effects of the drug displayed by the victim. They can further testify about how the drug may be distributed in a drink and how long it would be before the effects are felt, some of which can be corroborated by the victim herself. Most importantly, they can educate the jury regarding the physiologic and cognitive effects on a person who ingests such a drug, such as lack of capacity to consent, and its impact on their short-term memory during that time period.

A drug-facilitated sexual assault case is both difficult and frustrating for the investigator, the prosecutor, and the victim. Although the victim must be supported throughout the course of the investigation, it is also important to remain realistic throughout the process. Although there may be little doubt in everyone's mind that a sexual assault occurred, a prosecutor might need to consider other alternative charges if there is little or no corroboration to the sexual assault. Some other possibilities, depending upon the evidence, are drug possession, contributing to the delinquency of a minor, false imprisonment, and general assault.

MENTALLY RETARDED VICTIMS

Individuals with mental retardation or physical impairment are often the targets of sexual predators as a result of social and psychologic conditions, including short-term memory impairment, reduced language ability, difficulty with abstract thinking, reduced social skills, failure or inability to report, excessive obedience, and minimal sexual education. These conditions both promote victimization and make successful prosecution appear unlikely.

According to the *Diagnostic and Statistical Manual of Mental Disorders* (DSM-IV-TR, 2000), the diagnosis of "mental retardation" is made when a person meets the following qualifications:

1. Has an IQ of approximately 70 or below

2. Is unable to be independent in the activities of daily living commensurate with his or her chronological age

3. Experienced the onset of the disability before age 18 years (DSM-IV-TR, 2000)

General intellectual functioning can be determined through clinical assessment and 1 or more of the available standardized intelligence tests (e.g., Wechsler Intelligence Scales for Children–Revised, Stanford-Binet, Kaufman Assessment Battery for Children). Conditions such as autism, Down's syndrome or other chromosomal disorders, and traumatic brain injury may result in mental retardation.

Although some legal and technical issues are unique to cases involving victims with mental impairment, many of the issues mirror child sexual abuse prosecutions. For example, many jurisdictions have specific statutes that protect adult sexual assault victims with mental impairment from sexual abuse even if the perpetrator does not use "legal force or duress" (Cal Penal Code, 2002). These victims may be found to be incapable of legally consenting to the sexual conduct (*People v Whitten*, 1995; *State v Frost*, 1996; *People v Mobley*, 1999).

Furthermore, juror reluctance to believe the testimony of a person with mental impairment is not unlike juror reluctance to believe child victims in sexual abuse cases. As in child sexual abuse cases, proper investigation to develop corroboration, pretrial motions to limit the issues, and proper trial techniques are the key to success.

The Investigation

The Interview Procedure. Procedures adopted for child sexual abuse interviews can be employed in cases involving victims with mental impairment (APRI, 1993). These procedures include using a "victim-friendly" interview room, asking nonleading questions, and conducting a minimal number of victim interviews. Prior to the interview, an in-depth conversation should be conducted regarding the victim's impairment with a parent or guardian to learn about cognitive functioning, communication styles, and phobias. Psychologists and other professionals should be contacted to develop techniques to overcome the particular limitations that the victim's impairment presents.

Determining Competency to Consent. Evaluating a victim for competency to consent to sexual activity requires an in-depth understanding of forensic interview skills. The National Center for Prosecution of Child Abuse recommends the forensic interviewing course, "Finding Words," offered by American Prosecutors Research Institute. During the initial interview, the victim's knowledge level is appraised. In other words, does the victim understand the nature, quality and consequences of the act? Review local statutes to determine the requirements for competency to consent in your jurisdiction. Questions regarding the victim's true understanding of human reproduction and contraception are vital in this determination. For example, the questions, "where do babies come from?" or "how do babies get inside women?" and "why does the pill prevent a woman from getting pregnant?" are helpful. The answers should assist the prosecutor in determining whether the victim has a competent understanding of the consequences of engaging in sexual conduct.

Also, prior sexual conduct should be explored. The defense may attempt to present prior sexual conduct to establish that the victim consented in the past. Mere capitulation does not constitute competent consent. Be aware, the rape shield doctrine may not prevent admission of the victim's prior sexual conduct if proffered on the issue of competency to consent, rather than to impugn reputation (*State v Frost*, 1996).

Documenting the Physical Examination. A complete forensic examination and rape kit should be performed. All corroborating evidence is documented, including the victim's statements, demeanor, and any apparent difficulties understanding concepts or procedures during the examination. The examining professional should acquire a complete history of abuse or sexual conduct from the victim, if possible, or from another knowledgeable source. This information will assist in rendering an accurate opinion regarding the cause or timing of any physical findings.

The Police Investigation. A focus of the investigation is to find unbiased witnesses to enhance victim credibility and corroborate victim testimony. Optimal witnesses include teachers, friends, family, caretakers, bus drivers, neighbors, and employers. Pertinent interview topics include behavioral, physical, and social patterns. Behavior patterns that corroborate testimony or show emotional distress include daily routine; changes in routine before, during, or after the abuse; and reversion to childlike conduct such as bedwetting or nightmares. Changes in the victim's attitude such as perception of reality, aversion to trusted persons, or increased sexual knowledge or activity, corroborate abuse. Physical indications of abuse include refusal to undress or bathe; unusual walking or sitting; painful or itchy genital area; bruising, bleeding, stained or bloody clothing; pregnancy; or stress-related medical complaints.

Obtaining IQ Information. The IQ and mental age of the victim will be vital pieces of evidence during the criminal trial. A complete developmental history should be obtained at the outset of the investigation. Many states have Adult Protective Services or other agencies that maintain records on adults with the "mental retardation" diagnosis who are receiving assistance. If the victim attends or attended special education classes, the school district will maintain an Individual Educational Plan (IEP). The IEP contains information on the victim's educational level and social goals. The IEP provides a practical understanding of adaptive functioning, or "how effectively individuals cope with common life demands and how well they meet the standards of personal independence expected of someone in their particular age-group, sociocultural background, and community setting" (DSM-IV-TR, 2000). It should be determined if there is a school psychologist familiar with the victim and the victim's mental age and concrete thinking ability. The school psychologist may be a valuable, unbiased expert or lay witness.

A psychologist experienced in dealing with individuals meeting the DSM-IV-TR criteria for "mental retardation" and who is familiar with the victim's specific impairment and any cultural issues should be retained. The victim should be examined by the expert to determine (1) adaptive functioning to confirm that the victim meets the DSM-IV-TR definition of "mental retardation"; (2) IQ level and corresponding mental age; (3) confabulation (i.e., a behavioral reaction to memory loss in which the patient fills in memory gaps with inappropriate words); and (4) concrete thinking ability. The expert will be able to describe the victim's degree of mental retardation in terms of mild (IQ level from 50-55 to approximately 70), moderate (IQ level 35-40 to 50-55), severe (IQ level 20-25 to 35-40), or profound (IQ level below 20-25) (DSM-IV-TR, 2000, p. 41). This expert will be a vital witness at trial on the issue of the victim's ability to "consent" to sexual activity.

Getting To Know the Victim. Before going to court, it is important that the victim trust the prosecutor. By spending time with the victim, the prosecutor becomes familiar with the victim's body language, verbal expressions, and schedule. As a result, the prosecutor can alert the court when the victim is stressed, tired, agitated, or in need of medication.

Pretrial Motions

State and federal statutes exist to assist and protect child witnesses in court. "Child-friendly" statutes include closed courtroom during victim testimony; allowing leading questions during direct examination; use of anatomical dolls; limiting length of testimony and cross examination; support persons; preventing undue harassment; and accelerated court scheduling (18 USCA §3509, 1999; Department of Health and Human Services [DHHS], 1999a, 1999b; Fed R Evid 611; NY Exec Law § 642-a, 1999).

Child witnesses experience fear, embarrassment, exhaustion, short concentration spans, and inadequate vocabulary skills. Many difficulties that child witnesses encounter are also experienced by witnesses with mental impairment. Logically then, these "child-friendly" statutes should also be applicable to adult victims with mental impairment. It should be argued that "child-friendly" statutes, normally triggered by chronological age, should also be triggered by mental age. To support this argument, the prosecutor should offer in limine evidence via declaration, lay or expert testimony, witness examination, or generic psychologic studies **(Table 32-1)**.

Trial Considerations

Voir Dire. Jury selection is the prosecutor's first opportunity to promote the victim's credibility with the jury. In addition to standard child or sexual abuse questions, jurors should be asked about the following:

— Perceived credibility of mentally impaired persons

— Attitudes regarding mentally impaired persons

— The issue of incompetency to consent

— The fact that the state is not required to show force or duress if a victim is mentally incapable of giving meaningful consent to sexual activity

Competency To Testify. Care is taken not to confuse the fact that a victim is competent to be a witness in court with the fact that a victim is not competent to consent to sexual activity. Most jurisdictions agree that all persons are presumed competent to be a witness (Fed R Evid 601). To be competent, a witness must be capable of communicating relevant material and understanding the obligation to do so (*United States v Saenz*, 1985). The court decides the competency of a witness (*State v Briere*, 1994). The party challenging competency has the burden of proving incompetency through cross-examination (*Adamson v Department of Social Services*, 1988; *State v Watkins*, 1993; *State v Waugh*, 1989). Accordingly, courts should refuse defense requests to order a psychiatric examination to determine competency to testify (Fed R Evid 601; *United States v Gates*, 1993). Further, inconsistent statements do not make a witness incompetent to testify (*United States v Cook*, 1991).

The Oath. There is no special verbal formula required for an oath. The oath need only impress on the witness the duty to be truthful (Fed R Evid 603). Versatility is appropriate for children and witnesses who are mentally impaired (Fed R Evid 603

Key Point:
Many of the difficulties that child witnesses experience are also experienced by witnesses with mental impairments.

Key Point:
Considerations that must be addressed at trial include the following:
1. Promote the victim's credibility with the jury.
2. Make clear to the jury that competency to be a witness in court does not mean competency to consent to sexual activity.
3. The oath should be tailored to the witness's mental age and level of understanding.

Table 32-1. Rate of Maltreatment and Abuse of Young Persons with Mental and Physical Disabilities

In 1994 through 1995 a study involving Nebraska school children age 0 to 21 years old was conducted. Developmental disabilities were identified and maltreatment determined. Four databases were combined including more than 40,000 children from Omaha, Nebraska public and Catholic schools, Central Registry of Nebraska DSS, Nebraska Foster Care Review Board, and victim records from the combined data archive of Omaha Police Department and Sheriff (Summit, 1983, 1992). Eight percent of the total school population had a disability and met state and federal criteria for special education.

The results of the study easily identify the rate of maltreatment and abuse inflicted upon young persons with mental and physical disabilities.

Disability	School Population %	Maltreatment Prevalence %
Behavior disorder	20.7	53
Mental retardation	27.5	28
Health related	12.3	28
Speech/language	5.4	37
Orthopedics	2.6	13
Hearing disability	1.8	21
Visual disability	0.9	12
Autism	0.4	9
Learning disability	28.4	18

[ancillary laws and directives]). The trial judge should be encouraged to administer an oath appropriately tailored to the witness's mental age and level of understanding (Fed R Evid 603 [advisory committee's notes]; *United States v Allen J*, 1997).

Witness Order. A well-organized case-in-chief begins and finishes strongly. All weak or detrimental evidence is presented in the middle. Witnesses and evidence should be presented according to strength and relevance. A strong victim should testify early in the trial while the jurors are most attentive. However, a witness to educate the jury about the victim's impairment should precede the victim to the stand. Understanding how the victim thinks and acts will allow jurors to focus on the content of the victim's testimony and the issue of consent.

The retained psychologist is well suited for educating the jury. First, generic testimony regarding the victim's impairment is presented and the jury is educated on medical, psychologic, physical, and social issues. Second, evidence of the victim's mental age, language skills, concrete thinking ability, physical attributes, and other relevant issues is presented.

The victim should testify next, while the attributes of the victim's impairment are fresh in the jurors' minds. It is vital to establish the victim's reliability as a historian and credibility as a witness. Part of the direct examination is dedicated to developing information that can be corroborated by subsequent witnesses. Information is elicited regarding the victim's daily routine, transportation, and meal or school schedules. After establishing reliability, it is good to thoroughly explore the facts and details of the criminal conduct.

Photographs or other demonstrative evidence should be used during the victim's testimony. The victim's accurate identification of items, locations, and objects will further enhance reliability. The jury will have greater confidence in the victim's identification of the defendant, the crime scene, or other valuable items of evidence.

The prosecutor must be aware of the victim's special needs. Scheduling testimony around crucial activities such as meals, resting, and the taking of medication will maximize the quality of the testimony.

A witness who corroborates the victim's testimony should testify next. A parent, guardian, sibling, teacher, employer, daycare provider, or neighbor may be able to offer this evidence. Corroborating testimony may discuss the victim's daily routine, ability to perceive, personal habits, and character for truth and veracity.

Customary medical and scientific evidence, percipient witnesses, or investigative testimony should be presented around these core witnesses. Also, for issues such as unusual victim reaction or delayed or recanted disclosure, the prosecutor should consider presenting an expert on rape trauma syndrome or child sexual abuse accommodation syndrome (Summit, 1983, 1992).

Rebuttal Case. Expert and lay testimony is presented to contradict defense attempts to discredit the victim. Issues such as suggestibility, possible misidentification, and disability-related fabrication or fantasy are all fertile ground for rebuttal. The prosecution must try to anticipate the defense and consult an expert with some knowledge or understanding of the victim's issues. A knowledgeable professional can easily do away with a manufactured defense.

COMPUTER-ASSISTED SEXUAL EXPLOITATION OF ADULT VICTIMS

Computer-facilitated sexual assault and cyber stalking have become high-profile crimes. With the number of investigations and arrests increasing dramatically, the need to conduct skilled interviews of suspects is being recognized as a new area of expertise for law enforcement, as is forensic analysis of both the suspect's and victim's computers. Specifically, the new issues relevant to gathering computer evidence must be incorporated into the interview to give law enforcement the best chance of amassing the optimal amount of digital evidence from the suspect and, consequently, from the computer(s).

Preparing for the Interview

Investigators will find that during the interview phase, they are pitting their knowledge of computers and the Internet against that of the offenders, just as computer forensic examiners pit their knowledge against that of the offender in the areas of password protection, encryption, and the hiding of digital information.

Investigators should consider the following when determining what approach to use in interviewing a suspect in a computer-facilitated child sexual exploitation case:

— Assess their own computer knowledge to avoid trying to bluff a suspect who knows more than they do

— Assess the computer knowledge of the suspect from all other evidence to determine who you are up against

— Obtain as much information as possible concerning the hardware and software used by the suspect. Going into the suspect interview, the investigator may have obtained some of the following information: suspect's username or user ID; suspect's on-line profile; suspect's Internet service provider (ISP); suspect's account information; and the time of day or night the suspect is usually on-line.

It is best to conduct the suspect interview in a private room away from the location of the execution of the search warrant. The suspect interview should be audio and video recorded to protect the detective and his/her department, and to provide important evidence for later presentation at trial. Note of caution: Any telephone call the suspect is allowed to make may result in the removal or destruction of digital or other evidence. Many computers can be accessed remotely. Alternatively, the suspect may request the person called destroy the contents of the computer either by physically removing the computer(s) involved or by accessing the suspect's computer and destroying the evidence at the source.

Question Areas

The following questions should be prefaced with appropriate language consistent with the approach chosen. They should also be adapted to reflect the type of exploitation that occurred (e.g., date-rape vs. cyber stalking).

Search and Seizure Information. The initial interview is usually the best opportunity afforded to amass basic information from the suspect on the computer(s) used by him/her and how they may be protected from external scrutiny. By inquiring into what hardware and software the suspect used on a regular basis and how he/she used them, this information may assist the forensic examiner with his/her analysis of the computer(s). By inquiring into how many computers the suspect had access to and where they are located, probable cause may be gathered to search and seize additional computers or peripherals. The number and location of computers the victim used to receive e-mails from the suspect should also be asked. Additional questions in this area would include how many computers were used to correspond with the victim and how many individual e-mail accounts the victim and suspect each have.

Password and Encryption Issues. A password is a secret series of characters that enables a user to access a computer, program, or file. The password helps ensure that unauthorized users do not access these areas. The investigator should ask if the computer, programs, or files are password protected and, if so, what the passwords are and who else has knowledge or access to those passwords. If the password-protected information contains incriminating evidence, then this shows knowledge and intent on the suspect's part to hide or conceal the information. Encryption renders a message unintelligible by anyone other than the intended recipient. Encryption is the most effective way to achieve data security. To read an encrypted file, you must have access to a secret key or password that enables you to decrypt it. The investigator should ask if any of the computer files have been encrypted and, if so, what the names of the files are, what encryption software was used, and what the keys or passwords are to decrypt the files. This information can then be provided to the forensic examiner for the recovery of the encrypted files. Again, if the encrypted files contain incriminating evidence, this will show knowledge and intent on the suspect's part to hide or conceal the information.

Defeating the Some Other Dude Did It (SODDI) Defense. Attendant to the basic information already discussed, the next line of questions may preemptively preclude the defendant raising the mistaken identity defense. Questions within this area should include: "Who else uses the computer(s)?" "Who else goes on the Internet from the suspect's computer(s)?" "Who else goes on the Internet using the suspect's username?" By getting the defendant to admit exclusive dominion over the computer(s) and his username, later claims that another person was the wrongdoer may be avoided. By asking questions about when the suspect is normally on the computer, the answers may assist prosecutors in showing that the suspect was the person at the computer at the time in question.

Amassing Character Evidence. Because the defendant may choose to put his character and reputation at issue at trial, information should be solicited regarding the suspect's Internet usage and habits. Questions here include: "What do you do on the Internet?" "What Web sites do you visit?" "What news groups do you subscribe to?" "What chat rooms do you visit?" "Who do you chat with and about what topics?" "What Web sites or news groups do you have bookmarked or saved as a favorite?" By setting out this information now, later defenses that center around the concept of victim bashing may be precluded by the defendant's own statement.

Storage Location. One aspect that must be remembered is that not all images are necessarily stored on-site in the suspect's computer(s). It is entirely possible that off-site storage exists. The prosecutor must ask first about where the images are stored on the computer (which files, folders, and directories). The question "Where else do you store correspondence and where are these devices?" should also be asked. Answers might include floppy disks, CD-ROMs, or tapes.

Forensic Evaluation

Armed with whatever information was amassed during the suspect interview, investigators can begin the forensic analysis of the computer(s). It should be noted that a single stand-alone computer will take, on average, 40 hours to analyze. Thus, any information, such as passwords or encryption codes, that can assist the examiner should be turned over to the analyst immediately. The following areas must be addressed in the forensic examination(s).

Chat rooms, instant messaging, and other forms of communication and data sharing over the Internet, have become extremely popular. For this reason, it is vitally important to a proper investigation to search a suspect's computer. Although the crime of sexual assault does not directly involve the use of a computer, the information found on a computer can greatly aid in the prosecution of the crime. Therefore, the following paragraphs will provide a basic and general primer of computer terms and forensic techniques to incorporate into a thorough forensic examination of a suspect's computer. The information is very generalized, and technical exceptions to many of the ideas exist, so this section should be considered a brief introduction to the complex world of computer forensics.

Beginning the search. The most important axiom to remember when confronted with the seizure and search of a suspect's computer is "Cop first, nerd second" (Mills, 2002). Simply put, this means that a computer is like any other crime scene and should be treated as such. Because the computer itself is a complex machine and the forensic examiner may have a level of expertise sufficient to collect a great deal of information from it, accessing the computer's hard drive should be done only after a number of typical and procedural steps are taken (*Best Practices*, 2002).

First, if the computer is off, it should be left off. Turning it on may cause booby traps or destructive programs to begin. In addition, turning a computer on causes the computer to write over certain types of "temporary" computer memory, thus deleting potential information. Likewise, if a computer is on, it should be left on. The temptation to search the computer at that time must be resisted; extensive on-site searches of a running computer should be done with caution because the more done on a computer, the more likely those actions will appear in the "temporary" memory files than any incriminating evidence. The best course of action to take is to photograph the screen. Finally, when the computer must be turned off, it is important not to follow the normal shutdown procedures, but to simply disconnect the power cord from the back of the computer. This is important because properly shutting down a computer creates the possibility that some information, specifically that in "temporary" memory, might be lost. Also, some computers will start the normal shut down process if the power from the wall is interrupted. By pulling the plug from the computer, the computer does not take these steps (National Institute of Justice, 2001).

Second, once the decision to seize the computer is made, it is extremely important to remove the computer so that reconstructing it will be simple and exact. As with any crime scene, photography is crucial. Photographing the back of the computer hard drive to show where all the plugs were plugged in, and conversely which ports were empty, should be done at the start of the investigation. After the photographs are taken, it is necessary to isolate the computer from any telephone or cable connections. As remote access is a very real possibility, investigators must ensure that a suspect cannot alter evidence by accessing the seized computer from an off-site location. Next, all plugs and ports should be clearly marked so that they can be replaced once in custody. For example, a police officer would mark the power plug "A," then mark the slot into which it is inserted "A" also. If the computer has a great number of peripherals, such as printers, scanners, web cameras, speakers, or storage devices, this process can quickly get very complex, so a large number of labels is recommended.

Third, when transporting the seized items, great caution must be used. The items must be packed and cushioned well and each piece of hardware treated as extremely fragile. When transporting or storing, all items should be kept away from magnetic devices, microwaves, radio transmitters, and other sources of energy that might delete information. If possible, items should be transported on the floor of the back seat (National Cybercrime Training Partnership, 1999; National Institute of Justice, 2001).

As with any search and seizure, the success of recovering evidence depends on the meticulousness of the search. Therefore, a protocol should be developed describing the steps for proper seizure and proper search techniques. With a protocol, difficult seizures can be anticipated, and the process used to find evidence during complex searches can be easily explained in court.

What to Look for During the Search. Once the computer forensic examiner has the computer safely restarted in the laboratory, there are several different types of files and documents that can yield a great deal of useful evidence. Obviously, files, images, and saved e-mails can potentially contain information, correspondences, or writings that could reveal motive or planning. However, there are other types of files that can provide even greater evidence of where a suspect has been on-line, with whom he or she has been talking, how he or she has tried to create false identities, or when the suspect accessed, downloaded, or altered files on the hard drive.

Information from Websites. When a person logs onto the Internet, his or her computer begins a series of electronic transfers of information with the Internet service provider's (ISP) server. The transfers are the equivalent of the 2 machines talking with each other and are the source of the annoying screeching noise heard from modems. These transfers include information about the suspect's computer as well as information that is sent by the ISP about the websites the suspect is accessing. In addition to information being sent to the suspect's computer, however, the website's computer is also accessing information about the suspect's computer. The website's computer is getting information about the type, speed, and size of the suspect's computer and organizing that information in a file on the suspect's hard drive, commonly called a "cookie." Thus, when the suspect's computer logs back on to the website, the website's computer simply goes to the cookie file on the suspect's computer, finds the appropriate cookie, and can identify the computer as a past user. Because the cookies contain information accessed by websites, they can also be used by investigators to track where a suspect has been. By opening up a cookie, an investigator can tell the web address of the site and possibly even what pop-up ads were displayed on the screen.

Similar to cookies, computers keep a list of recently visited websites in a directory labeled history. The length of the history can be set, so website names can be saved for 1 day or longer. The site addresses show up in the address box on the computer screen and will also pop up in the box if prompted by typing them. Related to the history directory is the favorites directory. As counterintuitive as it may seem, some suspects are willing to make illegal or damaging websites favorites simply because it is easier to access them.

Finally, in the same directory as the cookies file is the "Temporary Internet Files" file. This file contains bits and pieces of downloads and website information from websites that were visited by the suspect's computer. These files can include partial images or documents accessed by the suspect's computer, as well as additional useful information. The Temporary Internet Files file is also another depository for cookies.

Information from E-mail. E-mail can provide a wealth of information, both from obvious sources and from those not readily apparent. When searching e-mail, the first place to look is at the file names under which the suspect might have the account divided. A scan of the sent items folder is also recommended, because suspects often fail to delete those items, not realizing that there are copies of e-mails there. Finally, a check of the Delete file is necessary because most programs require users to delete twice; a file is not deleted merely because it has been sent to the Delete file.

E-mail headers, the section of words and addresses preceding every e-mail message, can also provide a wealth of information if read properly. Although reading e-mail headers requires a fairly specialized amount of knowledge, this example offers a basic primer (*Best Practices*, 2002):

——Message header follows——

1. Return-path: jqpublic@email.com

2. Received: from ruguilty@netmail.com (4.1/SMI-4.1) id BB11011; Mon, 1 Mar 99 12:34 EST

3. Received: from localhost byjqpublic.email.com (4.1/SMI-4.1) id BB10011; Mon, 1 Mar 99 12:33 EST

4. Message-Id: <1234567890.BB1011@ruguilty.netmail.com>

5. Date: Mon, 1 Mar 1999 12:35 -0800 (EST)

6. From: "JQ Public" <jqpublic.email.com>

7. To: Joey Bagadonuts bagadonuts@internet.org

8. Cc: Reggie Osborn reggoz@law.fgu.edu

So what do these lines really mean? Basically, they all aid in the delivery process. However, be aware that with the exception of line 4, all of these can be altered in order to falsify or "spoof" who the real sender was and where he or she is located.

1. Informs receiving computer who sent the message and where to send error messages if the message doesn't go through.

2. Shows the route the message took from sending to reception. Every time a computer receives a message, it adds a "Received:" field with address and time stamp.

3. Same as line 2.

4. Message ID line is the only line that cannot be altered. The ID is logged by the computer and may be traced through the computers it has been sent from if needed.

5. Shows date, time, and time zone when the message was sent.

6. Gives e-mail address of sender.

7. Shows e-mail name and address of the recipient. In this case ".org" denotes an organization, ".com," a commercial vendor, and ".edu," an educational institution.

8. Shows names and addresses of any "Cc's." This can also be a "Bcc," or blind Cc, in which case the name and address would be hidden.

Created/Modified/Accessed Dates. Every file has 3 dates associated with it, and those dates can be very revealing. The 3 dates of interest are the "Created Date," the

the "Modified Date," and the "Accessed Date." Although it is possible to alter these dates by resetting the internal settings of the hard drive, for the purposes of this section it will be assumed that the time settings of the suspect's computer are accurate. The "Created Date" is the date that the file was created, first saved, or downloaded onto the suspect's hard drive. This date is important because it records the date when the file first appeared on the suspect's computer. This information can be used to show possession of a file, and also show that the suspect knew of its existence. For example, if a suspect claims that a file only recently appeared on the hard drive, or was accidentally placed there, a "Created Date" of any significant age would rebut that claim. Likewise, the "Modified Date" is of importance because it shows whether and when the suspect had altered or changed the file. This is useful because modification can imply knowledge of the file as well as use and affirmative possession of it. Finally, the "Access Date" is useful because it shows how recently the suspect opened the file. However, the Access Date only records when the most recent action was taken; therefore, if a forensic examiner is too hasty and opens a file before properly creating a duplicate copy of the hard drive, all the access dates will reflect the dates law enforcement accessed them, not the suspect.

Instant Messaging. Instant messaging is a service provided by most ISPs that allow subscribers to type conversations to each other in real time. The most common example of this is AOL's Instant Relay Chat (IRC). Instant messaging is a useful tool for investigators who are conducting on-line stings. The difficulty with the software, however, is that there is no automatic logging of conversations, nor are the chats saved. Therefore, investigators searching for records of instant message chats must hope that the suspect and/or victim either turned on the logging capabilities of the program or printed out or otherwise recorded the contents of the chat.

Where to Look During the Search. Once the investigator has properly seized the computer and has an understanding of the type of information that can be retrieved from the hard drive, he or she must know where on the hard drive or disks to look. This means that the investigator must be familiar with the different types of memory a computer uses to save information, how that memory functions, and the durability of those types of memory. Basically, there are 3 types of space on a hard drive or disk where files may be stored: allocated space, which is space that has data written to it; unallocated space, the space that is available for writing; and slack space, which is space left over from allocated space. However, before those 3 types of spaces can be explained, how a file is save must be explained.

Defining the Space on a Computer. A computer has a finite amount of memory. This is described in megabytes, megs, (mb), or often gigabytes, gigs, (gb), with a byte consisting of eight bits of data, roughly equivalent to a single character of information, like the letter "a." Internally, the hard drive orders bytes of memory into 2 units, the sector and the cluster. Both allocated and unallocated space are ordered in sectors and clusters. A sector is made up of 512 bytes, although the sector size may be altered, 512 is the standard size. Thus, when a file is created, it is allocated a certain number of sectors. For instance, if a document is 487 bytes, it partially fills 1 sector, and the remaining 25 bytes in the sector is what is called RAM slack. If a file is more than 512 bytes, it fills up as many sectors as needed; therefore, if a file is 1025 bytes, it takes up 3 sectors—two are completely full and one has 1 byte of information and 511 bytes of RAM slack.

Clusters are groups of sectors. For the sake of example, assume a cluster consists of 4 sectors. The computer creates clusters in order to maximize the space used by the computer for storing information. Conceptually, this is the same ordering of space as a closet; just as items placed in boxes make it easier to stack and organize clutter versus just throwing everything in and shutting the door quickly, clusters contain the various-size sectors of information so all the sectors fit efficiently together. However, just as there can be space left over in sectors when files are not large enough to fill them completely, there can be space left over in clusters if the sectors do not contain enough information to fill them. This type of slack space is known as disk slack.

Using the earlier example of a document 1025 bytes, large disk slack becomes easier to understand. The 1025-byte document spans 3 sectors in a cluster that is 4 sectors long. As stated earlier, the third sector contains 1 byte of information and 511 bytes of RAM slack. Leftover from that is an entire sector that is empty; that sector thus contains 512 bytes of disk slack.

Finally, the clusters that have information written and saved to them are known as the allocated space. The clusters that contain deleted information or have not yet been written to are considered the unallocated space. It is important to state that although the allocated space contains all of the easily accessible files and documents, it is the information on the unallocated space and slack space that can prove to be the most useful in investigations.

Searching the Unallocated and Slack Spaces. Unallocated space can contain information placed on it both intentionally and unintentionally. Intentionally placing information in unallocated space takes a great deal of knowledge and expertise, in addition to certain computer programs. Although hiding files in unallocated space is not very common, it is worth investigating. More common are the unintentionally remaining pieces of information present in RAM and disk slack resulting from deleting and rewriting sectors and clusters. Computers are logical and efficient machines; thus, when files are deleted what actually happens is that the computer merely renames the file. Therefore, if a person writes a letter that almost fills 1 cluster then deletes it, the computer simply renames the letter "unallocated." The letter does not disappear, the computer merely now looks at it and instead of thinking "letter," it thinks, "unallocated space." Therefore, when the computer user rewrites onto a cluster, he or she is actually writing over whatever was contained in the cluster, but then deleted. The computer does not try to match up file sizes, so an interesting result ensues. For example, a person writes a letter that is 1 cluster (4 sectors) in length. For whatever reason, the letter is deleted, but then the person decides to write a shorter letter that takes up only 2 sectors in a 4-sector cluster. The computer would take the short letter and write it over the longer letter. Although the letter would cover the first 2 sectors, there would be two sectors of slack space that contained almost half of the original letter. By using the proper software an investigator can recover that fragment of the original letter and thus preserve some potentially helpful evidence. The software of choice for most forensic examiners is Encase.

Along the same theoretical lines of recovering information from deleted files that are partially readable is the idea of recovering information stored in RAM and disk slack used temporarily by the computer to run larger, slower programs. When the hard drive is required to open a large or complex item, an image for example, it will often use RAM slack or disk slack to temporarily store the excess amounts of bytes of the item. By using RAM, the computer can more quickly and efficiently run demanding programs. Although RAM might seem like the jackpot in terms of discovering evidence, it is not always dependable because this use of space is very temporary, written over as soon as the computer needs additional memory. Information contained in RAM space can be lost if an investigator opens large files on the hard drive or reboots the computer. Likewise, this information can be lost if programs that depend on RAM space are run before the investigator has the opportunity to run the proper software to search it. Therefore, the investigator must first check all temporary files and run a thorough search of the RAM space in order to preserve any potentially useful information contained therein.

This has been a very brief and cursory discussion of some of the issues of computer forensic examinations. There are numerous exceptions and conditions to the general theories presented, and thus a trained computer forensic examiner should be consulted for both the computer seizure and its subsequent search. The evidence potentially available on a computer hard drive is great; however, the risk of losing it because of hasty examinations is also great. In addition to a trained forensic expert, every jurisdiction should have a clear, concise, and thorough protocol for handling computer evidence, and all investigators who potentially come in contact with computers should be familiar with it.

No 1 set of suggestions or guidelines can ever completely anticipate and respond to all circumstances that may arise during a suspect interview or forensic examination of a computer. However, by having a plan regarding the interview and the forensic examination of the computer(s), law enforcement will increase the effectiveness of these crucial aspects of investigating and prosecuting these crimes of violence against women. The American Prosecutors Research Institute's (APRI) National Center for Prosecution of Child Abuse can provide technical assistance to investigators and prosecutors to enhance their knowledge of both best investigative and forensic practices. Please contact the Center at 703-549-4253.

MARITAL RAPE AND DOMESTIC VIOLENCE

Any prosecutor who has handled domestic violence cases can explain the difficulty in prosecuting them. Domestic violence victims are situated differently from every other victim in our legal system. Domestic violence perpetrators greatly confuse our images of a violent criminal because the person causing harm is not some deranged stranger in an alley, but rather a beloved husband, wife, boyfriend, or girlfriend. For a variety of reasons, the victims of batterers have a great deal of difficulty cooperating with the prosecution of the crimes against them. In addition, it is extremely difficult for many victims of domestic violence to even recognize or acknowledge that they are "battered."

Key Point:
The victims of batterers have a great deal of difficulty cooperating with the prosecution of the crimes committed against them. It is often even difficult for victims of domestic violence to recognize or acknowledge that they are "battered."

Batterers seldom commit violence early in a relationship. Rather, they nurture the relationship and mold it into one in which they have total power and control over the victim. Batterers typically use a variety of tactics to obtain and retain this power and control over the victim. This creates in the victim the difficult conundrum: I love this person, but he or she hurts me. Often the parties will have children in common, property in common, and some amount of history together, including many periods of time in which the relationship is a warm and loving one. The batterer knows the victim well and knows what tactics work to keep him or her from testifying, whether by sympathy ploys, manipulation, or threats against the victim, children, or other family members. The victim knows the batterer well and is intimately aware of what kind of violence and vindictiveness the batterer is capable, which makes it extraordinarily difficult for a domestic violence victim to ignore threats made by the batterer, including those designed to make the victim afraid to cooperate with prosecution.

Rape is a crime that is grossly underreported as victims battle with feelings of guilt, shame, and fear. When a husband rapes his wife, all of the difficulties of both rape and domestic violence are combined. Victims feel ashamed, isolated, and frightened. They, like domestic violence victims, may also have a great deal of difficulty in defining the act committed against them as criminal. Therefore, although battered women are particularly vulnerable to being raped by their abusers, few will ever report the rape to authorities. Rape in the context of an ongoing relationship is a form of domestic violence. For some victims, it may be easier to succumb to the rape than to face a horrible beating. For others, the rape is the way that the batter knows he can hurt the victim the most, and he therefore rapes her to sadistically hurt her. Some batterers insist on having sexual relations with their victims after a beating as a way of "making up." Marital rapes reported to law enforcement are likely to be ones that accompany or follow a very severe domestic violence assault, and the injuries from the physical assault are likely to be viewed as more serious than the physical or emotional injury caused by the sexual assault.

When a victim does report a marital rape, the case must first overcome all of the stereotypes and myths held throughout the criminal justice system, from the law enforcement officers to the prosecutor to the grand jury and/or judge. For example, many criminal justice professionals have difficulty understanding how a woman can be raped by someone who she has had consensual sex with in the past, or how a woman can be raped and not have some sort of visible injury. These myths demonstrate that much education is needed in the criminal justice field about the psychologic and physical realities of rape.

If the case does make it to the courtroom for trial, it will be very difficult to prove because marital rape cases are further complicated by the great many myths about rape that society holds. The average person does not easily understand that the majority of rapists are not strangers, but rather acquaintances and even loved ones. Society has a tendency to engage in a great deal of victim blaming in rape cases: the victim must have done something to bring this on to herself. This serves to make each of us feel safer by allowing us to believe that, because we do not engage in the behavior that the victim engaged in, this crime could never happen to us. It also allows us to reconcile the nice guy image that many rapists have in public, because we cannot imagine that he could become some sort of monster in private.

As of 1993, marital rape is a crime in every state. In 33 of those states, however, there is some sort of exemption given to husbands in rape prosecutions (Bergen, 1999). For example, in Washington State a husband can be convicted of first-degree or second-degree rape, but not third-degree rape, which is defined as sexual intercourse with a person who did not consent, and the lack of consent was clearly expressed by the victim's words or conduct, or where there is a threat of substantial unlawful harm to property rights of the victim (Wash Rev Code §9A.44.060). The logic appears to be that if the victim is not physically harmed or threatened, then her spouse has not raped her. This obviously fails to consider the emotional harm caused by every rape.

In many respects, the legal system is just beginning to evolve in its handling of marital rape cases. A great deal of education is needed, both within and outside of the criminal justice system, before rape victims will truly receive justice and before rapists will truly be held accountable.

TRIAL STRATEGIES

VOIR DIRE

When prosecutors begin jury selection, they intend to accomplish 2 goals: to solicit enough information from a juror who is potentially harmful because of prejudice to have him or her stricken, and to persuade the jurors who are chosen that their case, the prosecution, is what the law forbids. Prosecutors have learned from experience that jurors regularly make up their minds early, some as early as at the end of jury selection. In addition, in certain types of cases, the subject matter awakens deep-seated personal values over which people adamantly disagree. Rape, the death penalty, politics, and racial prejudice are among these topics. In trials that involve these kinds of emotional issues, we have reason to believe that individual juror bias is a force to be reckoned with . . . it is clear that the ideal of an impartial jury rests heavily on the shoulders of an effective voir dire (Kassin & Wrightsman, 1988). Because rape, sexual assault, sexual battery, and other sexually related crimes are so emotionally charged, great care and subtlety are necessary to expose potential jurors' biases toward women and crimes committed against them. Compounding the prosecutors' challenge is that "empirical studies have shown that judges, jurors and the public know very little about rape, and what they believe about it is wrong" (Massaro, 1985).

Rape in America rarely fits the stereotype perception held by jurors, that rape is committed by a stranger who uses a weapon and chooses his victim randomly (Wright, 1995). The victim's relative, friend, neighbor, or other acquaintance commits 75% to 85% of sexual assaults (Wright, 1995). Nor do more than a small percentage of rapists use weapons in the commission of rape (Lisak, 2001a). Worse still, are the deep seated myths in jurors' views about women: (1) women are less credible community members; (2) women assume the risk of rape by their chosen behavior; and (3) women set and enforce limits upon men's sexual behavior (LaFree, 1989; Schafran, 1985; Wright, 1995). To ask jurors to overcome long-held mythical beliefs in the time taken for a prosecutor's portion of jury selection is akin to asking a cow to jump over the moon.

In efforts to ascertain enough information from potential jurors to discriminate between those who will not overcome their biases quickly enough to be a fair juror and those who will or those who do not hold them, prosecutors have developed questions that will expose the bias to the prosecutor. Most of these questions are so subtle that only the trained prosecutor may recognize that the answers indicate significant critical biases toward women. They may range from the less subtle question, "Do you know any woman who has falsely accused someone of rape," to "Have you done things in your life that, looking back on, you wish you could change?" The obvious and direct question, "Can a woman, who participates consensually in kissing say no to sexual intercourse?" exposes that the prospective juror associates kissing with foreplay, indicating that then a woman can no longer refuse.

In addition to accomplishing the first goal of exposing prejudices held by some that make them improper jurors for a rape case, prosecutors use jury selection to persuade potential jurors that the prosecution case is the law. "Rape," or the coercing of sexual intimacy against the victim's will, legally does not require the use of a weapon, some specific type of resistance, some magic words to communicate lack of consent, or some quantifiable amount of injury the rape survivor must sustain. In prosecutor parlance, these concepts are referred to as a lack of resistance, lack of consent, and lack of force. An attacker, who coerces a victim to surrender her body against her will, commits a crime by that very act, and does not need a weapon, physical struggle, or physical injury to be a rapist. Prosecutors know that these are not requirements necessary in order to convict the accused, although many lay people do not. A woman's resistance, in particular, is critical to potential jurors in determining a rapist's culpability (Feild & Bienen, 1980). Consequently, when prosecutors discuss these concepts, their purpose is to educate and persuade a potential juror that this is the law and the law is just. A successful approach is to follow up the question, "Do you expect to learn that the defendant used a gun or a knife in the assault?" with the question "Why?" Alternatively, "Do you expect to learn that the victim was beaten when she tried to fend off her attacker?" should be followed by the question "Why?" Another successful approach is to ask all the potential jurors to identify or describe the way people respond to trauma, violence, or attack, and then ask about the importance of availability of options one has when attacked.

Are there jurors, just by the obvious characteristics, who are good or bad jurors in a rape case, and if so, then, which ones? Prosecutors, particularly the inexperienced ones, ask those questions. A few, with more exposure, perhaps, will ask, "Are all women just bad jurors in rape cases?" If the answer was yes, then prosecutors would have another challenge because all lawyers are prohibited from striking a potential juror from the jury only because they belong to a certain race, ethnicity, or gender (*JEB v Alabama*, 1994). There is, however, the identification phenomenon that prosecutors must understand and use in their selection of a fair jury. The fear of being raped, especially in women, between age 19 and 35 years, is almost twice their fear of being murdered (*One night*, 1991). Those fears are warranted: the emotional and psychologic effects of rape are devastating (Fairstein, 1993). Women, when they become jurors, do not leave the fear at home, a long way from the courthouse. The identification phenomenon exists because women jurors do not want to accept that completely "normal" women are attacked. Accepting this would increase women's sense of their own vulnerability (Murphy, 1992). Linda Fairstein

Key Point:
There is no perfect way to pick jurors or perfect questions. Important factors to successful jury selection are the time and energy spent in preparation, the accuracy of the prosecutor's identification of the defense, and the ability to have gotten as close as possible to the whole truth and not run away from it.

Key Point:
The deciding factor in whether a prosecutor believes a case may be successfully prosecuted may be the presence of physical evidence of force or scientific evidence to prove the identity of the perpetrator. However, medical evidence is often lacking or inconclusive.

(1993), Chief of the Manhattan District Attorney's Sex Crimes Unit, has observed that, "for many women, the need to shield themselves from their own vulnerability is paramount. If they can insist that the victim's behavior was behavior they would never engage in, such as going to a man's apartment after meeting him in a bar, they can convince themselves that they are not at risk." Women with knowledge about rape know that any woman can be a rape survivor. A prosecutor's best tool to prevent women from successfully blaming the victim is to bring out into the open the identification and possible reaction. The prosecutor can then hope that, if not all jurors stop themselves from the phenomenon, some will stop the others. One example of a good question to elicit informative responses is to ask the panel of potential jurors to complete the following sentence: "I could never be raped because _____" (Wright, 1995). Supportive prosecution jurors will reply simply with, "I could be raped."

Prosecutors often hear that jury selection is not a science but an art. It is certainly the universal experience that there is no perfect way to pick jurors or perfect questions. Important factors in the success of a prosecutor's jury selection are the time and energy spent in preparation, the accuracy of a prosecutor's identification of the defense, and a prosecutor's ability to have gotten as close as possible to the whole truth and not run away from it. Rape is a crime of premeditation (Lisak, 2001b). Rapists target prey they believe to be the most vulnerable, or they target their prey when the prey is the most vulnerable. Rape survivors, all too often, are women who the rapists believe will never report or never be believed. There is power, however, in truth. The prosecutors in this country have made great strides, and will continue to make them, in insuring that the only one held accountable for the crime of rape is the rapist.

DIRECT EXAMINATION OF SEXUAL ASSAULT NURSE EXAMINERS (SANE)

When a prosecutor considers whether a sexual assault case can be successfully prosecuted, the deciding factor may be the presence of physical evidence of force or scientific evidence to prove identity of the perpetrator. Seasoned prosecutors recognize that many jurors often consider the presence of such evidence to be the cornerstone of a guilty verdict. However, the reality of sexual assault prosecution is that medical evidence is often lacking or inconclusive.

Being an effective witness in a sexual assault prosecution requires much more than simply performing the examination and then appearing in court to discuss the findings. The quality of the examination, understanding pertinent rules of evidence, understanding the needs of the prosecutor, preparing to testify, and providing testimony in an effective manner are all vital elements to being a strong witness.

Establishing a Protocol

Sexual assault examinations for the purpose of collecting forensic evidence to be used in a criminal proceeding must be conducted in a reliable and defensible manner. A protocol establishing a mandatory order and procedure should be in force. Every phase of the examination should be regulated by the protocol, including how a history will be obtained, collection of scientific evidence, and collection of the patient's clothing, as well as the examination itself.

The sexual assault professionals who work within the jurisdiction should create a protocol for a particular jurisdiction. Jurisdictional specific issues must be addressed and dealt with in the protocol. Local professionals will understand local resources, what the financial concerns may be, what agencies are in existence, and what local laws require. Protocols from foreign jurisdictions may be useful as a model to assist in creating the local protocol. However, because protocols are uniquely suited to a specific jurisdiction, it should not be assumed that a preestablished, well functioning protocol from a different jurisdiction will fulfill the needs elsewhere.

A multidisciplinary group of sexual assault professionals should participate in the creation of the protocol. This group should include medical professionals who will conduct the examination, law enforcement officials, prosecutors, therapists, counselors, crime laboratory personnel, and any other professional who has a role in the investigation and prosecution of a sexual assault case or treatment of the victims. Without the cooperation of all vital agencies in the jurisdiction, a successful criminal case is difficult to build.

There are many issues that need to be decided when a protocol is being created. One of the most difficult issues is the financial aspect of the examination. This issue must be confronted head on. Failure to decide who will bear the burden of the costs may prevent agencies from employing the services of the sexual assault examination facility. One must always consider the possibility of reimbursement from the defendant through a fine upon conviction and sentencing.

The authors of the protocol must decide if a single location will be established for conducting sexual assault examinations. If this is the case, a convenient location for the entire jurisdiction should be selected. Questions such as, "Who will staff the facility?" or "How will victims be transported to the facility?" and "Will the facility be open 24 hours a day?" should be considered and answered.

When writing the protocol, the manner in which the sexual assault examination should be conducted must be established. The format mandated must be well thought out and based on well-established medical information. Medical professionals who conduct the examinations must be thoroughly aware of the protocol requirements and understand why procedures were established. If called to court as an expert witness or a percipient witness (a person who has first-hand knowledge of events and testifies regarding their knowledge), the medical professional must be able to explain why a procedure was done in a certain manner, not just that the protocol "said so."

The protocol must also establish how a history should be taken. A history is a statement obtained from the patient regarding what happened during the sexual assault and any other events pertinent to the medical examination. Medical professionals who conduct sexual assault examinations are often highly trained and skilled regarding the medical procedure involved in conducting a thorough sexual assault examination and collection of relevant scientific evidence. However, extensive training regarding taking of history in accordance with applicable jurisdictional rules of evidence must also be provided.

There are numerous protocols available to be used as models in establishing a new protocol. The Office for Victims of Crime (US Department of Justice, Office of Justice Programs) publishes a Development and Operation guide. The American Prosecutor's Research Institute's National Center for Prosecution of Child Abuse maintains various protocols from around the country and makes them available upon request.

Rules of Evidence Every Sexual Assault Examiner Should Know and Understand

It is vital for medical professionals to understand their jurisdictional rules of evidence with respect to the admission of a statement acquired during a sexual assault medical examination. A majority of jurisdictions follow the Federal Rules of Evidence or have statutes that mirror the Federal Rules. Consequently, the rules and rationales stated here will apply to a majority of medical professionals.

Statements Made for Medical Diagnosis. The importance of verbatim and accurate documentation of statements made by the patient to the medical professional during the sexual assault examination cannot be sufficiently stressed.

Federal Rule of Evidence section 803(4), allows "statements made for purposes of medical diagnosis or treatment and describing medical history or past or present symptoms, pain, or sensations, or the inception or general character of the cause or external source thereof insofar as reasonably pertinent to diagnosis or treatment" to be admitted into evidence during a criminal trial.

Most jurisdictions admit statements of patients regarding their present medical condition if made to a physician for purposes of diagnosis and treatment. The basis of admissibility rests on the theory that a patient has a strong motivation to be truthful to a physician who is attempting to diagnose or provide treatment (McCormick §266, 1984). This guarantee of trustworthiness includes statements regarding past medical conditions and history provided to physicians for purposes of diagnosis or treatment. Also, a statement regarding the cause of a condition, if the statement is reasonably pertinent to diagnosis or treatment, is admissible as a statement of medical diagnosis (*Shell Oil v Industrial Commission*, 1954).

Frequently, courts will strike out information as to the identity of the perpetrator, while statements as to how an act was accomplished may be admissible. Regardless of the fact that the court may "modify" the statement, it remains vital for the medical professional to document the statement verbatim into the medical record.

If the patient is a young child, proof must be offered that the child was aware of the physician's capacity to provide medical care to the child. If a child does not understand the physician's purpose, the child will not have a "selfish" motive to be truthful (Zhender, 1994). The explanation to the child may be as simple as, "I am a doctor. My job is to check your body. I want to make sure your body is OK. You need to tell me if anything hurts on your body. Did anything happen to your body?" At trial, it is the prosecutor's job to establish the foundation that the child understood what the physician's job was at the time the statement was made (Fed R Evid 803(4), [advisory committee's comments]).

Excited Utterance. Patients undergoing a sexual assault examination are often emotional and suffering from the recent assault. Accurately and thoroughly documenting the demeanor of the patient in the medical record can be vital to assuring that a statement made by the patient be admissible in court.

Federal Rule of Evidence section 803(2) allows "[a] statement relating to a startling event or condition made while the declarant was under the stress of excitement caused by the event or condition" to be admissible into court. The circumstances that may produce a condition of excitement, which temporarily stills the capacity of reflection and produces utterances free of conscious fabrication, are considered to make these statements more reliable (6 Wigmore § 1747, p. 135).

To allow the admission of an "excited utterance" into evidence, proof that the statement was made while under the stress of excitement caused by the event must be proven. The witness to the statement must be able to testify about this type of information in court. Criminal cases may take up to a year or longer to come to trial. Sexual assault professionals may conduct dozens or even hundreds of sexual assault examinations every year. It is impossible to remember the details of every examination and the demeanor of each patient. Accordingly, the witness to an "excited utterance" is well served by recording in the medical record the speaker's emotions, demeanor, and verbatim words. A written record of the emotions can be used to refresh the witnesses recollection when called to testify.

Recording the demeanor, emotion, and statement of the patient in the medical record provides the information with an air of credibility. It is the responsibility of any medical professional to accurately record information in the medical record. The judge, jury, and defense attorney will have more confidence in the accuracy of information included in an official document.

Ten Tips for Being a Successful Expert Witness. Going to court can be a traumatic event—even for the medical expert witness. Several things can be done to reduce the stress of the event and increase the effectiveness of the information presented. Although sexual assault examiners are often highly trained and skilled in conducting a sexual assault examination, little if any training is provided on how to be an effective witness in the courtroom.

Regardless of whether the sexual assault examiner is called as an expert witness or a percipient witness, here are 10 helpful tips to being an effective witness.

1. ***Pretrial preparation***: Direct and cross-examination can be treacherous—especially without proper preparation. Preparation does not mean simply reading the medical report a couple of times before taking the witness stand. True preparation requires the medical witness to read and digest the entire medical record including the laboratory reports on all of the samples taken. It is important for the medical expert to have an overview of all of the information pertinent to the patient.

   Consider the following scenario. On cross-examination, the defense attorney asks if a medical finding of a sexually transmitted disease was present before the sexual assault. The medical witness responds that she does not know insofar as she never examined the patient's prior medical records and did not ask the patient during the examination. A juror's confidence in the medical witness's testimony is directly linked to the quality of information he or she possesses.

   Medical witnesses must prepare a curriculum vitae or resume before testifying. Of vital important are education, training, and experience. Even experienced witnesses often cannot recall all relevant training or experience while under the pressure of testifying. Preparing a comprehensive resume and providing it to the prosecutor and defense attorney before testifying is advised. All parties can use the curriculum vitae as a reference to allow the examination to progress with ease. The witness can, of course, reference the curriculum vitae during the examination to ensure no information has been overlooked.

2. ***Pretrial meeting with the prosecutor***: Every witness, especially an expert witness, should meet with the prosecutor before the day of testifying. Taking the stand blind is as dangerous as a game of Russian roulette. Numerous items should be discussed during this meeting.

   The prosecutor should outline the topics that will be discussed at trial. Often, prosecutors are unaware of the significance of certain medical evidence. This meeting should provide a time for the medical professional to educate the prosecutor about significant facts that will be of assistance at trial.

   Often, prosecutors are unaware of the appropriate question to be asked in order to elicit helpful information from the medical expert. The expert should assist the prosecutor in forming questions that will provide the expert with the right opportunity to testify to pertinent information.

   Possible topics of cross-examination should be discussed. These topics can range from mistakes or omissions in the medical report and biases of the witness, to potential defense theories regarding the medical testimony. The witness should ask the prosecutor if there is any additional information or reports available regarding the case. In this way, the witness can be as completely prepared as possible.

   Be aware that the defense attorney may ask to meet with you before testifying. Although you are not required to participate in such a meeting, it is necessary to be prepared to explain your decision on cross-examination. Meeting with the defense attorney may make you appear to be a neutral and unbiased witness in front of the jury. If you choose to meet with the defense attorney, keep in mind that you can bring the prosecutor or an investigator and can openly tape record the conversation. Always notify the prosecutor of the meeting and the content of the discussion.

3. ***Professionalism and promptness***: Court is where the phrase "hurry up and wait" certainly applies. It is easy to become frustrated if you are made to sit and

wait outside of a courtroom, only to learn your that testimony is not needed or that you need to return the following day. To mitigate these experiences, it is important to develop a good working relationship between prosecutors and medical professionals. The medical witness should call the day preceding the date of the subpoenaed appearance to determine if attendance is required. Prosecutors should promptly inform witnesses if they are not needed. Such simple courtesies will immediately improve or create a working relationship.

With a confirmed appearance schedule, medical professionals must be on time. Some judges are famous for taking no excuses as to why the next witness is not available. Not only may a judge publicly humiliate the prosecutor, but he or she may also force the prosecutor to conclude the case. Plan for traffic snarls, parking problems, and getting lost when going to court.

It is important to dress appropriately when going to court to testify, especially in a jury trial. Defense experts are often professionally trained and coached on their appearance and testimony. Jurors often make preliminary decisions on credibility based on the witness's appearance. Accordingly, what you wear and how you look does matter. Medical professionals should feel comfortable at any court appearance wearing a well-pressed traditional and conservative suit. Scrubs or traditional medical attire is not appropriate in the courtroom environment.

4. *Make it simple*. The average education level of a jury panel is eighth grade. Consequently, it is important to remember to structure answers in a simple and nontechnical fashion. For example, the word, "supine" should be replaced with "on her back." Before testifying, take a moment and consider all of the words used in daily conversation that can be considered technical language.

5. *Incorporate demonstrative aids*. It is important to incorporate demonstrative aids (exhibits) into testimony. We are a visual society. People are more accustomed to watching television than to sitting in a classroom type environment listening to a lecture. Hence, some jurors will lose interest if no photographs or other physical evidence is used. Also consider that jurors are more likely to remember evidence if it is communicated 3 times. Using demonstrative aids will allow for a repeated presentation of important facts.

For example, in a court case involving the rape of a young woman, first present the medical evidence of injuries by orally stating what was found. Second, use an anatomical diagram of the vaginal area. Mark on this board where the injuries were found. Third, present the colposcope photographs taken during the examination and indicate where in the photograph the injuries are located. If presented in this manner, the jurors are more likely to remember the evidence.

If demonstrative evidence is to be used in court, it is vital to practice. If you are speaking while facing the exhibit, it will be difficult for the jury to hear. Finally, consider how to incorporate the exhibit into the testimony. Often, a witness will need to leave the witness chair and approach an exhibit. Ask the questioning attorney or judge if this is possible. Permission will always be granted. Face the jury or have your side toward the jury. It is bad form to have your back to the jury. Do not worry if your back is toward the judge or even the prosecutor. Your audience is the jury. If possible, stand to the side of the exhibit. Obscuring the exhibit from the jury's sight during testimony destroys the benefit of a demonstrative aid.

Consider if a laser or wooden pointer will be helpful while at the exhibit. If you plan on using a felt marker, bring one to court with you and make sure it works. Also consider what color will be best visible when applied to the exhibit. It is helpful to practice testifying with an exhibit before coming to court. It can be difficult to talk, mark, stand correctly, and make sure that every member of the jury can see the exhibit during the testimony.

6. ***Be polite to the defense attorney.*** Defense attorneys are just doing their job. Regardless of the attitude of the defense attorney, medical witnesses must always remember that they are nonbiased, independent witnesses. Medical witnesses testify regarding the scientific findings that are not modified by whim or unfounded opinion. A defense attorney may attack the medical witness personally or professionally while on the witness stand. This is inappropriate, and prosecutors should object and attempt to halt this conduct. However, judges and prosecutors are not always sensitive to the attack. Sometimes, the objective of the defense attorney's attack is to unnerve the witness or cause him or her to become rude and aggressive and to appear biased.

It is important to keep your cool while on the witness stand. If the defense attorney is rude, condescending, or arrogant, do not react in kind. Be as polite and professional on cross-examination as during direct examination. Take comfort in knowing that the jury will acknowledge the attitude of the defense attorney.

7. ***Be aware of your body language.*** Body language is the silent witness. Many witnesses do not realize how differently they react to direct examination versus cross-examination. A witness who is comfortable on direct examination will sit back in the witness chair and answer questions in a cadence helpful to the jury. However, this well-composed witness can unknowingly become fidgety, fast speaking, and uncomfortable on cross-examination. Experience on the witness stand is not the only cure to these ills. By recognizing the existence of bad habits (ring twisting, rocking, arm crossing, or twisted facial gestures), a witness can begin to cease the nervous reaction.

It is vital that witnesses understand that a nervous reaction on cross-examination is noticed and distracting to jurors. It is reasonable that jurors might question the confidence a witness has in his or her opinion if he or she appears nervous on cross-examination.

8. ***Be assertive on cross-examination.*** On direct examination, witnesses are asked nonleading, usually open-ended questions that allow for a complete answer. Not so on cross-examination. Frequently, questions are couched to allow for a "yes" or "no" response. Often, the medical expert has a great deal of information to provide that would be helpful to the jury. Sadly, the prosecutor usually has no idea that the witness desires to provide a detailed answer.

It is exceptionally helpful to the prosecutor if the medical witness, when restricted to a "yes" or "no" response would simply state, "I would like to explain, but my answer would be yes/no." This statement notifies the prosecutor that a follow-up question should be asked on redirect examination. This also notifies the jury that there is additional relevant information that needs to be elicited.

9. ***Don't become a target.*** It is vital for medical witnesses to understand the parameters of their expertise. It is deadly for a witness to testify to expert information for which he or she is not qualified. It is inappropriate for prosecutors and defense attorneys to try to solicit expert testimony from an unqualified witness.

During the pretrial meeting, medical witnesses should explore all of the areas of information which the prosecutor intends to question. Defining this list will allow the medical witness to decide whether or not he or she is qualified to render testimony. Extending oneself further than his or her expertise allows questions that can destroy a person's credibility in the present case as well as all future cases.

10. ***Debrief with the prosecutor.*** A follow-up meeting with the prosecutor is beneficial to both the witness and the prosecutor. This meeting should be focused on each party providing kudos and constructive criticism to the other.

Key Point:
To be a successful expert witness, the following 10 factors are extremely helpful:
1. *Pretrial preparation*
2. *Pretrial meeting with the prosecutor*
3. *Professionalism and promptness*
4. *Make it simple*
5. *Incorporate demonstrative aids*
6. *Be polite to the defense attorney*
7. *Be aware of your body language*
8. *Be assertive on cross-examination*
9. *Don't become a target*
10. *Debrief with the prosecutor*

Table 32-2. The Direct Examination

PROSECUTOR QUESTIONS AND EXPERT WITNESS RESPONSE SUGGESTIONS

— Full name and spelling

— Current occupation
   State full title
   Duties and responsibilities in current position

— Prior occupation (if experience enhances credibility with the jury, such as rape crisis counselor, police officer, evidence technician, etc.)
   State full title
   Duties and responsibilities in past position
   Describe relevance of past position to current testimony

— Educational background
   Associate degree: date, institution, and discipline
   Undergraduate degree: date, institution, and discipline
   Graduate degree: date, institution, and discipline

— Medical training and experience
   Residency: date, institution, and specialty
   Internship: date, institution, and specialty
   Fellowship: date, institution, and specialty

— Specific sexual assault training
   Child sexual abuse training (be specific in amount and practicality of training)
   Physical abuse training (be specific in amount and practicality of training)
   Sexual assault training (be specific in amount and practicality of training)

— Peer review participation
   — What is peer review?
   — How often does peer review occur?
   — How is peer review conducted?
   — What is/are the benefits of peer review?
   — How often do you participate in peer review?
   — Describe your participation in peer review.

— Teaching
   — Do you train other professionals in the area of sexual assault examination?
   — What percentage of your current position involves training others in this expertise?
   — Does your teaching include lecturing or hand-on training also?
   — How long have you been responsible for training others in the area of sexual assault examinations?
   — Approximately how many other professionals have you trained?

— Continuing education
   —Do you participate in continuing education?
   —Define for the jury what constitutes continuing education.
   —How much continuing education do you receive on an annual basis?
   —How is the continuing education applicable to your expertise as a sexual assault examiner?

— Publications
   —Have you published any scholarly articles, studies, etc., in the area of sexual assault or abuse?
   —Have you published any scholarly articles, studies, etc., in any other areas of medical research?

(continued)

Table 32-2. *(continued)*

— Is there anything else that you should tell the jury about your training, experience, or background that would assist the jury in making a decision?

— In the course of your professional duties, have you ever performed a sexual assault examination to determine if a person was sexually assaulted?
    — How many sexual assault examinations have you personally performed?
    — How many sexual assault examinations have you observed being performed?

— Have you ever supervised the performance of a sexual assault examination?

— You stated earlier that you are involved in training other professionals in the performance of sexual assault examinations?
    — Who do you train to perform sexual assault examinations?
    — How do you perform this training?

— Have you previously qualified as an expert in the area of sexual assault forensic examination?
    — Which courts?
    — How many times have you qualified?
    — In what areas of expertise have you qualified as an expert?

— Is the manner in which a sexual assault examination is conducted regulated by a protocol?
    — What is a protocol for purposes of a sexual assault examination?

— Is there a protocol in place in your jurisdiction for sexual assault examination?
    — When was the protocol for sexual assault examination established?
    — Is the protocol ever evaluated and revised?
        History of protocol being reevaluated and revised.

— Please explain the procedure required in the protocol for sexual assault examination.
    This should include a short generalized answer, including information such as:
        Obtain a verbal history of the sexual assault.
        Conduct an external physical examination.
        Conduct a genital examination.

— What is a history?
    — Why do you obtain a history?
    — From whom do you obtain the history?
    — Why is a history obtained at the beginning of the examination?
    — Does a history assist you in forming your ultimate medical opinion or diagnosis?
    — How does the history assist you in forming a medical opinion?

— Do you document the history that you receive?
    — On what form do you document your findings?

— Does the protocol require this form to be completed?
    — Have you received training on how to correctly complete the form?
    — Approximately how many times have you completed this form?

— When do you document the information that you receive while obtaining the history?
    — Why do you document the information at this time?

— After obtaining and documenting the history received, what do you do next?

(continued)

Table 32-2. *(continued)*

— What is involved in performing the external examination?
> **This should outline the items to note during the examination, such as:**
>> **Temperature, blood pressure, weight, age, etc.**
>> **Demeanor and attitude of patient.**
>> **Bruising, scratches, etc.**

— Do you document the information and findings that you obtained during the external examination?
> — How?
> — When?
> — Where?

— After completing the external examination, what do you do next?

— Please explain how the genital examination is conducted.
> **Examination of external genitalia:**
>> **Labia majora**
> — Where is this?
> — What is the purpose of the labia majora?
>> **Labia minora**

— Where is this?
— What is the purpose of the labia minora?

— Continue through all parts of external genitalia
— I would assume that your next step is to conduct an examination of the internal genital area?
— Are there various positions used when conducting this part of the examination?
> — What are the different position(s) used to complete the examination?
> — Please describe the various positions used.

— Why are multiple positions used to complete the examination?

— What are the names of the body parts that are examined?
> **Vagina**
> **Hymen**

— What do you look for when examining the hymen?
> — Are all hymens shaped the same?
> — What are the different shapes possible?
> — What is the significance of the shape of a hymen?
> — Does the shape of the hymen affect your examination?
> — Does the shape of the hymen affect whether it can be injured?
> — Is the hymen located on the interior or exterior of the female body?
> — How far inside the female body is the hymen located?

— Continue with other significant body parts.

— Does the protocol require that you document these findings in a certain manner?
> — How?
> — When?
> — Where?

— How long does a typical sexual assault examination last?
> **Waiting time**
> **History**
> **Physical examination**

(continued)

Table 32-2. *(continued)*

— On _____, did you conduct a sexual assault examination on _____?

— In conducting this examination, was the protocol followed?

— In following the protocol, you obtained a history from the victim prior to conducting the examination. What is the history that you received?

— Did you receive additional historic information from any other source(s)?
Family members
Detectives, beat officers, social workers, etc.
Hearsay problems

— In accordance with the protocol, did you record the information that you received?

— While you were taking the history, did you have an opportunity to observe the victim's demeanor and attitude?

— What was her demeanor and attitude?
— Based on your training and experience, was her demeanor and attitude consistent with a person who has suffered a traumatic event?
— Why?

— Did you record her demeanor on the required form?
— When did you do this?

— Does the victim's demeanor affect your ultimate medical opinion?
— How?
— Why?

— After obtaining the history, your protocol requires an external examination to be conducted. Did you do this?

— Describe the examination that you conducted.

— What were your findings?
— Were your findings consistent with a person who has suffered a traumatic event?
— Why?
— How so?

— Did you document your findings from the external examination as required by protocol?
— When?
— How?

— What specifically did you document on the form?

— Did you do anything to visually document your findings from the external examination?
Hand-drawing on the required form.
Photographs:
   Make sure photographs have perspective.
   Use a ruler.
   Use a color scale.
— How do you identify the photographs as being of this victim if no face can be seen?
— Did you do this in this case?

— Is there anything else regarding the external examination that we have not discussed?

(continued)

Table 32-2. *(continued)*

— According to protocol, did you next conduct the genital examination?
— Did you follow the procedures as required by the protocol?
— How did you perform the examination?
— Please describe how the examination began.
    External genitalia
    Internal genital area
    Position(s) used to complete examination.
        Use diagram/board to demonstrate to jury.
        Define the different parts of genital area.
        Explain in plain English.
— What were your findings with respect to the examination of the external genitalia?
    Labia majora
    Labia minora
— Did you document your findings in accordance with protocol?
— Did you next conduct an examination of internal genital area?
— Did you examine the part(s) of the body that you earlier described to us:
    — Vagina?
    — Hymen?
    — Etc.

— What tools did you use to complete the examination?
    Swabs (size?)
    Speculum
    Colposcope
    — What is a speculum?
    — What is the purpose of a speculum?

— What did you discover during the internal genital examination?
    Vagina
    Hymen
    Injuries found:
        Type of injury
        Location of injury

— I am showing you what has been marked as _____; what is it?
— Please explain this diagram to the jury.
— Please explain the significance of the numbers.
— Please mark on the diagram the injuries that you found.
— You've placed a mark on the _____; what does that mark represent?

— Is the placement of an injury significant?
    — Why?
        Explain in detail.
— Were your findings different depending on the position of the victim?
    — Why is this significant?

— You stated earlier that you also used a colposcope during the examination. What is a colposcope?
    — Please explain what the function of a colposcope camera is during a sexual assault examination?
    — How is it used?
    — Does it actually touch the victim?

(continued)

Table 32-2. *(continued)*

— What is the benefit of using a colposcope rather than a traditional camera?
> **The subject matter is magnified by the colposcope.**
— Why are colposcopic photographs taken during the sexual assault examination?

— I am showing you what has been marked as _____; what is it?
— How do you recognize this as being a photograph of _____?
— Please identify the injuries that you have described finding on the victim.
— You earlier stated that the placement of the injury is significant. Using the photograph, demonstrate and explain why placement is significant.

— Were you able to determine the age of the injuries?
> — How is it possible to determine the age of an injury?
> — Do you have an opinion regarding the age of the injury?
> — What is your opinion?
> — What do you base your opinion on?

— Did you form an expert opinion regarding the cause of the genital injury?

— What is your expert opinion?

— What did you base your opinion on?
> **Examination, history by victim and others, experience, continuing education, etc.**
— Based on your examination, do you have an opinion as to whether your findings are consistent with the victim's history of sexual assault?
— What is your opinion?
— What do you base your opinion on?

For example, this is the perfect opportunity for the prosecutor to critique nervous habits a witness displayed on cross-examination, or for the witness to express why the question the prosecutor posed did not allow for the necessary information to be provided.

Direct Examination: What to Expect. There are of course many variations on the order of questions of a direct examination. It is important to be familiar with the type of questions that will be posed in order to prepare complete and accurate answers. Witnesses must be prepared to discuss at length their education, training, and experience as well as the facts of the specific case. It is the extent of the education, training, and experience that gives the jury the ability to put weight on the opinions expressed by the expert witness. Often, the trial boils down to a "competition of the experts," and whoever testifies more professionally and completely wins (**Table 32-2**).

Surviving Cross-Examination

Once you have completed direct examination, you will undoubtedly face a rigorous cross-examination. There are 6 basic areas of attack that a medical professional should be prepared to handle.

1. ***Expertise***: Are you truly qualified to testify as an expert in the areas questioned by the prosecutor? One goal of cross-examination is to give the appearance that you are not. Hence, make sure you are adequately qualified. Do not testify outside your area of expertise. Be prepared with facts to support your expertise.

2. ***Basis of conclusion***: It is reasonable to inquire into the facts that allow an expert to form an opinion. It is also reasonable to question whether or not the

Key Point:
The 6 basic areas of attack that a medical professional should be prepared to handle are as follows:
1. Expertise
2. Basis of conclusion
3. Age of information
4. Source of facts
5. Conclusion
6. Prejudice

expert has considered the theory propounded by the defense. Even if the theory is untenable, it is unprofessional for an expert to dismiss the defense theory without giving it adequate consideration. It is important to be prepared to explain to the jury why a theory can be easily dismissed. In this way, the expert is truly unbiased and open-minded.

3. *Age of information*: Again, an important part of preparing to go to court is to assure that you have the most recent information available regarding the facts. If reports were generated after your examination, it is incumbent upon you to obtain this information and be prepared. Don't let yourself be criticized on cross-examination for not having current and complete information.

4. *Source of facts*: What are your sources of information? Because defense witnesses usually have no ability to be professionally involved in the medical care of the victim, they are often supplied all relevant information by the defense attorney. Their knowledge of the case is solely from review of the records. This is a very dangerous situation for an expert to occupy. Medical experts testifying solely based on review of records need to assure themselves that all information has been provided. Innocent mistakes can easily be made, records can be misplaced or lost. If possible, review the original records contained in the court file or if possible, obtain permission to review the medical file at the hospital or medical office where the original is located.

5. *Conclusion*: All trial lawyers dream of their "Perry Mason" moment in which, after a rigorous cross-examination, the witness admits guilt. When an expert witness is on the stand, this moment is achieved when he or she realizes his or her opinion is mistaken and admits this fact. Much effort will be expended to achieve this scenario. To prevent this situation, experts must listen very carefully to the information presented to them on cross-examination. Do not agree to discuss a study you have not personally read. Do not take the word of a defense attorney as to what a study says or stands for. Always ask to see a copy of the study the defense attorney is referring to, and ask the judge for time to read it before commenting. Listen carefully to facts included in a hypothetical question. Speak up if the hypothetical question is not relevant to the facts in the particular case. The key to success on cross-examination is to be aware of misinterpretation and misstatement of facts.

6. *Prejudices*: "So, how much are you being paid to testify here today?" "Have you ever testified for the defense in a sexual assault case?" and "Why didn't you return my telephone call?" are just a few of the questions that can be posed to demonstrate prejudice on behalf of the sexual assault examiner.

These questions and others like them are easily handled if you are prepared for them to be posed. Think about why you have never testified for the defense before you find yourself in the witness chair. Is it that cases with no medical evidence are not prosecuted? Have you consulted with the defense, and after hearing your opinion has the defendant pled guilty? Would you be willing to testify for the defense if called? Do you change your testimony depending on which side calls you to testify? If asked, "Have you ever testified for the defense?" do not simply say no. Respond, "I have never been called by the defense, but would gladly testify." It is important to take control, especially when your impartiality is being questioned.

CROSS-EXAMINATION OF DEFENDANT

Cross-examination of witnesses in open court begins after the prosecutor has rested her "case-in-chief" or her production of the evidence against the defendant. A prosecutor cross-examines the defendant or the defendant's witnesses, who testify after the prosecution finishes its case. Preparation for cross-examination, however, must begin months in advance of trial. Specifically, whenever the defense to the charges is identified or known, preparation for cross-examination should begin then. Prosecutors may cross-examine, categorically, expert witnesses for the defendant, defense lay witnesses, or the defendant. In the prosecution of sexual assault crimes, the applicable defenses are identity, consent, or the defendant's mental impairment that prevents the rapist from forming the requisite criminal intent to be held accountable for his conduct.

As soon as the defense is known (by way of the defendant's statements, the other facts, or the defense attorney's statements or motions) the prosecutor must evaluate the facts in light of the pertinent jury instructions. That evaluation enables the prosecutor to decide whether the facts or the applicable laws are the best tools to use to defeat the defense, in the case. Generally, the facts are the best tools to defeat a consent defense, whereas the laws are the best tools to defeat an impairment defense. Most commonly, the facts, as proven by physical evidence and forensic analysis, provide the requisite proof of identification accurately and beyond successful challenge. Occasionally, the identity defense will involve defense expert witnesses to challenge the forensic analysis. Complete familiarity with both the facts and the law is key to choosing which will be the primary subject of a cross-examination. Then the prosecutor tailors and executes the examination in a way that remains true to the choice between facts or law.

When cross-examining defense expert witnesses, early preparation includes obtaining background materials pertinent to the witness. These materials are not only resumes and publications but also transcripts of prior testimony; news articles or industry publications about the witness; the witness's fee and cost rates; other cases the expert has been involved in; and the relationship between the defense attorney and the witness, the defense bar, or other pertinent professional or personal relationships of the witness. What is most important to remember regarding an expert witness is that the expert cannot change the facts or the laws. Both are what they are for the expert as well as the lawyers; all an expert can do is interpret the facts or the laws. An interpretation, even founded in education or experience, is always a subjective interpretation.

Knowing that an expert provides only an interpretation, the expert's paradigm is examined. An expert, by employer, by personal belief, or by both, will have biases and agendas. A prosecutor finds them and exploits them. An expert, as does every other human being, has some motivation for testifying. A defense expert has motivation for testifying for the defendant, someone accused of sexual criminal behavior. Whatever that expert's motive is, the prosecutor can find it. Defense experts in the forensic analysis of DNA, the most common type of defense expert in an identity defense, are never employed by the government or the law enforcement agency; their motivation is never to maintain the integrity of the criminal justice system. If that was their motivation, then the expert should work for the government to ensure integrity by being a part of the process affecting all of the cases. Because the expert has a private employer, the expert is either motivated by greed or too incompetent to work for the government. (An expert for the defendant will always testify, if cornered, that they are motivated by greed and prosecutors know it.)

After identifying the expert's motivation, biases, and history, prosecutors examine the information that was given to the expert to assist her in forming her expert opinion. Specifically, the prosecutor examines the facts of the case that were given to the expert and in what form or method they were given to her. Opinions, given by experts, are based, theoretically, on facts. Prosecutors know the true facts. They know what facts should have been given to the expert to be truthful about the case. A prosecutor obtains confirmation of what facts were provided to the expert. Then she reviews to find what, if any, facts were not given to the expert and learns why. Was the expert not given facts or given incorrect facts in order to manipulate the opinion the expert could provide? Or was the expert not given facts because the evidence was not collected or preserved? Was the expert given all of the facts but is ignoring some or many of them? Questions regarding which facts the expert relied upon or did not rely upon are crucial questions to establish the absolute dependency between that opinion and some facts. Experts must concede that facts determine opinion—change the facts and that given opinion must fail.

The same is true of the pertinent laws. An expert's opinion is helpful to a defendant only if the law recognizes the opinion as creating a legitimate defense. Rarely are experts fluent in the law. Prosecutors exploit the expert's ignorance of the materiality, significance, or conformity to the laws of the jurisdiction. Finally, prosecutors should not, and rarely do, attempt to defeat or discredit an expert's opinion by becoming an expert and engaging in a personal quarrel with the expert. In the odd case when a prosecutor decides to challenge the expert's interpretation as unsound, she will do so only after receiving assistance, education, and direction from other experts in that field.

In cross-examination, less is always more persuasive. A prosecutor narrows, sharpens, and limits questions to bring clarity to the structure of the cross-examination. Less is always more.

In most ways, preparation for the cross-examination of other lay witnesses, the defendant or defense witnesses, is the same as for expert witnesses. Knowing the facts of the case is crucial; after all, the defendant knows all of the facts of his crimes, and so should the prosecutor. Prosecutors review everything regarding the defendant or his witnesses they can obtain, far beyond the reports regarding the primary case: medical, educational, employment, financial records as well as anything written or said by others who know the defendant.

Again, prosecutors identify the defense and tailor their examination accordingly. If identity is the defense, there should be an alibi the prosecutor will break. If the defense is mental impairment, the cross-examination will highlight all of the defendant's statements, actions, or both that will demonstrate the defendant's functional, purposeful mind. If the defense is that the victim's consent excuses his conduct, then the cross-examination will establish 2 things: the prosecutor will establish through the defendant and/or his witnesses the vast number of facts are exactly as the victim testified them to be and that there is only a single fact, the victim's consent, in dispute. The corroboration of the victim regarding a majority of facts demonstrates the victim's accuracy and credibility. The defendant has everything to gain and nothing to lose by disputing the victim's accuracy about the ultimate issue of consent; but jurors understand that when the defendant admits the victim is correct (and therefore truthful) about all of the facts save one, it is the defendant who is not to be believed. Conversely, if the defendant knows absolutely nothing about many facts such as the temperature, the smells, the sounds, the lighting, but the victim does, her heightened sense of awareness, her acute observations and recollections are consistent with her refusal and the consequent acts against her will that terrified her. The victim had every reason to pay the utmost attention to her surroundings—she wanted to save her dignity and her life.

Cross-examination of the defendant follows the pattern of eliciting the defendant's confirmation of as much of the victim's testimony as possible followed by clearly isolating him in his claim of the victim's consent to the acts. In addition, that corroboration will include the planning and the purpose behind the defendant's conduct: to facilitate the rape of the victim. The defendant will admit a number of facts that undermine his consent defense, such as the disparate size, height, and weight differences between himself and the victim, that his holding of her caused bruises, or that her clothes were not torn before the assault. Slowly, the cross-examination will emphasize that many of the case facts are not in dispute—only consent. He is then limited in his dispute to a dispute of only a single element of the charge against him. Less is more.

Defendants always have bias and motive behind their testimony; prosecutors will always find and exploit them. The defendant has known what the trial date will be in time for preparation. He knows the charges, the penalties, and he has heard all of the witnesses' testimony throughout the trial.

Finally, all cross-examination questions should be closed—completely closed. Cross-examination by a prosecutor is not when the prosecutor allows a defendant to tell his story; it is when the prosecutor identifies the facts and obtains, unwillingly, the defendant's concession to the truth. The prosecutor knows what the answers will be and structures the questions to elicit those answers. Prosecutors know to listen, however, because desperate defendants do desperate things; the defendant's answers may become more fantastical, more impossible, more defensive, and more absurd.

Successful cross-examination exposes and defeats unsuccessful defenses precisely, methodically, and quickly after preparation and design.

OPENING STATEMENTS

The importance of the opening statement cannot be overlooked. Studies have confirmed that a great majority of jurors make up their minds following opening statements in a case. In addition, after an especially lengthy jury selection process, this is the time that the jurors are anxious to finally hear what the case is all about. It may, therefore, be a time of great juror attention.

Establish Goals

The goals that the prosecutor establishes for the opening statement are going to primarily depend on the type of case being tried, as well as its strengths and weaknesses. To the extent the prosecutor may have been unable to do so during jury selection, he or she may need to educate the jury with regard to issues such as a developmentally delayed or retarded victim, the fact that the victim recanted, or perhaps delayed reporting the assault. Other goals may include things such as preparing jurors for sexual language, or for a victim who is over- or under-emotional on the stand. If the victim is hostile toward the prosecutor, it will be necessary to prepare jurors for that emotion as well.

It is important that the prosecutor does not lose sight of the fact that jurors are forming an impression of him or her during the opening statement. In those jurisdictions that follow the federal model and use primarily judge-conducted jury selection, this is the prosecutor's first opportunity to speak face to face with the jurors. It is good to be conversational, yet professional in delivery. As in jury selection, eye contact and body language are important.

The Importance of the Theme and Theory

The theme is the emotional context surrounding the entire trial process. The theme should begin in jury selection, weave through the opening statement, be reinforced through the state's witnesses, and culminate with the closing argument. The theme should explain how the event took place. The theory, on the other hand, is the legal basis for prosecution. In some cases, the theme and theory are one and the same.

It may be helpful to think of the theme as a newspaper headline. It should be 1 line, phrase, or saying that simplifies the case. It should be memorable and easy to relate and remember. The theme, ideally, will be parroted back multiple times during jury deliberations as the jurors piece together the evidence produced in the case.

Related to the theme is the importance of telling the story. A good story, in the form of a narrative, will help to simplify the case for the jurors. A good narrative also makes otherwise mundane and dull facts interesting. It should be clear, easy to follow, and compelling.

It is good to begin using the theme as early as jury selection. For those jurisdictions who utilize attorney-conducted jury selection, this process will be much easier than those who follow either judge-conducted or the federal model of jury selection.

However, whichever model of jury selection is followed, the importance of weaving the theme throughout the opening statement cannot be underestimated.

Covering the Issues

The prosecution, especially in cases of sexual assault, must often deal with various issues that are not present in other types of prosecutions. There may be issues pertaining to the victim regarding her continued contact with the defendant, for example, writing a love letter to the defendant after the assault or failing to report the assault in a timely fashion. Other issues that often arise in sexual assault cases are drug and alcohol problems, sexual lifestyle issues, and sexual preferences. It is important to not hide these potentially negative facts, but to weave these negative facts into the opening statement in a positive way. As an example, it may be helpful to talk about these facts in such a way as to coincide with the theme of manipulation and control on the part of the defendant. By picturing the defendant as a manipulating and controlling individual, the prosecutor has not only defined the defendant to the jury, but has also helped to explain the weaknesses in the prosecution's case with regard to the victim's behaviors and reactions. It then explains and simplifies these issues for the jury.

Another way to explain problem issues in the prosecution's case is to find ways to personalize the victim. By talking about the human side of a person's life, the jury will perhaps empathize or identify with the person.

Paint a Picture

Unlike other times during the trial, the attorney can control the use of words. The prosecutor should strive to use those words to paint a picture for the jury that they will be able to take into the deliberation room with them. Opening with a gripping fact that will capture the attention of the jury and then weaving the other facts around it is a useful technique.

Although an opening statement is not an argument, it can be equally as persuasive. Powerful, descriptive language should be used. The use of adverbs rather than adjectives can assist in painting a more descriptive picture of the event (e.g., viciously, not viscous; savagely, not savage; brutally, not brutal).

It is important to avoid using legal terms in the opening statement or getting bogged down in the elements of the crime(s) charged. If legal terms must be used, the prosecutor should take the time to explain them to the jury.

CLOSING ARGUMENT

The time when an attorney can be most creative is also when he or she can commit the most errors. Because sexual assault trials are generally very emotional by nature, emotional arguments are often used in closing arguments. Emotional arguments, however, can easily run afoul of the rules of summation and may be counter-productive with the jury. Goals of the closing argument should be to (1) reiterate the theme; (2) deal with the defense case; and (3) show corroboration of the state's case.

Reiterate the Theme

This is the time to give a sound summation that will make the jury feel good about rendering a guilty verdict. The same theme that was developed through jury selection and opening statement and carried through the trial testimony should be reiterated 1 more time for the jury to hear and remember. Now that the case has been completed, the theme should be more understandable for the jury, because they have heard all of the evidence to corroborate the theme.

Deal with the Defense Case

No matter how absurd the defense case may be, it must be dealt with in the closing argument. The unreasonableness of the defense case cannot be assumed to be apparent to the jury. The state should talk about it, and, if applicable, show how even the defense case corroborates the victim's testimony. If the defense case does not corroborate the victim's testimony, the unreasonableness of such a defense should be argued.

Show Corroboration of the State's Case

Showing corroboration of the state's case can be done through a multitude of means. Perhaps the defendant's own admissions can corroborate the state's version of the events. Even if the defendant fails to admit the ultimate criminal act, perhaps the defendant admitting less significant events will allow the state to be able to argue the accuracy of the historian (the victim). Corroboration can be shown through the testimony of other witnesses, by the victim's intimate details of the attack, and by any prior consistent statements of the victim. If other victims of the defendant were found, perhaps those "other acts" can serve as corroboration of the victim's testimony. Obviously, any and all physical evidence of the crime serves as corroboration of the rape, as well as actions by the victim that can be attributed to posttraumatic stress disorder or rape trauma syndrome.

Sexual assault crimes are among the most difficult to prove to a jury. Ending a closing argument on these corroborative points is a positive finish for the state's case.

REFERENCES

6 John H. Wigmore, Evidence in Trials at Common Law § 1747 James H. Chadbourn rev ed. Boston: Little, Brown & Co.; 1978:135.

18 USCA Child victims' and child witnesses' rights §3509 (West 1999).

124 Cong Rec 34,913 (1978).

Adamson v Department of Social Services, 254 Cal Rptr 667 (Cal Ct App 1988).

American Prosecutors Research Institute (APRI). *Investigation and Prosecution of Child Abuse*. 2nd ed. Alexandria, Va: APRI; 1993.

American Prosecutors Research Institute (APRI). *Date rape drugs*. In: The Prosecution of Rohypnol and GHB Related Sexual Assaults. Alexandria, Va: APRI; 1999:7.

Ark Code Ann 16-42-101. Admissibility of evidence of victim's prior sexual conduct. 2002.

Baumgarden J. Burden of proof. *Harper's Magazine*. October 2001:303(1817);72-73.

Bergen RK. Marital rape. March 1999. Violence against Women On-line Resources. Available at: http://www.vaw.umn.edu/Vawnet/mrape.htm. Accessed October 24, 2001.

Best Practices for Seizing Electronic Evidence. Washington DC: US Secret Service, International Association of Chiefs of Police, National Institute of Justice; 2002.

Briddell DW, Rimm DC, Caddy GR, Krawitz G, Sholis D, Wunderlin RJ. Effects of alcohol and cognitive set on sexual arousal to deviant stimuli. In: Kramer KM. Rule by myth: the social and legal dynamics governing alcohol-related acquaintance rapes. *Stanford Law Rev*. 1994;47:115, 119-120, 123-124.

Brown v State, 280 So 177, 179 (Ala App 1973).

Browning MD, Hoffer BJ, Dunwiddie TV. Alcohol, memory, and molecules: research on memory loss. *Alcohol Health Res World*. 1992:16;280.

California Evidence Code §.

California Penal Code § 13823.11(a-g) 2001. Minimum standards for examination and treatment of sexual assault victims.

California Penal Code § 261(a)(1). 2002 Rape.

Daubert v Merrell Dow Pharmaceutical, Inc, 509 US 579 (1993).

Department of Health and Human Services (DHHS). Authorization for special support persons in criminal child abuse proceedings. Vol 4. *Child Witnesses*. Washington DC: National Clearinghouse on Child Abuse and Neglect Information; 1999a. Child Abuse and Neglect State Statute Series; No. 26.

Department of Health and Human Services (DHHS). Special procedures in criminal child abuse cases. Vol 4. *Child Witnesses*. Washington DC: National Clearinghouse on Child Abuse and Neglect Information; 1999b. Child Abuse and Neglect State Statute Series; No. 28.

Diagnostic and Statistical Manual of Mental Disorders (DSM-IV-TR). 4th ed, text rev. Washington, DC: American Psychiatric Association (APA); 2000:46.

Drug Enforcement Administration (DEA). *Intelligence report on Rohypnol*. Washington DC: DEA Resources for Law Enforcement Officers; July 1995.

Drug Enforcement Administration (DEA). *Rohypnol fact sheet*. Washington DC; Drug Policy Information Clearinghouse, White House Office of National Drug Control Policy; September 1996.

Fairstein LA. *Sexual Violence: Our War against Rape*. New York, NY: Berkley Publishing Group; 1993:132.

Fed R Evid 601. [advisory committee's note]. 2002 General Rule of Competency.

Fed R Evid 603. [advisory committee's notes]. [ancillary laws and directives].

Fed R Evid 611. 2002 Mode and Order of Interrogation and Presentation.

Fed R Evid 803(4). [advisory committee's comments]. 2002 Hearsay Exceptions, Statements for Purposes of Medical Diagnosis or Treatment.

Feild HS, Bienen LB. *Jurors and Rape: A Study in Psychology and Law*. New York, NY: The Free Press; 1980:88-89, 1047.

Fishman CS. Consent, credibility, and the constitution: evidence relating to sex offense complainant's past sexual behavior. *Catholic Univ Law Rev*. 1995:44;711, 715, 721-723, 725-726.

Frye v United States, 293 F2d 1013 (2d Cir 1923).

Galvin HR. Shielding rape victims in the state and federal courts: a proposal for the second decade. *Minn L Rev*. 1986;70:765, 782, 787.

Harvey SM, Beckman LJ. Alcohol consumption, female sexual behavior and contraceptive use. In: Kramer KM. Rule by myth: the social and legal dynamics governing alcohol-related acquaintance rapes. *Stanford Law Rev*. 1994;47:115, 119-120, 123-124.

Hughes K. Bill would provide funding for rape kits. *The State News*. July 31, 2001. Available at www.statenews.com. Accessed October 24, 2001.

JEB v Alabama ex rel TB, 114 SCt 1419, 1421 (1994).

Johnson SD, Gibson L, Linden R. Alcohol and rape in Winnipeg 1966-1975. In: Collins JJ. *Alcohol Use and Criminal Behavior: An Executive Summary*. Washington, DC: US Department of Justice: 1981:3.

Kassin SM, Wrightsman LS. *The American Jury on Trial: Psychological Perspectives*. New York, NY: Hemisphere Publishing Corporation; 1988:31.

LaFree GD. *Rape and Criminal Justice: The Social Construction of Sexual Assault*. Belmont, Calif: Wadsworth; 1989.

LeBeau M. Recommendations for toxicological investigations of drug facilitated sexual assaults. *J Forensic Sci*. 1999;44:227-230.

Ledray LE. Forensic evidence collection and care of the sexual assault survivor: the SANE–SART response. *Violence Against Women Online Resources*. August 2, 2001. Available at: www.vaw.umn.edu. Accessed May 24, 2002.

Liles RE, Childs D. Similarities in family dynamics of incest and alcohol abuse. *Alcohol Health Res World*. 1986;2:66-67.

Lisak D. Offenders: myths and realities–overview. In: *Understanding Sexual Violence: Response to Stranger and Nonstranger Rape and Sexual Assault*. Alexandria, Va: American Prosecutors Research Institute and National Judicial Education Program; 2001a.

Lisak D. The undetected rapists. In: *Understanding Sexual Violence: Response to Stranger and Nonstranger Rape and Sexual Assault*. Alexandria, Va: American Prosecutors Research Institute and National Judicial Education Program; 2001b.

Lisak D & Ivan C. Deficits in intimacy and empathy in sexually aggressive men. *J Interpers Violence*. 1995:10;296-308.

Massaro TM. Experts, psychology, credibility, and rape: the rape trauma syndrome issue and its implications for expert psychological testimony. *Minn Law Rev*. 1985;69:395, 404.

Mayfield D. Alcoholism, alcohol intoxication and assaultive behavior. In: Collins JJ. *Alcohol Use and Criminal Behavior: An Executive Summary*. Washington, DC: US Department of Justice; 1981:3.

McCormick on Evidence §266 at 563-564. Edward W. Cleary, ed. St. Paul, Minn; 1984.

McGovern G. *Terry*. New York, NY: Villiard; 1996:64.

Mich Comp Laws Ann 750.520j (Lexis 2001).

Michigan v Lucas, 500 US 145, 149 (1991).

Mills J. Turning the juries on to computer evidence: strategies for forensic examiners and prosecutors preparing for trial. *Update*. APRI's National Center for Prosecution of Child Abuse; 2002:15(8).

Mosher D, Anderson RD. Macho personality, sexual aggression, and reactions to guided imagery of realistic rape. In: Kramer KM. Rule by myth: the social and legal dynamics governing alcohol-related acquaintance rapes. *Stanford Law Rev*. 1994;47:115, 119-120, 123-124.

Murphy S. Assisting the jury in understanding victimization: expert psychological testimony on battered woman syndrome and rape trauma syndrome. *Columbia J Law Soc Problems*. 1992;25:277-278.

Myers JEB, Goodman GS, Saywitz K. Psychological research on children as witnesses: practical implications for forensic interviews and courtroom testimony. *Pacific Law J*. 1996:28;22-27.

National Cybercrime Training Partnership. *Cyber Crime Fighting: The Law Enforcement Officer's Guide to Online Crime*. Washington, DC: Computer Crimes and Intellectual Property Section, US Department of Justice; 1999.

National Institute of Justice. *Electronic Crime Scene Investigation: A Guide for First Responders*. Washington, DC: National Institute of Justice, US Department of Justice; 2001.

Nelson T, McSpadden M, Marlatt G. Effects of alcohol intoxication on metamemory and on retrieval from long term memory. *J Exp Psychol Gen*. 1986;115:247-254.

NY Exec Law §642-a (Lexis 1999).

One night, a stranger . . ., *New Statesman Soc*. October 1991: 25.

People v Collins, 186 NE2d 30, 33 (Ill 1962).

People v Kelly, 17 Cal 3d 24 (1976).

People v Mobley, 85 Cal Rptr 2d (Cal Ct App 1999) (discussing Cal Penal Code § 261(a)(1)).

People v Whitten, 647 NE2d 1062 (Ill App Ct 1995).

Price JM. Sex, lies and rape shield statutes: the constitutionality of interpreting rape shield statutes to exclude evidence related to the victim's motive to fabricate. *W New Engl Law Rev*. 1996;18:541, 542, 547.

Privacy Protection for Rape Victims Act of 1978, Pub. L. No. 95-540 (1978), (which enacted Fed R Evid 412).

Reno J. Introductory remarks. *The Prosecution of Rohypnol and GHB Related Sexual Assaults*. [videotape]. Washington, DC: American Prosecutors Research Institute's Violence Against Women Program; January 1999.

Scarborough Hospital Sexual Assault Care Center. It just happened—what now? Available at: www.sacc.to. Accessed May 15, 2002.

Schafran LH. How stereotypes about women influence judges. *Judges' J*. 1985;24:12.

Schiro G. Special considerations for sexual assault evidence. Available at: www.crime-scene-investigator.net. Accessed October 24, 2002.

Sexual Assault Evidence Collection Kits (Rape Kits). Available at: www.state.ma.us. Accessed October 24, 2002.

Shell Oil Co. v Industrial Commission, 2 Ill2d 590, 119 NE2d 224 (1954).

State v Briere, 644 A2d 551, 554 (NH 1994).

State v Frost, 686 A2d 1172 (NH 1996) (discussing NH Rev Stat § 632-A:2).

State v Love, 936 SW2d 236 (Mo Ct App 1997).

State v Watkins, 857 P2d 300 (Wash Ct App 1993).

State v Waugh, 771 P2d 949 (Kan Ct App 1989).

Strong J, Broun K, Dix G, et al. *McCormick on Evidence*, 4th ed. Eagan, Minn: West Group; 1997:345.

Summit RC. The child sexual abuse accommodation syndrome. *Child Abuse Negl*. 1983;7:177.

Summit RC. Abuse of the child sexual abuse accommodation syndrome. *J Child Sexual Abuse*. 1992;4(1);153.

Tully LA, Jones JP, Kaas LM, Forman L. *Funding Update from the National Institute of Justice*. Washington, DC: Investigative and Forensic Sciences Division, Office of Science and Technology, National Institute of Justice, Office of Justice Programs, US Department of Justice; November 2000.

United States v Allen J, 127 F3d 1292 (10th Cir 1997), cert denied, 523 US 1013 (1998).

United States v Cook, 949 F2d 289 (10th Cir 1991).

United States v Gates, 10 F3d 765 (11th Cir 1993), aff'd on reh'g, 20 F3d 1550 (1994).

United States v Saenz, 747 F2d 930 (5th Cir), reh'g denied, en banc, 752 F2d, and cert. denied, 473 US 906 (1985).

Van der Kolk BA, Fisler R. Dissociation and the fragmentary nature of traumatic memories: overview and exploratory study. In: Myers JEB, Goodman GS, Saywitz K. Psychological research on children as witnesses: practical implications for forensic interviews and courtroom testimony. *Pacific Law J*. 1996:32; 22-27.

Wash Rev Code §9A.44.060.

Wolfgang ME. Patterns in criminal homicide. In: Collins JJ. *Alcohol Use and Criminal Behavior: An Executive Summary*. Washington, DC: US Department of Justice; 1981:3.

Wright JA. Using the female perspective in prosecuting rape cases. [also appendix]. *The Prosecutor.* January/February 1995:28(1).

Zhender MM. A step forward: Rule 803(25). A new approach to child hearsay statements, 20 Wm. Mitchell L. Rev 875, 911 (1994).

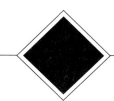

INDEX

A